# Radiobiology for the Radiologist

Fourth Edition

# *Radiobiology for the Radiologist*

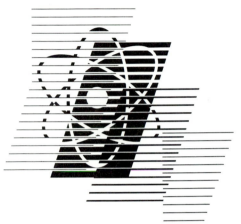

## Eric J. Hall, D.PHIL., D.Sc., F.A.C.R.

*Professor of Radiation Oncology and Radiology*
*Director, Center for Radiological Research*
*College of Physicians & Surgeons*
*Columbia University*
*New York, New York*

**J.B. Lippincott Company**
Philadelphia

*Acquiring Editor:* James D. Ryan
*Sponsoring Editor:* Kimberley Cox
*Project Editor:* Dina Papadopoulos
*Indexer:* Sandi Schroeder
*Designer:* Doug Smock
*Cover Designer:* Russell Rollins
*Production Manager:* Caren Erlichman
*Production Coordinator:* Sharon McCarthy
*Compositor:* Graphic Sciences Corporation
*Printer/Binder:* Arcata Graphics/Kingsport

4th Edition

6 5 4 3 2 1

Library of Congress Cataloging-in-Publication Data
Hall, Eric J.
    Radiobiology for the radiologist / Eric J. Hall. — 4th ed.
        p.      cm.
    Includes bibliographical references and index.
    ISBN 0-397-51248-1
    1. Radiology, Medical.   2. Radiobiology.   3. Medical physics.
    I. Title.
    [DNLM: 1. Radiobiology.   2. Radiotherapy.   3. Radiation Effects.
    WN 610 H175rb 1993]
    R895.H34   1994
    616.07'57—dc20
    DNLM/DLC
    for Library of Congress                           93-22626
                                                        CIP

The author and publisher have exerted every effort to ensure that drug selection and dosage set forth in this text are in accord with current recommendations and practice at the time of publication. However, in view of ongoing research, changes in government regulations, and the constant flow of information relating to drug therapy and drug reactions, the reader is urged to check the package insert for each drug for any change in indications and dosage and for added warnings and precautions. This is particularly important when the recommended agent is a new or infrequently employed drug.

# Preface

This revised fourth edition of *Radiobiology for the Radiologist* represents my effort (frantic at times) to retain an overall view of advances in the whole field of radiation biology, while still remaining an active laboratory researcher in a few specialized areas.

The motivation for the revision was the encouragement of students and teachers alike who found the earlier editions of some use.

Up to now, each successive revision resulted in a thicker book, crammed with more information. This is inevitable to some extent in a field that is in an exponential phase of growth. However, this time I went through the previous edition and the accumulated new material ruthlessly, asking the questions: "What does the student really need to know?," "What are the guiding principles?," "What are the exciting new insights?" I have, reluctantly and with great personal pain, deleted much historical detail chronicling the development of the field, recognizing that my increasing preoccupation with history is a sure sign of impending senility! It is of little interest to the new generation of radiologists and radiation oncologists. This urge to be brief, to summarize, and to pick out the vital information was further prompted to some extent by observing my own son, a resident in a different medical field, struggling to digest the accumulated stores of human knowledge.

The overall plan of the book retains the format introduced in the second edition: areas of interest to radiation oncology, diagnostic radiology, and nuclear medicine are clearly delineated.

To meet the needs of residents in nuclear medicine and in diagnostic radiology (or imaging, as many now prefer to call it), the chapters on carcinogenesis, hereditary effects of radiation, and the effects on the developing embryo and fetus have been updated to reflect advances in molecular genetics. These are surely the areas of principal concern to students in imaging, because the doses of radiation involved will never be enough to kill many cells.

The most far-reaching revision of concern to the radiation oncologist involves the discussion of fractionation. Altered patterns of fractionation represent one of the most exciting areas of clinical investigation, and it all started from radiobiological considerations in the laboratory. The section on high-LET radiations has been shortened to reflect the consensus view that their place in radiotherapy is clearly limited. At the time of writing, hypoxic cell sensitizers have not proved their usefulness in the clinic, but research in this area has shifted to bioreductive drugs that are hypoxic cytotoxins and markers of hypoxia.

The chapter on hyperthermia has been retained to reflect the continuing conviction that the biology of heat appears favorable for its use to treat cancer, though improvements in equipment to produce uniform regions of elevated temperature at a depth in the body are disappointing and must limit the clinical utility of this new modality.

The only new chapter added is a summary of the techniques of molecular biology that are used increasingly in radiation biology. This chapter is clearly optional for residents whose only concern is to pass the boards, but for anyone contemplating a career in academic radiation oncology, molecular biology is here to stay and the terms and techniques need to be learned.

*Eric J. Hall,* D.PHIL., D.Sc., F.A.C.R.

# *Preface to the First Edition*

This book, like so many before it, grew out of a set of lecture notes. The lectures were given during the autumn months of 1969, 1970, and 1971 at the Columbia-Presbyterian Medical Center, New York City. The audience consisted primarily of radiology residents from Columbia, affiliated schools and hospitals, and various other institutions in and around the city.

To plan a course in radiobiology involves a choice between, on the one hand, dealing at length and in depth with those few areas of the subject in which one has personal expertise as an experimenter or, on the other hand, surveying the whole field of interest to the radiologist, necessarily in less depth. The former course is very much simpler for the lecturer and in many ways more satisfying; it is, however, of very little use to the aspiring radiologist who, if this course is followed, learns too much about too little and fails to get an overall picture of radiobiology. Consequently, I opted in the original lectures, and now in this book, to cover the whole field of radiobiology as it pertains to radiology. I have endeavored to avoid becoming evangelical over those areas of the subject which interest me, those to which I have devoted a great deal of my life. At the same time I have attempted to cover, with as much enthusiasm as I could muster and from as much knowledge as I could glean, those areas in which I had no particular expertise or personal experience.

This book, then, was conceived and written for the radiologist—specifically, the radiologist who, motivated ideally by an inquiring mind or more realistically by the need to pass an examination, elects to study the biological foundations of radiology. It may incidentally serve also as a text for graduate students in the life sciences or even as a review of radiobiology for active researchers whose viewpoint has been restricted to their own area of interest. If the book serves these functions, too, the author is doubly happy, but first and foremost it is intended as a didactic text for the student of radiology.

Radiology is not a homogeneous discipline. The diagnostician and therapist have divergent interests; indeed it sometimes seems that they come together only when history and convenience dictate that they share a common course in physics or radiobiology. The bulk of this book will be of concern, and hopefully of interest, to all radiologists. The diagnostic radiologist is commended particularly to Chapters 11, 12, and 13 concerning radiation accidents, late effects, and the irradiation of the embryo and fetus. A few chapters, particularly Chapters 8, 9, 15, and 16, are so specifically oriented towards radiotherapy that the diagnostician may omit them without loss of continuity.

A word concerning reference material is in order. The ideas contained in this book represent, in the author's estimate, the consensus of opinion as expressed in the scientific literature. For ease of reading, the text has not been broken up with a large number of direct references. Instead a selection of general references has been included at the end of each chapter for the reader who wishes to pursue the subject further.

I wish to record the lasting debt that I owe to my former colleagues at Oxford and my present colleagues at Columbia, for it is in the daily cut and thrust of debate and discussion that ideas are formulated and views tested.

Finally, I would like to thank the young men and women who have regularly attended my classes. Their inquiring minds have forced me to study hard and reflect carefully before facing them in a lecture room. As each group of students has grown in maturity and understanding, I have experienced a teacher's satisfaction and joy in the belief that their growth was due in some small measure to my efforts.

*E. J. H.*

*New York*
*July 1972*

# *Acknowledgments*

I would like to thank the many colleagues who generously and willingly gave permission for diagrams and illustrations from their published work to be reproduced in this book.

While the ultimate responsibility for the content of this book must be mine, I acknowledge with gratitude the help of a number of friends who read chapters relating to their own areas of special expertise and made invaluable suggestions and additions. With each successive revision, this list grows longer and now includes Drs. Ged Adams, Philip Alderson, Joel Bedford, Roger Berry, Max Boone, Victor Bond, J. Martin Brown, Bill Dewey, Frank Ellis, Stan Field, Greg Fryer, Charles Geard, Eugene Gerner, Julian Gibbs, George Hahn, Tom Hei, Robert Kallman, Howard Lieberman, Philip Lorio, Edmund Malaise, Mortimer Mendelsohn, George Merriam, Gillies McKenna, Jim Mitchell, Anthony Nias, Ray Oliver, Julian Preston, Harald Rossi, Roberts Rugh, Robert Sutherland, Len Tolmach, Liz Travis, John Ward, Barry Winston, Rod Withers, Basil Worgul, Stanley Order, Dennis Leeper, and James Cox.

Without their help this volume would be much the poorer.

The principal credit for this book must go to the successive classes of residents in radiology, radiation oncology, and nuclear medicine that I have taught over a period of almost 40 years. Their perceptive minds and searching questions have kept me on my toes. Their impatience to learn what was needed of radiobiology, and to get on with being doctors, has continually prompted me to summarize, be brief, and get to the point!

I am deeply indebted to the United States Department of Energy and the National Cancer Institute, who have generously supported my work and indeed much of the research, performed by numerous investigators, described in this book.

Finally, I thank my wife, Bernice, who has been most patient and gave me every encouragement when I needed it most. She also spent many hours proofreading the manuscript and galleys.

# Contents

**NOTE:** *D* indicates relevance to Diagnostic Radiology, *N* to Nuclear Medicine, and *T* to Radiation Therapy.

**NOTE:** *D* indicates relevance to Diagnostic Radiology, *N* to Nuclear Medicine, and *T* to Radiation Therapy.

# Radiobiology for the Radiologist

*Radiobiology for the Radiologist, Fourth Edition*, by Eric J. Hall
J. B. Lippincott Company, Philadelphia © 1994.

# 1

# *The Physics and Chemistry of Radiation Absorption*

**TYPES OF IONIZING RADIATIONS**
**ABSORPTION OF X-RAYS**
**DIRECT AND INDIRECT ACTION OF RADIATION**
**ABSORPTION OF NEUTRONS**
**CONTRAST BETWEEN NEUTRONS AND PHOTONS**
**SUMMARY OF PERTINENT CONCLUSIONS**

Diagnostic Radiology
Nuclear Medicine
Radiation Therapy

In 1895 the German physicist Wilhelm Conrad Röntgen discovered "a new kind of ray," emitted by a gas discharge tube, that could blacken photographic film contained in light-tight containers. He called these rays *x-rays*, in his first announcement in December 1895—the *x* representing the unknown. In demonstrating the properties of x-rays at a public lecture, Röentgen asked Rudolf Albert von Kölliker, a prominent Swiss professor of anatomy, to put his hand in the beam and so produced the first radiograph (Fig. 1-1). The first medical use of x-rays was reported in the *Lancet* of January 23, 1896. In this report, x-rays were used to locate a piece of a knife in the backbone of a drunken sailor, who was paralyzed until the fragment was removed following its localization. The new technology spread rapidly through Europe and the United States, and the field of diagnostic radiology was born. There is some debate about who first used x-rays therapeutically, but, by 1897, Wilhelm Alexander Freund, a German surgeon, demonstrated, before the Vienna Medical Society, the disappearance of a hairy mole following treatment with x-rays. Antoine Henri Becquerel discovered radioactivity in 1898, and radium was isolated by Pierre and Marie Curie in the same year.

The first recorded experiment in radiobiology was performed by Becquerel when he inadvertently left a radium container in his vest pocket. He subsequently described the skin erythema that appeared 2 weeks later and the ulceration that developed and required several weeks to heal. It is said that Pierre Curie repeated the experiment in 1901 by deliberately producing a radium "burn" on his own forearm (Fig. 1-2). From these early beginnings just before the turn of the century, the study of radiobiology began.

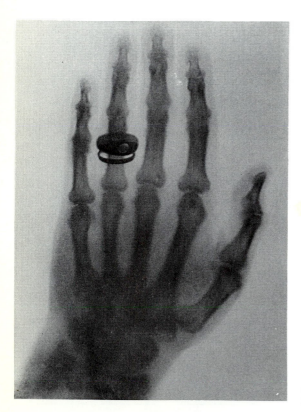

**Figure 1-1.** The first radiograph of a living object, taken in January 1896—just a few months after the discovery of x-rays. (Courtesy of Röntgen Museum, Würzburg, Germany)

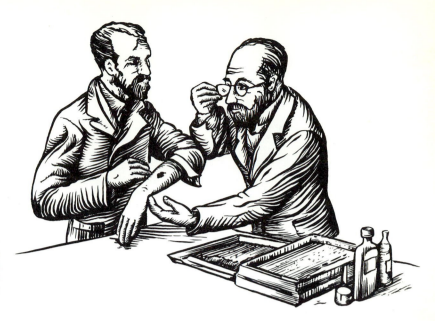

**Figure 1-2.** The first radiobiology experiment. Pierre Curie is said to have used a radium tube to produce a radiation ulcer on his arm. He charted its appearance and subsequent healing.

**Radiobiology** is the study of the action of ionizing radiations on living things. As such, it inevitably involves a certain amount of radiation physics. The purpose of this chapter is to present, in summary form and with a minimum of mathematics, a listing of the various types of ionizing radiations and a description of the physics and chemistry of the processes by which radiation is absorbed.

## TYPES OF IONIZING RADIATIONS

The absorption of energy from radiation in biological material may lead to *excitation* or to *ionization*. The raising of an electron in an atom or molecule to a higher energy level without actual ejection of the electron is called *excitation*. If the radiation has sufficient energy to eject one or more orbital electrons from the atom or molecule, the process is called *ionization,* and that radiation is said to be *ionizing radiation.* The important characteristic of ionizing radiations is the localized release of large amounts of energy. The energy dissipated per ionizing event is about 33 eV, which is more than enough to break a strong chemical bond; for example, the energy associated with a C=C bond is 4.9 eV. For convenience it is usual to classify ionizing radiations as *electromagnetic* or *particulate*.

### Electromagnetic Radiations

Most experiments with biological systems have involved x- or γ-rays, two forms of electromagnetic radiation. X- and γ-rays do not differ in nature or in properties; the designation x or γ reflects the way in which they are produced. X-rays are produced extranuclearly, while γ-rays are produced intranuclearly. In practical terms this means that x-rays are produced in an electrical device that accelerates electrons to high energy and then stops them abruptly in a target, usually made of tungsten or gold. Part of the kinetic energy (the energy of motion) of the electrons is converted into x-rays. On the other hand, γ-rays are emitted by radioactive isotopes; they represent excess energy that is given off as the unstable nucleus breaks up and decays in its efforts to reach a stable form. Everything that is stated of x-rays in this chapter will apply equally well to γ-rays.

X-rays may be considered from two different standpoints. First, they may be thought of as a wave of electrical and magnetic energy. The magnetic and electrical fields, in planes at right angles to one another, vary with time so that the wave moves forward in much the same way as ripples move over the surface of a pond when a stone is dropped into the water. The wave moves with a velocity, c, which in a vacuum has a value of $3 \times 10^{10}$ cm/s. The distance between succes-

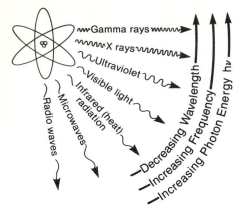

**Figure 1-3.** Illustration of the electromagnetic spectrum. X-rays and γ-rays have the same nature as visible light, radiant heat, and radio waves; however, they have a shorter wavelength and consequently a larger photon energy. As a result, x- and γ-rays can break chemical bonds and produce biological effects.

sive peaks of the wave, λ, is known as the wavelength. The number of waves passing a fixed point per second is the frequency, ν. The product of frequency times wavelength gives the velocity of the wave; that is, $\lambda\nu = c$.

A helpful, if trivial, analogy is to liken the wavelength to the length of a man's stride when walking; the number of strides per minute is the frequency. The product of the length of stride times the number of strides per minute then gives the speed, or velocity, of the walker.

Like x-rays, radio waves, radar, radiant heat, and visible light are forms of electromagnetic radiation. They all have the same velocity, c, but they have different wavelengths and therefore different frequencies. To extend the previous analogy, different radiations may be likened to a group of men, some tall, some short, walking together at the same speed. The tall men will take long measured strides but will make few strides per minute; to keep up, the short men will compensate for the shortness of their stride by increasing the frequency of their stride. A radio wave may have a distance between successive peaks (ie, wavelength) of 300 m, while for a wave of visible light the corresponding distance is about five hundred thousandths of a centimeter ($5 \times 10^{-5}$ cm). The wavelength for x-rays may be one hundred millionth of a centimeter ($10^{-8}$ cm). X- and γ-rays, then, occupy the short wavelength end of the electromagnetic spectrum (Fig. 1-3).

Alternatively, x-rays may be thought of as a stream of **photons,** or "packets" of energy. Each energy packet contains an amount of energy

equal to hν, where h is known as Planck's constant and ν is the frequency. If a radiation has a *long wavelength*, it will have a *small frequency*, and so the energy per photon is small. Conversely, if a given radiation has a *short wavelength*, the *frequency* will be large and the energy per photon is large. There is a simple numerical relationship between the photon energy (in kiloelectron volts*) and the wavelengths (in angstroms†):

$$\lambda(\text{Å}) = \frac{12.4}{\text{E(keV)}}$$

For example, x-rays with a wavelength of 1/10 Å correspond to a photon energy of 124 keV.

The concept of x-rays being composed of photons is very important in radiobiology. When x-rays are absorbed in living material, energy is deposited in the tissues and cells. This energy is deposited unevenly in discrete packets. The energy in a beam of x-rays is quantized into large individual packets, each of which is big enough to break a chemical bond and initiate the chain of events that culminates in a biological change. The critical difference between nonionizing and ionizing radiations is the size of the *individual* packets of energy, not the *total* energy involved. A simple calculation will illustrate this point. It

---

*The kiloelectron volt (keV) is a unit of energy. It is the energy possessed by an electron that has been accelerated through 1000 volts. It corresponds to $1.6 \times 10^{-9}$ ergs.

†The angstrom (Å) is a unit of length equal to $10^{-8}$ cm.

will be seen later that a total-body dose of about 4 Gy (400 rads)‡ of x-rays given to a human is lethal in many cases. This dose represents an absorption of energy of only about 67 calories, assuming the person to be a "standard man," weighing 70 kg. The smallness of the amount of energy involved can be illustrated in many ways. Converted to heat it would represent a temperature rise of 0.002°C, which would do no harm at all; the same amount of energy in the form of heat is absorbed when drinking one sip of warm coffee. Alternatively, the energy inherent in a lethal dose of x-rays may be compared with mechanical energy or work: it would correspond to the work done in lifting a man about 16 inches from the ground (Fig. 1-4).

Energy in the form of heat or mechanical energy is absorbed uniformly and evenly, and much greater quantities of energy in these forms are required to produce damage in living things. The potency of x-rays, then, is a function not so much of the total energy absorbed as of the size of the individual energy packets. In their biological effects, electromagnetic radiations are usually considered to be ionizing if they have a photon energy in excess of 124 eV, which corresponds to a wavelength shorter than about $10^{-6}$ cm.

## Particulate Radiations

Other types of radiation used experimentally and used or contemplated for radiotherapy are electrons, protons, α-particles, neutrons, negative π-mesons, and heavy charged ions. Some may also have a potential in diagnostic radiology not yet exploited.

**Total-Body Irradiation**

Mass = 70 kg
LD/50/60 = 4 Gy
Energy absorbed =

$$70 \times 4 = 280 \text{ joules}$$
$$= \frac{280}{4.18} = 67 \text{ calories}$$

X-ray

**A**

**Drinking Hot Coffee**

Excess temperature (°C) = 60° − 37° = 23°
Volume of coffee consumed to
equal the energy in the LD/50/60 = $\frac{67}{23}$
$$= 3 \text{ mL}$$
$$= 1 \text{ sip}$$

**B**

**Mechanical Energy: Lifting a Person**

Mass = 70 kg
Height lifted to equal
the energy in the

LD/50/60 = $\frac{280}{70 \times 0.0981}$
$$= 0.4 \text{ m (16 inches)}$$

**C**

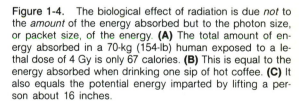

**Figure 1-4.** The biological effect of radiation is due *not* to the *amount* of the energy absorbed but to the photon size, or packet size, of the energy. **(A)** The total amount of energy absorbed in a 70-kg (154-lb) human exposed to a lethal dose of 4 Gy is only 67 calories. **(B)** This is equal to the energy absorbed when drinking one sip of hot coffee. **(C)** It also equals the potential energy imparted by lifting a person about 16 inches.

‡Quantity of radiation is expressed in roentgens, rads, or gray. The roentgen (R) is the unit of exposure and is related to the ability of x-rays to ionize air. The rad is the unit of absorbed dose and corresponds to an energy absorption of 100 ergs/g. In the case of x- and γ-rays an exposure of 1 R results in an absorbed dose in water or soft tissue roughly equal to 1 rad. Officially, the rad has been replaced as a unit by the gray (Gy), which corresponds to an energy absorption of 1 joule/kg. Consequently, 1 Gy = 100 rads. Although the gray is now commonly used in Europe, it is slow to be adopted in everyday practice in the United States. Often centigray (cGy) is used; thus, 1 cGy = 1 rad.

**Electrons** are small, negatively charged particles that can be accelerated to high energy to a speed close to that of light by means of an electrical device, such as a betatron.

**Protons** are positively charged particles and are relatively massive, having a mass almost 2000 times greater than an electron. Because of their mass they require more complex and more expensive equipment to accelerate them to useful energies.

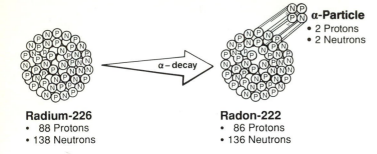

**Figure 1-5.** Illustration of the decay of a heavy radionuclide by the emission of an α-particle. An α-particle is a helium nucleus consisting of two protons and two neutrons. The emission of an α-particle decreases the atomic number by two and the mass number by four. Note that the radium has changed to another chemical element, radon, as a consequence of the decay.

**α-Particles** are nuclei of helium atoms and consist of two protons and two neutrons in close association. They have a net positive charge and can therefore be accelerated in large electrical devices similar to those used for protons. They are also emitted during the decay of some heavy, naturally occurring radionuclides (eg, uranium, thorium, radium, and radon). This is illustrated in Figure 1-5.

**Neutrons** are particles with a mass similar to that of a proton, but they carry no electrical charge. Because they are electrically neutral, they cannot be accelerated in an electrical device. They are produced when a charged particle, such as a deuteron, is accelerated to high energy and then made to impinge on a suitable target material. (A **deuteron** is a nucleus of deuterium and consists of a proton and a neutron in close association.) Neutrons are also emitted as a by-product when heavy radioactive atoms undergo **fission,** that is, split to form two smaller atoms.

**Heavy charged ions** are nuclei of elements, such as carbon, neon, silicon, or argon, that are positively charged since some or all of the planetary electrons have been stripped from them. To be useful, they must be accelerated to energies of hundreds or thousands of millions of volts and can therefore be produced in only a very limited number of laboratories. In the United States, heavy ions for radiotherapy were available for some years at the Lawrence Berkeley Laboratory in California, but facilities are being constructed in Europe and Japan.

## ABSORPTION OF X-RAYS

Radiation may be classified as *directly* or *indirectly* ionizing. All of the charged particles previously discussed are **directly ionizing;** that is, provided the individual particles have sufficient kinetic energy, they can directly disrupt the atomic structure of the absorber through which they pass and produce chemical and biological changes. Electromagnetic radiations (x- and γ-rays) are **indirectly ionizing.** They do not produce chemical and biological damage themselves, but when they are absorbed in the material through which they pass they give up their energy to produce fast-moving charged particles.

The process by which x-ray photons are absorbed depends on the energy of the photons concerned and the chemical composition of the absorbing material. At high energies, characteristic of a cobalt-60 unit or a linear accelerator used for radiotherapy, the **Compton process** dominates. In this process the photon interacts with what is usually referred to as a "free" electron, an electron whose binding energy is negligibly small compared with the photon energy. Part of the energy of the photon is given to the electron as kinetic energy; the photon, with whatever energy remains, continues on its way, deflected from its original path (Fig. 1-6). In place of the incident photon there is a fast electron and a photon of reduced energy, which may go on to take part in further interactions. In any given case the photon may lose a little energy or a lot; in fact, the fraction lost may vary from 0% to 80%. In practice, when an x-ray beam is absorbed by tissue, a vast number of photons interact with a vast number of atoms, and on a statistical basis all possible energy losses will occur. The net result is the production of a large number of fast electrons, many of which can ionize other atoms of the absorber, break vital chemical bonds, and initiate the change of events that ultimately is expressed as biological damage.

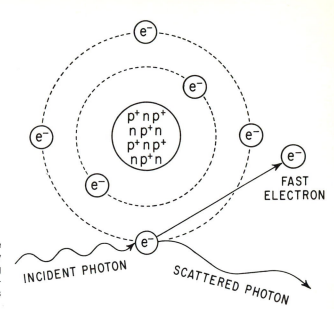

**Figure 1-6.** Absorption of an x-ray photon by the Compton process. The photon interacts with a loosely bound planetary electron of an atom of the absorbing material. Part of the photon energy is given to the electron as kinetic energy. The photon, deflected from its original direction, proceeds with reduced energy.

For photon energies characteristic of diagnostic radiology, both Compton and photoelectric absorption processes occur, the former dominating at the higher end of the energy range and the latter being most important at lower energies. In the **photoelectric process** (Fig. 1-7) the x-ray photon interacts with a bound electron in, for example, the K, L, or M shell of an atom of the absorbing material. The photon gives up all of its energy to the electron; some is used to overcome the binding energy of the electron and release it from its orbit, while the remainder is given to the electron as kinetic energy of motion. The kinetic energy (KE) of the ejected electron is, therefore, given by the expression

$$KE = h\nu - E_B$$

where $h\nu$ is the energy of the incident photon and $E_B$ is the binding energy of the electron in its orbit. The vacancy left in the atomic shell as a result of the ejection of an electron must then be filled by another electron falling in from an outer shell of the same atom or by a conduction electron from outside the atom. The movement of an electron from one shell to another represents a change of energy states. Because the electron is negatively charged, its movement from a loosely bound to a tightly bound shell represents a *decrease* of potential energy; this energy change is balanced by the emission of a photon of "characteristic" electromagnetic radiation. In soft tissue, this characteristic radiation has a low energy, typically 0.5 kV, and is of little biological consequence.

The Compton and photoelectric absorption processes differ in several respects that are vital in the application of x-rays to diagnosis and therapy. The mass absorption coefficient for the Compton process is independent of the atomic number of the absorbing material. By contrast, the mass absorption coefficient for photoelectric absorption varies rapidly with atomic number $(Z)$[1] and is, in fact, about proportional to $Z^3$.

For diagnostic radiology, photons are used in the energy range in which photoelectric absorption is as important as the Compton process. Because the mass absorption coefficient varies critically with Z, the x-rays are absorbed to a greater extent by bone because bone contains elements with a high atomic number, such as calcium. This differential absorption in materials of

---

[1]Z, the atomic number, is defined as the number of positive charges on the nucleus; it is therefore the number of protons in the nucleus.

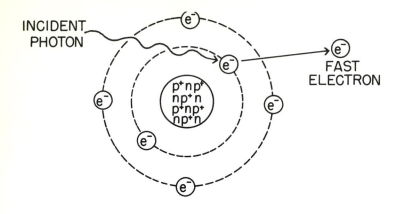

INCIDENT PHOTON

FAST ELECTRON

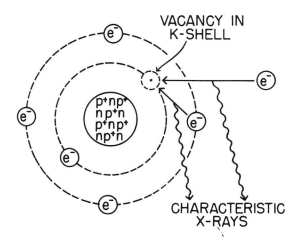

VACANCY IN K-SHELL

CHARACTERISTIC X-RAYS

**Figure 1-7.** Absorption of a photon of x- or γ-rays by the photoelectric process. The interaction involves the photon and a tightly bound orbital electron of an atom of the absorber. The photon gives up its energy entirely; the electron is ejected with a kinetic energy equal to the energy of the incident photon less the binding energy that previously held the electron in orbit (*upper panel*). The vacancy is filled either by an electron from an outer orbit or by a free electron from outside the atom (*lower panel*). When an electron changes energy levels, the difference in energy is emitted as a photon of characteristic x-rays. For soft tissue these x-rays are of very low energy.

high Z is one reason for the familiar appearance of the radiograph. On the other hand, for radiotherapy high-energy photons in the megavoltage range are preferred, because the Compton process is overwhelmingly important. As a consequence, the absorbed dose is about the same in soft tissue, muscle, and bone, so that differential absorption in bone, which posed a problem in the early days when lower energy photons were used for therapy, is avoided.

Although the differences between the various absorption processes are of practical importance in radiology, the consequences for radiobiology are minimal. Whether the absorption process is the photoelectric or the Compton process, much of the energy of the absorbed photon is converted into the kinetic energy of a fast electron.

## DIRECT AND INDIRECT ACTION OF RADIATION

The biological effects of radiation result principally from damage to DNA, which is the critical target.

When any form of radiation—x- or γ-rays, charged or uncharged particles—is absorbed in biological material, there is a possibility that it will interact directly with the critical targets in the cells. The atoms of the target itself may be ionized or excited, thus initiating the chain of events that leads to a biological change. This is the so-called **direct action** of radiation (Fig. 1-8); it is the dominant process when radiations with high linear energy transfer (LET), such as neutrons or α-particles, are considered.

Alternatively, the radiation may interact with

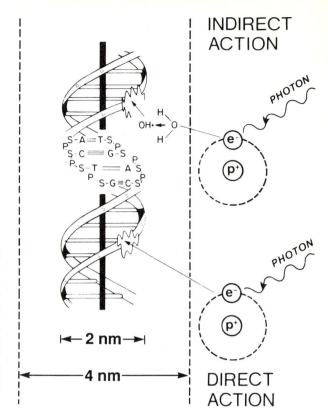

INDIRECT
ACTION

DIRECT
ACTION

|← 2 nm →|

|←——— 4 nm ———→|

**Figure 1-8.** Direct and indirect actions of radiation. The structure of DNA is shown schematically; the letters S, P, A, T, G, and C represent sugar, phosphorus, adenine, thymine, guanine, and cytosine, respectively. In direct action a secondary electron resulting from absorption of an x-ray photon interacts with the DNA to produce an effect. In indirect action the secondary electron interacts with, for example, a water molecule to produce a hydroxyl radical (OH·), which in turn produces the damage to the DNA. The DNA helix has a diameter of about 20Å (2 nm). It is estimated that free radicals produced in a cylinder with a diameter double that of the DNA helix can affect the DNA. Indirect action is dominant for sparsely ionizing radiation, such as x-rays.

other atoms or molecules in the cell (particularly water) to produce free radicals that are able to diffuse far enough to reach and damage the critical targets. This is called the **indirect action** of radiation. A free radical is a free (not combined) atom or molecule carrying an unpaired orbital electron in the outer shell. An orbital electron not only revolves around the nucleus of an atom but also spins around its own axis. The spin may be clockwise or counterclockwise. In an atom or molecule with an even number of electrons, spins are paired; that is, for every electron spinning clockwise there is another one spinning counterclockwise. This state is associated with a high degree of chemical stability. In an atom or molecule with an odd number of electrons there

is one electron in the outer orbit for which there is no other electron with an opposing spin; this is an unpaired electron. This state is associated with a high degree of chemical reactivity.

For simplicity, we will consider what happens when radiation interacts with a water molecule, since 80% of a cell is composed of water. As a result of the interaction of a photon of x- or $\gamma$-rays or a charged particle, such as an electron or proton, the water molecule may become ionized. This may be expressed as

$$H_2O \rightarrow H_2O^+ + e^-$$

$H_2O^+$ is an ion radical. An **ion** is an atom or molecule that is electrically charged because it has lost an electron. A **free radical** contains an unpaired electron in the outer shell, as a result of which it is highly reactive. $H_2O^+$ is charged and has an unpaired electron; consequently, it is both an ion and a free radical. Ion radicals have an extremely short lifetime, on the order of $10^{-10}$ second. They decay to form free radicals, which

---

It is important to avoid confusion between directly and indirectly ionizing radiation, on the one hand, and the direct and indirect actions of radiation on the other.

are not charged but which still have an unpaired electron. In the case of water, the ion radical reacts with another water molecule to form the highly reactive hydroxyl radical (OH·):

$$H_2O^+ + H_2O \rightarrow H_3O^+ + OH·$$

The hydroxyl radical possesses nine electrons, so one of them is unpaired. It is a highly reactive free radical and can diffuse a short distance to reach a critical target in a cell. For example, it is thought that free radicals can diffuse to DNA from within a cylinder with a diameter about twice that of the DNA double helix. It is estimated that about two thirds of the x-ray damage to DNA in mammalian cells is due to the hydroxyl radical. The best evidence for this estimate comes from experiments using free radical scavengers, which can reduce the biological effect of sparsely ionizing radiations, such as x-rays, by a factor of close to 3. This is discussed further in Chapter 11. Indirect action is illustrated in Figure 1-8.

For the indirect action of x-rays, the chain of events, from the absorption of the incident photon to the final observed biological change, may be described as follows:

Incident x-ray photon
↓
Fast electron (e⁻)
↓
Ion radical
↓
Free radical
↓
Chemical changes from
the breakage of bonds
↓
Biological effects

There are vast differences in the time scale involved in these various events. The physics of the process, the initial ionization, may take only $10^{-15}$ second. The ion radicals have a lifetime of about $10^{-10}$ second, and the free radicals perhaps $10^{-5}$ second. The step between the breakage of chemical bonds and the expression of the biological effect may be hours, days, months, or years, depending on the consequences involved. If cell killing is the result, the biological effect may be expressed hours to days later, when the damaged cell attempts to divide. If the radiation damage is oncogenic, its expression as an overt cancer may be delayed 40 years. If it is a mutation, in a germ

cell leading to heritable changes, it may not be expressed for many generations.

## ABSORPTION OF NEUTRONS

Neutrons are uncharged particles. For this reason they are highly penetrating compared with charged particles of the same mass and energy. They are indirectly ionizing and are absorbed by elastic or inelastic scattering.

Fast neutrons differ basically from x-rays in the mode of their interaction with tissue. *X-ray photons* interact with the *orbital electrons* of atoms of the absorbing material by the Compton or photoelectric process and set in motion *fast electrons. Neutrons,* on the other hand, interact with the *nuclei* of atoms of the absorbing material and set in motion *fast recoil protons, α-particles*, and *heavier nuclear fragments.*

In the case of intermediate fast neutrons, *elastic scattering* is the dominant process. The incident neutron collides with the nucleus of an atom of the absorber; part of its kinetic energy is transferred to the nucleus and part is retained by the deflected neutron, which may go on to make further collisions.

In soft tissues, the interaction between incident neutrons and hydrogen nuclei—which are, of course, single protons—is the dominant process of energy transfer. There are several reasons for this. First, a large proportion of energy is transferred when a neutron interacts with a proton, because the particles are of similar mass. Second, hydrogen is the most abundant atom in tissue. Third, the collision cross section for hydrogen is large. This process is illustrated in Figure 1-9. The recoil protons that are set in motion lose energy by excitation and ionization as they pass through the biological material. These recoil protons deposit much of their energy at an LET of less than 30 keV/μm, and the maximum LET associated with protons as they come to rest is about 100 keV/μm. (See Chapter 9 for a discussion of LET.) Elastic collisions of neutrons with heavier elements in tissue make small contribution to the dose, although the energy is deposited at high LET.

At energies above about 6 MeV, *inelastic scattering* begins to take place and assumes increasing importance as the neutron energy rises.

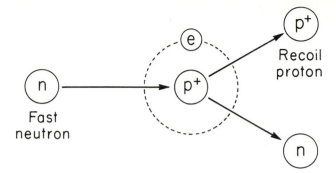

**Figure 1-9.** Interaction of a fast neutron with the nucleus of a hydrogen atom of the absorbing material. Part of the energy of the neutron is given to the proton as kinetic energy. The neutron, deflected from its original direction, proceeds with reduced energy.

The neutron may interact with a carbon nucleus to produce three α-particles or with an oxygen nucleus to produce four α-particles (Fig. 1-10). These are the so-called spallation products, which become very important at higher energies. The α-particles produced in this way represent a relatively modest proportion of the total absorbed dose, but they are densely ionizing and have an important effect on the biological characteristics of the radiation.

## CONTRAST BETWEEN NEUTRONS AND PHOTONS

X- and γ-rays are indirectly ionizing and give rise to fast-moving secondary electrons. *Fast neutrons* are also indirectly ionizing but give rise to recoil protons, α-particles, and heavier nuclear fragments.

The electrons that are set in motion when x-rays are absorbed are very light, negatively

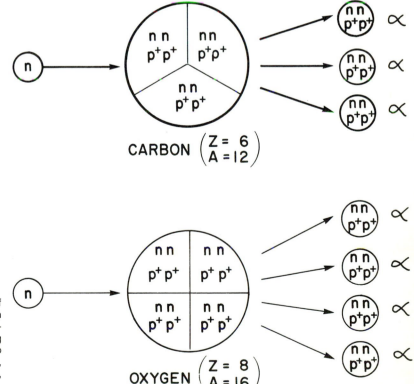

**Figure 1-10.** The production of spallation products. As the neutron energy rises, the probability increases of a neutron interacting with a carbon or oxygen nucleus to produce three or four α-particles, respectively. (Z, atomic number; A, mass number)

## Neutrons

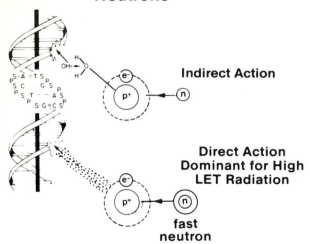

**Indirect Action**

**Direct Action
Dominant for High
LET Radiation**

**fast
neutron**

Figure 1-11. Direct action dominates for more densely ionizing radiations, such as neutrons, since the secondary charged particles produced (protons, α-particles, and heavier nuclear fragments) result in a dense column of ionizations more likely to interact with the DNA. Free radicals are still produced, but they are not needed to kill the cell.

charged particles. By contrast, the particles set in motion when neutrons are absorbed are heavy and densely ionizing. They also, for the most part, carry a positive charge, but this difference appears to be relatively trivial biologically. What is important is that they are *heavy* compared with the electron. A proton, for example, has a mass almost 2000 times greater than an electron; an α-particle has a mass four times larger still; and nuclear fragments may occur that are an order of magnitude larger in mass again. The pattern of ionizations and excitations along the tracks of these various charged particles is very different; in particular, the *density* of ionization is

### ► *Summary of Pertinent Conclusions*

- X- and γ-rays are *indirectly* ionizing; the first step in their absorption is the production of fast recoil *electrons*.
- Neutrons are also *indirectly* ionizing; the first step in their absorption is the production of fast recoil protons, α-particles, and heavier nuclear fragments.
- Biological effects of x-rays may be due to *direct action* (the recoil electron directly ionizes the target molecule) or to *indirect action* (the recoil electron interacts with water to produce an hydroxyl radical, which diffuses to the target molecule).
- About two thirds of the biological damage by x-rays is due to indirect action.
- Indirect action can be modified by chemical sensitizers or protectors.
- High-LET radiations produce most biological damage by the direct action, which cannot be modified by chemical sensitizers and protectors.
- The physics of the absorption process is over in $10^{-15}$ second; the chemistry takes longer, since the lifetime of the free radicals is about $10^{-5}$ second; the biology takes days to months for cell killing, years for carcinogenesis, and generations for heritable damage.

greater for neutrons, pions, and heavy ions than is the case for x- or γ-rays, and this accounts for the dramatic differences in the biological effects observed. This will be discussed further in Chapter 9.

For heavy particles, as for x-rays, the mechanism of biological effect may be by *direct* or *indirect* action, but there is a shift in the balance between the two modes of action (Fig. 1-11). For x-rays, indirect action is dominant; for the heavy particles set in motion by neutrons, direct action assumes a greater importance, which increases with the density of ionization. As the density of ionization increases, the probability of a direct interaction between the particle track and the target molecule (possibly the DNA) increases.

## BIBLIOGRAPHY

Goodwin PN, Quimby EH, Morgan RH: Physical Foundations of Radiology. New York, Harper & Row, 1970

Johns HE, Cunningham JR: The Physics of Radiology. Springfield, IL, Charles C Thomas, 1969

Rossi HH: Neutron and heavy particle dosimetry. In Reed GW (ed): Radiation Dosimetry: Proceedings of the International School of Physics, pp 98–107. New York, Academic Press, 1964

Smith VP (ed): Radiation Particle Therapy. Philadelphia, American College of Radiology, 1976

*Radiobiology for the Radiologist, Fourth Edition*, by Eric J. Hall
J. B. Lippincott Company, Philadelphia © 1994.

# 2

# *DNA Strand Breaks and Chromosomal Aberrations*

Diagnostic Radiology
Nuclear Medicine
Radiation Therapy

# DNA STRAND BREAKS

There is strong circumstantial evidence to indicate that DNA is the principal target for the biological effects of radiation, including cell killing, mutation, and carcinogenesis. A consideration of the biological effects of radiation must therefore begin logically with a description of the breaks in DNA caused by charged particle tracks and by the chemical species produced.

DNA consists of two strands that form a double helix. Each strand is composed of a series of deoxynucleotides, the sequence of which contains the genetic code (Fig. 2-1A). Sugar moieties and phosphate groups form the backbone of the double helix. The bases on opposite strands must be complementary; adenine pairs with thymine, while guanine pairs with cytosine. When cells are irradiated with x-rays, many breaks of a single strand occur. These can be observed and scored as a function of dose if the DNA is denatured and the supporting structure stripped away. In intact DNA, however, single-strand breaks are of little biological consequence as far as a cell killing is concerned because they are readily repaired using the opposite strand as a template (see Fig. 2-1B). If the repair is incorrect (misrepair), it may result in a mutation. If both strands of the DNA are broken, and the breaks are well separated (see Fig. 2-1C), repair again occurs readily since the two breaks are handled separately.

By contrast, if the breaks in the two strands are opposite one another, or separated by only a few base pairs (see Fig. 2-1D), this may lead to a double-strand break; that is, the piece of chromatin snaps into two pieces. A double-strand break is believed to be the most important lesion produced in chromosomes by radiation; as is described in the next section, the interaction of two double-strand breaks may result in cell killing, mutation, or carcinogenesis.

In practice, the situation is probably much more complicated than illustrated in Figure 2-1D, since both free radicals and direct ionizations may be involved. As described in Chapter 1, the en-

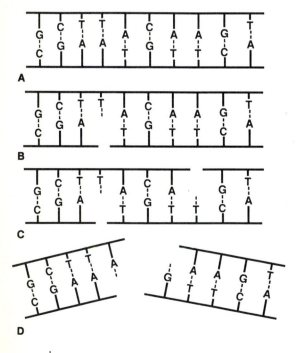

**A**

**B**

**C**

**D**

**Figure 2-1.** Diagrams of single- and double-strand DNA breaks caused by radiation. **(A)** Two-dimensional representation of the normal DNA double helix. The base pairs carrying the genetic code are complementary (ie, adenine pairs with thymine, guanine pairs with cytosine). **(B)** A break in one strand is of little significance because it is readily repaired, using the opposite strand as a template. **(C)** Breaks in both strands, if well separated, are repaired as independent breaks. **(D)** If breaks occur in both strands and are directly opposite or separated by only a few base pairs, this may lead to a double-strand break where the chromatin snaps into two pieces. (Courtesy of Dr. John Ward)

ergy from ionizing radiations is not deposited uniformly in the absorbing medium but is located along the tracks of the charged particles set in motion—electrons in the case of x- or γ-rays; protons and α-particles in the case of neutrons. Radiation chemists speak in terms of "spurs, blobs, and short tracks." There is, of course, a full spectrum of energy event sizes, and it is quite arbitrary to divide them into just three categories, but it turns out to be instructive. A spur contains up to 100 eV of energy and involves, on average, three ion pairs. In the case of x- or γ-rays, 95% of the energy deposition events are spurs, which have a diameter of about 4 nm, which is about twice the diameter of the DNA double helix (Fig. 2-2). Blobs are much less frequent for x- or γ-rays; they have a diameter of about 7 nm and contain on average about twelve ion pairs (see Fig. 2-2). Since spurs and blobs have dimensions similar to the DNA double helix, multiple radical attack will occur if they overlap the DNA helix. There are likely to be a wide variety of complex lesions, including base damage as well as double-strand breaks. The term *locally multiply damaged site* has been coined by John Ward to describe this phenomenon. Given the size of a spur and the diffusion distance of hydroxyl free radicals, the multiple damage could be spread out up to 20 base pairs. This is illustrated in Figure 2-2, where a double-strand break is accompanied by base damage and the loss of genetic information.

In the case of densely ionizing radiations, such as neutrons or α-particles, a greater proportion of blobs are produced. The damage produced, therefore, is qualitatively different to that produced by x-or γ-rays and much more difficult for the cell to repair.

## MEASURING DNA STRAND BREAKS

Both single-strand and double-strand DNA breaks can be measured readily by isolating the DNA from irradiated cells and causing the pieces to pass through a porous substrate, such as a gel or a filter. The DNA pieces move either under the influence of flow through the filter or electric field in the gel (using the fact that DNA is positively charged). Smaller pieces move faster and farther than larger pieces of DNA and can thus be separated and counted. The larger the dose of radiation, the more the DNA is broken up. DNA is denatured and lysed by a strong alkaline preparation so that single-strand breaks are measured. Double-strand breaks are measured in a neutral preparation.

## CHROMOSOMES AND CELL DIVISION

The backbone of DNA is made of molecules of sugar and phosphates, which serve as a framework to hold the bases that carry the genetic code. Attached to each sugar molecule is a base—thymine, adenine, guanine, or cytosine. This whole configuration is coiled tightly in a double helix.

Figure 2-3 is a highly schematized illustration of the way in which an organized folding of the long DNA helix might be achieved as a closely packed series of looped domains wound in a tight helix. The degree of packing is also illustrated by the relative dimensions of the DNA helix and the condensed metaphase chromosome.

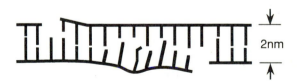

2nm

**Figure 2-2.** Illustration of a locally multiply damaged site. Energy from x-rays is not absorbed uniformly but tends to be localized along the tracks of charged particles. Radiation chemists speak in terms of spurs and blobs, which contain a number of ion pairs and which have dimensions comparable to the DNA double helix. A double-strand break is likely to be accompanied by extensive base damage. John Ward coined the term *locally multiply damaged site* (LMDS) to describe this phenomenon.

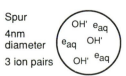

Spur
4nm diameter
3 ion pairs

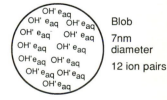

Blob
7nm diameter
12 ion pairs

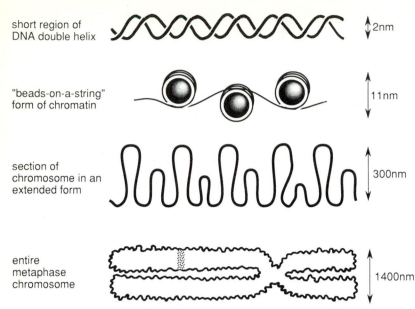

short region of
DNA double helix

↕2nm

"beads-on-a-string"
form of chromatin

↕11nm

section of
chromosome in an
extended form

↕300nm

entire
metaphase
chromosome

↕1400nm

**Figure 2-3.** Illustration of the relative sizes of the DNA helix, the various stages of folding and packing of the DNA, and an entire chromosome condensed at metaphase.

The largest part of the life of any somatic cell is spent in **interphase,** during which the nucleus, in a stained preparation, appears as a lacework of fine, lightly stained material in a translucent, colorless material surrounded by a membrane. In the interphase nucleus of most cells, one or more bodies of various sizes and shapes, called *nucleoli,* will be seen. In most cells, little more than this can be identified with a conventional light microscope. In fact, a great deal is happening during this time: the quantity of DNA in the nucleus doubles as each chromosome lays down an exact replica of itself next to itself. When the chromosomes become visible at mitosis, they are each present in duplicate.

The various events that occur during **mitosis** will first be reviewed. The first phase of division is called **prophase.** The beginning of this phase is marked by a thickening of the chromatin and an increase in its stainability as the chromosomes condense into light coils. By the end of prophase each chromosome has a lightly staining constriction known as a **centromere;** extending from the centromere are the arms of the chromosome. Prophase ends when the chromosomes reach maximal condensation and the nuclear membrane disappears, as do any nucleoli.

With the disappearance of the nuclear membrane the nuclear plasm and the cytoplasm mix. **Metaphase** then follows, in which two events occur simultaneously. The chromosomes move to the center of the cell (ie, to the cell's equator), while the spindle forms. The spindle is composed of fibers that cross the cell, linking its poles. Once the chromosomes are stabilized at the equator of the cell, their centromeres divide, and metaphase is complete.

The phase that follows, **anaphase,** is characterized by a movement of the chromosomes on the spindle to the poles. Chromosomes appear to be pulled toward the poles of the cell by fibers attached to the centromeres. The arms, particularly the long arms, tend to trail behind.

Anaphase is followed by the last step of the process of mitosis, **telophase.** In this phase the chromosomes, congregated at the poles of the cell, begin to uncoil. The nuclear membrane reappears, as do the nucleoli; and as the phase progresses, the chromosome coils unwind until the nucleus regains the appearance characteristic of interphase.

## RADIATION-INDUCED CHROMOSOME ABERRATIONS

In the traditional study of chromosome aberrations, the effects of ionizing radiations is described in terms of their appearance when a preparation is made at the first metaphase after exposure to radiation. This is the time when the structure of the chromosomes can be discerned.

The study of radiation damage in mammalian cell chromosomes is hampered by the large number of mammalian chromosomes per cell and by their small size. Most mammalian cells currently available for experimental purposes have a diploid complement of 40 or more chromosomes. There are exceptions, such as the Chinese hamster, with 22 chromosomes, and various marsupials, such as the rat kangaroo and woolly opossum, which have chromosome complements of 12 and 14, respectively. Many plant cells, however, contain fewer and generally much larger chromosomes; consequently, until recently, information on chromosomal radiation damage accrued principally from studies with plant cells.

When cells are irradiated with x-rays, breaks are produced in the chromosomes. The broken ends appear to be "sticky" and can rejoin with any other sticky end. It would appear, however, that a broken end cannot join with a normal, unbroken chromosome end. Once breaks are produced, different fragments may behave in a variety of ways:

1. The breaks may restitute, that is, rejoin in their original configuration. In this case, of course, nothing amiss will be visible at the next mitosis.
2. The breaks may fail to rejoin and give rise to an aberration, which will be scored as a deletion at the next mitosis.
3. Broken ends may reassort and rejoin other broken ends to give rise to chromosomes that appear to be grossly distorted when viewed at the following mitosis.

This is an oversimplified account; whether actual breaks occur in the chromosomes at the time of irradiation is not known, nor is the biological significance of "stickiness" understood.

The aberrations seen at metaphase are of two classes: *chromosome* aberrations and *chromatid* aberrations. **Chromosome aberrations** result if a cell is irradiated early in interphase, before the chromosome material has been duplicated. In this case the radiation-induced break will be in a single strand of chromatin; during the DNA synthetic phase that follows, this strand of chromatin will lay down an identical strand next to itself and will replicate the break that had been produced by the radiation. This will lead to a chromosome aberration visible at the next mitosis, because

there will be an identical break in the corresponding points of a pair of chromatin strands. If, on the other hand, the dose of radiation is given later in interphase, after the DNA material has doubled and the chromosomes consist of two strands of chromatin, then the aberrations produced are called **chromatid aberrations.** In regions removed from the centromere, chromatid arms may be fairly well separated, and it is reasonable to suppose that the radiation might break one chromatid without breaking its sister chromatid, or at least not in the same place. A break that occurs in a single chromatid arm after chromosome replication and leaves the opposite arm of the same chromosome undamaged leads to chromatid aberrations.

## EXAMPLES OF RADIATION-INDUCED ABERRATIONS

Many types of chromosomal aberrations and rearrangements are possible, but an exhaustive analysis is beyond the scope of this book. Three types of aberrations that are *lethal* to the cell will be described, followed by two common rearrangements that are consistent with cell viability but are involved in carcinogenesis as described in a Chapter 19. The three lethal aberrations are the ring and the dicentric, which are chromosome aberrations, and the anaphase bridge, which as described is a chromatid aberration. All three represent gross distortions and are clearly visible. Many other aberrations are possible but are not described here.

The formation of a **dicentric** is illustrated in diagrammatic form in Figure 2-4*A*. This aberration involves an interchange between two separate chromosomes. If a break is produced in each one early in interphase and the sticky ends are close to one another, they may rejoin as shown. This bizarre interchange will replicate during the DNA synthetic phase, and the result will be a grossly distorted chromosome with two centromeres (hence, *dicentric*). There will also be a fragment that has no centromere (*acentric fragment*). The appearance at metaphase is shown in the bottom panel of Figure 2-4*A*. An example of a dicentric and fragment in a metaphase human cell is shown in Figure 2-5*B*.

(text continues on page 22)

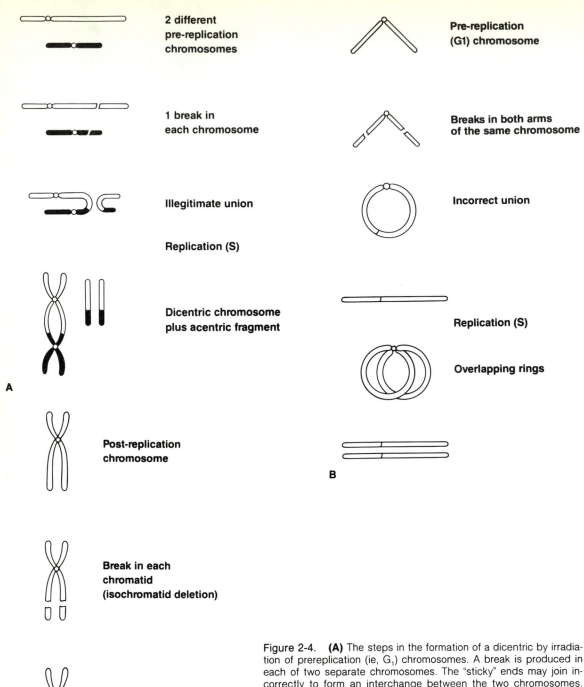

**A**

2 different
pre-replication
chromosomes

1 break in
each chromosome

Illegitimate union

Replication (S)

Dicentric chromosome
plus acentric fragment

Post-replication
chromosome

Break in each
chromatid
(isochromatid deletion)

Sister union

Dicentric chromatid,
N.B. symmetrical plus
acentric chromatid fragment

**C**

Pre-replication
(G1) chromosome

Breaks in both arms
of the same chromosome

Incorrect union

Replication (S)

Overlapping rings

**B**

Figure 2-4. **(A)** The steps in the formation of a dicentric by irradiation of prereplication (ie, $G_1$) chromosomes. A break is produced in each of two separate chromosomes. The "sticky" ends may join incorrectly to form an interchange between the two chromosomes. Replication then occurs in the DNA synthetic period. One chromosome has two centromeres, a dicentric. The other is an acentric fragment, which will be lost at a subsequent mitosis, since, lacking a centromere, it will not go to either pole at anaphase. **(B)** The steps in the formation of a ring by irradiation of a prereplication (ie, $G_1$) chromosome. A break occurs in each arm of the same chromosome. The sticky ends rejoin incorrectly to form a ring and an acentric fragment. Replication then occurs. **(C)** The steps in the formation of an anaphase bridge by irradiation of a postreplication (ie, $G_2$) chromosome. Breaks occur in each chromatid of the same chromosome. Incorrect rejoining of the sticky ends then occurs in a sister union. At the next anaphase the acentric fragment will be lost, while one centromere of the dicentric will go to each pole, and the chromatid will be stretched between the poles. Separation of the daughter cells will not be possible; this aberration is likely to be lethal. (Courtesy of Dr. Charles Geard)

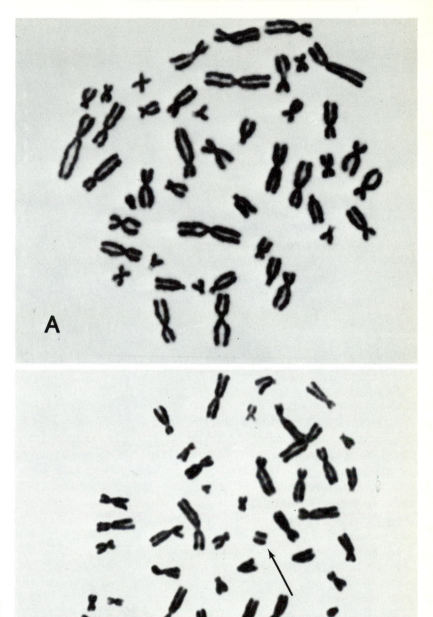

Figure 2-5. Radiation-induced chromosome aberrations in human leukocytes viewed at metaphase. **(A)** Normal metaphase. **(B)** Dicentric and fragment (*arrows*). **(C)** Ring (*arrow*). (Courtesy of Drs. Brewen, Luippold, and Preston)

*(continued)*

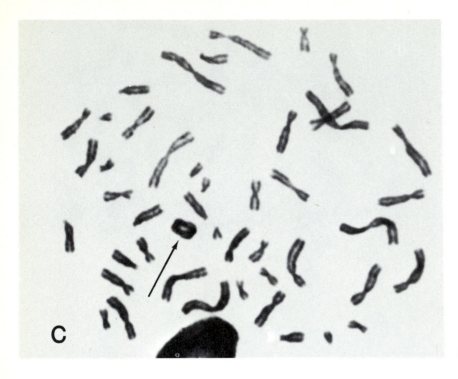

C

Figure 2-5. *(Continued)*

The formation of a **ring** is also illustrated in diagrammatic form in Figure 2-4B. A break is induced by radiation in each arm of a single chromatid early in the cell cycle. The sticky ends may rejoin to form a ring and a fragment. Later in the cycle, during the DNA synthetic phase, the chromosome replicates. The ultimate appearance at metaphase is shown in the lower panel of Figure 2-4B. The fragment has no centromere and probably will be lost at mitosis because it will not be pulled to either pole of the cell. An example of a ring chromosome in a human cell at metaphase is illustrated in Figure 2-5C.

An **anaphase bridge** may be produced in a variety of ways. As illustrated in Figure 2-6, it results from breaks that occur late in the cell cycle (in $G_2$), after the chromosomes have replicated. Breaks may occur in both chromatids of the same chromosome, and the sticky ends may rejoin incorrectly to form a sister union. At anaphase, when the two sets of chromosomes move to opposite poles, the section of chromatin between the two centromeres is stretched across the cell between the poles, hindering the separation into two new daughter cells, as illustrated in the bottom panel of Figure 2-6. The two fragments may

join as shown, but since there is no centromere it will probably be lost at the first mitosis. This type of aberration occurs in human cells and is essentially always lethal. It is hard to demonstrate because preparations of human chromosomes are usually made by accumulating cells at metaphase while the bridge is only evident at anaphase. Figure 2-6 is an anaphase preparation of *Tradescantia paludosa,* a plant used extensively for cytogenetic studies because of the small number of large chromosomes. The anaphase bridge is clearly seen as the replicate sets of chromosomes move to opposite poles of the cell.

Gross chromosome changes of the types discussed earlier inevitably lead to the reproductive death of the cell.

Two important types of chromosomal changes that are *not* lethal to the cell are a symmetrical translocation and a small deletion. The formation of a symmetrical translocation is illustrated in Figure 2-7. It involves a break in two prereplication (ie, $G_1$ phase) chromosomes, with the broken ends being exchanged between the two chromosomes as illustrated. An aberration of this type is difficult to see in a conventional preparation but is easy to observe with the

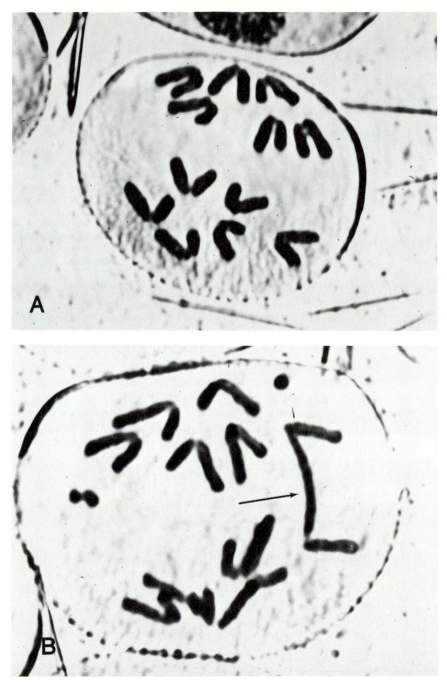

Figure 2-6. Anaphase chromosome preparation of *Tradescantia paludosa*. **(A)** Normal anaphase. **(B)** Bridge and fragment resulting from radiation (*arrow*). (Courtesy of Drs. Brewen, Luippold, and Preston)

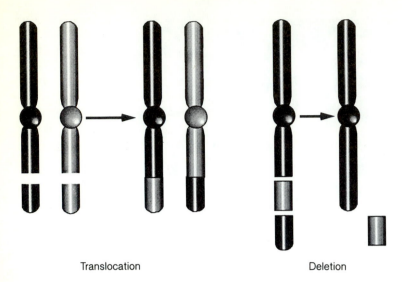

Translocation

Deletion

**Figure 2-7.** (*Left*) Illustration of the formation of a symmetrical translocation. Radiation produces breaks in two different prereplication chromosomes. The broken pieces are exchanged between the two chromosomes, and the "sticky" ends rejoin. This aberration is not necessarily lethal to the cell. There are examples in which an exchange aberration of this type leads to the activation of an oncogene. See Chapter 19 on radiation carcinogenesis. (*Right*) Diagram of a deletion. Radiation produces two breaks in the same arm of the same chromosome. What actually happens is illustrated more clearly in Figure 2-8.

technique of fluorescent in situ hybridization (FISH), or chromosome painting as it is commonly called. Probes are available for many human chromosomes that make them fluoresce in a bright color. Exchange of material between two different chromosomes is then readily observable. A translocation is associated with several human malignancies owing to the activa-

tion of an oncogene. Burkitt's lymphoma is an example.

The other type of nonlethal chromosomal change is a small interstitial deletion. This is also illustrated in Figure 2-7 and may result from two breaks in the same arm of the same chromosome, leading to the loss of the genetic information between the two breaks. The actual se-

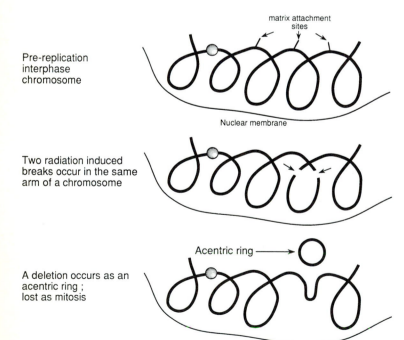

Pre-replication interphase chromosome

matrix attachment sites

Nuclear membrane

Two radiation induced breaks occur in the same arm of a chromosome

A deletion occurs as an acentric ring ; lost as mitosis

Acentric ring

**Figure 2-8.** Illustration of the formation of a deletion by ionizing radiation in an interphase chromosome. It is easy to imagine how two breaks may occur (by a single or two different charged particles) in such a way as to isolate a loop of DNA. The "sticky" ends rejoin, and the deletion is lost at a subsequent mitosis since it has no centromere. This loss of DNA may include the loss of a suppressor gene and lead to a malignant change. See Chapter 19 on radiation carcinogenesis.

quence of events in the formation of a deletion is easier to understand from Figure 2-8, which shows an interphase chromosome. It is a simple matter to imagine how two breaks may isolate a loop of DNA—an acentric ring—which will be lost at a subsequent mitosis. A deletion may be associated with carcinogenesis if the lost genetic material includes a suppressor gene. This will be discussed further in Chapter 19 on radiation carcinogenesis.

## CHROMOSOME ABERRATIONS IN HUMAN LYMPHOCYTES

Chromosomal aberrations in peripheral lymphocytes have been widely used as biomarkers of radiation exposure. When blood samples are obtained for cytogenetic evaluation within a few days to a few weeks after total-body irradiation, the frequency of asymmetrical aberrations in the lymphocytes (dicentrics and rings) reflects the dose received. Lymphocytes in the blood sample are stimulated to divide with a mitogen such as phytohemagglutinin and are arrested at metaphase, and the incidence of rings and dicentrics is scored. The dose can be estimated by comparison with in vitro cultures exposed to known doses. Figure 2-9 shows a dose–response curve

for aberrations in human lymphocytes produced by γ-rays. The data are fitted by a linear-quadratic relationship, as would be expected since rings and dicentrics result from the interaction of two chromosome breaks as previously described. The **linear** component is a consequence of the two breaks resulting from a single charged particle. If the two breaks result from different charged particles, the probability of an interaction will be a **quadratic** function of dose. This is also illustrated for the formation of a dicentric in Figure 2-9.

When a sufficient number of metaphases are scored, cytogenetic evaluations in cultured lymphocytes can readily detect recent total-body exposures of 10 to 20 rem in the exposed person. Such studies are useful in distinguishing between "real" and "suspected" exposures, particularly in those instances involving "black film badges" or in potential accidents when it is not certain whether persons who were at risk for exposure actually received a radiation dose.

Mature T lymphocytes have a finite life span of about 1500 days and are slowly eliminated from the peripheral lymphocyte pool. Consequently, the yield of dicentrics observed in peripheral lymphocytes will decline in the months and years after a radiation exposure.

During in vivo exposures to ionizing radiation,

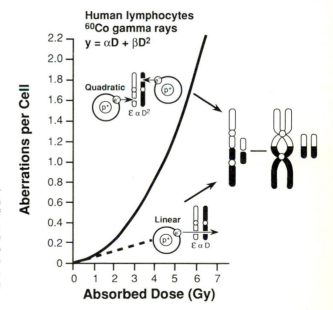

**Figure 2-9.** The frequency of chromosomal aberrations (dicentrics and rings) is a linear-quadratic function of dose because the aberrations are the consequence of the interation of two separate breaks. At low doses, both breaks may be caused by the same electron; the probability of an exchange aberration is proportional to dose (D). At higher doses, the two breaks are more likely to be caused by separate electrons. The probability of an exchange aberration is proportional to the square of the dose (D²)

chromosome aberrations are induced not only in mature lymphocytes but also in lymphocyte progenitors in marrow, nodes, or other organs.

The stem cells that sustain asymmetrical aberrations (such as dicentrics) will die in attempting a subsequent mitosis, but those that sustain a symmetrical nonlethal aberration (such as a translocation) will survive and pass on the aberration to their progeny. These persistent stable aberrations can be detected in persons exposed to radiation many years before. Until recently, translocations were much more difficult to observe than dicentrics, but now the technique of fluorescent in situ hybridization, or "chromosome painting" as it is commonly called, makes the scoring of such symmetrical aberrations a relatively simple matter. The frequency of translocations assessed in this way correlates with total-body dose, even in exposed persons after more than 40 years, as has been shown from a recent study of the survivors of the A-bomb attacks on Hiroshima and Nagasaki in 1945.

► *Summary of Pertinent Conclusions*

- Many single-strand breaks are produced in DNA by radiation but are readily repaired using the opposite DNA strand as a template.
- Breaks in both strands, if well separated, are also readily repaired since they are handled individually.
- Breaks in both strands that are opposite, or separated by only a few base pairs, may lead to a double-strand break.
- Energy from x-rays is deposited unevenly in "spurs" and "blobs." This may lead to *multiply damaged sites*, that is, a combination of a double-strand break and base damage.
- Radiation-induced breakage and incorrect rejoining in prereplication chromosomes ($G_1$ phase) may lead to *chromosome aberrations*.
- Radiation-induced breakage and incorrect rejoining in postreplication chromosomes (S or $G_2$ phase) may lead to *chromatid aberrations*.
- Principal aberrations include *dicentrics, rings, acentric fragments*, and *anaphase bridges*.
- The incidence of most radiation-induced aberrations is a linear-quadratic function of dose.
- Scoring aberrations in lymphocytes from peripheral blood may be used to estimate total-body doses in humans accidentally irradiated. The lowest single dose that can be detected readily is 25 rads (0.25 Gy).
- Aberrations can still be detected in irradiated persons up to 40 years after exposure.
- There is a good correlation between cells killed and cells with an asymmetrical exchange aberration (ie, a dicentric or a ring).

# BIBLIOGRAPHY

Alper T, Fowler JF, Morgan RL, Vonberg DD, Ellis F, Oliver R: The characterization of the "type C" survival curve. Br J Radiol 35:722–723, 1962

Andrews JR, Berry RJ: Fast neutron irradiation and the relationship of radiation dose and mammalian cell reproductive capacity. Radiat Res 16:76–81, 1962

Barendsen GW, Beusker TLJ, Vergroesen AJ, Budke L: Effects of different ionizing radiations on human cells in tissue culture: II. Biological experiments. Radiat Res 13:841–849, 1960

Bender M: Induced aberrations in human chromosomes. Am J Pathol 43:26a, 1963

Carrano AV: Chromosome aberrations and radiation-induced cell death: II. Predicted and observed cell survival. Mutat Res 17:355–366, 1973

Cornforth MN, Bedford JS: A quantitative comparison of potentially lethal damage repair and the rejoining of interphase chromosome breaks in low passage normal human fibroblasts. Radiat Res 111:385–405, 1987

Cornforth MN, Bedford JS: X-ray-induced breakage and rejoining of human interphase chromosomes. Science 222:1141–1143, 1983

Elkind MM, Sutton H: Radiation response of mammalian cells grown in culture: I. Repair of x-ray damage in surviving Chinese hamster cells. Radiat Res 13:556–593, 1960

Evans HJ: Chromosome aberrations induced by ionizing radiation. Int Rev Cytol 13:221–321, 1962

Frankenberg D, Frankenberg-Schwager M, Harbich R: Split-dose recovery is due to the repair of DNA double-strand breaks. Int J Radiat Biol 46:541–553, 1984

Gasser SM, Laemmli UK: A glimpse at chromosomal order. Trends Genet 3:16–22, 1987

Geard CR: Effects of radiation on chromosomes. In Pizzarello D (ed): Radiation Biology, pp 83–110. Boca Raton, FL, CRC Press, 1982

Georgiev GP, Nedospasov SA, Bakayev VV: Supranucleosomal levels of chromatin organization. In

Busch H (ed): The Cell Nucleus, vol 6, pp 3–34. New York, Academic Press, 1978

Grell RF: The chromosome. J Tenn Acad Sci 37:43–53, 1962

Ishihara T, Sasaki MS (eds): Radiation-Induced Chromosome Damage in Man. New York, Alan R. Liss, 1983

Lea DEA: Actions of Radiations on Living Cells, 2nd ed. Cambridge, England, Cambridge University Press, 1956

Littlefield LG, Kleinerman RA, Sayer AM, Tarone R, Boice JD Jr: Chromosome aberrations in lymphocytes—biomonitors of radiation exposure. In Barton L, Gledhill I, Francesco M (eds): New Horizons in Biological Dosimetry, pp 387–397. New York, Wiley-Liss, 1991

Littlefield LG, Lushbaugh CC: Cytogenetic dosimetry for radiation accidents—"The good, the bad, and the ugly." In Ricks RC, Fry SA (eds): The Medical Basis for Radiation Accident Preparedness, Vol II, Clinical Experience and Follow-up Since 1979, pp 461–478. New York, Elsevier, 1990

Marsden M, Laemmli UK: Metaphase chromosome structure: Evidence for a radial loop model. Cell 17:849–858, 1979

Moorhead PS, Nowell PC, Mellman WJ, Battips DM, Hungerford DA: Chromosome preparation of leukocytes cultured from human peripheral blood. Exp Cell Res 20:613–616, 1960

Munro TR: The relative radiosensitivity of the nucleus and cytoplasm of the Chinese hamster fibroblasts. Radiat Res 42:451–470, 1970

Puck TT, Markus PI: Action of x-rays on mammalian cells. J Exp Med 103:653–666, 1956

Revell SH: Relationship between chromosome damage and cell death. In Ishihara T, Sasaki MS (eds): Radiation-Induced Chromosome Damage in Man, pp 215–233. New York, Alan R. Liss, 1983

Ris H: Chromosome structure. In McElroy WD, Glass B (eds): Chemical Basis of Heredity. Baltimore, Johns Hopkins University Press, 1957

Spear FG: On some biological effects of radiation. Br J Radiol 31:114–124, 1958

*Radiobiology for the Radiologist, Fourth Edition,* by Eric J. Hall
J. B. Lippincott Company, Philadelphia © 1994.

# 3

# *Cell Survival Curves*

Diagnostic Radiology
Nuclear Medicine
Radiation Therapy

# REPRODUCTIVE INTEGRITY

A **cell survival curve** describes the relationship between the radiation dose and the proportion of cells that survive. What is meant by "survival"? Cell survival, or its converse, **cell death,** may mean different things to different persons; therefore, a precise definition is essential. For differentiated cells that do not proliferate, such as nerve, muscle, or secretory cells, death can be defined as the loss of a specific function. For proliferating cells, such as hematopoietic stem cells or cells growing in culture, loss of the capacity for sustained proliferation—that is, loss of *reproductive integrity*—is an appropriate definition. This is sometimes called **reproductive death.**

This definition reflects a narrow view of radiobiology. A cell may still be physically present and apparently intact, may be able to make proteins or synthesize DNA, and may even be able to struggle through one or two mitoses; but if it has lost the capacity to divide indefinitely and produce a large number of progeny, it is by definition dead; it has not survived. A survivor that has retained its reproductive integrity and is able to proliferate indefinitely to produce a large clone or colony is said to be **clonogenic**.

This definition is generally relevant to the radiobiology of whole animals and plants and their tissues. It has particular relevance to the radiotherapy of tumors. For a tumor to be eradicated, it is only necessary that cells be "killed" in the sense that they are rendered unable to divide and cause further growth and spread of the malignancy. For cells in culture, death while attempting mitosis appears to be dominant. It is not, however, the only form of cell death. Programmed cell death, or apoptosis, occurs in tumors and normal tissues and is described in Chapter 4.

In general, a dose of 100 Gy (10,000 rads) is necessary to destroy cell function in nonproliferating systems. By contrast, the mean lethal dose for loss of proliferative capacity is usually less than 2 Gy (200 rads).

# THE IN VITRO SURVIVAL CURVE

The capability of a single cell to grow into a large colony, which can easily be seen with the naked eye, is a convenient proof that it has retained its reproductive integrity. The loss of this ability as a function of radiation dose is described by the dose survival curve.

With modern techniques of tissue culture it is possible to take a specimen from a tumor or from many normal regenerative tissues, chop it into small pieces, and prepare a single-cell suspension by the use of the enzyme trypsin, which dissolves and loosens the cell membrane. If these cells are seeded into a culture dish, covered with an appropriate complex growth medium, and maintained at 37°C under aseptic conditions, they attach to the surface, grow, and divide.

In practice, most fresh explants grow well for a few weeks but subsequently peter out and die. A few pass through a crisis and then continue to grow for many years. Every few days the culture must be "farmed": the cells are removed from the surface with trypsin, most of the cells are discarded, and the culture flask is reseeded with a small number of cells, which quickly repopulate the culture flask. These are the so-called **established cell lines,** which have been used extensively in experimental cellular radiobiology.

Survival curves are so basic to an understanding of much of radiobiology that it is worthwhile to go through the steps involved in a typical experiment using an established cell line in culture.

Cells from an actively growing stock culture are prepared into a suspension by the use of trypsin, which causes the cells to round up and detach from the surface of the culture vessel. The number of cells per unit volume of this suspension is counted in a hemocytometer or with an electronic counter. In this way, for example, 100 individual cells may be seeded into a dish; if this dish is incubated for 1 to 2 weeks, each single cell will divide many times and form a colony that is easily visible with the naked eye, especially if it is fixed and stained (Fig. 3-1). All cells

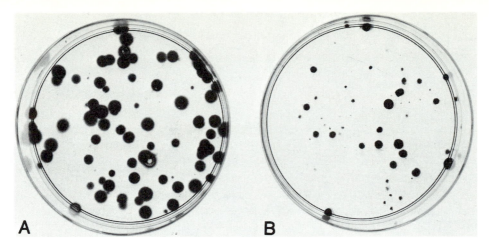

**Figure 3-1.** Colonies obtained with Chinese hamster cells cultured in vitro. **(A)** In this unirradiated control dish 100 cells were seeded and allowed to grow for 7 days before being stained. There are 70 colonies; therefore the plating efficiency is 70/100, or 70%. **(B)** Two thousand cells were seeded, then exposed to 800 rads (8 Gy) of x-rays. There are 32 colonies on the dish. Thus

$$\text{Surviving fraction} = \frac{\text{Colonies counted}}{\text{Cells seeded} \times (\text{PE}/100)}$$

$$= \frac{32}{2000 \times .70}$$

$$= 0.023$$

comprising each colony are the progeny of a single ancestor. For a nominal 100 cells seeded into the dish, the number of colonies counted may be expected to be in the range of 50 to 90. Ideally, it should be 100, but it seldom is for a variety of reasons, including suboptimal growth medium, errors and uncertainties in counting the cell suspension, and the trauma of trypsinization and handling. The term **plating efficiency** (PE) indicates the percentage of cells seeded that grow into colonies. There are 70 colonies on the control dish in Figure 3-1*A*; therefore the PE is 70%.

When a parallel dish is seeded with cells, exposed to a dose of 8 Gy (800 rads) of x-rays, and incubated for 1 to 2 weeks before being fixed and stained, then the following may be observed: (1) some of the seeded single cells are still single and have not divided; (2) some cells have managed to complete one or two divisions to form a tiny abortive colony; and (3) some cells have grown into large colonies that differ little from the unirradiated controls, although they may vary more in size. These cells are said to have survived, since they have retained their reproductive integrity.

In the example shown in Figure 3-1*B*, 2000 cells had been seeded into the dish exposed to 8 Gy (800 rads). Since the PE is 70%, 1400 of the 2000 cells plated would have grown into colonies if the dish had not been irradiated. In fact, there are only 32 colonies on the dish in Figure 3-1*B*; the fraction of cells surviving the dose of x-rays is thus

$$\frac{32}{1400} = 0.023$$

In general, the surviving fraction is given by

$$\text{Surviving fraction} = \frac{\text{Colonies counted}}{\text{Cells seeded} \times (\text{PE}/100)}$$

This process is repeated so that estimates of survival are obtained for a range of doses. The number of cells seeded per dish is adjusted so that a countable number of colonies results; too few would reduce statistical significance, while too many could not be counted accurately because they tend to merge into one another. The technique is illustrated in Figure 3-2.

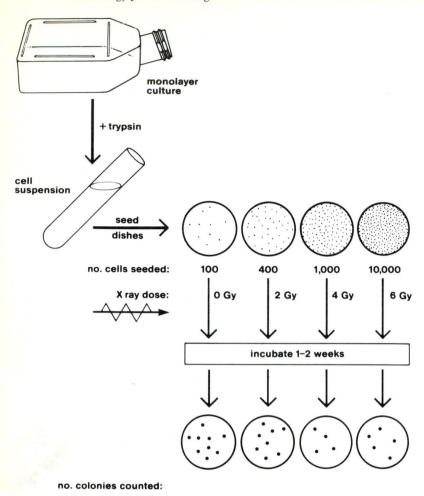

**Figure 3-2.** The cell culture technique used to generate a cell survival curve. Cells from a stock culture are prepared into a single-cell suspension by trypsinization, and the cell concentration is counted. Known numbers of cells are inoculated into petri dishes and irradiated. They are then allowed to grow until the surviving cells produce macroscopic colonies that can be readily counted. The number of cells per dish initially inoculated varies with the dose so that the number of colonies surviving is in the range that can be counted conveniently. Surviving fraction is the ratio of colonies produced to cells plated, with a correction necessary for plating efficiency (ie, for the fact that not all cells plated grow into colonies, even in the absence of radiation).

## THE SHAPE OF THE SURVIVAL CURVE

Survival curves for mammalian cells are usually presented in the form shown in Figure 3-3, with dose plotted on a linear scale and surviving fraction on a logarithmic scale. Qualitatively, the shape of the survival curve can be described in relatively simple terms. At "low doses" for sparsely ionizing (low linear energy transfer) radiations, such as x-rays, the survival curve starts out straight on the log-linear plot with a finite initial slope; that is, the surviving fraction is an exponential function of dose. At higher doses, the curve bends. This bending or curving region extends over a dose range of a few Gy (few hundred rads). At very high doses the survival curve often tends to straighten again; the surviving fraction returns to being an exponential function of dose. In general, this does not occur until doses in excess of those used as daily fractions in radiotherapy have been reached.

By contrast, for densely ionizing (high linear energy transfer) radiations, such as α-particles or low-energy neutrons, the cell survival curve is a straight line from the origin; that is, survival approximates to an exponential function of dose (see Fig. 3-3).

Although it is a simple matter to qualitatively describe the shape of the cell survival curve, finding an explanation of the biological obervations in terms of biophysical events is another matter. Many biophysical models and theories have been proposed to account for the

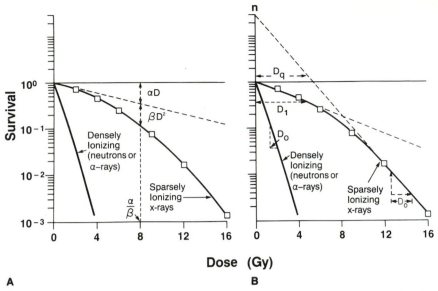

**Figure 3-3.** Shape of survival curve for mammalian cells exposed to radiation. The fraction of cells surviving is plotted on a logarithmic scale against dose on a linear scale. For $\alpha$-particles or low-energy neutrons (said to be densely ionizing) the dose–response curve is a straight line from the origin (ie, survival is an exponential function of dose). The survival curve can be described by just one parameter, the slope. For x- or $\gamma$-rays (said to be sparsely ionizing), the dose–response curve has an initial linear slope, followed by a shoulder; at higher doses the curve tends to become straight again. **(A)** The experimental data are fitted to a linear-quadratic function. There are two components of cell killing: one is proportional to dose ($\alpha D$), while the other is proportional to the square of the dose ($\beta D^2$). The dose at which the linear and quadratic components are equal is the ratio $\alpha/\beta$. The linear-quadratic curve bends continuously but is a good fit to experimental data for the first few decades of survival. **(B)** The curve is described by the initial slope ($D_1$), the final slope ($D_0$), and a parameter that represents the width of the shoulder, either $n$ or $D_q$.

shape of the mammalian cell survival curve. Almost all can be used to deduce a curve shape that is consistent with experimental data, but it is never possible to choose among different models or theories on the basis of goodness of fit to experimental data. The biological data are not sufficiently precise nor are the predictive theoretical curves sufficiently different for this to be possible.

Two descriptions of the shape of survival curves are discussed briefly with a minimum of mathematics (see Fig. 3-3). First, the multitarget model that was widely used for many years still has some merit. In this model, the survival curve is described in terms of an initial slope, $D_1$, due to single-event killing, a final slope, $D_0$, due to multiple-event killing, and some quantity (either $n$ or $D_q$) to represent the size or width of the shoulder of the curve. The quantities $D_1$ and $D_0$ are the reciprocals of the initial and final slopes. In each case it is the dose required to reduce the

fraction of surviving cells to 37% of its previous value. As illustrated, $D_1$, the initial slope, is the dose required to reduce the fraction of surviving cells to 0.37 on the initial straight portion of the survival curve. The final slope, $D_0$, is the dose required to reduce survival from 0.1 to 0.037, or from 0.01 to 0.0037. Since the surviving fraction is on a logarithmic scale and the survival curve becomes straight at higher doses, the dose required to reduce the cell population by a given factor (to 0.37) is the same at all survival levels. It is, on average, the dose required to deliver one inactivating event per cell.

The *extrapolation number*, $n$, is a measure of the width of the shoulder. If $n$ is large (eg, 10 or 12), the survival curve has a broad shoulder. If $n$ is small (eg, 1.5 to 2), the shoulder of the curve is narrow. Another measure of shoulder width is the *quasi-threshold dose*, shown as $D_q$ in Figure 3-3. This sounds like a term invented by a committee, which in a sense it is! An easy way to remember its meaning is to think of the hunchback of Notre Dame. When the priest was handed the badly deformed infant who was to grow up to be the hunchback, he cradled him in his arms and said, "We will call him Quasimodo—he is almost a person!" Similarly, the quasi-threshold dose is almost a threshold dose. It is defined as the dose at which the straight portion of the survival curve, extrapolated backward, cuts the dose axis drawn through a survival fraction of unity. A threshold dose is the dose below which there is no effect. There is no dose below which radiation produces *no* effect, so there can be no true threshold dose; $D_q$, the quasi-threshold dose, is the closest thing.

At first sight this might appear to be a most awkward parameter, but in practice it has certain merits that will become apparent later. The three parameters, n, $D_0$, and $D_q$ are related by the expression

$$\log_e n = D_q/D_0$$

The linear-quadratic model has now taken over as the model of choice to describe survival curves. It is a direct development of the relation used to described exchange-type chromosome aberrations which are clearly the result of an interaction between two separate breaks. This is discussed in some detail in Chapter 2.

The linear-quadratic model assumes that there are two components to cell killing by radiation, one that is proportional to dose and one that is proportional to the square of the dose. The notion of a component of cell inactivation that varies with the square of the dose introduces the concept of *dual-radiation action*. This idea goes back to the early work with chromosomes in which many chromosome aberrations are clearly the result of two separate breaks. (Examples discussed in Chapter 2 were rings, dicentrics, and anaphase bridges, all of which are likely to be lethal to the cell.)

By this model the expression for the cell survival curve is

$$S = e^{-\alpha D - \beta D^2}$$

where S is the fraction of cells surviving a dose D, and $\alpha$ and $\beta$ are constants. The components

of cell killing that are proportional to dose and to the square of the dose are equal when

$$\alpha D = \beta D^2,$$

or

$$D = \alpha/\beta$$

This is an important point that bears repeating: the linear and quadratic contributions to cell killing are equal at a dose that is equal to the ratio of $\alpha$ to $\beta$. This is illustrated in Figure 3-3A.

A characteristic of the linear-quadratic formulation is that the resultant cell survival curve is continuously bending; there is no final straight portion. This does not coincide with what is observed experimentally when survival curves are determined down to 7 or more decades of cell killing, when the dose–response relationship closely approximates to a straight line in a log-linear plot; that is, cell killing is an exponential function of dose. In the first decade or so of cell killing and up to any doses used as daily fractions in clinical radiotherapy, however, the linear-quadratic model is an adequate representation of the data. It has the distinct advantage of having only two adjustable parameters, $\alpha$ and $\beta$.

Figure 3-4 illustrates, in a much oversimplified way, the relationship between chromosome aberrations and cell killing. As explained in Chapter 2, cells in which there is an asymmetrical exchange-type aberration (such as a dicentric or a ring) lose their reproductive integrity. Exchange-type aberrations require *two* chromosome breaks. At low doses, the two breaks may result from the passage of a single electron set in motion by the absorption of a photon of x- or $\gamma$-rays. The probability of an interaction between the two breaks to form a lethal exchange-type aberration is proportional to dose. Consequently, the survival curve is linear at low doses. At higher doses the two chromosome breaks may result from two *separate* electrons. The probability of an interaction between the two breaks is then proportional to (dose)$^2$. When this quadratic component dominates, the survival curve bends over and becomes curved. Thus, the linear-quadratic relationship characteristic of the induction of chromosome aberrations is carried over to the cell survival curve.

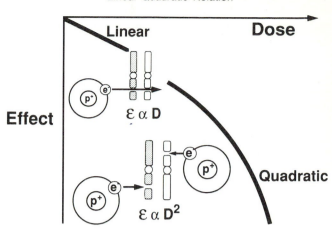

**Figure 3-4.** Relationship between chromosome aberrations and cell survival. Cells that suffer exchange-type chromosome aberrations (such as a dicentric) are unable to survive and continue to divide indefinitely. At low doses, the two chromosome breaks are the consequence of a single electron set in motion by the absorption of x- or γ-rays. The probability of an interaction between the breaks is proportional to dose; this is the linear portion of the survival curve. At higher doses, the two chromosome breaks may result also from two separate electrons. The probability of an interaction is then proportional to (dose)$^2$. The survival curve bends when the quadratic component dominates.

## SURVIVAL CURVES FOR VARIOUS MAMMALIAN CELLS IN CULTURE

Survival curves have been measured for many established cell lines grown in culture. These cell lines have been derived from the tissues of humans or other mammals, such as small rodents. In some cases the parent tissue has been neoplastic, and in other cases it has been normal. The first in vitro survival curve for mammalian cells irradiated with x-rays is shown in Figure 3-5. All mammalian cells studied to date, normal or malignant, regardless of their species of origin, exhibit x-ray survival curves similar to those in Figure 3-5; there is an initial shoulder followed by a portion that tends to become straight on a log-linear plot. The size of the initial shoulder is extremely variable. For some cell lines the survival curve appears to bend continuously so that the linear-quadratic relationship is a better fit and n has no meaning. The $D_0$ of the x-ray survival

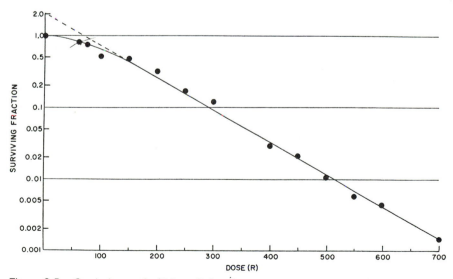

**Figure 3-5.** Survival curve for HeLa cells in culture exposed to x-rays. Characteristically, this cell line has a small initial shoulder. (From Puck TT, Marcus PI: J Exp Med 103:653, 1956; courtesy of the author and Rockefeller University Press)

curves for most cells cultured in vitro fall in the range of 1 to 2 Gy (100 to 200 rads). The exceptions are cells from patients with cancer-prone syndromes, such as ataxia-telangiectasia; these cells are much more sensitive to ionizing radiations, with a $D_0$ for x-rays of about 0.5 Gy (50 rads). This in vitro sensitivity correlates with a hypersensitivity to radiotherapy found in these persons.

The first in vitro survival curve was reported in 1956 and generated great excitement in the field of radiobiology. It was thought that at last, with a quantitative system available to relate absorbed dose with surviving fraction of cells, great strides would be made in understanding the effect of ionizing radiation on biological materials. In particular, it was anticipated that significant contributions would be made toward understanding radiotherapeutic practice. This enthusiasm was not shared by everyone. Some researchers were skeptical that these in vitro techniques, which involved growing cells in petri dishes in very artificial conditions, would ever benefit clinical radiotherapy. The fears of these skeptics were eloquently voiced by Dr. F. G. Spear in the MacKenzie Davidson Memorial Lecture given to the British Institute of Radiology in 1957:

> An isolated cell *in vitro* does not necessarily behave as it would have done if left *in vivo* in normal association with cells of other types. Its reactions to various stimuli, including radiations, however interesting and important in themselves, may indeed be no more typical of its behaviour in the parent tissue than Robinson Crusoe on his desert island was representative of social life in York in the mid-seventeenth century.

The appropriate answer to this charge was given by Dr. David Gould, then Professor of Radiology at the University of Colorado. He pointed out that the in vitro culture technique measured the reproductive integrity of cells and that there was no reason to suppose that Robinson Crusoe's reproductive integrity was any different on his desert island from what it would have been had he remained in York; all that Robinson Crusoe lacked was the opportunity! The opportunity to reproduce to the limit of their capability is afforded to cells cultured in vitro when they find themselves in the petri dish, with temperature and humidity controlled, and with an abundant supply of nutrients.

At the time it required a certain amount of faith and optimism to believe that survival curves determined with the in vitro technique could indeed be applied to the complex in vivo situation. Such faith and optimism were, however, completely vindicated by subsequent events. When techniques became available to measure cell survival in vivo, the parameters of the dose–response relationships were shown to be similar to those in vitro.

In more recent years, extensive studies have been made of the radiosensitivity of cells of human origin, both normal and malignant, grown and irradiated in culture. In general, cells from a given normal tissue show a narrow range of radiosensitivities when many hundreds of persons are studied (Fig. 3-6). By contrast, cells from human tumors show a very broad range of $D_0$ values; some cells such as those from squamous carcinomas tend to be more radioresistant, while sarcomas are somewhat more radiosensitive. Each tumor type, however, has a broad spectrum of radiosensitivities that tend to overlap. Tumor cells bracket the radiosensitivity of cells from normal tissues; that is, some are more sensitive, while others are more resistant.

## INTRINSIC RADIOSENSITIVITY AND PREDICTIVE ASSAYS

Predictive assays of individual tumor radiosensitivity require cells to be grown from fresh explants of human tumor biopsies. These do not grow well as attached cells in regular clonogenic assays. Better results have been obtained with the Courtenay assay, in which cells grow in a semisolid agar gel supplemented with growth factors. In addition, a number of nonclonogenic assays have been developed based on cell growth in a multi-well plate. Growth is assessed in terms of the ability of cells to reduce a compound that can be visualized by staining or is based on total DNA or total RNA content of the well. These endpoints are surrogates from clonogenicity or reproductive integrity. See Chapter 15 for a discussion of predictive assays.

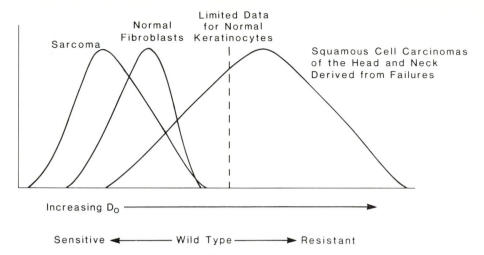

**Figure 3-6.** Summary of $D_0$ values for cells of human origin grown and irradiated in vitro. Cells from human tumors tend to have a wide range of radiosensitivities, which brackets the radiosensitivity of normal human fibroblasts. In general, squamous cell carcinoma cells are more resistant than sarcoma cells, but the spectra of radiosensitivities are broad and overlap. (Courtesy of Dr. Ralph Wechselbaum)

## THE EFFECTIVE SURVIVAL CURVE FOR A MULTIFRACTION REGIMEN

Since multifraction regimens are most often used in clinical radiotherapy, it is frequently useful to think in terms of an effective survival curve.

When radiation dose is delivered in a series of equal fractions, separated by sufficient time for repair of sublethal damage to occur between doses, the effective dose survival curve becomes an exponential function of dose. The shoulder of the survival curve is repeated many times so that the effective survival curve is a straight line from the origin through a point on the single-dose survival curve corresponding to the daily dose fraction. This is illustrated in Figure 3-7. The effective survival curve will be an exponential function of dose whether the single-dose survival curve has a constant terminal slope (as shown) or whether it is continuously bending as implied by the linear-quadratic relation. The $D_0$ of the effective survival curve (ie, the reciprocal of the slope), defined to be the dose required to reduce the fraction of cells surviving to 37%, has a value close to 300 cGy for cells of human origin. This is an average value and can differ significantly for different tumor types.

For calculation purposes, it is often useful to use the $D_{10}$, the dose required to kill 90% of the population. For example,

$$D_{10} = 2.3 \times D_0$$

where 2.3 is the natural logarithm of 10.

## CALCULATIONS OF TUMOR CELL KILL

The concept outlined earlier of an effective survival curve for a multifraction radiation treatment may be used to perform simple calculations of tumor cell kill after radiotherapy. Although such calculations are greatly oversimplified, they are nevertheless instructive. Four examples are given here.

PROBLEM 1: A tumor consists of $10^9$ clonogenic cells. The effective dose–response curve, given in daily dose fractions of 2 Gy, has no shoulder and a $D_0$ of 3 Gy. What total dose is required to give a 90% chance of tumor cure?

ANSWER: To give a 90% probability of tumor control in a tumor containing $10^9$ cells requires a cellular depopulation of $10^{-10}$. The dose to result in 1 decade of cell killing ($D_{10}$) is given by

$$D_{10} = 2.3 \times D_0 = 2.3 \times 3 = 6.9 \text{ Gy}$$

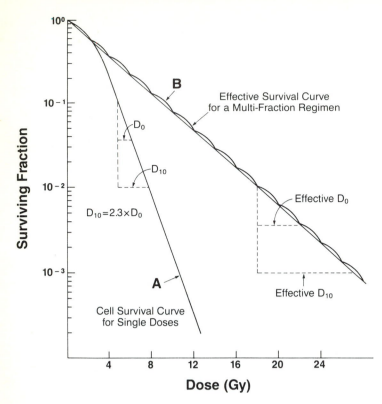

**Figure 3-7.** The concept of an "effective" survival curve for a multifraction regimen is illustrated. When the radiation dose is delivered in a series of equal fractions separated by time intervals sufficiently long for the repair of sublethal damage to be complete between fractions, the shoulder of the survival curve is repeated many times. The effective dose survival curve is an exponential function of dose, that is, a straight line from the origin through a point on the single dose survival curve corresponding to the daily dose fraction (eg, 2 Gy). The dose required to result in 1 decade of cell killing ($D_{10}$) is related to the $D_0$ by the expression $D_{10} = 2.3 \times D_0$.

Total dose for 10 decades of cell killing, therefore, is $10 \times 6.9 = 69$ Gy.

PROBLEM 2: Suppose that, in the previous example, the clonogenic cells underwent *three* cell doublings during treatment. About what total dose would then be required to achieve the same probability of tumor control?

ANSWER: Three cell doublings would increase the cell number by

$$2 \times 2 \times 2 = 8$$

Consequently about 1 extra decade of cell killing would be required, corresponding to an additional dose of 6.9 Gy. Total dose is $69 + 6.9 = 75.9$ Gy.

PROBLEM 3: During the course of radiotherapy, a tumor containing $10^9$ cells receives 40 Gy. If the $D_0$ is 2.2 Gy, how many tumor cells will be left?

ANSWER: If the $D_0$ is 2.2 Gy, the $D_{10}$ is given by

$$D_{10} = 2.3 \times D_0$$
$$= 2.3 \times 2.2 = 5 \text{ Gy}$$

Since the total dose is 40 Gy, the number of decades of cell killing = $40 \div 5 = 8$

Number of cells remaining = $10^9 \times 10^{-8}$
$$= 10$$

PROBLEM 4: If $10^7$ cells are irradiated according to single-hit kinetics so that the average number of hits per cell is one, how many cells will survive?

ANSWER: A dose that gives an average of one hit per cell is the $D_0$; that is, the dose that on the exponential region of the survival curve reduces the number of survivors to 37%; the number of surviving cells will therefore be

$$10^7 \times \frac{37}{100} = 3.7 \times 10^6$$

## ONCOGENES AND RADIORESISTANCE

Numerous reports have appeared in the literature that transfection of activated oncogenes into cells cultured in vitro increases their radioresistances as defined by clonogenic survival. Reports include the transfection of activated N-*ras*, *raf*, or *ras* + *myc*, a combination that is particularly effective in transforming primary explants of rodent embryo cells to a malignant state. Results, however, are equivocal and variable. The change of radiosensitivity did not correlate with cell cycle distribution or double-strand DNA breaks or their repair; the best correlation was with the length of the $G_2$ phase delay induced by radiation. It is by no means clear that oncogene expression is directly involved in the induction of radioresistance, and it is far less clear that oncogenes play any major role in radioresistance in human tumors.

## THE MECHANISM OF CELL KILLING

Abundant evidence shows that the sensitive sites for radiation-induced cell lethality are located in the nucleus as opposed to the cytoplasm.

Early experiments with nonmammalian systems, such as frog's eggs, amebae, and algae, were designed so that either the cell nucleus or the cytoplasm could be selectively irradiated with a microbeam. The results indicated that the nucleus was very much more radiosensitive than the cytoplasm.

More recently, Munro irradiated mammalian cells with short-range α-particles from polonium (Fig. 3-8). Individual cells attached to a glass coverslip were studied. A large proportion of the cytoplasm could be irradiated by locating a polonium microneedle at a known distance from the cell; the α-particles from the polonium have a definite well-defined range, and it is possible to ensure that the α-particles irradiate the cytoplasm without reaching the nucleus. By the same token it was possible to position the α source above the cell and to irradiate the nucleus with α-particles, while irradiating a minimal amount of cytoplasm. It was found that large numbers of α-particles,

corresponding to a dose in excess of 250 Gy (25,000 rads), if delivered to the cytoplasm, had no effect on cell proliferation. By contrast, the penetration of a few α-particles a distance of 1 or 2 μm into the nucleus could prove to be lethal.

Evidence for chromosomal DNA as the principal target for cell killing is circumstantial but overwhelming. There is evidence that the nuclear membrane may be involved, too; indeed, the one does not exclude the other, since some portion of the DNA may be intimately involved with the membrane during some portions of the cell cycle.

The evidence implicating the chromosomes, specifically the DNA, as the primary target for radiation-induced lethality may be summarized as follows:

1. Cells are killed by radioactive tritiated thymidine incorporated into the DNA. The radiation dose is due to short-range β-particles and is therefore very localized.

2. Certain structural analogues of thymidine, particularly the halogenated pyrimidines, are selectively incorporated into DNA in place of thymidine when substituted in cell-culture growth medium. This substitution dramatically increases the radiosensitivity of the mammalian cells to a degree that increases as a function of the amount of the incorporation. Substituted deoxyuridines, which are not incorporated into DNA, have no such effect on cellular radiosensitivity.

3. Factors that modify cell lethality, such as variation in the type of radiation, oxygen concentration, or dose rate, also affect the production of chromosome damage in a fashion qualitatively and quantitatively similar. This is at least prima facie evidence to indicate that

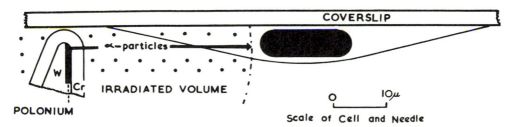

**Figure 3-8.** Irradiation of part of the cytoplasm of a cultured Chinese hamster cell by α-particles from a polonium-tipped microneedle. The irradiated volume is limited by the range of the particles. (From Munro TR: Radiat Res 42:451, 1970)

damage to the chromosomes is implicated in cell lethality.

4. Early work showed a relationship between virus size and radiosensitivity; later work showed a better correlation with nucleic acid volume. The radiosensitivity of a wide range of plants has been correlated with the mean interphase chromosome volume, which is defined as the ratio of nuclear volume to chromosome number. The larger the mean chromosome volume, the greater the radiosensitivity.

5. A direct correlation has been observed in hamster cells between aberrant chromosomes at the first postirradiation division and the failure of the cell to form a colony. Also, a correlation has been observed between chromosome fragments in irradiated plants and the failure of the pollen grain to germinate.

This accumulated evidence strongly indicates that chromosomal DNA is the principal target for radiation-induced lethality.

## EXCHANGE-TYPE CHROMOSOMAL ABERRATIONS AND CELL LETHALITY

Many authors have reported a close quantitative relationship between cell killing and the induction of specific chromosomal aberrations. The results of one of the most elegant studies, that by Cornforth and Bedford, are shown in Figure 3-9. The log of the surviving fraction is plotted against the average number of putative "lethal" aberrations per cell, that is, asymmetrical exchange-type aberrations such as rings and dicentrics. There is virtually a one-to-one correlation. In addition, there is an excellent correlation between the fraction of cells surviving and the fraction of cells without visible aberrations.

Data such as these provide strong circumstantial evidence to support the notion that asymmetrical exchange-type aberrations represent the principle mechanism for radiation-induced lethality in mammalian cells.

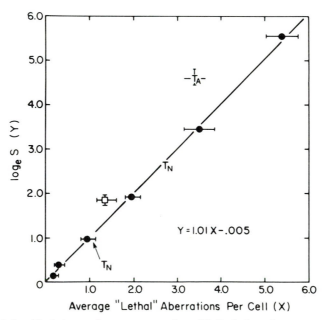

**Figure 3-9.** Relationship between the average number of "lethal" aberrations per cell (ie, asymmetrical exchange-type aberrations such as dicentrics and rings) and the log of the surviving fraction in AC 1522 normal human fibroblasts exposed to x-rays. There is virtually a one-to-one correlation. (From Cornforth MN, Bedford JS: Radiat Res 111:385–405, 1987)

► *Summary of Pertinent Conclusions*

- Cells from tumors and many normal regenerative tissues will grow and form colonies in vitro.
- Fresh explants of normal tissues often grow well in culture for a few weeks before they peter out and die. A few pass through a "crisis" and become immortal; these are the established cell lines.
- A cell is said to have retained its *reproductive integrity* if it is capable of sustained proliferation, that is, if it can grow into a macroscopic colony.
- A survivor that has retained its reproductive integrity is said to be *clonogenic*.
- The percentage of untreated cells seeded that grow into macroscopic colonies is known as the *plating efficiency* (PE). Thus

$$PE = \frac{\text{Number of colonies counted}}{\text{Number of cells seeded}} \times 100$$

- The PE may be close to 100% for some established cell lines but 1% or less for fresh explants of human cells.
- The fraction of cells surviving (SF) a given dose is determined by counting the number of macroscopic colonies as a fraction of the number of cells seeded. Allowance must be made for the PE. Thus

$$SF = \frac{\text{Number of colonies}}{\text{Number of cells seeded} \times PE / 100}$$

- A *cell survival curve* is the relationship between the fraction of cells retaining their reproductive integrity and absorbed dose.
- Conventionally, surviving fraction on a logarithmic scale is plotted on the ordinate against dose on the abscissa. The shape of the survival curve is important.
- The cell survival curve for α-particles and low-energy neutrons (densely ionizing radiations) is a straight line on a log-linear plot; that is, survival approximates to an exponential function of dose.
- The cell survival curve for x- or γ-rays (sparsely ionizing radiations) has an initial slope, followed by a bending region or shoulder, after which it tends to straighten again at higher doses.
- Survival data are adequately fitted by many models and theories. The data are never sufficiently precise nor are the models sufficiently different for experimental results to discriminate among models.
- For the first 1 or 2 decades of survival and up to doses used in single fractions in radiotherapy, survival data are adequately represented by the linear-quadratic relationship.

$$S = e^{-\alpha D - \beta D^2}$$

where S is the fraction of cells surviving a dose D and α and β are constants representing the linear and quadratic components of cell killing.
- The initial slope of the cell survival curve is determined by α; the quadratic component of cell killing (β) causes the curve to bend at higher doses.
- The ratio α/β is the dose at which linear and quadratic components of cell killing are equal.

*(continued)*

► *Summary of Pertinent Conclusions* (Continued)

- Cells cultured from different tumors in humans show a broad range of radiosensitivities that bracket the sensitivity of normal cells from different persons.
- Predictive assays for intrinsic radiosensitivity of tumor cells from individual patients require special assays. This is discussed in Chapter 15.
- The effective survival curve for a multifraction regimen is an exponential function of dose: a straight line from the origin through a point on the single-dose survival curve corresponding to the daily dose fraction.
- The average value of the effective $D_0$ for the multifraction survival curve for human cells is about 3 Gy.
- The $D_{10}$, the dose to result in 1 decade of cell killing is related to the $D_0$ by the expression

$$D_{10} = 2.3 \times D_0$$

- Calculations of tumor cell kill can be performed for fractionated clinical radiotherapy regimens using the concept of effective survival curve.
- There is some evidence in cells cultured in vitro that transfection of activated oncogenes in cells increases their radioresistance. It is not clear that oncogenes play a role in the resistance of human tumors in vivo.
- There is good evidence that the nucleus, specifically the DNA, is the principal target for radiation-induced cell lethality. Membrane damage may also be a factor.
- There is a one-to-one correlation between cell survival and the average number of putative "lethal" chromosomal aberrations per cell, that is, asymmetrical exchange-type aberrations such as dicentrics and rings.

# BIBLIOGRAPHY

Alper T, Fowler JF, Morgan RL, Vonberg DD, Ellis F, Oliver R: The characterization of the "type C" survival curve. Br J Radiol 35:722–723, 1962

Andrews JR, Berry RJ: Fast neutron irradiation and the relationship of radiation dose and mammalian cell reproductive capacity. Radiat Res 16:76–81, 1962

Barendsen GW, Beusker TLJ, Vergroesen AJ, Budke L: Effects of different ionizing radiations on human cells in tissue culture: II. Biological experiments. Radiat Res 13:841–849, 1960

Bender M: Induced aberrations in human chromosomes. Am J Pathol 43:26a, 1963

Carrano AV: Chromosome aberrations and radiation-induced cell death: II. Predicted and observed cell survival. Mutat Res 17:355–366, 1973

Cornforth MN, Bedford JS: X-ray-induced breakage and rejoining of human interphase chromosomes. Science 222:1141–1143, 1983

Cornforth MN, Bedford JS: A quantitative comparison of potentially lethal damage repair and the rejoining of interphase chromosome breaks in low passage normal human fibroblasts. Radiat Res 111:385–405, 1987

Elkind MM, Sutton H: Radiation response of mammalian cells grown in culture: I. Repair of x-ray damage in surviving Chinese hamster cells. Radiat Res 13:556–593, 1960

Evans HJ: Chromosome aberrations induced by ionizing radiation. Int Rev Cytol 13:221–321, 1962

Frankenberg D, Frankenberg-Schwager M, Harbich R: Split-dose recovery is due to the repair of DNA double-strand breaks. Int J Radiat Biol 46:541–553, 1984

Geard CR: Effects of radiation on chromosomes. In Pizzarello D (ed): Radiation Biology, pp 83–110. Boca Raton, FL, CRC Press, 1982

Grell RF: The chromosome. J Tenn Acad Sci 37:43–53, 1962

Ishihara T, Sasaki MS (eds): Radiation-Induced Chromosome Damage in Man. New York, Alan R. Liss, 1983

Lea DEA: Actions of Radiations on Living Cells, 2nd ed. Cambridge, England, Cambridge University Press, 1956

Moorhead PS, Nowell PC, Mellman WJ, Battips DM, Hungerford DA: Chromosome preparation of leukocytes cultured from human peripheral blood. Exp Cell Res 20:613–616, 1960

Munro TR: The relative radiosensitivity of the nucleus and cytoplasm of the Chinese hamster fibroblasts. Radiat Res 42:451–470, 1970

Puck TT, Markus PI: Action of x-rays on mammalian cells. J Exp Med 103:653–666, 1956

Ris H: Chromosome structure. In McElroy WD, Glass B (eds): Chemical Basis of Heredity. Baltimore, John Hopkins University Press, 1957

Spear FG: On some biological effects of radiation. Br J Radiol 31:114–124, 1958

*Radiobiology for the Radiologist, Fourth Edition,* by Eric J. Hall
J. B. Lippincott Company, Philadelphia © 1994.

# 4

# *Dose–Response Relationships for Normal Tissues*

Radiation Therapy

## MITOTIC DEATH AND APOPTOSIS: HOW AND WHY CELLS DIE

Cells cultured in vitro die a mitotic death after irradiation; that is, they die while attempting to divide. This does not necessarily occur at the first postirradiation mitosis; the cell may struggle through one, two, or more mitoses before the damaged chromosomes cause it to die in attempting the complex task of cell division. Time-lapse films of irradiated cells cultured in vitro clearly show this process of mitotic death, which is the dominant cause of death when reproductive integrity is assessed in vitro as described in Chapter 3.

It is not, however, the only form of cell death. Programmed cell death, or *apoptosis*, occurs in normal tissues and neoplasms, in mammals and amphibians, in the embryo and in the adult. It is implicated, for example, in tissue involution such as the regression of the tadpole tail during metamorphosis. It is the programmed cell death that is common during embryonic development. It can also occur after irradiation. Apoptosis, like mitosis, comes from the Greek and means "falling off" as of petals from flowers or leaves from trees.

Apoptosis is characterized by a stereotyped sequence of morphologic events, which take place in two discrete phases. In the first phase, cells condense and bud to produce many membrane-enclosed bodies. In the second phase these bodies are phagocytized and digested by nearby tissue cells. Apoptosis characteristically affects scattered individual cells. When apoptosis affects cells in tissues, the resulting apoptotic bodies are squeezed along the intercellular spaces and are either shed from the epithelial surface or rapidly phagocytized by nearby cells. The cells surrounding those being deleted merely close ranks, and there is no tissue disorganization such as occurs after necrosis.

## ASSAYS FOR DOSE–RESPONSE RELATIONSHIPS

A number of experimental techniques are available to obtain dose–response relationships for the cells of normal tissues. First, there are a limited number of clonogenic assays—techniques in which the endpoint observed depends directly on the reproductive integrity of individual cells. These systems are directly analogous to cell survival in vitro. The techniques developed by Withers and his colleagues are based on the observation of a clone of cells regenerating in situ in irradiated tissue. The skin colony, testes, kidney tubule, and regenerating crypts in the jejunum systems are briefly described. It is also possible to obtain dose–response curves for the cells of the epithelial lining of the colon or stomach, but the method used is essentially the same as for the jejunum. Kember described a system for scoring regenerating clones in cartilage at about the same time as the Withers' skin colony system, but it has not been used widely and is not discussed here.

The assay system for the stem cells in the bone marrow or cells of the thyroid and mammary gland depends on the observation of the growth of clones of cells taken from a donor animal and transplanted into a different tissue in a recipient animal. In Till and McCulloch's bone marrow assay, colonies of bone marrow cells are counted in the spleens of recipient animals. Dose–response curves for mammary and thyroid cells have been obtained by Clifton and Gould by observing colonies growing from cells transplanted into the fat pad of recipient animals.

Second, dose–response relationships can be obtained that are repeatable and quantitative but that depend on functional endpoints. These include skin reactions in rodents or pigs (eg, erythema and desquamation), pneumonitis or fibrosis in mouse lungs reflected in an increased breathing rate, myelopathy of the hind limbs from damage to the spinal cord, and deformities to the feet of mice. The endpoints observed tend to reflect the minimum number of functional cells remaining in a tissue or organ, rather than the fraction of cells retaining their reproductive integrity.

Finally, one can *infer* a dose–response curve for a tissue in which it cannot be observed directly by assuming the form of the dose–response curve (linear-quadratic) and performing a series of multifraction experiments. This procedure, first suggested by Douglas and Fowler, has been widely used to infer values for α and β in the dose–response relationships for normal tissues in which the parameters cannot be directly measured.

This chapter includes assays for both early- and late-responding tissues. The skin, intestinal epithelium, and bone marrow cells, for example, are all rapidly dividing self-renewal tissues. The spinal cord, lung, and kidney, by contrast, are late-responding tissues. This reflects the current philosophy that the radiation response of *all* tissues is due to the depletion of the critical parenchymal cells and that the difference in time at which early- and late-responding tissues express radiation damage is a function simply of different cell turnover rates. Many papers in the older literature ascribe the response of late-responding tissues to vascular damage, rather than to depletion of parenchymal cells, but this thesis is becoming increasingly difficult to accept.

The various types of normal tissue assay systems are described briefly. The reader who is content with the previous summary may wish to skip the remainder of this chapter.

## CLONOGENIC ENDPOINTS

### Clones Regrowing in Situ

#### Skin Colonies

Withers developed an ingenious technique (Fig. 4-1) to determine the survival curve for mouse skin cells. The hair was plucked from an area on the back of the mouse, and a superficial x-ray machine was used to irradiate an annulus of skin to a massive dose of 30 Gy (3000 rads). This produced a "moat" of dead cells, in the center of which was an isolated island of intact skin that had been protected during the first exposure to low-voltage x-rays by a small metal sphere. This small area of intact skin was then given a test dose, D rads, and subsequently observed for regrowth of skin. If one or more stem cells survived in this small area, nodules of regrowing skin could be seen some days later. If no cells survived in this small area, the skin would heal much later by infiltration of cells crossing the moat. Figure 4-2 shows nodules regrowing in

**3000 RADS TO MOAT**

**TEST DOSE D TO CENTRAL AREA**

**OBSERVED REGROWTH OF SKIN NODULE IN CENTRAL AREA**

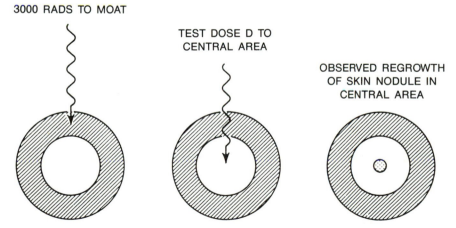

**Figure 4-1.** Technique used to isolate an area of skin for experimental irradiation. A superficial (30-kV) x-ray machine is used to irradiate an annulus of skin to a massive dose of about 3000 rads (30 Gy). An isolated island of intact skin in the center of this "moat" is protected from the radiation by a metal sphere. The intact skin is then given a test dose and observed for nodules of regrowing skin. (Redrawn from Withers HR: Br J Radiol 40:187, 1967)

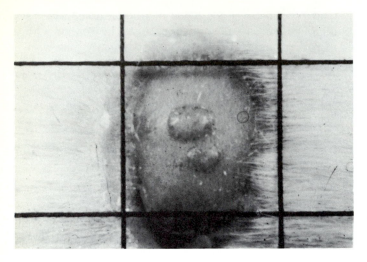

**Figure 4-2.** Photograph of a nodule of mouse skin regrowing from a single surviving cell in the treated area. (Courtesy of Dr. H. R. Withers)

mouse skin. To obtain a survival curve, it was necessary to repeat this operation with a number of different areas of skin. A range of ball bearings was used to shield a small area of skin in the middle of the "moat." The resulting survival data are shown in Figure 4-3, in which the dose is plotted against the number of surviving cells per square centimeter of skin.

There are practical limits to the range in which the dose–response relationship could be

determined. At one extreme, it is not possible to irradiate too large an area on the back of the mouse to produce the moat of sterilized skin. At the other extreme, the smallest area that can be used is determined by the fact that even 30-kV radiation scatters laterally to some extent. As can be seen from Figure 4-3, the technique results in a single-dose survival curve that extends from 8 to 25 Gy (800 to 2500 rads); over this range, with dose plotted on a linear scale and the number of

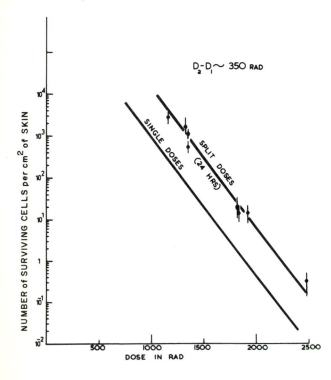

**Figure 4-3.** Single-dose and two-dose survival curves for epithelial cells of mouse skin exposed to 29-kVp x-rays. The 37% dose slope ($D_0$) is 1.35 Gy (135 rads). The ordinate is not the surviving fraction, as in the survival curves for cells cultured in vitro but is the number of surviving cells per square centimeter of skin. In the two-dose survival curve the interval between dose fractions was always 24 hours. The curves are parallel, their horizontal separation being equal to 3.5 Gy (350 rads); this corresponds to $D_q$. From a knowledge of $D_q$ and the slope of the survival curve, $D_0$, the extrapolation number, n, may be calculated. (From Withers HR: Radiat Res 32:227, 1967 and Withers HR: Br J Radiol 40:187, 1967)

surviving cells per square centimeter plotted on a logarithmic scale, the survival curve is straight and has a $D_0$ of 1.35 Gy (135 rads). This $D_0$ value is very similar to that obtained with mammalian cells cultured in vitro.

The extrapolation number cannot be obtained directly with this technique because the ordinate is the number of surviving cells per square centimeter of skin; this cannot be converted to the surviving fraction because it is not known with any accuracy how many skin stem cells there are per unit area. It is, however, possible to make an indirect estimate of the extrapolation number by obtaining the survival curve for doses given in two fractions separated by 24 hours. The survival curve obtained in this way is also shown in Figure 4-3. It is parallel to that obtained for single doses but is displaced from it toward higher doses. As explained in Chapter 3, this lateral displacement in a direction parallel to the dose axis is a measure of *Dq*, the *quasi-threshold dose*. The Dq for mouse skin is 3.5 Gy (350 rads), which is very

similar to the value for human skin estimated from split-dose experiments.

### Crypt Cells of the Mouse Jejunum

A technique perfected by Withers and Elkind makes it possible to obtain the survival characteristics of the crypt cells of the mouse jejunum. The lining of the jejunum is a classic example of a self-renewal system. The cells in the crypts divide rapidly and provide a continuous supply of cells that move up the villi, differentiate, and become the functioning cells. The cells at the top of the folds of the villi are slowly but continuously sloughed off in the normal course of events and are continuously replaced by cells that originate from mitoses in the crypts. Figure 4-4, an electron micrograph, dramatically shows the three-dimensional structure of the lining of the intestinal epithelium in the mouse. Mice are given a total-body dose of 11 to 16 Gy (1100 to 1600 rads), which sterilizes a significant proportion of

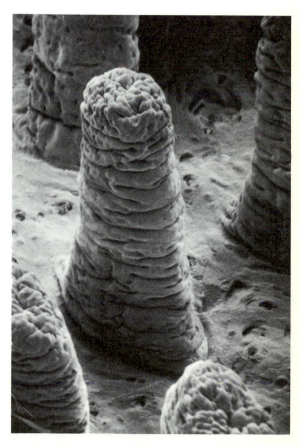

**Figure 4-4.** Scanning electron micrograph that allows three-dimensional visualization of the jejunal villi from the hamster. (x 175) (From Taylor AB, Anderson JH: Micron 3:430–453, 1972)

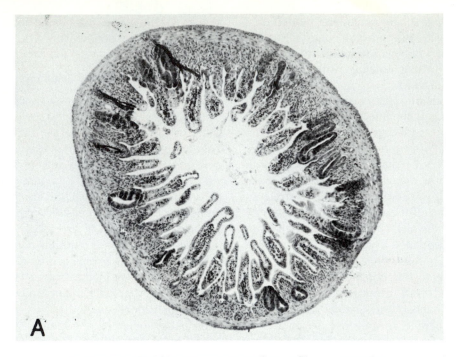

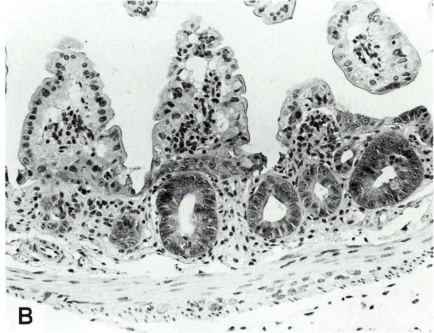

Figure 4-5. **(A)** Section of mouse jejunum taken $3\frac{1}{2}$ days after a total-body dose in excess of 10 Gy. Note the shortened villi and the regenerating crypts. **(B)** Regenerating crypts shown at a higher magnification. (From Withers HR: Cancer 28:78–81, 1971)

the dividing cells in the crypts but has essentially no effect on the differentiated cells in the villi. Consequently, crypt degeneration appears early after irradiation, while the villi remain long and their epithelial covering of differentiated cells shows little change. With the further passage of time, the tips of the villi continue to be sloughed away by normal use but no replacement cells are available from the depopulated crypts, and so the villi begin to shorten and shrink. At sufficiently high doses the surface lining of the jejunum is completely denuded of villi. To obtain a survival curve for the jejunal crypt cells, groups of animals are exposed to graded total-body doses of radiation. After 3 days, each animal is sacrificed and sections are made of the jejunum (Fig. 4-5*A*). At this time, crypts are just beginning to regenerate and it is relatively simple to identify them. Figure 4-5*B* shows a number of regenerating crypts at a higher magnification. These pictures also show the shortened villi and the greatly reduced density of cells lining the surface. The score of radiation damage is the *number of regenerating crypts per circumference* of the sectioned jejunum. This quantity is plotted as a function of dose and yields a survival curve as shown in Figure 4-6. The single-dose survival curve has a $D_0$ (for γ-rays) of about 1.3 Gy (130 rads). Also shown in Figure 4-6 are survival curves for radiation delivered in multiple fractions, from 2 to 20. The separation between the single- and two-dose survival curves gives a measure of Dq, which has the very large value of between 4 and 4.5 Gy (400 to 450 rads).

This technique has two limitations. First, the quantity plotted on the ordinate is the number of surviving crypts per circumference, *not* the surviving fraction. Second, experiments can be done only at doses of about 10 Gy (1000 rads) or more, at which there is a sufficient level of biological damage for individual regenerating crypts to be identified. The doses can, however, be delivered in a number of smaller fractions, as long as the total results in enough biological damage to be scored. The shape of the entire survival curve can then be reconstructed from the multifraction data, if it is assumed that in a fractionated regimen each dose produces the same amount of cell killing and if an estimate is made of the number of clonogens at risk per crypt. This has been done by Withers and his colleagues; the resultant survival curve is shown in Figure 4-7.

### Testes Stem Cells

A technique to measure the radiation response of testicular cells capable of sustaining spermatogenesis (ie, the stem cells) was devised by Withers and his colleagues. About 6 weeks after irradiation, mouse testes are sectioned and examined histologically. Sections of normal and irradiated testes are shown in Figure 4-8. The proportion of tubules containing spermatogenic epithelium is counted and plotted as a function of dose in Figure 4-9. As in many in vivo assays, relatively high single doses of 8 to 16 Gy (800 to 1600 rads) are necessary, so that the level of damage is sufficient to be scored. In this dose range the $D_0$ is about 1.68 Gy (168 rads). When the split-dose technique is used, the Dq is about 2.7 Gy (270 rads) (see Fig. 4-9). It is possible to estimate the effect of small doses and reconstruct a complete survival curve by giving large doses in multiple small fractions and *assuming* that the response to each fraction is the same. The result of this reconstruction is shown in Figure 4-10.

### Kidney Tubules

A technique using kidney tubules, again developed by Withers and his colleagues, is the first clonal assay for a late-responding tissue. One kidney per mouse is irradiated with a small field and removed for histologic examination 60 weeks later. Figure 4-11 shows sections of normal and irradiated kidneys. For ease of scoring, only those tubules touching the renal capsule are scored, and a tubule is considered fully regenerated only if it is lined with well-differentiated cuboidal or columnar cells with a large amount of eosinophilic cytoplasm. By 60 weeks, tubules either have no surviving epithelial cells or are completely lined with epithelium that has regenerated from a small number of surviving cells, usually one. The number of tubules regenerating in an arbitrary number of sections counted is plotted as a function of radiation dose. The result is shown in Figure 4-12; the $D_0$ is about 1.53 Gy (153 rads).

*(text continues on page 56)*

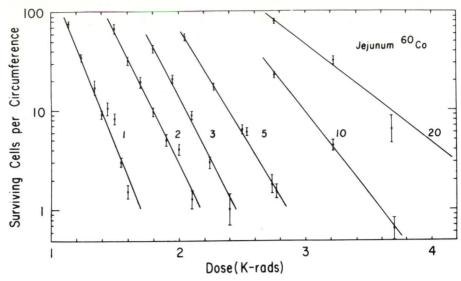

**Figure 4-6.** Survival curves for crypt cells in the mouse jejunum exposed to single or multiple doses of γ-rays (1 to 20 fractions). The score of radiation damage is the number of surviving cells per circumference (ie, the number of regenerating crypts per circumference of the jejunum) counted from sections such as those shown in Figure 4-5. This quantity is plotted on a logarithmic scale against radiation dose on a linear scale. The $D_0$ for the single-dose survival curve is about 1.3 Gy (130 rads). The shoulder of the survival curve is very large. The separation between the single- and two-dose survival curves indicates that the $D_q$ is 4 to 4.5 Gy (400 to 450 rads). From Withers, HR, Mason K, Reid BO, Dubrasky N, Barkley HT, Brown W, Smathers JB: Cancer 34:39–47, 1974)

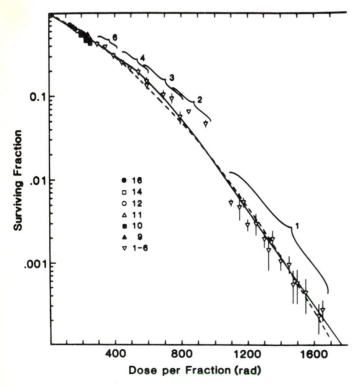

**Figure 4-7.** Effective single-dose survival curve reconstructed from multifraction experiments for clonogenic cells of the jejunal crypts of mice. The numbers on the curve refer to the number of fractions used to reconstruct that part of the curve. The initial and final slopes are about 3.57 and 1.43 Gy (357 and 143 rads), respectively. The quasi-threshold dose is 4.3 Gy (430 rads). The data are equally well fitted by the linear-quadratic formulation. (From Thames HD, Withers HR, Mason KA, Reid BO: Int J Radiat Oncol Biol Phys 7:1591–1597, 1981)

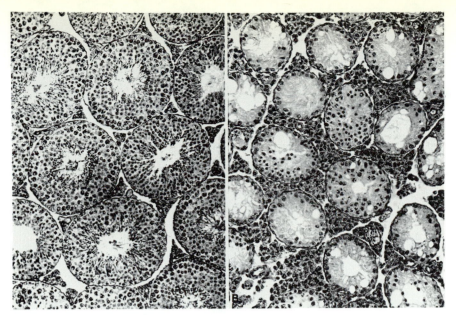

**Figure 4-8.** **(A)** Histology of normal testis. **(B)** Histology of testis 35 days after a dose of 9 Gy (900 rads) of γ-radiation. Some tubules are completely devoid of spermatogenic epithelium and some are not. (Sertoli's cells persist in the tubules sterilized of spermatogenic cells.) Foci of spermatogenesis can be derived from single surviving stem cells. (× 200) (From Withers HR, Hunter N, Barkley HT Jr, Reid B: Radiat Res 57:88–103, 1974)

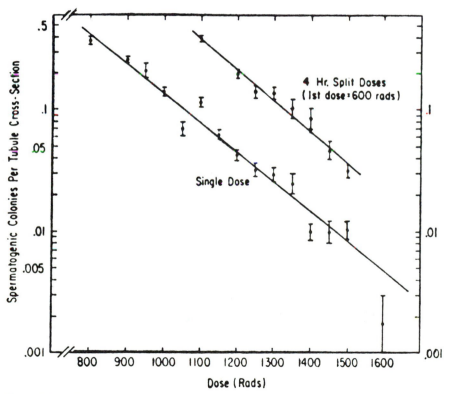

**Figure 4-9.** Single- and split-dose survival curves for spermatogenic stem cells of the mouse testis. The $D_0$ is about 1.68 Gy (168 rads). The $D_q$, assessed from the horizontal separation of the single- and split-dose curves, is about 2.7 Gy (270 rads). (From Withers HR, Hunter N, Barkley HT Jr, Reid B: Radiat Res 57:88–103, 1974)

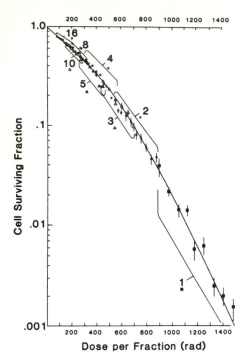

Figure 4-10. Survival curve for testis stem cells reconstructed from multifraction experiments, assuming that each fraction produces the same biological effect. The numbers on the curve refer to the number of fractions used to reconstruct that portion of the curve. The $D_0$ is about 1.6 Gy (160 rads), and the $D_q$ is about 3.92 Gy (392 rads). (From Thames HD Jr, Withers HR: Br J Radiol 53:1071–1077, 1980)

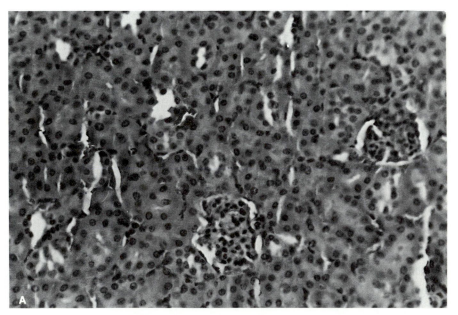

Figure 4-11. Photomicrographs of mouse kidney. **(A)** Normal, showing proximal tubules in contact with capsule. (H&E, × 400) **(B)** Sixty weeks after 13 Gy (1300 rads). Note normal proximal tubules and glomeruli amid ghosts of de-epithelialized tubules. One epithelialized tubule is in contact with capsule. (H&E, × 200) (From Withers HR, Mason KA, Thames HD Jr: Br J Radiol 59:587–595, 1986)

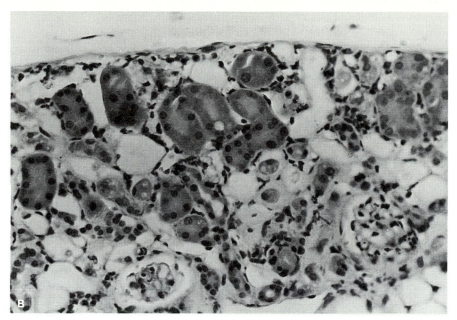

**Figure 4-11.** *(Continued)*

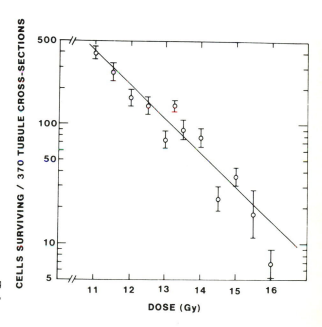

**Figure 4-12.** Dose-survival curve for tubule-regenerating cells. The $D_0$ is 1.53 Gy (153 rads). (From Withers HR, Mason KA, Thames HD Jr: Br J Radiol 59:587–595, 1986)

The radiosensitivity of the cells of this late-responding tissue is not very different from that of early-responding tissues, such as the skin or intestinal epithelium. The *rate* of response, however, is quite different. The time required for depletion of the epithelium after a single dose of 14 Gy (1400 rads) is about 3 days in the jejunum, 12 to 24 days in the skin, and 30 days in the seminiferous tubules of the testes, but 300 days in the kidney tubules. These results argue strongly that radiation injury in the kidney results from depletion of parenchymal cells and that the slow expression of injury reflects merely the slow turnover of this cell population. Vascular injury is unlikely to be the mechanism underlying the destruction of renal tubules.

## Cells Transplanted to Another Site

### Bone Marrow Stem Cells

Till and McCulloch developed a system to determine a survival curve for colony-forming bone marrow cells (Fig. 4-13). Recipient animals are first supralethally irradiated with a dose of 9 to 10 Gy (900 to 1000 rads), which sterilizes their spleens. Nucleated isologous bone marrow cells taken from another animal are then injected intravenously into the recipient animals. Some of these cells lodge in the spleen, where they form nodules, or colonies, 10 to 11 days later because the cells of the recipient animal's spleen have previously been sterilized by the large dose of radiation. At about 10 days, therefore, the animals' spleens are removed and the colonies counted. Figure 4-14 is a photograph of a spleen showing the colonies to be counted.

About $10^4$ cells must be injected into a recipient animal to produce one spleen colony, since the majority of the cells in the nucleated isologous bone marrow are fully differentiated cells and would never be capable of forming a colony. To obtain a surviving fraction for bone marrow cells, a donor animal is irradiated to some test dose, D, and the suspension of cells from the bone marrow is inoculated into groups of recipient animals that had previously been supralethally irradiated. By counting the colonies in the spleens of the recipient animals and with a knowledge of the number of cells required to produce a colony in an unirradiated animal (plating efficiency), the surviving fraction may be simply calculated as follows:

$$\text{Surviving fraction for a dose D} = \frac{\text{Colonies counted}}{\text{Cells inoculated} \times \text{PE}}$$

This procedure is repeated for a range of doses, and a survival curve is obtained (Fig. 4-15). These bone marrow stem cells are the

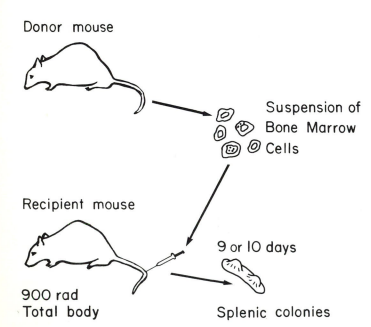

**Donor mouse**

**Suspension of Bone Marrow Cells**

**Recipient mouse**

**9 or 10 days**

**900 rad Total body**

**Splenic colonies**

**Figure 4-13.** Till and McCulloch's technique. From the donor mouse a cell suspension is made of nucleated isologous bone marrow. A known number of cells is injected into recipient mice previously irradiated with 9 Gy (900 rads) total-body dose. The spleen is removed from each recipient mouse 9 or 10 days later, and the number of nodules are counted. (Redrawn from Till JE, McCulloch EA: In Cameron IL, Padilla GM, Zimmerman AM (eds): Developmental Aspects of the Cell Cycle, pp 297–313. New York, Academic Press, 1971)

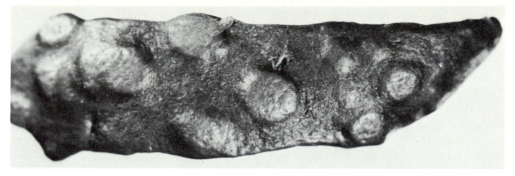

**Figure 4-14.** Photograph of a mouse's spleen. The mouse was supralethally irradiated to sterilize all the cells of the spleen. The nodules of regrowth originate from intravenously injected bone marrow cells from another animal. (Courtesy of Dr. A. Carsten)

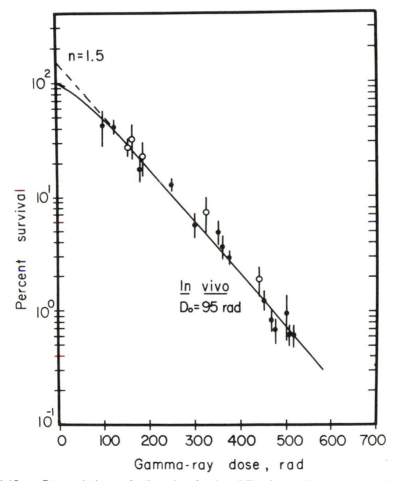

**Figure 4-15.** γ-Ray survival curve for the colony-forming ability of mouse bone marrow cells. The cells are irradiated in vivo in the donor animal and grow into colonies in the spleens of supralethally irradiated recipient animals. (Redrawn from McCulloch EA, Till JE: Radiat Res 16:822, 1962)

most sensitive mammalian cells to die a mitotic death, with a $D_0$ of about 0.95 Gy (95 rads) and little or no shoulder to the survival curve.

### Mammary and Thyroid Cells

Clifton and Gould and their colleagues developed very useful clonogen transplant assays for epithelial cells of the mammary and thyroid glands. They have been used largely for cell survival studies, described later, but the initial motivation for their development was to study carcinogenesis in a quantitative system. Most in vitro transformation assays involve fibroblasts, while the bulk of human cancers arise in epithelial cells, hence the importance and interest in these two systems.

The techniques for the two cell systems are much the same. To generate a survival curve for mammary or thyroid gland cells in the rat, cells may be irradiated in vivo before the gland is removed from donor animals and treated with enzymes to obtain a monodispersed cell suspension. Known numbers of cells are injected into the inguinal or interscapular white fat pad of recipient animals.

Under appropriate host conditions and grafted cell numbers, the injection of mammary cells gives rise to mammary structures that are morphologically and functionally normal. One such mammary structure may develop from a single cell. By 3½ weeks after the injection of mammary cells, positive growth is indicated by alveolar units. An example of a milk-filled alveolar unit is shown as an inset in Figure 4-16. When thyroid cells are injected, thyroid follicular units develop (Fig. 4-17).

With either type of cell, a larger number must be injected to produce a growing unit if the cells are first irradiated to a given dose, D. In practice, some fancy statistics are involved, a discussion of which is beyond the scope of this chapter; in essence, the ratio of the number of irradiated to unirradiated cells required to produce one growing unit (thyroid follicular unit or alveolar unit) is a measure of the cell-surviving fraction corresponding to the dose, D. This procedure must be repeated for a range of graded doses to generate a survival curve. The resultant survival curve for mammary cells is shown in Figure 4-16. The characteristics of the curve are unremarkable—the $D_0$ is about 1.27 Gy (127 rads), while the extrapolation number (n) is about 5, quite typical of rodent cells cultured in vitro. The corresponding survival curve for thyroid cells is shown in Figure 4-17. The $D_0$ is a little larger than for mammary glands assayed in a similar way, implying that the cells are a little more resistant. Figures 4-16 and 4-17 also show data for cells left in situ for 24 hours after irradiation before being removed and assayed. When this is done, the shoulder of the survival curve is larger because of the repair of potentially lethal damage. This is discussed in more detail in Chapter 7.

An interesting use of these clonogen transplant assays is that the physiological state of either donor or recipient animals can be hormonally manipulated. For the mammary cell assay, cells may be taken from inactive, slowly dividing

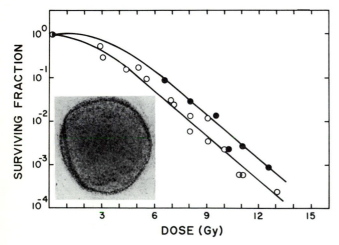

Figure 4-16. Dose–response relationship for rat mammary cells assayed by transplantation into the fat pad of recipient animals. (Redrawn from Gould MN, Clifton K: Radiat Res 77:149–155, 1979) The inset shows a milk-filled spherical alveolar unit developed from a transplanted cell. (From Gould MN, Biel WF, Clifton KH: Exp Cell Res 107:405–416, 1977)

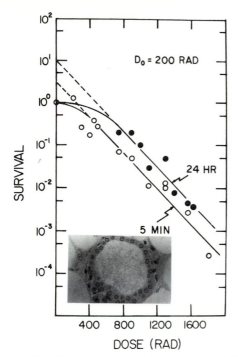

**Figure 4-17.** Dose–response relationship for rat thyroid cells assayed by transplantation into the fat pad of recipient animals. (From Mulcahy RT, Gould MN, Clifton KH: Radiat Res 84:523–528, 1980) The inset shows a single thyroid follicle that developed 4 weeks after the inoculation of thyroid cells into the fat pad of recipient animals. (From Clifton KH, Gould MN Potten CS, Hendry J [eds]: Cell Clones, pp 128–138. New York, Churchill Livingstone, 1985)

glands of virgin rats, from rapidly dividing glands of rats in midpregnancy, or from milk-producing glands of lactating rats. For the thyroid cell assay, the physiological states of both donor and recipient can be manipulated by control of the diet or by partial thyroidectomy.

## SUMMARY OF DOSE–RESPONSE CURVES FOR CLONOGENIC ASSAYS IN NORMAL TISSUES

The survival curves for all of the clonogenic assays in normal tissues are plotted together in Figure 4-18. There is a substantial range of radiosensitivities, with shoulder width being the principal variable. In vitro curves for cells from patients with ataxia-telangiectasia are also shown, since these are probably the most radiosensitive mammalian cells.

## DOSE–RESPONSE RELATIONSHIPS FOR FUNCTIONAL END POINTS

### Pig Skin

Pig skin has been widely used in radiobiological studies because it has many features in common with human skin, such as color, hair follicles, sweat glands, and a layer of subcutaneous fat. In view of these structural similarities it is not surprising that the response of pig skin to radiation closely resembles that of human skin, both qualitatively and quantitatively.

Fowler and his colleagues pioneered the use of pig skin as a radiobiological test system. A number of small rectangular fields on the pig's flank were irradiated with graded doses of x-rays, and the reactions were scored daily using the arbitrary scale shown in Table 4-1. After a single dose of radiation, the reaction becomes apparent after about 15 days and develops as shown in Figure 4-19.

Two phases of the reaction can be distinguished. First, an early wave of erythema occurred (at 10 to 40 days), which was variable from one animal to another. This represents the uncomfortable "acute" reaction sometimes seen in patients on radiotherapy at about the end of a course of treatment. Second, a more gradual increase to a second broad wave of moderately severe reactions took place (between 50 and 100 days), representing a more permanent kind of damage. This second wave shows the tolerance of skin to a more serious type of long-term damage and is also a more repeatable and consistent index of radiation damage. It was subsequently found to correlate well with longer term damage (up to 2 years) and with subcutaneous damage.

The "score" of radiation damage is taken to be the average skin reaction occurring between certain time limits that encompass the medium-term reactions. After a single dose, this might be a 35-day period between 50 and 85 days after irradiation. For a protracted fractionated regimen, this period of reaction may come later, between days 65 and 100. The average skin reaction in the chosen time period is then plotted as a function of dose; examples of dose–response curves obtained this way are shown in

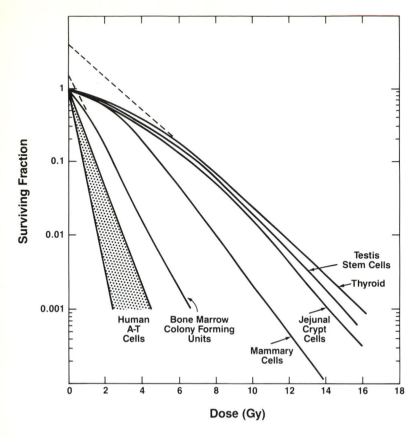

**Figure 4-18.** Summary of survival curves for clonogenic assays of cells from normal tissues. The human ataxia-telangiectasia (A-T) cells are included because they are the most sensitive mammalian cells. The bone marrow colony-forming units, together with the mammary and thyroid cells, represent systems in which cells are irradiated and assayed by transplantation into a different tissue in recipient animals. The jejunal crypt and testis stem cells are examples of systems in which cells are assayed for regrowth in situ after irradiation.

Figure 4-20 for single and fractionated dose schedules.

Late effects have also been studied in pig skin by measuring the contraction that results from fibrosis a year or more after irradiation. A square is tattooed on the skin of the animal in the irradiated field, and the dimensions of this square are recorded as a function of dose as the contraction occurs. This is a primitive but effective measure of late effects.

Many of the important early studies on the fractionation effects of x-rays and the comparison of x-rays with fast neutrons were performed with this biological system. One overwhelming advantage is that data obtained this way can be extrapolated to the human with a high degree of confidence. The balancing disadvantage is that the animals are large and awkward to work with, and their maintenance involves a considerable expense.

Table 4-1.
**Radiation Reactions in Pig Skin**

| ARBITRARY SCORE | REACTION |
| --- | --- |
| 0 | No visible reaction |
| 1 | Faint erythema |
| 2 | Erythema |
| 3 | Marked erythema |
| 4 | Moist desquamation of less than half the irradiated area |
| 5 | Moist desquamation of more than half the irradiated area |

*(From Fowler JF, Morgan RL, Silvester JA, Bewley DK, Turner BA: Br J Radiol 36:188–196, 1963)*

## Rodent Skin

Because of the inconvenience and expense of using pigs, the skin of the mouse leg and foot is commonly used instead. One hind leg of each animal is irradiated; the other serves as a control. The skin response is observed each day for about 30 days after irradiation and is scored according

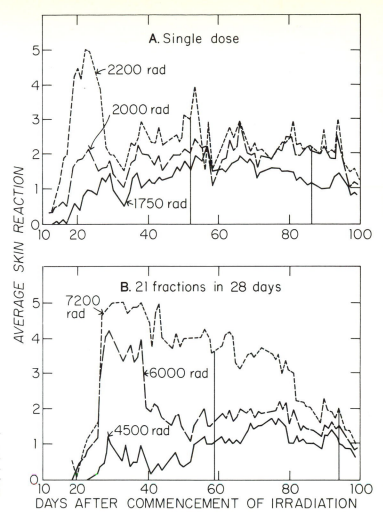

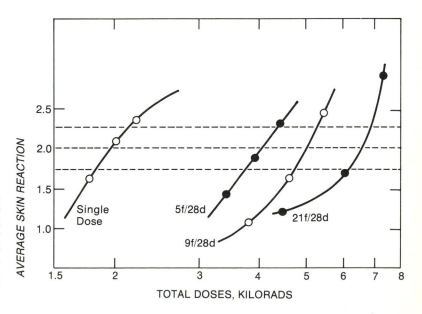

Figure 4-19. Development of skin reactions in the pig after graded doses of x-rays, delivered **(A)** as a single exposure or **(B)** as multiple fractions spaced over time. (Redrawn from Fowler JF, Morgan RL, Silvester JA, Bewley DK, Turner BA: Br J Radiol 36:188–196, 1963)

Figure 4-20. Average skin reaction as a function of total dose for medium-term skin reactions in pigs exposed to a single dose of x-rays or to fractionated doses given over 28 days. (Redrawn from Fowler JF, Morgan RL, Silvester JA, Bewley DK, Turner BA: Br J Radiol 36:188–196, 1963)

Table 4-2.
Radiation Reactions in Mouse Leg Skin

| ARBITRARY SCORE* | OBSERVATIONS |
| --- | --- |
| 0.5 | 50/50; doubtful if any difference from normal or not |
| 1− | † |
| 1 | Definite abnormality; definite reddening, top or bottom of leg; "clean" appearance means not greater than 1 |
| 1+ | Severe reddening or reddening with definite white marks in creases under foot; query breakdown; query puffiness |
| 1.5 | Some breakdown of skin (usually seen on bottom of foot first); scaly or crusty appearance; definite puffiness, plus (query) breakdown; very marked white marks in creases plus puffiness and/or severe redness |
| 1.5+ | Query possibly moist desquamation in small areas |
| 2 | Breakdown of large areas of skin and/or toes stuck together; possibly moist in places but not all moist |
| 2.5 | Breakdown of large areas of skin with definite moist exudate |
| 3 | Breakdown of most of skin with moist exudate |
| 3.5 | Complete necrosis of limb (rarely seen so far) |

* + and − are equivalent to 0.25.
† Since 1 covers a wide range of reddening, even before reaching the severity or additional factors requiring 1+, it is necessary to have 1− for "definite reddening (ie, definitely not normal), but only to a very slight degree."
(From Fowler JF, Kragt K, Ellis RE, Lindop PJ, Berry RJ: Int J Radiat Biol 9:241–252, 1965)

to the arbitrary scale shown in Table 4-2. Various doses are used. The progressive development of the reaction after 10 doses of 6 Gy (600 rads) each is illustrated in Figure 4-21; each point represents the mean of several animals. Reactions appear by about the 10th day, peak by 15 to 20 days, and then subside. The second wave of the reaction, noted for pig skin, is not seen in mice but is observed in rats.

A dose–response curve is obtained by averaging the skin reaction in the first 30 days and plotting this average as a function of dose. An example is shown in Figure 4-22.

**Early and Late Response to the Lung Based on Breathing Rate**

Travis and her colleagues developed a noninvasive assay of breathing frequency to assess both early and late damage in mouse lungs. Breathing frequency increases progressively with dose after a threshold of about 11 Gy (1100 rads) (Fig. 4-23). The increased breathing frequency in ro-

dent lungs between 14 and 24 weeks is associated with the early response (ie, pneumonitis); by 52 weeks, the elevated breathing frequency is associated with the late response (ie, fibrosis). This is a simple but highly quantitative and reproducible system.

**Spinal Cord Myelopathy**

A dose–response relationship can be determined for late damage caused by local irradiation of the spinal cord of rats. A number of investigators have worked with this system, notably van der Kogel. After latent periods of 4 to 12 months, symptoms of myelopathy develop, the first signs of which are palpable muscle atrophy, followed some time later by impaired use of the hind legs. This type of damage has been described for rats, rabbits, and monkeys. The cell at risk is probably the oligodendrocyte. Some investigators believe that the symptoms observed at doses in the therapeutic range are due to late vascular damage, rather than to the depletion of parenchymal

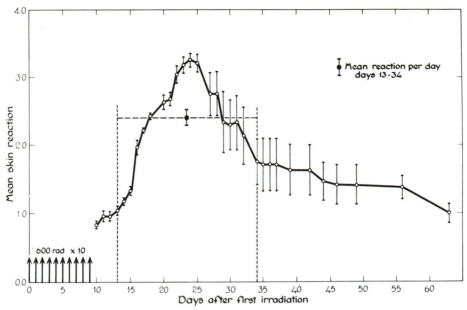

Figure 4-21. Daily skin reaction scores for mice receiving 60 Gy (6000 rads) in 10 equal fractions to the right hind leg. Each point represents the mean score of six animals; the vertical lines represent the standard errors of the mean. (From Brown JM, Goffinet DR, Cleaver JE, Kallman RF: JNCI 47:75–89, 1971)

**60 | Radiobiology for the Radiologist**

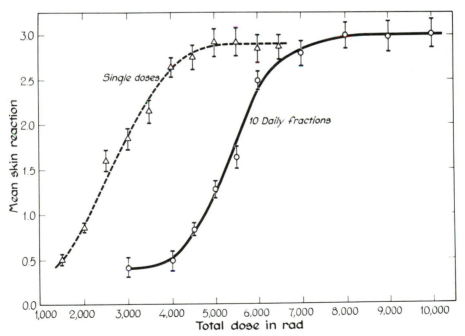

Figure 4-22. Dose–response curves for skin reactions in the mouse foot for single doses and for 10 daily fractions. The mean skin reaction for single doses was obtained by averaging the daily skin reaction scores for the 8th to 29th postirradiation days. The scores for the fractionated treatment were averaged over 13 to 34 days from the start of treatment (as shown in Fig. 4-21). This shift of 5 days between the starting periods for averaging the reactions for single-dose and 10 daily fraction data was done to match the leading edges of skin reaction versus time plots. (From Brown JM, Goffinet DR, Cleaver JE, Kallman RF: JNCI 47:75–89, 1971)

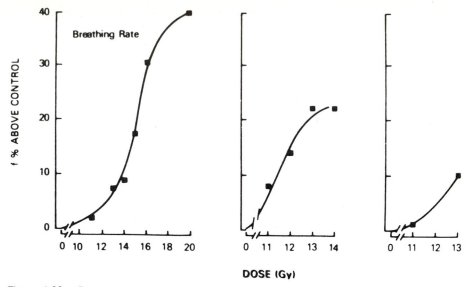

**Figure 4-23.** Breathing frequency in mice as a function of dose measured (*left to right*) 16, 36, and 52 weeks after irradiation with x-rays. Breathing frequency is expressed as a percentage increase above the age-related control value. (From Travis EL, Down JD, Holmes SH, Hobson B: Radiat Res 84:133–143, 1980)

cells. This is unlikely, but the question is controversial.

Much larger doses can be tolerated by the spinal cord if the radiation is divided into two fractions. This reflects the accumulation and repair of a large amount of sublethal damage. The significance of this will become apparent in later chapters.

## INFERRING THE RATIO α/β FROM MULTIFRACTION EXPERIMENTS IN NONCLONOGENIC SYSTEMS

The parameters of the dose–response curve for any normal tissue system for which a functional endpoint can be observed may be *inferred* by performing a multifraction experiment. Take, for example, an experiment in which mouse foot skin reaction is scored. Doses that result in the same skin reaction (eg, moist desquamation over 50% of the area irradiated) when delivered as a single exposure in a multifraction regimen (eg, 5, 10, 20 fractions) must be determined experimentally. A number of assumptions must be made:

1. The dose–response relationship is adequately represented by the linear-quadratic formulation:

$$S = e^{-\alpha D - \beta D^2}$$

where S is the fraction of cells surviving in a dose, D, and α and β are constants.

2. Each dose in a fractionated regimen produces the same biological effect.

3. Full repair of sublethal damage takes place between dose fractions, but no cell proliferation occurs.

Suppose the total dose, D, is divided into n equal fractions of dose d. The previous equation can then be rewritten:

$$S = (e^{-\alpha d - \beta d^2})^n$$

or

$$\frac{-\log_e S}{nd} = \alpha + \beta d$$

If the reciprocal of the total dose (1/nd) is plotted against the dose per fraction (d), a straight line will result, as shown in Figure 4-24. The intercept on the ordinate gives $\alpha/\log_e S$, while the slope gives $\beta/\log_e S$. In general, the value of $\log_e S$ is not known unless other cell survival studies are available, but the ratio of the intercept to the slope provides an estimate of α/β.

Multifraction experiments have been performed and estimates of α/β made for essentially

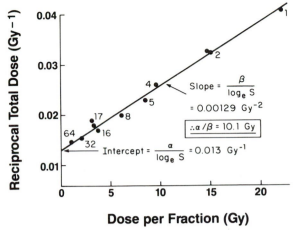

**Figure 4-24.** Reciprocal of the total dose required to produce a given level of injury (acute skin reaction in mice) as a function of dose per fraction in multiple equal doses. The overall time of these experiments was sufficiently short so that proliferation could be neglected; numbers of fractions are shown by each point. From the values of the "intercept" and "slope" of the best-fit line, the values of $\alpha$ and $\beta$ and the ratio $\alpha/\beta$ for the dose–response curve for organ function can be determined. (Redrawn from Douglas BG, Fowler JR: Radiat Res 66:401, 1976)

all of the normal tissue endpoints described in this chapter. One of the important conclusions arrived at is that the value of $\alpha/\beta$ tends to be larger for early-responding tissues, about 10 Gy (1000 rads) than for late-responding tissues, about 2 Gy (200 rads).

Since $\alpha/\beta$ is the dose at which cell killing by linear and quadratic components is equal (see Chapter 3), the implication is that dose–response relationships for late-responding tissues are "curvier" than for early-responding tissues. The importance of this conclusion will become evident in the discussion of fractionation in radiotherapy in Chapter 13.

## FUNCTIONAL SUBUNITS IN NORMAL TISSUES

The killing of individual cells is the basic effect of importance to radiotherapy. The fraction of cells surviving determines the success or failure of a treatment regimen as far as the tumor is concerned, but for normal tissues it is not the whole story. The tolerance of normal tissues to radiation depends on the ability of the clonogenic cells to maintain a sufficient number of mature cells suitably structured to maintain organ function. The relationship between the survival of clonogenic cells and organ function, or failure, depends on the structural organization of the tissue. Tissues may be thought of as consisting of functional subunits (FSUs). A concept proposed to link the survival of clonogenic cells and functional survival is the tissue-rescue unit (TRU), defined to be the minimum number of FSUs required to maintain tissue function. This model assumes that the number of TRUs in a tissue is proportional to the number of clonogenic cells, that FSUs contain a constant number of clonogens, and that FSUs can be repopulated from a single surviving clonogen.

In some tissues, the FSUs are discrete, anatomically delineated structures whose relationship to tissue function is clear. Obvious examples are the nephron in the kidney, the lobule in the liver, and perhaps the acinus in the lung. In other tissues, the FSUs have no clear anatomical demarcation. Examples include the skin, the mucosa, and the spinal cord. The response to radiation of these two types of tissue—with structurally defined or structurally undefined FSUs—is quite different.

The survival of structurally defined FSUs depends on the survival of one or more clonogenic cells within them, and tissue survival in turn depends on the number and radiosensitivity of these clonogens. Although such tissues are composed of a large number of FSUs, each is a small self-contained entity independent of its neighbors. Surviving clonogens cannot migrate from one to the other. Because each FSU is both small and autonomous, low doses deplete the clonogens in it. Each kidney, for example, is composed of a large number of relatively small FSUs, each of which is a self-contained structural entity independent of its neighbors. Consequently survival of a nephron after irradiation depends on the survival of at least one clonogen within it, and therefore on the initial number of renal tubule cells per nephron and their radiosensitivity. Since this FSU is relatively small, it is completely depleted of clonogens by low doses, which accounts for the low tolerance to radiation of the kidney. Other organs that resemble the kidney in having structurally defined FSUs not repopulated from adjacent FSUs, may be those with a branching tree-like system of ducts and vasculature that ultimately terminate in "end structures" or lobules of parenchymal cells. These can be visualized as independent structurally defined FSUs. Examples of organs with this tissue architecture include the lung, liver, and exocrine organs. At least some of these also have low tolerance to radiation.

By contrast, the clonogenic cells that can repopulate the structurally *undefined* FSUs after depletion by radiation are not confined to one particular FSU itself. Rather, clonogenic cells can migrate from one FSU to another and allow repopulation of a depleted FSU. For example, reepithelialization of a denuded area of skin can occur either from surviving clonogens within the denuded area or by migration from adjacent areas.

Some tissues defy classification by this system. The crypts of the jejunum for example are structurally well-defined subunits, but, in fact, surviving crypt cells can and do migrate from one crypt to another to repopulate depleted neighbors.

## THE VOLUME EFFECT IN RADIOTHERAPY: TISSUE ARCHITECTURE

It is generally observed in clinical radiotherapy that the total dose that can be tolerated depends on the volume of tissue irradiated. Tolerance dose has been defined as that dose that produces an acceptable probability of a treatment complication. This definition includes objective criteria such as the radiobiology involved and subjective factors that may be socioeconomic, medicolegal, or psychological.

The spatial arrangement of the FSUs in the tissue is critical. In the case of tissue where the FSUs are arranged in series, like the links of a chain, the integrity of each is critical to organ function and the elimination of any one results in a measurable probability of a complication. The spinal cord is the clearest example where specific functions are controlled by specific segments arranged linearly. Because impulses must pass along the cord, death of critical cells in any one segment will result in complete failure of the organ. The effect on the probability of development of a threshold-binary or quantum response in a serial FSU tissue is illustrated in Figure 4-25. As the field size increases to include a greater number of FSUs, 1, 4 or 16 in this example, the curve relating probability of a complication to dose rises much more steeply with dose and moves to lower doses. This explains the important volume effect found in, for example the spinal cord, where FSUs are arranged in series and loss of any one may result in myelopathy.

By contrast, tissues in which the FSUs are *not* arranged serially show a graded dose response and do not show a volume effect at lower levels of injury when healing can occur from surviving clonogens scattered throughout the treatment volume. This would be true for the skin or mucosa, where a volume effect would not be expected on radiobiological grounds. This is never quite true in practice since when a larger area of skin or mucosa is ulcerated, the prolonged healing time plus the increased potential for infection are more debilitating than similarly severe ulceration in a smaller area. In other words, while the severity of a skin reaction is relatively independent of the area irradiated, because healing occurs by regeneration of surviving clonogens scattered throughout the treated area, the tolerability is not. Therefore, there is a volume effect in clinical practice, but it is not based on an increased probability of injury as it is in tissues where FSUs are arranged serially.

## RADIATION PATHOLOGY OF TISSUES

The response of a tissue or organ to radiation depends primarily on two factors: (1) the inherent sensitivity of the individual cells and (2) the kinetics of the population as a whole of which the cells are a part. These factors combine to account for the substantial variation in response to radiation characteristic of different tissues.

In the case of tissues composed of highly differentiated cells that are performing specialized functions, cell-survival curves are largely irrelevant, since these cells have no mitotic future. Little information is available at the cellular level

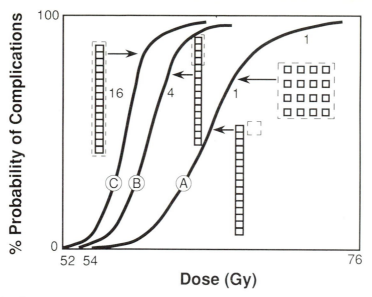

**Figure 4-25.** Relationship between dose and probability of complications for different types of normal tissues. Curve A relates to a normal tissue in which the functional subunits are *not* arranged serially regardless of whether one or all subunits are exposed (ie, regardless of field size). It also applies to a normal tissue in which functional subunits *are* arranged serially if only one subunit is exposed (ie, if the field is small). Note that the curve is relatively shallow (ie, the probability of a complication rises relatively slowly with dose. Curves B and C refer to a tissue with serially arranged functional subunits; the complication curve gets steeper and moves to lower doses as the treatment field size increases. For example, curves B and C relate to 4 or 16 functional subunits exposed. (Note that the position of the curves in relation to the abscissae is arbitrary, resulting from two assumptions: (1) an effective $D_0$ of 4 Gy for a survival curve for cells exposed to multiple doses of 2 Gy and (2) 58 Gy in 2-Gy fractions sterilizes 10% of the functional subunits) (Adapted and redrawn from Withers HR, Taylor JMG, Maciejewski B: Int J Radiat Oncol Biol Phys 14:751–759, 1988)

concerning the effects of radiation on differentiated cells. All that can be said is that, in general, the amount of radiation needed to destroy the functioning ability of a differentiated cell is far greater than that necessary to stop the mitotic activity of a dividing cell.

A closed static population, composed entirely of mature differentiated cells, therefore, is very resistant to radiation. In the case of self-renewing tissues the Achilles heel is the dividing cell; loss of reproductive ability in an appreciable fraction of these cells occurs after a moderate dose of a few Gy (a few hundred rads). Whether the tissue or organ as a whole appears to be affected to a small or large extent—and is consequently labeled as sensitive or resistant—depends on the extent to which the tissue involved can continue to function adequately with a reduced number of cells.

Another factor that is evident from even this most elementary consideration of population kinetics is that the time interval between the delivery of the radiation insult and its expression in tissue damage will be very variable for different populations. This time interval is determined by the normal life span of the mature functional cells and the time it takes for a cell "born" in the stem cell compartment to mature to a functional state. For example, the mature cells in circulating blood have a relatively long life span and are separated from the primitive stem cell compartment by a number of transit compartments, and time is required for a cell to pass through the various stages of differentiation and maturation. Consequently, a considerable time interval will elapse between the depopulation of the stem cell compartment and the final expression of this injury in terms of a reduced peripheral blood cell count. By contrast, in the case of the intestinal epithelium, the mature functional cells on the surface of the villi have a short life span and the time interval between the "birth" of a new cell in the stem compartment of the crypt and its appearance as a mature functional cell is very short, on the order of a few days. As would be expected, therefore, radiation damage is expressed correspondingly quickly in this tissue.

## RESPONSE TO HYPERTHERMIA RELATIVE TO X-RAYS

In the context of this discussion, which is concerned principally with the response of organized tissues, there are two big differences between hyperthermia and ionizing radiations:

1. Cells killed by heat are removed from a tissue promptly, whereas cells lethally damaged by radiation die in attempting the next or some subsequent mitosis, which may be much later. Put another way, apoptosis is much more dominant for hyperthermia but is only part of the story for x-rays.
2. Heat affects differentiated as well as dividing cells. Consequently, the kinetic factors described earlier for x-rays do not apply to heat. The time interval between the delivery of a radiation insult and its expression in tissue damage reflects the normal life span of the mature functional cells and the time taken for a cell "born" in the stem cell compartment to mature into a differentiated functional cell, since for practical purposes only dividing cells are vulnerable to modest doses of radiation. Heat makes no such distinction and may affect differentiated as well as dividing cells.

As a consequence of both of these differences, heat damage is expressed early compared with radiation. For example, heat damage to the gut includes damage to differentiated as well as dividing cells, and the villi collapse quickly. This rapid expression is due to the death of both nonproliferating and dividing cells, leading to stromal injury, including the vasculature. Assays based solely on clonogenicity may therefore greatly underestimate the early effects of heat on normal tissues. Another obvious consequence of these basic differences is that the time interval between treatment and the expression of injury, which is so variable for x-rays because of differences in the rate of differentiation among various tissues, is much less variable for heat.

## CASARET'S CLASSIFICATION OF TISSUE RADIOSENSITIVITY

The limitations of our knowledge of cellular population kinetics is remedied to some extent by a wealth of information on the relative sensitivities of various tissues based on histopathologic observations. It must be emphasized that these data are based on entirely different endpoints from those with which previous chapters have been concerned. To score a cell as "dead" by observing a fixed and stained section of tissue through a microscope is quite different from the experimental test of cell death in terms of loss of reproductive capacity, which has been used previously. Nevertheless, the study of radiation pathology provides data that are highly relevant to clinical radiotherapy.

Casaret has suggested a classification of mammalian cell radiosensitivity based on histologic observation of early cell death. He divided parenchymal cells into four major categories, numbered I to IV (Table 4-3). The supporting structures, such as the connective tissue and the endothelial cells of small blood vessels, are regarded as intermediate in sensitivity between groups II and III of the parenchymal cells.

One of the most sensitive cells to radiation in fact defies all the "laws" and systems of classification; it is the small lymphocyte. This cell, it is believed, never divides at all, or at least only in exceptional circumstances. Small lymphocytes disappear from circulating blood after very small doses of radiation, and it is believed that they suffer an interphase death. Most sensitive cells die a mitotic death after irradiation; most cells that never divide require very large doses to kill them. The small lymphocyte breaks both of these rules, inasmuch as it does not usually divide, dies an interphase death, and at the same time is one of the most sensitive mammalian cells.

Group I of Casaret's classification, the most sensitive group, includes the stem cells of the classic self-renewing systems, such as the basal layers of the epidermis of the skin and the intestine, the erythroblasts or precursors of the red blood cell, and the primitive cells of the spermatogenic series. The stem cells divide regularly and provide a steady and abundant supply of daughter cells, some of which differentiate and

Table 4-3.
## Categories of Mammalian Cell Sensitivity

| CELL TYPE | PROPERTIES | EXAMPLES | SENSITIVITY* |
|---|---|---|---|
| I Vegetative intermitotic cells | Divide regularly; no differentiation | Erythroblasts<br>Intestinal crypt cells<br>Germinal cells of epidermis | High |
| II Differentiating intermitotic cells<br><br>Connective tissue cells† | Divide regularly; some differentiation between divisions | Myelocytes | |
| III Reverting postmitotic cells | Do not divide regularly; variably differentiated | Liver | |
| IV Fixed postmitotic cells | Do not divide; highly differentiated | Nerve cells<br>Muscle cells | Low |

*Sensitivity decreases for each successive group.*
†*Intermediate in sensitivity between groups II and III.*
*(Based on Casaret G in Harris RJC (ed): Cellular Basis and Aetiology of Late Somatic Effects of Ionizing Radiations. New York, Academic Press, 1963; and Rubin R, Casaret GW: Clinical Radiation Pathology, vol 1. Philadelphia, WB Saunders, 1968)*

mature into functioning cells. A reservoir of primitive dividing stem cells is maintained and in some cases can be triggered to divide more rapidly in response to a need. The primitive dividing stem cells are vulnerable to radiation; a moderate dose will cause a proportion of them to "die" in attempting the next or a subsequent mitosis. The time of crisis for the organism as a whole occurs when the supply of functioning cells is inadequate: a shortage of circulating red and white blood cells in the case of the blood and a shortage of mature covering dermal cells in the case of the skin. The time interval between irradiation and the crisis is about equal to the life span of the mature functioning cells. As the functioning cells die off at the end of their natural life span, there are none to take their place if a dose of radiation has previously depopulated the stem cell compartment. Depending on the size of the dose, the organ or tissue may not survive the critical time when the number of functioning cells reaches a minimum value.

Group II consists of cells that divide regularly but that also mature and differentiate between divisions. Cells in this category are relatively short-lived as individuals and are produced by division of vegetative intermitotic cells. These cells usually complete a limited number of divisions and differentiate to some extent between successive mitoses. This group includes cells of the hematopoietic series in the intermediate stages of differentiation and likewise the more differentiated spermatogonia and spermatocytes.

Group III, the reverting postmitotic cells, are relatively resistant and as individuals have a relatively long life. Ordinarily, they do not undergo mitosis but are capable of dividing under the appropriate stimulus, which is usually a damage to or loss of many of their own kind. The liver cells are a good example of cells of this category. In the adult, there is normally little or no cell division, but if a large part of the liver is removed by surgery, the remaining cells are triggered to divide and make good the loss. Other examples in this category include the cells of the kidney and pancreas and cells of various glands, such as the adrenal, thyroid, and pituitary.

Group IV consists of the fixed postmitotic cells. These are generally considered to be the most resistant to radiation. They are highly differentiated and appear to have lost the ability to divide. Some have a long life span, such as the neurons. Others have a short life span, such as the granulocytes, which have to be continually replaced by the division of more primitive cells. The superficial epithelial cells of the gut also fall into this category. In the normal course of events they are sloughed off the tops of the villi and replaced by cells dividing in the crypts.

## PARENCHYMAL CELLS AND CONNECTIVE TISSUE

The *parenchymal* cells perform the unique functions of a particular tissue, but they are supported and held in place by *connective tissue* and are supplied with oxygen and nutrients by the *blood vessels*. According to Casaret's classification, connective tissue and blood vessels are intermediate in sensitivity between the most sensitive and most resistant parenchymal cells.

When a tissue or organ is exposed to a dose of radiation, the course of events will be determined by radiation effects on both parenchymal and connective tissue elements. The parenchymal cells may be more sensitive than the connective tissue or vice versa, depending on the organ involved. There is a long-standing dispute, unresolved at the present time, as to whether late effects of radiotherapy are due primarily to damage to parenchymal cells or to damage to the vasculature.

► *Summary of Pertinent Conclusions*

- In general after irradiation, cells die a *mitotic death*, that is, they die in attempting the next or a later mitosis. In some tissues cells die by *apoptosis*, which is a programmed cell death.
- Systems involving clonogenic endpoints (ie, cell survival) for cells of normal tissues include some in which cells regrow in situ and some in which cells are transplanted to another site.
- In situ regrowth techniques include the skin, crypt cells in the jejunum or colon, testes stem cells, and kidney tubules. Single-dose experiments can yield the slope ($D_0$) of the dose–response curve over a range of high doses. Multifraction experiments allow the whole dose–response curve to be reconstructed.
- Systems in which cell survival is assessed by transplantation into another site include bone marrow stem cells, thyroid cells, and mammary cells.
- A dose–response curve for bone marrow stem cells can be obtained by allowing cells from the donor animal to lodge and grow in the spleen of recipient animals. These are the most sensitive normal mammalian cells that die a mitotic death; $D_0$ is close to 1 Gy (100 rads), with little or no shoulder.
- Dose–response curves for mammary and thyroid cells can be obtained by transplanting them into a fat pad of recipient animals.
- The radiosensitivity of cells from normal tissues varies widely. The width of the shoulder of the curve is the principal variable. Jejunal crypt cells have a very large shoulder; bone marrow stem cells have little, if any, shoulder. Most other cell types studied in clonogenic assays fall in between.
- Dose–response curves for functional endpoints, distinct from cell survival, can be obtained for:

*(continued)*

► **Summary of Pertinent Conclusions**   *(Continued)*

1. Pig skin and rodent skin by measuring skin reactions
2. Early and late response of the lung by measuring breathing rate
3. Spinal cord by observing myelopathy

- The shape of the dose–response relationship for functional endpoints, obtained from multifraction experiments, is more pertinent to radiotherapy than clonogenic assays.
- The ratio α/β (the dose at which the linear and quadratic components of radiation damage are equal) may be inferred from multifraction experiments in systems scoring nonclonogenic endpoints.
- Spatial arrangement of functional subunits (FSUs) is critical to the tolerance of some normal tissues.
- In some tissues (eg, spinal cord), the FSUs are arranged serially (like links in a chain) and the integrity of each is critical to organ function.
- Tolerance depends more critically on volume irradiated for tissues where FSUs are arranged serially.

### Organized Tissues

- Apparent radioresponsiveness of a tissue depends on

  1. Inherent sensitivity of cells
  2. Kinetics of the cell population

- Sensitivity of actively dividing cells is expressed by their survival curve for reproductive integrity.
- Radiation dose needed to destroy the functioning ability of a differentiated cell is *far greater than* that necessary to stop the mitotic activity of a dividing cell.
- The time interval between irradiation and its expression in tissue damage depends on the life span of mature functional cells and the time it takes for a cell born in the stem compartment to mature.
- Hyperthermia damage is expressed early compared with radiation damage because

  1. Heat kills differentiated as well as dividing cells.
  2. Heat-killed cells can die in interphase, whereas radiation-killed cells die at the next or a subsequent mitosis.

- Our limited knowledge of population kinetics is remedied by a wealth of histopathologic observations.
- In terms of radiosensitivity, based on histologic observation of cell death, parenchymal cells fall into four categories, from most sensitive to most resistant:

  I. Stem cells of classic self-renewal tissues, which divide regularly
  II. Differentiating intermitotic cells, which divide regularly but in which there is some differentiation between divisions
  III. Reverting postmitotic cells, which do not divide regularly but can divide under the appropriate stimulus
  IV. Fixed postmitotic cells, which are highly differentiated and appear to have lost the ability to divide

*(continued)*

► *Summary of Pertinent Conclusions* *(Continued)*

- Connective tissue and blood vessels are intermediate in radiosensitivity between groups II and III. There is a long-standing dispute as to whether the late effects of radiotherapy are due principally to damage to parenchymal cells or to damage to the vasculature.

# BIBLIOGRAPHY

Andrews JR: The Radiobiology of Human Cancer Radiotherapy. Philadelphia, WB Saunders, 1968

Barendsen GW, Broerse JJ: Experimental radiotherapy of a rat rhabdomyosarcoma with 15 MeV neutrons and 300 kV x-rays: I. Effects of single exposures. Eur J Cancer 5:373–391, 1969

Casaret G: Concept and criteria of radiologic ageing. In Harris RJC (ed): Cellular Basis and Aetiology of Late Somatic Effects of Ionizing Radiations. New York, Academic Press, 1963

Clifton KH, Briggs RC, Stone HB: Quantitative radiosensitivity studies of solid carcinomas in vivo: Methodology and effect of anoxia. JNCI 36:965–974, 1966

DeMott RK, Mulcahy RT, Clifton KH: The survival of thyroid cells following irradiation: A directly generated single-dose survival curve. Radiat Res 77:395–403, 1979

Field SB, Jones T, Thomlinson RH: The relative effects of fast neutrons and x-rays on tumor and normal tissue in the rat. Br J Radiol 40:834–842, 1967

Fowler JF, Denekamp J, Page AL, Begg AC, Field SB, Butler K: Fractionation with x-rays and neutrons in mice: Response of skin and C3H mammary tumors. Br J Radiol 45:237–249, 1972

Fowler JF, Morgan RL, Silvester JA, Bewley DK, Turner BA: Experiments with fractionated x-ray treatment of the skin of pigs: I. Fractionation up to 28 days. Br J Radiol 36:188–196, 1963

Gould MN, Clifton KH: The survival of mammary cells following irradiation in vivo: A directly generated single-dose survival curve. Radiat Res 72:343–352, 1977

Hendry JH, Thames HD: The tissue-rescuing unit. Br J Radiol 59:628–630, 1986

Hermens AF, Barendsen GW: Cellular proliferation patterns in an experimental rhabdomyosarcoma in the rat. Eur J Cancer 3:361–369, 1967

Hermens AF, Barendsen GW: Changes of cell proliferation characteristics in a rat rhabdomyosarcoma before and after irradiation. Eur J Cancer 5:173–189, 1969

Hewitt HB: Studies on the quantitative transplantation of mouse sarcoma. Br J Cancer 7:367–383, 1953

Hewitt HB, Chan DPS, Blake ER: Survival curves for clonogenic cells of a murine keratinizing squamous carcinoma irradiated in vivo or under hypoxic conditions. Int J Radiat Biol 12:535–549, 1967

Hewitt HB, Wilson CW: A survival curve for mammalian leukaemia cells irradiated in vivo. Br J Cancer 13:69–75, 1959

Hewitt HB, Wilson CW: Survival curves for tumor cells irradiated in vivo. Ann NY Acad Sci 95:818–827, 1961

Hill RP, Bush RS: A lung colony assay to determine the radiosensitivity of the cells of a solid tumor. Int J Radiat Biol 15:435–444, 1969

Hume SP, Marigold JCL, Field SB: The effect of local hyperthermia on the small intestine of the mouse. Br J Radiol 52:657–662, 1979

Kerr JFR, Searle J: Apoptosis: Its nature and kinetic role. In Meyn RE, Withers HR (eds): Radiation Biology in Cancer Research, pp 367–384. New York, Raven Press, 1980

McNally NJ: Recovery from sublethal damage by hypoxic tumor cells in vivo. Br J Radiol 45:116–120, 1972

McNally NJ: A comparison of the effects of radiation on tumor growth delay and cell survival: The effect of oxygen. Br J Radiol 46:450–455, 1973

Peters LJ, Brock WA, Travis EL: Radiation biology at clinically relevant doses. In DeVita VT, Hellman S, Rosenberg SA (eds): Important Advances in Oncology, pp 65–83. Philadelphia, JB Lippincott, 1990

Reinhold HS: Quantitative evaluation of the radiosensitivity of cells of a transplantable rhabdomyosarcoma in the rat. Eur J Cancer 2:33–42, 1966

Rockwell SC, Kallman RF: Cellular radiosensitivity and tumor radiation response in the EMT6 tumor cell system. Radiat Res 53:281–294, 1973

Rockwell SC, Kallman RF, Fajardo LF: Characteristics of a serially transplanted mouse mammary tumor and its tissue-culture-adapted derivative. JNCI 49:735–749, 1972

Rubin R, Casaret GW: Clinical Radiation Pathology, vol 1. Philadelphia, WB Saunders, 1968

Stephen LC, Arg KK, Schultheiss TE, Milas L, Meyn R: Apoptosis in irradiated murine tumors. Radiat Res 127:308–316, 1991

Suit HD, Maeda M; Hyperbaric oxygen and radiobiology of the C3H mouse mammary carcinoma. JNCI 39:639–652, 1967

Suit H, Wette R: Radiation dose fractionation and tumor control probability. Radiat Res 29:267–281, 1966

Suit HD, Wette R, Lindberg R: Analysis of tumor-recurrence times. Radiology 88:311–321, 1967

Sutherland RM, Durand RE: Radiation response of multicell spheroids: An in vitro tumor model. Curr Top Radiat Res Q 11:87–139, 1976

Sutherland RM, McCredie JA, Inch WR: Growth of multicell spheroids in tissue culture as a model of nodular carcinomas. JNCI 46:113–120, 1971

Tannock IF: The relation between cell proliferation and the vascular system in a transplanted mouse mammary tumour. Br J Cancer 22:258–273, 1968

Thames HD, Withers HR: Test of equal effect per fraction and estimation of initial clonogen number in microcolony assays of survival after fractionated irradiation. Br J Radiol 53:1071–1077, 1980

Thames HD, Withers R, Mason KA, Reid BO: Dose survival characteristics of mouse jejunal crypt cells. Int J Radiat Oncol Biol Phys 7:1591–1597, 1981

Travis EL: The tissue rescuing unit. In Fielden EM, Fowler JF, Hendry JH, Scott D (eds): Proceedings of the 8th International Congress of Radiation Research, Edinburgh, July 1987. Radiat Res 2:795–800, 1987

Travis EL, Down JD, Holmes SJ, Hobson B: Radiation pneumonitis and fibrosis in mouse lung assayed by respiratory frequency and histology. Radiat Res 84:133–142, 1980

Travis EL, Vojnovic B, Davies EE, Hirst DG: A plethysmographic method for measuring function in locally irradiated mouse lung. Br J Radiol 52:67–74, 1979

Van der Kogel AJ: Mechanisms of late radiation injury in the spinal cord. In Meyn RE, Withers HR (eds): Radiation Biology in Cancer Research, pp 461–470. New York, Raven Press, 1980

Wara WM, Phillips TL, Margolis LW, Smith V: Radiation pneumonitis: A new appraoch to the derivation of time–dose factors. Cancer 32:547–552, 1973

Williams GT: Programmed cell death: Apoptosis and oncogenesis. Cell 65:1097–1098, 1991

Withers HR, Hunter N, Barkley HT Jr, Reid BO: Radiation survival and regeneration characteristics of spermatogenic stem cells of mouse testis. Radiat Res 57:88–103, 1974

Withers HR, Mason KA, Thames HD: Late radiation response of kidney assayed by tubule cell survival. Br J Radiol 59:587–595, 1986

Withers HR, Taylor JMG, Maciejewski B: Treatment volume and tissue tolerance. Int J Radiat Oncol Biol Phys 14:751–759, 1988

Withers HR, Thames HD, Peters LJ, Fletcher GH: Keynote address: Normal tissue radioresistance in clinical radiotherapy. In Fletcher GH, Nervi C, Withers HR (eds): Biological Bases and Clinical Implications of Tumor Radioresistance, pp 139–152. New York, Masson, 1983

*Radiobiology for the Radiologist, Fourth Edition*, by Eric J. Hall
J. B. Lippincott Company, Philadelphia © 1994.

# 5

# *Model Tumor Systems*

Radiation Therapy

## TRANSPLANTABLE SOLID TUMOR SYSTEMS IN EXPERIMENTAL ANIMALS

A wide range of experimental tumors of various histologic types have been developed for radiobiological studies. To produce a large number of virtually identical tumors, propagation by transplantation from one generation of animals to the next is used, which makes it mandatory that the animals be isologous. In practice, pure inbred strains of rats or mice are used and are maintained by brother–sister mating, which also serves the function of reducing the variability between animals to a minimum.

The tumor from a donor animal is aseptically removed and when possible is prepared into a single cell suspension; this is accomplished by separating the cells with an enzyme such as trypsin and then forcing them through a fine wire mesh. To effect a transplant, $10^4$ to $10^6$ cells are inoculated subcutaneously into each of a large group of recipient animals of the same strain. The site of transplantation varies widely; the flank or back is commonly used, but sometimes a special tumor requires a particular site, such as the brain. Some tumors cannot be handled in this way and must be propagated by transplanting a small piece of tumor rather than a known number of single cells; this is obviously less quantitative. Within days or weeks, depending on the type of tumor and the strain of animals, palpable tumors appear in the recipient animals that are uniform in size, histologic type, and so on. Hundreds to thousands of animals can be used, which makes it possible to design highly quantitative studies of tumor response to different radiations, fractionation regimens, sensitizers, and combinations of radiation and chemotherapeutic agents.

There are five commonly used techniques to assay the response of solid tumors to a treatment regimen:

**1.** Tumor growth measurements
**2.** Tumor cure (TCD$_{50}$)

**3.** Tumor cell survival determined in vivo by the dilution assay technique
**4.** Tumor cell survival assayed by the lung colony system
**5.** Tumor cell survival—in vivo treatment followed by in vitro assay

These methods are each discussed briefly.

## TUMOR GROWTH MEASUREMENTS

Tumor growth measurement is possibly the simplest endpoint to use and involves the daily measurement of each tumor to arrive at a mean diameter. For tumor growth experiments a large number of transplanted tumors are prepared as previously described. When they have grown to a specified size (eg, a diameter of 8 to 10 mm in rats or 2 to 4 mm in mice), they are treated according to the plan of the particular experiment. Figure 5-1 illustrates the variation of tumor size with time for unirradiated controls and tumors given a single dose of x-rays. The untreated tumors grow rapidly at a relatively uniform rate, while the radiation treatment causes a temporary shrinkage of the tumor, followed by regrowth.

Two different methods have been used to score the tumor response. Barendsen and his colleagues have used growth delay, illustrated in Figure 5-1, as the time taken after irradiation for the tumor to regrow to the size it was at the time of irradiation. Clearly, this index of response is only suitable for tumors that shrink significantly after irradiation. For tumors that do not shrink so obviously, a more convenient measure of growth delay is the time taken for the irradiated tumor to grow to some specified size after exposure, compared with controls. In the figure these quantities are labeled T$_{X-RAY}$ and T$_{CON}$ Either index of growth delay will increase as a function of dose. Figure 5-2A shows growth curves for a rat rhabdomyosarcoma irradiated with various doses of x-rays or fast neutrons. In Figure 5-2B, growth delay is expressed as a function of radiation dose.

76

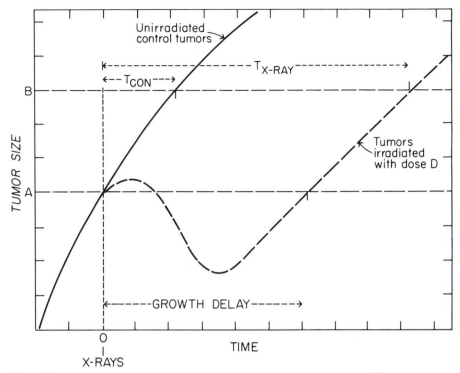

**Figure 5-1.** The pattern of response of a tumor to a dose (D) of x-rays. The size of the tumor, either the mean diameter or the volume, is plotted as a function of time after irradiation. Two different indices of tumor responses have been used by different investigators. Growth delay represents the time after irradiation that it takes for the tumor to regrow to the size at the time of irradiation. Alternatively, the index of radiation damage may be the time taken for the tumor to grow from a specified size A at the time of irradiation to some specified larger size B. Typically, this may be from 9 to 25 mm in diameter for rat tumors. This quantity is shown as $T_{CON}$ for unirradiated control animals and $T_{X-RAY}$ for tumors irradiated with a dose (D) of x-rays. Either index of tumor response may be plotted as a function of radiation dose.

## TCD$_{50}$ ASSAY

Tumor control provides data of most obvious relevance to radiotherapy. In experiments of this kind a large number of animals with tumors of uniform size are divided into separate groups, and the tumors are irradiated locally with graded doses. The tumors are subsequently observed regularly for recurrence or local control. The proportion of tumors that are locally controlled can be plotted as a function of dose, and data of this kind are amenable to a sophisticated statistical analysis to determine the TCD$_{50}$, the dose at which 50% of the tumors are locally controlled. This quantity is highly repeatable from one experiment to another in an inbred strain of animals. Suit and his colleagues, over more than 30 years, have made an extensive study of the response to radiation of a mammary carcinoma in

C$_3$H mice. Data from a typical experiment are presented in Figure 5-3. Tumors were propagated by transplanting $4 \times 10^4$ cells into the outer portion of the mouse ear, and irradiations were performed when the tumors had grown to a volume of about 4 mm$^3$. A brass circular clamp was fitted across the base of the ear and maintained for at least a minute before the initiation of the irradiation, so that the tumors were uniformly hypoxic. Single-dose, 2-dose, and 10-dose experiments were performed, with a 24-hour interval between dose fractions. Tumor control results are shown in Figure 5-3. The TCD$_{50}$ for a single treatment is 45.75 Gy (4575 rads), rising to 51.1 Gy (5110 rads) for 2 fractions and to 84 Gy (8400 rads) if the radiation is delivered in 10 equal fractions. This indicates that a marked and extensive repair of sublethal damage has taken place during a multifraction regimen. Other ex-

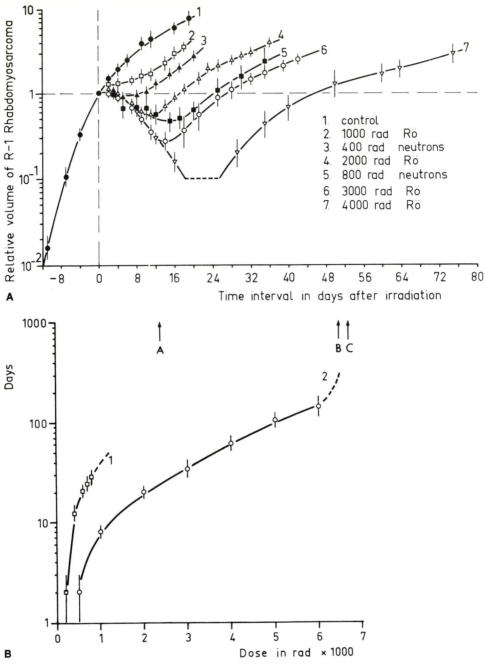

**Figure 5-2.** **(A)** Volume changes of rhabdomyosarcomas in rats after irradiation. Curve 1 represents the growth of the unirradiated control tumors. Curves 2, 4, 6, and 7 refer to tumors irradiated with 10 to 40 Gy (1000–4000 rads) of 300-kV x-rays, respectively. Curves 3 and 5 refer to tumors irradiated with 4 and 8 Gy (400 and 800 rads) of 15-MeV d$^+$ →T fast neutrons. **(B)** Growth delay of rhabdomyosarcomas in rats as a function of dose of x-rays (*curve 2*) or fast neutrons (*curve 1*). A and C indicate the doses of neutrons and x-rays required to "cure" 90% of the tumors, calculated on the basis of cell-survival curves. B indicates the observed TCD$_{90}$ for x-rays. Note the good agreement between calculated and observed values of the TCD$_{90}$ for x-rays. (From Barendsen GW, Broerse JJ: Eur J Cancer 5:373–391, 1969)

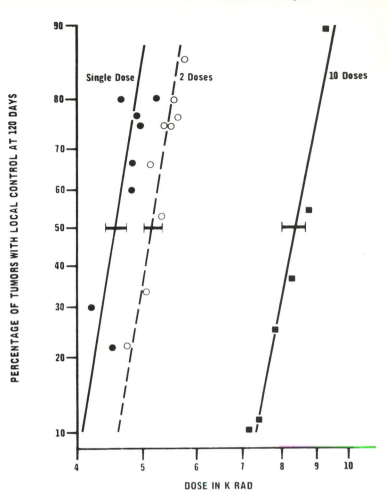

**Figure 5-3.** Percentage of mouse mammary tumors locally controlled as a function of x-ray dose, for single exposures and for two different fractionation patterns. The tumors were isotransplants derived from a spontaneous mammary carcinoma in a $C_3H$ mouse. The transplantation was made into the outer portion of the ear with $4 \times 10^4$ viable cells. The tumors were treated when they reached a diameter of 2 mm (ie, a volume of about 4 mm³). (From Suit HD, Wette R: Radiat Res 29:267–281, 1966)

amples of the use of this system are discussed in later chapters.

## DILUTION ASSAY TECHNIQUE

The dilution assay technique was devised by Hewitt and Wilson, who used it to produce the first in vivo survival curve in 1959. They used a lymphocytic leukemia of spontaneous origin in mice. A single cell suspension can be prepared from the infiltrated liver of an animal with advanced disease and the tumor transplanted by injecting known numbers of cells into the peritoneal cavities of recipient mice, which subsequently develop a leukemia. The leukemia can be transmitted, on average, by the injection of only two cells; this quantity—the number of cells re-

quired to transmit the tumor to 50% of the animals—is known as the $TD_{50}$. The **dilution assay technique** became the basis for obtaining an in vivo cell survival curve.

The procedure used, illustrated in Figure 5-4, is as follows. An animal containing the tumor may be irradiated to a given dose of radiation, for example, 10 Gy (1000 rads). A single cell suspension is then prepared from the infiltrated liver, the cells are counted and diluted, and various numbers of these cells are injected intraperitoneally into groups of recipient animals. It is then a matter of observation and calculation to determine how many irradiated cells are required to produce a tumor in half of the animals inoculated with that given number of cells. Suppose, for instance, that it takes 20 irradiated cells, on the average, to transmit the tumor; since it is

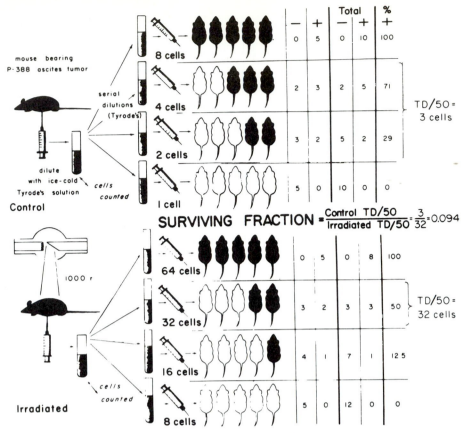

**Figure 5-4.** Schematic representation to show the general features of the dilution assay technique. Various numbers of tumor cells from the donor animal are injected into groups of recipients, and a determination is made of the number of cells required for a tumor to take in half of the animals of the group ($TD_{50}$). The ratio of this quantity for control and irradiated donors is the surviving fraction. (From Andrews JR, Berry RJ: Radiat Res 16:76, 1962)

known that only 2 clonogenic cells are needed to transmit the tumor, it is a simple matter to decide that in the irradiated population of cells 2 of 20, or 10%, were clonogenic and survived the dose of 10 Gy (1000 rads).

$$\text{ie, Surviving fraction} = \frac{TD_{50} \text{ controls}}{TD_{50} \text{ irradiated}}$$

If this process is repeated for a number of doses of radiation and the corresponding surviving fractions are determined by this assay technique, a survival curve for cells irradiated and assayed in vivo can be constructed.

This technique is a true in vivo system, but it involves a leukemia as opposed to a solid tumor. The cells, when reinoculated into the mouse, grow in the peritoneal cavity in much the same

way that the cells grow in a petri dish in the in vitro technique; the mice are in fact being used as small portable incubators.

Since these pioneering efforts, the dilution assay technique has been applied by many different workers to measure survival curves for a number of leukemias and solid tumors when the tumors can be removed and prepared into a single cell suspension; some collected results are shown in Figure 5-5. The survival curves obtained have a $D_0$ of about 4 Gy (400 rads), because the cells in the peritoneal cavity of the mouse are so numerous and so closely packed that they are deficient in oxygen. This technique, therefore, produces a "hypoxic" survival curve. To obtain a survival curve characteristic of aerated conditions, it is necessary either to remove the cells from the donor animal and irradiate them in a petri dish where they are in contact with air or to inject hydrogen peroxide into the peritoneal cavity of the mouse before irradiation so that oxygen is available to the tumor cells during the irradiation. When this is done, the $D_0$ is about 1.3 to 1.6 Gy (130 to 160 rads).

## LUNG COLONY ASSAY

Hill and Bush have devised a technique to assay the clonogenicity of the cells of a solid tumor irradiated in situ by injecting them into recipient animals and counting the number of lung colonies produced. The general principles of the method are illustrated in Figure 5-6. The tumor used in these studies was the KHT sarcoma, which is a transplantable tumor that arose originally in a $C_3H$ mouse, and which has been

serially propagated through many generations. Tumors are irradiated in situ, after which they are removed and made into a preparation of single cells by a combined trypsinization and mechanical procedure. A known number of cells is then mixed with a large number of heavily irradiated tumor cells and injected intravenously into recipient mice. About 3 weeks later these mice are sacrificed, and the colonies formed in the lungs are readily countable. The number of lung colonies is a measure of the number of surviving clonogenic cells in the injected suspension.

This technique was used for studies of dose rate described in Chapter 7. The lung colony technique is not confined to the KHT sarcoma but has been used with other tumor cells. For example, the demonstration of the absence of repair of potentially lethal damage after neutron irradiation involved the use of the Lewis lung carcinoma, and the fraction of surviving cells was assayed by counting lung colonies.

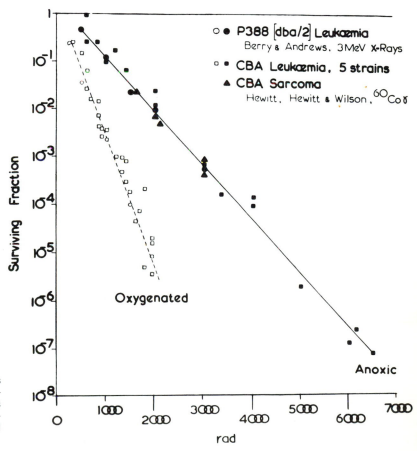

Figure 5-5. Dose–response curves in vivo, using the dilution assay technique, for various murine tumors under oxygenated and hypoxic conditions. (From Berry RJ: Br J Radiol 37:948, 1964)

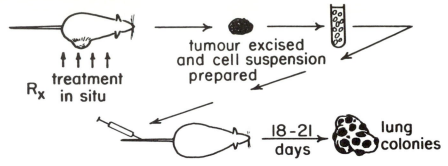

**Figure 5-6.** The lung colony assay system. The tumor is irradiated in situ, after which it is excised and made into a single-cell suspension. A known number of cells is then injected intravenously into recipient animals. About 3 weeks later the recipient animals are sacrificed, and the colonies that have formed in the lungs are counted. The number of lung colonies is a measure of the number of surviving clonogenic cells in the injected suspension. (From Hill RP, Bush RS: Br J Radiol 46:167–174, 1973)

## IN VIVO/IN VITRO TECHNIQUE

A limited number of cell lines have been adapted so that they will grow either as a transplantable tumor in an animal or as clones in a petri dish. These cells can be readily transferred from in vivo to in vitro and back. In one generation they may be growing as a solid tumor in an animal and in the next as a monolayer in a petri dish. The three most commonly used systems are a rhabdomyosarcoma in the rat (Hermens and Barendsen), a fibrosarcoma in the mouse (McNally), and the EMT6 mammary tumor also in the mouse (Rockwell and Kallman).

The steps involved in this method are illustrated in Figure 5-7. It combines many of the advantages of the in vitro and in vivo techniques. The tumors are treated in vivo in a natural environment, so that the cellular response is modified by the various factors that are important in determining gross tumor response. After treatment, each tumor is removed and prepared into a single cell suspension, and the cell concentration is counted in a hemocytometer or electronic cell counter. Known numbers of cells can then be transferred to petri dishes containing fresh growth medium, and the proportion of clonogenic cells can be determined by counting colonies 10 days later. The speed, accuracy, and relative economy of the in vitro system replaces the expense and inconvenience of the recipient animals in the dilution assay technique.

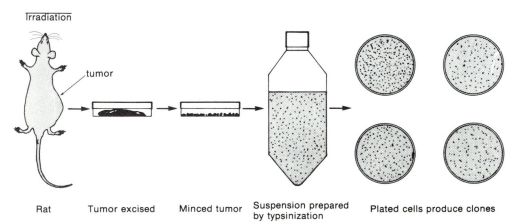

| Rat | Tumor excised | Minced tumor | Suspension prepared by typsinization | Plated cells produce clones |

**Figure 5-7.** The principle of the in vivo/in vitro assay system using the rhabdomyosarcoma in the rat. The solid tumor in the animal can be removed and the tumor cells assayed for colony formation in petri dishes. This cell line can be transferred to and fro between the animal and the petri dish. (Courtesy of Drs. G. W. Barendsen and J.J. Broerse)

# XENOGRAFTS OF HUMAN TUMORS

A wide variety of human tumor cells can be grown as xenografts in immune-deficient animals. Steel has estimated that more than 300 individual human tumors have been investigated in this way. Breast and ovarian tumors have generally been difficult to graft, with melanomas and tumors of the colon and bronchus being relatively successful. Most often, the animals used for xenografts are "nude" mice (ie, mice that are genetically athymic). Some investigators have used animals in which the immune response is suppressed by drugs, total-body irradiation, or a combination of both. The objective, of course, is to maintain the response characteristic of the source tumor.

Xenografts retain human karyotypes through serial passages and maintain some of the response characteristics of the individual source human tumors; to this extent, they have great advantages over mouse tumors. There are, however, certain drawbacks. First, there is a tendency for the tumor to be rejected, so that observing tumor control as an end point can be misleading. Growth delay and cell-survival studies, on the other hand, are probably less affected. Second, human tumor cells do undergo kinetic changes and cell selection when transplanted into mice. For example, xenografts commonly have doubling times about one fifth of the values observed in humans, so that increased responsiveness should be expected to proliferation-dependent chemotherapeutic agents. Third, while the histologic characteristics of the human source tumors are usually well maintained by xenografts, the stromal tissue is of mouse origin. Consequently, xenografts of human tumor cells are not much more valid than murine tumors for any studies in which the vascular supply plays an important role. For example, the fraction of hypoxic cells in xenografts is much the same as in mouse tumors.

Steel and colleagues reviewed the field in 1983 and concluded that xenografts generally maintain the chemotherapeutic response characteristics of the class of tumors from which they are derived. There is good evidence, too, for individuality of response among xenografts. For example, in studying melanomas, one was responsible clinically, while the other was not, and the cell survival curve after therapy with melphalan was twice as steep in the xenograft of the cells from the responsive tumor.

Figure 5-8 summarizes the correlation between growth delay in the xenograft and clinical remission of the donor patient. In the figure the growth delay in xenografts for maximum tolerated treatment with the single agents that are in common clinical use against the disease is plotted against clinical complete response rate for that category of tumor. The correlation between these parameters is good. Testicular tumors were the most responsive in xenografts or in the clinic; small cell lung cancer and breast tumors occupied an intermediate position; and the other three tumor types were unresponsive, either clinically or experimentally. This consistency of agreement between patient and xenograft responses to chemotherapeutic agents is encouraging for a variety of human tumor types tested. Similarly, studies of radiation response indicate that measurements of growth delay in xenografts rank tumors in the same order as clinical responsiveness: testicular teratoma is greater than pancreatic carcinoma, which is greater than bladder carcinoma, for example.

**Figure 5-8.** Correlation between response of human tumor xenografts and clinical complete remission rates to chemotherapy. Ordinate is growth delay observed in 3 to 10 xenograft lines treated with the clinically used drugs that proved most effective in the xenografts. (Steel GG: How well do xenografts maintain the therapeutic response characteristics of the source tumor in the donor patient? In Kallman RF (ed): Rodent Tumors in Experimental Cancer Therapy. New York, Pergamon, 1987)

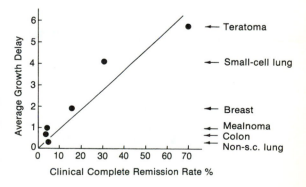

# SPHEROIDS: AN IN VITRO MODEL TUMOR SYSTEM

Mammalian cells in culture may be grown either as a monolayer attached to a glass or plastic surface or in suspension, where they are prevented from settling out and attaching to the surface of the culture vessel by continual gentle stirring. Most cells in suspension, or in "spinner culture" as it is often called, remain as single cells; at each mitosis the daughter cells separate and the cell concentration increases with time but consists of individual, separate cells.

However, some cells, notably several rodent tumor cell lines, such as Chinese hamster V79 lung cells, mouse EMT6 mammary and R1F fibrosarcoma cells, and rat 9L brain tumor cells, do not behave in this way but instead grow as spheroids. At each successive division the daughter cells stick together, and the result is a large spherical clump of cells that grows bigger and bigger with time. A photograph of a large spheroid consisting of about $8 \times 10^4$ cells is shown in Figure 5-9. Five days after the seeding of single cells into suspension culture, the spheroids have a diameter of about 200 μm; by 15 days the diameter may exceed 800 μm. Oxygen and nutrients must diffuse into the spheroids from the surrounding tissue culture medium. In the center of a spheroid there is a deficiency of oxygen and nutrients and a buildup of waste products because of diffusion limitations. Eventually, central necrosis appears and the mean cell cycle lengthens. Mature spheroids contain a heterogeneous population of cells resulting from many of the same factors, as in a tumor in vivo.

The spheroid system is simpler, more reproducible, less expensive, and easier to manipulate than animal tumors, and yet the cells can be studied in an environment that includes the complexities of cell-to-cell contact and nutritional stress from diffusion limitations that are characteristic of a growing tumor. Spheroids are irradiated intact and then separated into single cells

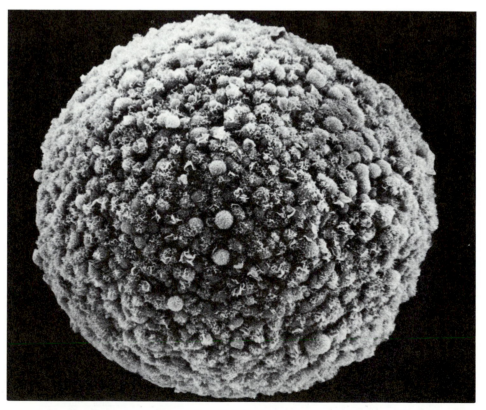

**Figure 5-9.** Photograph of an 800-μm spheroid containing about $8 \times 10^4$ cells. (Courtesy of Dr. R.M. Sutherland)

by the use of trypsin and gentle agitation before being plated out into petri dishes to be assayed for the reproductive integrity of individual cells.

Mature spheroids consist of three populations of cells with varying radiosensitivity; starting from the outside and working toward the center, they are (1) asynchronous, aerobic cycling cells; (2) noncycling $G_1$-like cells; and (3) noncycling $G_1$-like hypoxic cells. Very large spheroids may contain about 20% hypoxic cells, similar to many animal tumors. By gently trypsinizing the spheroids for varying periods of time, the spheroid can be peeled like an onion and these three cell populations separated out. Using more sophisticated methods, such as centrifugal elutriation and flow cytometry, it is possible to separate many more cell subpopulations based on location in the spheroid, cell cycle, or other parameters. Figure 5-10 is a cross-section through a large spheroid, showing clearly the development of a central necrotic area when its size is such that oxygen and other nutrients cannot diffuse into the center.

The spheroid system has been applied to a number of problems in radiobiology and in the study of pharmacologic agents, such as radiosensitizers or chemotherapeutic agents. A major problem in the application of these drugs to human tumors is the presence of resistant cells that are resting or noncycling, often located away from blood vessels. Drugs are required to diffuse

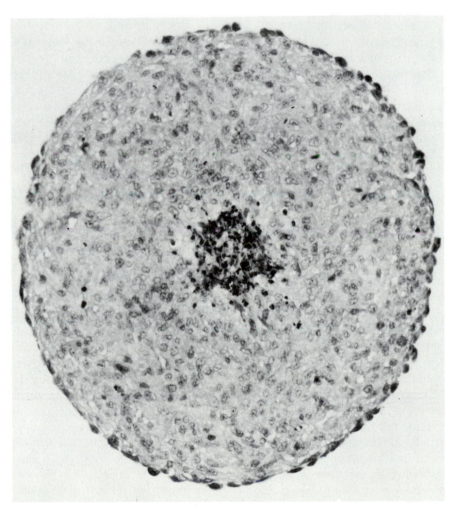

**Figure 5-10.** Photomicrograph of a spheroid. Note the area of central necrosis. The spheroid was grown 15 days and was 520 μm in diameter; the viable rim had an average thickness of about 200 μm. (Courtesy of Dr. R.M. Sutherland)

in effective concentration to these cells through layers of growing actively dividing cells, which may inactivate the drug through their metabolism. The spheroid system mimics many of these tumor characteristics and provides a rapid, useful, and economic method for screening sensitizers and chemotherapeutic agents because it is intermediate in complexity between single-cell in vitro culture and tumors in experimental animals.

## SPHEROIDS OF HUMAN TUMOR CELLS

Many types of human tumor cells can be cultured as spheroids, with a wide spectrum of morphologic appearances and growth rates. In general, cells from disaggregated surgical specimens form spheroids when cultured in liquid suspension above a nonadhesive surface, which can be a thin layer of agar or agarose gel or the bottom of a culture dish not prepared for cell culture.

Only when the spheroid is formed and grown to a certain size can it be transferred to a spinner culture vessel and grown in the same way as spheroids of established rodent cell lines. Human tumors successfully grown as spheroids include thyroid cancer, renal cancer, squamous carcinoma, colon carcinoma, neuroblastoma, human lung cancer, glioma, lymphoid tumors, melanoma, and osteosarcoma. There appears to be no general pattern. One glioma line might form and grow as spheroids, while another might not. The same applies to other tumor types. Thus it seems that the capacity to form and grow as spheroids is not a general property of tumor cells. Many nontumor cells also form spheroids, but only the spheroids of lymphoid origin will continue to grow to any size.

Morphologic studies of spheroids of human tumor cells show that they maintain many characteristics of the original tumor specimens taken from the patient and of the cells when grown as a xenograft in nude mice. Radiobiological studies show that, in addition to maintaining histologic characteristics of individual tumors, spheroids of human cells preserve characteristic radiosensitivity, since dose–response curves for spheroids are virtually identical to those for cells growing as xenografts in nude mice.

## COMPARISON OF THE VARIOUS MODEL TUMOR SYSTEMS

In all five transplantable systems described the tumor is treated in situ with all of the realism and complexities of the in vivo milieu, such as cell-to-cell contact and the presence of hypoxic cells, factors that can never be fully simulated in a petri dish. The tumor cure ($TCD_{50}$) and growth delay systems share the additional advantage that they are left in situ undisturbed after treatment. In the other three techniques the tumor must be removed, minced, and prepared into a single cell suspension by the use of an enzyme, such as trypsin, before survival is assessed. Although this step does not appear to affect the assessment of the effects of radiation, it can result in artifacts in the case of other agents, such as chemotherapeutic drugs or hyperthermia, in which the cell membrane may be involved in the cellular response. The procedure of breaking up the tumor and partially dissolving the cell membrane with a digestive enzyme may influence results. For this reason, in the testing and evaluation of a new drug, one tumor system involving the determination of growth delay or $TCD_{50}$ is always included. By the same token, these same systems are very expensive, since they require a large number of animals for the amount of information produced. The determination of $TCD_{50}$ is perhaps ideal for producing data relevant to clinical radiotherapy. It is certainly the most expensive; to produce a single $TCD_{50}$ value for one of the lines in Figure 5-3, six to eight groups of up to 10 animals that must be kept and observed for weeks are required. The same information can be obtained in 10 days with one or two mice and six petri dishes using the in vivo/in vitro technique.

The dilution assay technique allows clonogenic cell survival to be assessed over a large range of doses and for tumors that cannot be grown in culture. It, too, is relatively expensive, since a whole group of recipient animals must be used and kept for weeks to obtain the same information as obtained from one petri dish. Unquestionably, the most rapid and efficient technique is the in vivo/in vitro technique, which combines the realism of irradiation in vivo with the speed and efficiency of in vitro plating to assess clonogenic survival. The concomitant disadvantage is that any tumor that can be switched from petri dish to animal in alternate passages is so undifferentiated and anaplastic that it bears little resemblance to a spontaneous tumor in the human.

To some extent, the same criticism can be levied at all transplantable tumor systems. They are highly quantitative, but they are also very artificial. Having been passaged for many generations, they tend to be highly undifferentiated, and they grow as encapsulated tumors in a muscle or beneath the skin rather than in the tissue of origin. In addition, some have produced misleading results because they are highly antigenic, which, in general, human tumors are not.

In short, transplantable tumors in laboratory animals are model systems; they must be used with care, and the results must not be overinterpreted. If used with caution, these systems have provided invaluable quantitative data and helped to establish important radiobiological principles. They have also, however, "led us up the garden path" on several occasions in the past (Fig. 5-11). For all of the reasons listed earlier, they differ in important ways from spontaneous human tumors, and for the testing of drugs at the National Cancer Institute they have been largely replaced by a battery of cells of human origin cultured in vitro.

Xenografts of human tumors have so far been used on a much more limited scale. Since they are grown in the absence of an immune response, it could be argued that they are the epitome of artificiality. They do, however, allow a comparison to be made of the intrinsic sensitivity to radiation or chemotherapeutic agents of fresh explants of human tumors. As in vitro culture techniques improve and better growth media are developed, xenografts may be less necessary.

Spheroids represent a most important intermediate model between monolayers of cells in culture and tumors in vivo. A number of important radiobiological principles have been established using spheroids of rodent cells, in which the various populations of cells, aerated versus hypoxic, cycling versus noncycling, can be separated out. Human cell spheroids have only been used on a limited scale, but it is clear that the cells retain many of the characteristics of the tumor from which they were taken. Spheroids are much less expensive than xenografts in immunosuppressed animals and perform much the same function.

## APOPTOSIS IN TUMORS

It is generally thought that irradiated cells die in attempting the next or a subsequent mitosis. This

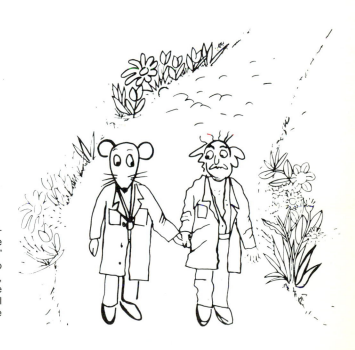

**Figure 5-11.** Transplantable tumors in small laboratory animals have provided invaluable quantitative data, but they have also "led us up the garden path" on several occasions. Transplantable tumors tend to be fast growing, undifferentiated, highly antigenic, and growing as an encapsulated tumor in a muscle or beneath the skin, not in their site of origin. For all of these reasons they are highly artificial, and care must be used in interpreting results.

is not the only form of cell death, however. Programmed cell death, or apoptosis, occurs in both normal tissues and tumors.

In a later chapter on tumor kinetics, it will be pointed out that tumors grow much more slowly than would be predicted from the cell cycle time of the individual cells and the fraction of cells actively dividing. One of the reasons for this "cell loss," as it is called, is random cell death due to apoptosis.

Studies with transplanted mouse tumors, as well as human tumors growing as xenografts in nude mice, have shown that the importance of apoptosis as a mechanism of cell death after x-irradiation varies substantially. Apoptosis was most important in lymphomas, essentially absent in sarcomas, and intermediate and very variable for carcinomas. In a mouse lymphoma, for example, 50% to 60% of the cells may show signs of dying an apoptotic death by 3 hours after irradiation, whereas in a sarcoma there may be so few apoptotic cells that the process is of little significance. If a tumor responds rapidly to a relatively low dose of radiation, it generally means that apoptosis is involved, since the process peaks at 3 to 5 hours after irradiation. Susceptibility to the induction of apoptosis may also be an important factor determining radiosensitivity, since programmed cell death appears to be a prominent early effect in radiosensitive mouse tumors and essentially absent in radioresistant tumors. It has been suggested that apoptosis is the dominant form of cell death in lymphoma cells treated with photodynamic therapy and that the process occurs more rapidly than after x-rays. It is also involved in cell death by a range of cytotoxic drugs used in cancer therapy.

## ► Summary of Pertinent Conclusions

- A wide range of tumors of different histologic types can be grown in laboratory animals and propagated by transplantation.
- Transplanted tumor systems can be highly quantitative, but in general the more quantitative the system, the more artificial it is, because the tumors are highly undifferentiated and encapsulated.
- The five assays in common use are tumor cure; tumor growth delay; and tumor cell survival determined by the dilution assay technique, the production of lung colonies, or colonies in vitro.
- In all five assays the cells can be irradiated in situ with all the realism and complexity of in vivo conditions.
- When tumor "cure" ($TCD_{50}$) or growth delay are scored, the tumor is left undisturbed after treatment. This avoids artifacts involved in disaggregating the tumor, especially in the study of some chemicals or hyperthermia, in which cell membrane effects are important.
- The dilution assay technique, the lung colony assay, and the in vivo/in vitro assay all measure cell surviving fraction; that is, they are clonogenic assays.
- They require fewer animals and are therefore more efficient than the scoring of tumor cure or growth delay. All three assays require, however, that a single cell suspension be prepared from the tumor, and this may result in artifacts.
- Transplantable tumors in small laboratory animals have been used to establish many radiobiological principles; but they are highly artificial and must be used with care. They have "led us up the garden path" on several occasions.
- Many human tumor cells can be grown as xenografts in immune-deficient animals.

*(continued)*

► *Summary of Pertinent Conclusions* *(Continued)*

- While the histologic characteristics of the human source tumor are maintained, the stroma is of mouse origin.
- Xenografts of human tumor cells are not much better than mouse tumors for studies in which the vascular supply is important.
- Human tumor cells undergo kinetic changes and selection when transplanted into immune-deficient mice.
- Xenografts generally maintain the chemotherapeutic response characteristics of the class of tumors from which they are derived. There is evidence, too, of individuality of response.
- Spheroids of established rodent cells can be grown in suspension culture (ie, "spinner culture"). Oxygen and nutrients must diffuse into the spheroid from the surrounding culture medium. Oxygen deficiency and a buildup of waste products result, just as in a tumor.
- Mature spheroids contain a heterogeneous population of cells, much like a tumor, but are more quantitative and more economical to work with.
- Starting from the outside and working toward the center, spheroids consist of (1) asynchronous aerated cells, (2) noncycling $G_1$-like aerated cells, (3) noncycling $G_1$-like hypoxic cells, and (4) necrotic cells.
- Spheroids are intermediate in complexity between monolayer cell cultures in vitro and transplantable tumors in animals.
- Many types of human tumor cells will grow as spheroids and maintain many characteristics of the original tumor from the patient or of the same cells grown as xenografts.
- Programmed cell death, or apoptosis, occurs in many animal tumors after irradiation, as well as mitotic death.
- When it occurs, cells may show signs of dying an apoptotic death by 3 hours after irradiation.
- Apoptosis is most important in lymphomas, essentially absent in sarcomas, and intermediate and variable in carcinomas.

# BIBLIOGRAPHY

Acker H, Carlsson J, Durand R, Sutherland R (eds): Spheroids in Cancer Research. Berlin, Springer-Verlag, 1984

Barendsen GW, Broerse JJ: Experimental radiotherapy of a rat rhabdomyosarcoma with 15 MeV neutrons and 300 kV x-rays: I. Effects of single exposures. Eur J Cancer 5:373–391, 1969

Clifton KH, Briggs RC, Stone HB: Quantitative radiosensitivity studies of solid carcinomas in vivo: Methodology and effect of anoxia. JNCI 36:965–974, 1966

Dertinger H, Guichard M, Malaise EP: Relationship between intercellular communication and radiosensitivity of human tumor xenografts. Eur J Cancer Clin Oncol 20:561–566, 1984

Fowler JF: Biological foundations of radiotherapy. In Turano L, Ratti A, Biagini C (eds): Progress in Radiology, vol 1, pp 731–737. Amsterdam, Excerpta Medica, 1967

Hermens AF, Barendsen GW: Cellular proliferation patterns in an experimental rhabdomyosarcoma in the rat. Eur J Cancer 3:361–169, 1967

Hermens AF, Barendsen GW: Changes of cell proliferation patterns in an experimental rhabdomyosarcoma in the rat. Eur J Cancer 5:173–189, 1969

Hewitt HB: Studies on the quantitative transplantation of mouse sarcoma. Br J Cancer 7:367–383, 1953

Hewitt HB, Chan DPS, Blake ER: Survival curves for clonogenic cells of a murine keratinizing squamous carcinoma irradiated in vivo or under hypoxic conditions. Int J Radiat Biol 12:535–549, 1967

Hewitt HB, Wilson CW: A survival surve for mammalian leukaemia cells irradiated in vivo. Br J Cancer 13:69–75, 1959

Hewitt HB, Wilson CW: Survival curves for tumor cells irradiated in vivo. Ann NY Acad Sci 95:818–827, 1961

Hill RP, Bush RS: A lung colony assay to determine the radiosensitivity of the cells of a solid tumor. Int J Radiat Biol 15:435–444, 1969

Hill RP, Bush RS, Yeung P: The effect of anemia on the fraction of hypoxic cells in an experimental tumor. Br J Radiol 44:299–304, 1971

Kerr JFR, Searle J: Apoptosis: Its nature and kinetic role. In Meyn RE, Withers HR (eds): Radiation Biology in Cancer Research, pp 367–384, New York, Raven Press, 1980

McNally NJ: Recovery from sublethal damage by hypoxic tumor cells in vivo. Br J Radiol 45:116–120, 1972

Pourreau-Schneider N, Malaise EP: Relationship between surviving fractions using the colony method, the $LD_{50}$, and the growth delay after irradiation of human melanoma cells grown as multicellular spheroids. Radiat Res 85:321–332, 1981

Reinhold HS: Quantitative evaluation fo the radiosensitivity of cells of a transplantable rhabdomyosarcoma in the rat. Eur J Cancer 2:33–42, 1966

Rockwell SC, Kallman RF: Cellular radiosensitivity and tumor radiation response in the EMT6 tumor cell system. Radiat Res 53:281–294, 1973

Rockwell SC, Kallman RF, Fajardo LF: Characteristics of a serially transplanted mouse mammary tumor and its tissue-culture-adapted derivative. JNCI 49:735–749, 1972

Steel GG, Courtenay VC, Beckjam MJ: The response to chemotherapy of a variety of human tumour xenografts. Br J Cancer 47:1–13, 1983

Stephens LC, Ang KK, Schultheiss TE, Milas L, Meyn R: Apoptosis in irradiated murine tumors. Radiat Res 127:308–316, 1991

Suit HD, Maeda M: Hyperbaric oxygen and radiobiology of the $C_3H$ mouse mammary carcinoma. JNCI 39:639–652, 1967

Suit H, Wette R: Radiation dose fractionation and tumor control probability. Radiat Res 29:267–281, 1966

Suit HD, Wette R, Lindberg R: Analysis of tumor-recurrence times. Radiology 88:311–321, 1967

Sutherland RM, Durand RE: Radiation response of multicell spheroids: An in vitro tumor model. Curr Top Radiat Res Q 11:87–139, 1976

Sutherland RM, McCredie JA, Inch WR: Growth of multicell spheroids in tissue culture as a model of nodular carcinomas. JNCI 46:113–120, 1971

Sutherland RM, Sordat B, Bamat J, Gabbert H, Bourrat B, Mueller-Klieser W: Oxygenation and differentiation in multicellular spheroids of human colon carcinoma. Cancer Res 46:5320–5329, 1986

Tannock IF: The relation between cell proliferation and the vascular system in a transplanted mouse mammary tumour. Br J Cancer 22:258–273, 1968

Thomlinson RH, Craddock EA: The gross response of an experimental tumour to single doses of x-rays. Br J Cancer 21:108–123, 1967

Williams GT: Programmed cell death: Apoptosis and oncogenesis. Cell 65:1097–1098, 1991

Yuhas JM, Blake S, Weichselbaum RR: Quantitation of the response of human tumor spheroids to daily radiation exposures. Int J Radiat Oncol Biol Phys 10:2323–2327, 1984

Yuhas JM, Tarleton AE, Molzen KB: Multicellular tumor spheroid formation by breast cancer cells isolated from different sites. Cancer Res 38:2486–2491, 1978

*Radiobiology for the Radiologist, Fourth Edition*, by Eric J. Hall
J. B. Lippincott Company, Philadelphia © 1994.

# 6

# *Radiosensitivity and Cell Age in the Mitotic Cycle*

THE CELL CYCLE
SYNCHRONOUSLY DIVIDING CELL CULTURES
THE EFFECT OF X-RAYS ON SYNCHRONOUSLY
  DIVIDING CELL CULTURES
MOLECULAR CHECKPOINT GENES
THE EFFECT OF OXYGEN AT VARIOUS PHASES
  OF THE CELL CYCLE
THE AGE–RESPONSE FUNCTION FOR A TISSUE IN VIVO
VARIATION OF SENSITIVITY WITH CELL AGE FOR
  NEUTRONS
MECHANISMS FOR THE AGE–RESPONSE FUNCTION
THE POSSIBLE IMPLICATIONS OF THE AGE–RESPONSE
  FUNCTION IN RADIOTHERAPY
SUMMARY OF PERTINENT CONCLUSIONS

Diagnostic Radiology
Nuclear Medicine
Radiation Therapy

# THE CELL CYCLE

Mammalian cells propagate and proliferate by mitosis (see Chapter 2). When a cell divides, two daughter cells are produced, each of which carries a chromosome complement identical to that of the mother cell. After an interval of time has elapsed, each of the daughter cells may undergo a further division. The time between successive divisions is known as the **mitotic cycle time,** or, as it is commonly called, the **cell cycle time.**

When a population of dividing cells is observed with a conventional light microscope, the only event in the entire cell cycle that can be identified and distinguished is mitosis or division itself. Just before the cell divides to form two daughter cells, the chromosomes (which are diffuse and scattered in the cell in the period between mitoses) condense into clearly distinguishable forms. In addition, in monolayer cultures of cells, just before mitosis, the cells round up and become loosely attached to the surface of the culture vessel. This whole process of mitosis—in preparation for which the cell rounds up, the chromosome material condenses, the cell divides into two and then stretches out again and attaches to the surface of the culture vessel—lasts only about 1 hour. The remainder of the cell cycle, the interphase, occupies all of the intermitotic period. No events of interest can be identified with a conventional microscope during this time.

Since cell division is a cyclic phenomenon, repeated in each generation of the cells, it is usual to represent it as a circle, as shown in Figure 6-1. The circumference of the circle represents the full mitotic cycle time for the cells ($T_c$); the period of mitosis is represented by M. The remainder of the cell cycle can be further subdivided by the use of **autoradiography.** This technique was first introduced by Howard and Pelc in 1953 and has revolutionized the study of cell biology.

The basis of the technique, illustrated in Figure 6-2, is to feed the cells thymidine, a basic building block used for making a new set of chromosomes, which has been labeled with radioactive tritiated thymidine ($^3$H TdR). Cells that are actively synthesizing new DNA as part of the process of replicating their chromosome complement will incorporate the radioactive thymidine. The surplus radioactive thymidine is then flushed from the system, the cells are fixed and stained so that they may be viewed easily, and the preparation of cells is coated with a very thin layer of nuclear (photographic) emulsion.

β-Particles from cells that have incorporated radioactive thymidine pass through the nuclear emulsion and produce a latent image. When the emulsion is subsequently developed and fixed, the area through which a β-particle has passed appears as a black spot. It is then a comparatively simple matter to view the preparation of cells and to observe that some of the cells have black spots or "grains" over them, which indi-

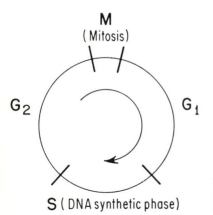

**Figure 6-1.** The stages of the mitotic cycle for actively growing mammalian cells. (M, mitosis; S, DNA synthetic phase; $G_1$ and $G_2$, "gaps" or periods of apparent inactivity between the major discernible events in the cycle)

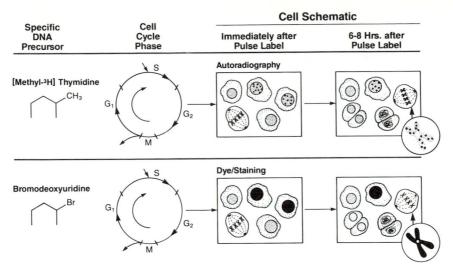

**Figure 6-2.** Cell labeling techniques, (*Left panels*) The principle of autoradiography, which may be applied to cells in culture growing as a monolayer on a glass microscope slide or to thin sections cut from a tumor or normal tissue. Cells in the DNA synthetic phase (S) take up tritiated thymidine. After the cells are fixed and stained so that they are visible by light microscopy, they are covered with a layer of nuclear (photographic) emulsion and left for several weeks in a cool refrigerator. As β-particles from the tritiated thymidine pass through the emulsion, they form latent images that appear as black grains when the emulsion is subsequently developed and fixed. If cells are stained and autoradiographed immediately after incorporation of the tritiated thymidine, cells that are labeled are in S phase. If the staining and autoradiography is delayed for hours after the flash-label (*right panels*), some cells may move from S to M, and labeled mitotic cells will be observed. The lengths of the various phases of the cycle can be determined in this way. (*lower panels*) The principle of cell cycle analysis using 5-bromodeoxyuridine as the DNA precursor instead of radioactively labeled thymidine. The bromodeoxyuridine is incorporated into cells in S. It can be recognized by the use of a specific stain or a monoclonal antibody to bromodeoxyuridine-substituted DNA. The antibody is tagged with a fluorescing dye (eg, fluorescein), which shows up bright green under a fluorescence microscope. If cells are stained immediately after labeling with bromodeoxyuridine, those staining darkly are in S phase. If staining is delayed for 6 to 8 hours, cells incorporating bromodeoxyuridine may move from S to M, and a darkly staining mitotic cell will be seen (*right panel*), (Courtesy of Dr. Charles Geard)

cates that they were actively synthesizing DNA at the time radioactive thymidine was made available. Other cells do not have any grains over their nuclei; this is interpreted to mean that the cells were not actively making DNA when the radioactive label was made available to them. Examples of labeled cells are shown in Figure 6-3. If the cells are allowed to grow for some time after labeling with tritiated thymidine so that they move into mitosis before being fixed, stained, and autoradiographed, then a labeled mitotic cell may be observed (see Fig. 6-3*A*).

In recent years the use of tritiated thymidine to identify cells in the DNA synthetic phase (S) has been replaced largely with 5-bromodeoxyuridine, which differs from thymidine only by the substitution of a bromine atom for a methyl group. If this halogenated pyrimidine is fed to the

cells, it is incorporated into DNA in place of thymidine and its presence can be detected by using an appropriate stain (see Fig. 6-2). In a black and white print, cells incorporating bromodeoxyuridine appear darkly stained. In practice they are easier to recognize because the stain is brightly colored. To even more readily identify cells that are in S phase and have incorporated bromodeoxyuridine, one can use an antibody against bromodeoxyuridine-substituted DNA, which fluoresces brightly under a fluorescence microscope. Examples of stained and unstained cells are shown in Figure 6-3*B*. If time is allowed between labeling with bromodeoxyuridine and staining, then a cell may move from S to M phase, and a stained mitotic cell is observed (see Fig. 6-3*B*). If the cell is in the first mitosis after bromodeoxyuridine incorporation, both chroma-

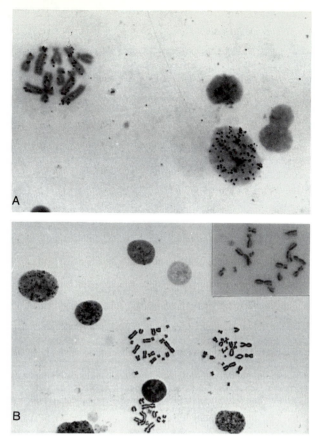

**Figure 6-3.** **(A)** Autoradiograph of Chinese hamster cells in culture flash-labeled with tritiated thymidine. The black grains over some cells indicate that they were synthesizing DNA when they were labeled. Also shown is a labeled mitotic cell. This cell was in S phase when the culture was flash-labeled but moved to M phase before it was stained and autoradiographed. **(B)** Photomicrograph showing cells labeled and unlabeled with bromodeoxyuridine. Cells were grown in the presence of bromodeoxyuridine, then fixed and stained 20 hours later. Incorporated bromodeoxyuridine stains purple, which shows up dark in this black and white print; the rest of the cell is light blue. The stained interphase cell indicates that it was in S phase during the time the bromodeoxyuridine was available. Also shown is a first-generation mitotic cell, which had been in S phase at the time the bromodeoxyuridine was available and had moved to M phase by the time it was fixed and stained. It can be identified as first generation because both chromatids of each chromosome are uniformly stained. The inset shows a second-generation mitotic cell, which passed through two S phases during bromodeoxyuridine availability. One chromatid of each chromosome is darker because both strands of the DNA double helix have incorporated bromodeoxyuridine. One chromatid is lighter because only one strand of the DNA has incorporated bromodeoxyuridine. (Courtesy of Dr. Charles Geard)

tids of each chromosome will be equally stained, as shown in the figure, but by the second mitosis, one chromatid will be stained darker than the other (illustrated in the inset, Fig. 6-3B).

The use of bromodeoxyuridine has two advantages over conventional autoradiography using tritiated thymidine. First, it does not involve radioactive material. Second, it greatly shortens the time to produce a result, since, when cells are coated with emulsion to produce an autoradio-

graph, they must be stored in a refrigerator for about 1 month to allow β-particles from the incorporated tritium to produce a latent image in the emulsion.

By using either of these techniques it can be shown that cells synthesize DNA only during a discrete well-defined fraction of the cycle known as the DNA synthetic phase (S). There is an interval between mitosis and DNA synthesis in which no label is incorporated. This first "gap" in activity was named $G_1$ by Howard and Pelc, and the nomenclature is still used today. After DNA synthesis has been completed, there is a second gap before mitosis, $G_2$.

All proliferating mammalian cells, whether in culture or growing normally in a tissue, have a mitotic cycle of mitosis (M), followed by $G_1$, a period of DNA synthesis (S), and $G_2$, after which mitosis occurs again. The relative lengths of these various constituent parts of the cell cycle vary according to the particular cells studied.

The characteristics of two cell lines commonly used for in vitro culture are summarized in Table 6-1. HeLa cells have a total cell cycle of about 24 hours, which is more than double that of the Chinese hamster cell, with a cell cycle time of about 11 hours. Mitosis lasts only a relatively short time, about 1 hour, and is not very different for those two cell lines or for most others. The S phase is 8 hours for HeLa cells and 6 hours for hamster cells; in all cell lines studied in culture or growing in vivo the S phase never exceeds about 15 hours. The $G_2$ period is very similar in HeLa and hamster cells, too; in fact, the difference in the total cell cycle time between these two cell lines is accounted for almost entirely by the difference in the length of the $G_1$ period.

This is an important point: the difference among mammalian cell cycle times in different circumstances, varying from about 10 hours for a hamster cell grown in culture to hundreds of hours for stem cells in some self-renewal tissues, is the result of a dramatic variation in the length of the $G_1$ period. The remaining components of the cell cycle, M, S, and $G_2$, vary comparatively little between different cells in different circumstances.

Table 6-1.
**Phases of the Cell Cycle for Two Commonly Used Cell Lines Cultured in Vitro**

|  | HAMSTER CELLS (HOURS) | HeLa CELLS (HOURS) |
| --- | --- | --- |
| $T_C$ | 11 | 24 |
| $T_M$ | 1 | 1 |
| $T_S$ | 6 | 8 |
| $T_{G2}$ | 3 | 4 |
| $T_{G1}$ | 1 | 11 |

# SYNCHRONOUSLY DIVIDING CELL CULTURES

In the discussion of survival curves in Chapter 3 the assumption was implicit that the population of irradiated cells was asynchronous; that is, it consisted of cells distributed throughout all phases of the cell cycle. A study of the variation of radiosensitivity with the position or age of the cell in the cell cycle was only made possible by the development of techniques to produce synchronously dividing cell cultures—populations of cells in which all of the cells occupy the same phase of the cell cycle at a given time.

There are essentially two techniques that have been used to produce a synchronously dividing cell population. The first is the **mitotic harvest** technique, first described by Terasima and Tolmach. This technique can only be used for cultures that grow in monolayers attached to the surface of the growth vessel. It exploits the fact that when such cells are close to mitosis, they round up and become loosely attached to the surface. If at this stage the growth medium over the cells is subjected to gentle motion (by shaking), the mitotic cells become detached from the surface and float in the medium. If this medium is then removed from the culture vessel and plated out into new petri dishes, the population consists almost entirely of mitotic cells. Incubation of these cell cultures at 37°C then causes the cells to move together synchronously in step through their mitotic cycle. By delivering a dose of radiation at various times after the initial harvesting of mitotic cells, one can irradiate cells at various phases of the cell cycle.

An alternative method for synchronizing cells, which is applicable to cells in a tissue as well as cells grown in culture, involves the use of a drug. A number of different substances are possible. One of the most widely applicable is hydroxyurea. When this drug is added to a population of dividing cells, it has two effects on the cell population. First, all cells that are synthesizing DNA take up the drug and are killed. Second, the drug imposes a block at the end of the $G_1$ period; cells that occupy the $G_2$, M, and $G_1$ compartments when the drug is added progress through the cell cycle and accumulate at this block.

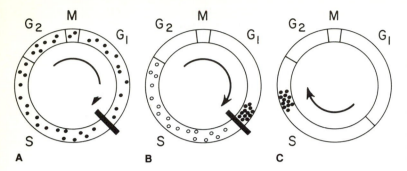

**Figure 6-4.** Mode of action of hydroxyurea as an agent to induce synchrony. This drug kills cells in S phase and imposes a "block" at the end of $G_1$ phase. Cells in $G_2$, M, and $G_1$ phases accumulate at this block when the drug is added. When the block is removed, the synchronized cohort of cells moves on through the cycle.

The dynamics of the action of hydroxyurea are illustrated in Figure 6-4. The drug is left in position for a period equal to the combined lengths of $G_2$, M, and $G_1$ for that particular cell line. By the end of the treatment period, all of the viable cells left in the population will be situated in a narrow "window" at the end of $G_1$, poised and ready to enter S. If the drug is then removed from the system, this synchronized cohort of cells will proceed through the cell cycle. For example, in hamster cells, 5 hours after the removal of the drug, the cohort of synchronized

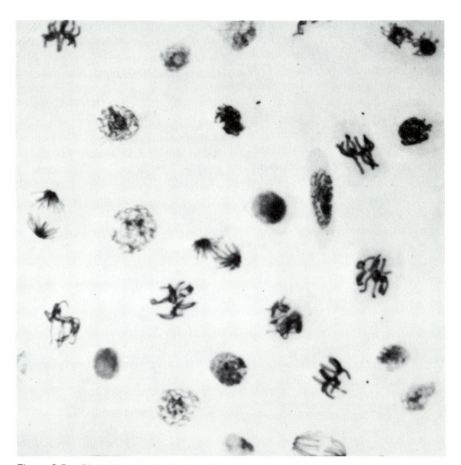

**Figure 6-5.** Photomicrograph of a squash preparation of the root tip of a *Vicia* seedling 11 hours after synchrony was induced with hydroxyurea. Note the large proportion of cells in mitosis. (From Hall EJ, Brown JM, Cavanagh J: Radiosensitivity and the oxygen effect measured at different phases of the mitotic cycle using synchronously dividing cells of the root meristem of *Vicia faba*. Radiat Res 35:622–634, 1968)

cells will occupy a position late in the S phase. Some 9 hours after the removal of the drug, the cohort of cells will be at, or close to, mitosis.

Techniques involving one or another of a wide range of drugs have been used to produce synchronously dividing cell populations in culture, in organized tissues (in a limited number of cases), and even in the whole animal. Figure 6-5 is a photomicrograph of a squash preparation of the root tip of a *Vicia* seedling 11 hours after synchrony was induced with hydroxyurea. A very large proportion of the cells are in mitosis.

## THE EFFECT OF X-RAYS ON SYNCHRONOUSLY DIVIDING CELL CULTURES

Figure 6-6 shows results of an experiment in which mammalian cells, harvested at mitosis, were irradiated with a single dose of 6.6 Gy (660 rads) at various times afterward, corresponding to different phases of the cell cycle. The data (from Sinclair) were obtained using Chinese hamster cells in culture. As can be seen from the figure, 1 hour after the mitotic cells were seeded into the petri dishes, when the cells were in $G_1$, a dose of 6.6 Gy (660 rads) resulted in a surviving fraction of about 13%. The proportion of cells that survive the dose increases rapidly with time as the cells move into S; by the time the cells near the end of S, 42% of the cells survive this same dose. When the cells move out of S into $G_2$

and subsequently to a second mitosis, the proportion of surviving cells falls again. This pattern of response is characteristic for most lines of Chinese hamster cells and has been reported by a number of independent investigators.

Complete survival curves at a number of discrete points during the cell cycle were measured by Sinclair. The results are shown in Figure 6-7. Survival curves are shown for mitotic cells (M), for cells in $G_1$ and $G_2$, and for cells in early and late S. It is at once evident that the most sensitive cells are those in M and $G_2$, which are characterized by a survival curve that is steep and has no shoulder. At the other extreme, cells in the latter part of S phase exhibit a survival curve that is less steep, but the essential difference is that the survival curve has a very broad shoulder. The other phases of the cycle, such as $G_1$ and early S, are intermediate in sensitivity between the two extremes.

The broken line in Figure 6-7 is the calculated survival curve that would be expected to apply for mitotic cells under conditions of hypoxia; that is, the slope is two and a half times shallower than the solid line for mitotic cells, which applies to the aerated condition. This line is included in the figure to show that the range of sensitivity between the most sensitive cells (mitotic) and the most resistant cells (late S) is of the same order of magnitude as the oxygen effect.

The experiments of Terasima and Tolmach with HeLa cells are shown in Figure 6-8, in which a dose of 3Gy (300 rads) was delivered to cul-

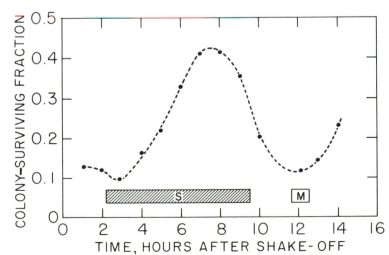

**Figure 6-6.** Fraction of Chinese hamster cells surviving a dose of 6.6 Gy (660 rads) of x-rays as a function of time. Time zero corresponds to the harvesting of mitotic cells. The cell-surviving fraction increases to a maximum late in S phase. (Redrawn from Sinclair WK, Morton RA: Radiat Res 29:450–474, 1966)

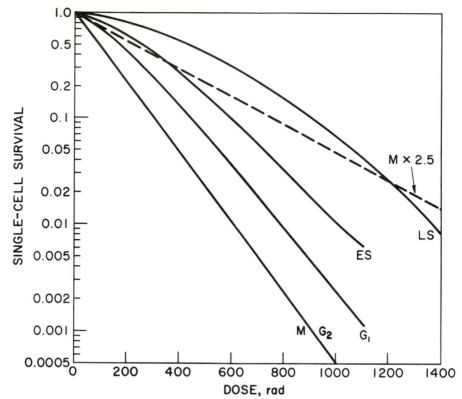

**Figure 6-7.** Cell survival curves for Chinese hamster cells at various stages of the cell cycle. The survival curve for cells in mitosis is steep and has no shoulder. The curve for cells late in S phase is shallower and has a large initial shoulder. $G_1$ and early S phases are intermediate in sensitivity. The broken line is a calculated curve expected to apply to mitotic cells under hypoxia. (From Sinclair WK: Radiat Res 33:620–643, 1968)

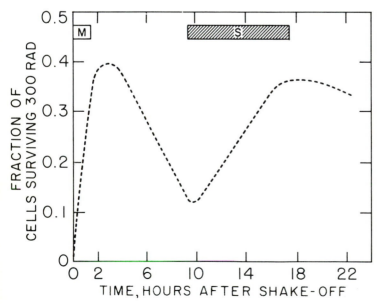

**Figure 6-8.** Fraction of HeLa cells surviving a dose of 3 Gy (300 rads) of x-rays administered at different times in the division cycle. Time zero represents mitosis. (Redrawn from Terasima T, Tolmach LJ: Biophys J 3:11–33, 1963)

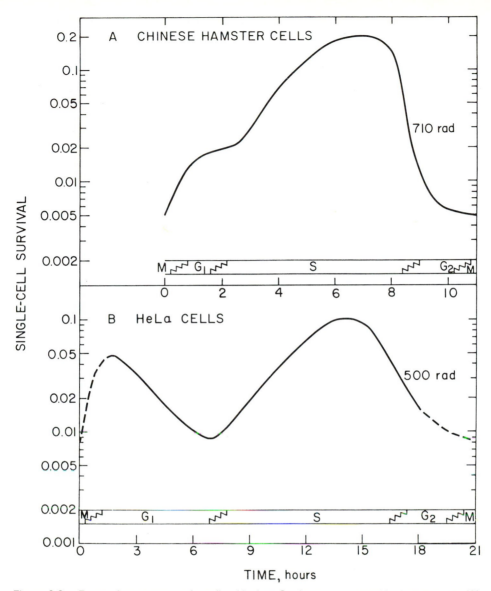

**Figure 6-9.** Forms of age response for cells with short $G_1$ phase, represented by hamster cells **(A)**, and cells with long $G_1$ phase, represented by HeLa cells **(B)**. The time scales have been adjusted so that S phase has a comparable length on the figure for both cell lines. (From Sinclair WK: Dependence of radiosensitivity upon cell age. In: Proceedings of the Carmel Conference on Time and Dose Relationships in Radiation Biology as Applied to Radiotherapy, pp 97–107. Upton, NY, BNL Report 50203 [C-57], 1969)

tures at various intervals after mitotic harvesting of the cells. From the beginning of S phase onward, the pattern of sensitivity is very similar to that of hamster cells: the cells become progressively more resistant as they proceed toward the latter part of S, and after the cells move from S into $G_2$, their sensitivity increases rapidly as they approach mitosis. The important difference between HeLa and hamster cells is the length of the $G_1$ phase. The $G_1$ of HeLa cells is appreciably long, and there appears to be a fine structure in the age–response function during this period. At the beginning of $G_1$ there is a resistant peak, followed by a sensitive trough toward the end of $G_1$. This pattern cannot be distinguished in the hamster cell because $G_1$ is too short.

Figure 6-9 compares the forms of the age response for cells with short $G_1$, represented by

V79 hamster cells, with cells with a long $G_1$, represented by HeLa cells. When the time scales are adjusted so that S phase has a comparable length for both cell lines, it is evident that the general pattern of cyclic variation is very similar, the only important difference being the extra structure during $G_1$ in the HeLa cells. In later experiments other sublines of hamster cells were investigated for which $G_1$ had an appreciable length; an extra peak of resistance was noted for hamster cells that was similar to the one observed for HeLa cells.

A number of investigators have performed comparable experiments with various sublines of hamster and HeLa cells and have obtained similar results. The following is a summary of the main characteristics of the variation of radiosensitivity with cell age in the mitotic cycle:

1. Cells are most sensitive at or close to mitosis.
2. Resistance is usually greatest in the latter part of S phase.
3. If $G_1$ phase has an appreciable length, a resistant period is evident early in $G_1$ phase, followed by a sensitive period toward the end of $G_1$ phase.
4. $G_2$ phase is usually sensitive, perhaps as sensitive as M phase.

A number of cells lines other than HeLa and hamster have been investigated, some of which tend to agree with these results and some of which are contradictory. The summary points listed here are widely applicable, but exceptions to every one of these generalizations have been noted for one cell line or another.

## MOLECULAR CHECKPOINT GENES

Cell cycle progression is controlled by a family of genes known as molecular checkpoint genes. It has been known for many years that mammalian cells exposed to a small dose of radiation tend to experience a block in the $G_2$ phase of the cell cycle. For example, the inverse dose-rate effect reported for cells of human origin, whereby over a limited range of dose rates around 0.30 to 0.40 Gy/h cells become *more* sensitive to radiation-induced cell killing as the dose rate is reduced, is due to the piling up of cells in $G_2$, which is a radiosensitive phase of the cell cycle. This is described in Chapter 7. The mechanisms for this observation in human cells are not understood in detail, but the molecular genetics in yeast have been worked out and the search is on for homology in mammalian cells.

In several strains of yeast, mutants have been isolated that are more sensitive than the wild type both to ionizing radiation and ultraviolet light, by a factor between 10 and 100. The mutant gene has been cloned and sequenced and found to be a "molecular checkpoint gene." In the most general terms, the function of checkpoint genes is to ensure the correct order of cell cycle events, that is, to ensure that the initiation of later events is dependent on the completion of earlier events. The particular genes involved in radiation effects halts cells in $G_2$, so that an inventory of chromosome damage can be taken, and repair initiated and completed, before the complex task of mitosis is attempted (Fig. 6-10).

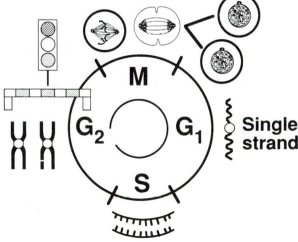

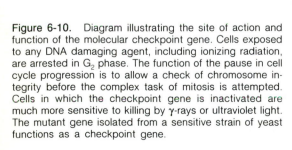

**Figure 6-10.** Diagram illustrating the site of action and function of the molecular checkpoint gene. Cells exposed to any DNA damaging agent, including ionizing radiation, are arrested in $G_2$ phase. The function of the pause in cell cycle progression is to allow a check of chromosome integrity before the complex task of mitosis is attempted. Cells in which the checkpoint gene is inactivated are much more sensitive to killing by γ-rays or ultraviolet light. The mutant gene isolated from a sensitive strain of yeast functions as a checkpoint gene.

Mutant cells that lose this gene function move directly into mitosis with damaged chromosomes and are therefore at a higher risk of dying, hence their greater sensitivity to radiation, or for that matter to any DNA damaging agent.

It has been proposed that a checkpoint control monitors spindle function during mitosis. If the spindle is disrupted by a microtubular poison, progression through mitosis is blocked. The checkpoint control is involved in this dependency of mitosis on spindle function. It is thought that the mechanism of action of checkpoint genes involves p 34 protein kinase, levels of which control passage thorough mitosis. It is likely that mammalian cells that lack checkpoint genes would be sensitive, not only to radiation-induced cell killing but also to carcinogenesis. Cells with damaged chromosomes that survive mitosis are likely to give rise to errors in chromosome segregation at mitosis, and this is one of the hallmarks of cancer.

## THE EFFECT OF OXYGEN AT VARIOUS PHASES OF THE CELL CYCLE

By combining the most sophisticated techniques of flow cytometry to separate cells into different phases of the cycle, with the most sensitive assays for cell survival, it has been shown that the oxygen enhancement ratio (OER) varies significantly through the cycle, at least when measured for fast-growing proliferating cells cultured in vitro. The OER was measured to be 2.3 to 2.4 for $G_2$ phase cells, compared with 2.8 to 2.9 for S phase, with $G_2$ phase cells showing an intermediate value.

For any given single phase of the cell cycle, oxygen was purely dose modifying, that is, the value of the OER was the same for all dose levels. For an *asynchronous* population of cells, however, the OER does vary slightly with dose or survival level. This is illustrated in Figure 8-1. The OER appears to be *smaller* at high levels of survival, where the survival curve is dominated by the killing of the most sensitive moieties of the population, while the OER appears to be larger at higher doses and lower levels of survival, where the response of the most resistant (S phase) cells

dominate, which also happen to exhibit the largest OER.

This is an interesting radiobiological observation, but the small change of OER is of little or no clinical significance in radiation therapy.

## THE AGE–RESPONSE FUNCTION FOR A TISSUE IN VIVO

Most studies of the variation in radiosensitivity with phase of the mitotic cycle have been done with mammalian cells cultured in vitro because of the ease with which they can be made to divide synchronously. The mitotic harvest technique is clearly only applicable to monolayer cultures, but techniques that involve a drug, such as hydroxyurea, to produce a synchronously dividing population can be applied to some organized tissues.

The crypt cells in the mouse jejunum are a classic self-renewal tissue (the technique used to obtain a survival curve for these cells was described in Chapter 3). The rapidly dividing crypt cells can be synchronized by giving each mouse five intraperitoneal injections of hydroxyurea every hour. The rationale for this regimen is that all S cells are killed by the drug, and cells in other phases of the cycle are accumulated at the $G_1$–S boundary for at least 4 hours (the overall time of the five injections). Figure 6-11, from Withers and his colleagues, shows the response of the jejunal crypt cells to a single dose of 11 Gy (1100 rads) of $\gamma$-rays (uppermost curve) delivered at various times after the synchronizing action of the five injections of hydroxyurea. The number of crypt cells per circumference of the sectioned jejunum varies by a factor of 100, according to the phase in the cycle at which the radiation is delivered, ranging from about two survivors per circumference for irradiation 2 hours after the last injection of hydroxyurea to about 200 survivors per circumference by 6 hours. The DNA synthetic activity of the synchronized jejunal mucosa was monitored by injecting groups of mice with tritiated thymidine at hourly intervals after the last injection of hydroxyurea and subsequently removing a sample of the jejunum and assaying the radioactive content. The bot-

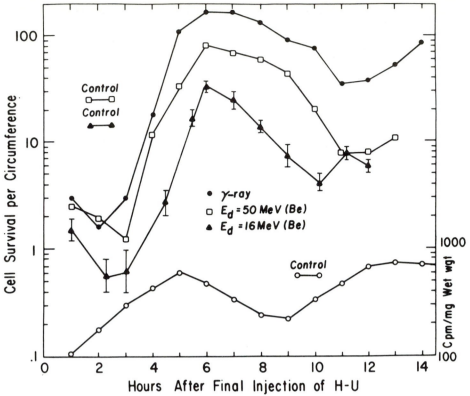

**Figure 6-11.** The upper three curves represent fluctuations in the survival of jejunal crypt cells exposed to γ-rays or neutrons as they pass through the cell cycle after synchronization with hydroxyurea (H-U). The doses were 11 Gy (1100 rads) of γ-rays; 7 Gy (700 rads) of neutrons generated by 50-MeV d⁺ →Be; and 6 Gy (600 rads) of neutrons generated by 16-MeV d⁺ →Be. The lower curve represents the uptake of tritiated thymidine (expressed as counts per minute) per wet weight of jejunum as a function of time after the last injection of hydroxyurea. The first wave indicates crypt stem cells passing through S phase after synchronization at $G_1$-S phase by hydroxyurea. (From Withers HR, Mason K, Reid BO, Dubravsky N, Barkley HT, Brown BW, Smathers JB: Cancer 34:39–47, 1974)

tom curve of Figure 6-11 shows the variation of thymidine uptake with time. The first wave of the thymidine uptake represents the period of DNA synthesis of the synchronized crypt cells. The peak coincides closely with the period of maximum resistance to x-rays (about 5 hours after the last injection of hydroxyurea).

These data indicate clearly that the radiosensitivity of crypt cells in the mouse jejunum varies substantially with the phase of the cell cycle at which the radiation is delivered. Further, the *pattern* of response in this organized normal tissue, with a sensitive period between $G_1$ and S and maximum radioresistance late in S, is very similar

to that characteristic of many cell lines cultured in vitro.

## VARIATION OF SENSITIVITY WITH CELL AGE FOR NEUTRONS

With the introduction of neutrons for use in radiotherapy in place of conventional modalities, such as x- or γ-rays, all possible radiobiological parameters of the two types of radiation were compared.

It was found that the variation in radiosensitivity as a function of cell age was qualitatively similar for neutrons and x-rays; that is, with both types of radiation maximum sensitivity is noted at or close to mitosis, while maximum resistance is evident late in S phase. There are, however, quantitative differences between neutrons and x-rays in this respect, as in every other. The range of radiosensitivity between the most resistant and the most sensitive phases of the cell cycle is much less for fast neutrons than for x-rays. While the variation of sensitivity with cell age is reduced in the case of neutrons compared with x-rays, it is still very evident and cannot by any means be ignored.

Figure 6-11 shows the fluctuations in survival of jejunal crypt cells in the mouse after irradiation with γ-rays or neutrons. The neutron beams studied were produced by 50-MeV deuterons bombarding a beryllium target. Both of these energies have been used for clinical neutron radiotherapy. The *pattern* of response as a function of cell age is similar for γ-rays and neutrons, with maximum resistance occurring in late S phase for both types of radiation. The *magnitude* of the variation is, however, less for neutrons than for γ-rays. There is a 100-fold fluctuation in cell survival through the division cycle for γ-rays, a 70-fold fluctuation for neutrons generated by 50-MeV d$^+$ → Be, and a 60-fold fluctuation for neutrons generated by 16-MeV d$^+$ → Be.

It has been argued that the reduced cycle-related fluctuations in radiation response that occur with neutrons could represent an advantage over conventional therapeutic radiation modalities, such as x- or γ-rays. There could be an important difference in the response of normal tissues and of neoplastic tissues to neutrons if the age-density distributions of normal and neoplastic tissues were dissimilar as a consequence of different rates of proliferation. At all events the reduced age–response function seen with neutrons represents a difference between this relatively densely ionizing radiation and x-rays over and above the oxygen effect.

## MECHANISMS FOR THE AGE–RESPONSE FUNCTION

The reasons for the sensitivity changes through the cell cycle are not at all understood. Several correlations have been proposed, of which two

will be mentioned. First, if DNA is the primary target for radiation-induced cell lethality, as is commonly supposed, then changes in the amount or form of the DNA might be expected to result in variations in sensitivity. During S phase the DNA content doubles as the genome is replicated; just before mitosis the chromosome material appears to condense into discrete entities. These two events coincide with the periods of minimum and maximum radiosensitivity. The nature of any cause-and-effect relationship is not clear; all that is observed is really a correlation. Second, there is also a correlation between changing radiosensitivity through the cell cycle and varying levels of naturally occurring sulfhydryl compounds in the cell. As is noted in Chapter 11, these compounds are powerful radioprotectors.

Either or both of these factors may be at the root of the important and substantial changes in radiosensitivity that cells exhibit as they progress through their generation cycle.

## THE POSSIBLE IMPLICATIONS OF THE AGE–RESPONSE FUNCTION IN RADIOTHERAPY

When a single dose of radiation is delivered to a population of cells that are asynchronous—that is, distributed throughout the cell cycle—the effect will be different on cells occupying different phases of the cell cycle at the time of the radiation exposure. A greater proportion of cells will be killed in the sensitive portions of the cell cycle, such as those at or close to mitosis, while a smaller proportion of those in the DNA synthetic phase will be killed. The overall effect is that a dose of radiation will, to some extent, tend to synchronize the cell population, leaving the majority of cells in a resistant phase of the cycle. Between dose fractions, movement of cells through the cycle into more sensitive phases may be an important factor in "sensitizing" a cycling population of tumor cells to later doses in fractionated regimen. This is termed *sensitization due to reassortment*. It results in a therapeutic gain since sensitization by this mechanism occurs only in rapidly dividing cells and not in late responding normal tissues.

## ► *Summary of Pertinent Conclusions*

- The cell cycle for mammalian cells can be divided into four phases: mitosis (M), followed by $G_1$, followed by the DNA synthetic phase (S), then $G_2$, and into mitosis again.
- The fastest cycling mammalian cells in culture, and crypt cells in the intestinal epithelium, have a cycle time as short as 9 to 10 hours. Stem cells in resting mouse skin may have a cycle time of more than 200 hours. Most of this difference is due to the varying length of $G_1$, the most variable phase of the cycle. M and S phases do not vary much.
- In general, cells are most radiosensitive in M and $G_2$ phases and most resistant in late S phase.
- For cells with longer cell cycle time and a significantly long $G_1$ phase, there is a second peak of resistance early in $G_1$.
- Molecular checkpoint genes stop cells in $G_2$ when exposed to x-rays or any other DNA-damaging agent, to allow the chromosomes to be checked for integrity before the complex task of mitosis is attempted.
- The oxygen enhancement ratio (OER) varies little with phase of the cell cycle but may be slightly lower for cells in $G_1$ than for cells in S.
- The age–response function for crypt cells in the mouse jejunum is similar to that for cells in culture. This is the only tissue that has been studied.
- The age–response function for neutrons is qualitatively similar to that for x-rays, but the magnitude of changes through the cycle is smaller.
- The pattern of resistance and sensitivity correlates with the level of sulfhydryl compounds in the cell. Sulfhydryls are natural radioprotectors and tend to be at their highest levels in S phase and at their lowest near mitosis.
- Variations in sensitivity through the cell cycle may be important in radiation therapy because they lead to "sensitization due to reassortment" in a fractionated regimen.

## BIBLIOGRAPHY

Dolbeare F, Beisker W, Pallavicini M, Vanderlaan M, Gray JW: Cytochemistry for BrdUrd/DNA analysis: Stoichiometry and sensitivity. Cytometry 6:521–530, 1985

Dolbeare F, Gratzner H, Pallavicini M, Gray JW: Flow cytometric measurement of total DNA content and incorporated bromodeoxyuridine. Proc Natl Acad Sci USA 80:5573–5577, 1983

Freyer JP, Jarrett K, Carpenter S, Raju MR: Oxygen enhancement ratio as a function of dose and cell cycle phase for radiation-resistant and sensitive CHO cells. Radiat Res 127:297–307, 1991

Gray JW: Quantitative cytokinetics: Cellular response to cell cycle specific agents. Pharmacol Ther 22:163–197, 1983

Gray JW, Dolbeare F, Pallavicini MG, Beisker W, Waldman F: Cell cycle analysis using flow cytometry. Int J Radiat Biol 49:237–255, 1986

Hall EJ: Radiobiological measurements with 14-MeV neutrons. Br J Radiol 42:805–813, 1969

Hall EJ, Brown JM, Cavanagh J: Radiosensitivity and the oxygen effect measured at different phases of the mitotic cycle using synchronously dividing cells of the root meristem of *Vicia faba*. Radiat Res 35:622–634, 1968

Hartwell LH, Weiner TA: Checkpoints: Controls that ensure the order of cell cycle events. Science 246:629–634, 1989

Hoshino T, Yagashima T, Morovic J, Livin E, Livin V: Cell kinetic studies of in situ human brain tumors with bromodeoxyuridine. Cytometry 6:627–632, 1985

Howard A, Pelc SR: Synthesis of deosyribonucleic acid in normal and irradiated cells and its relation to chromosome breakage. Heredity 6(suppl):261–273, 1953

Hoyt MA, Totis L, Roberts BT: *S. cerevisiae* genes required for cell cycle arrest in response to loss of microtubule function. Cell 66:507–517, 1991

Legrys GA, Hall EJ, The oxygen effect and x-ray sensitivity in synchronously dividing cultures of Chinese hamster cells. Radiat Res 37;161–172, 1969

Li R, Murray AW: Feedback control of mitosis in budding yeast. Cell 66:519–531, 1991

Lieberman HB, Hopkins KM, Laverty M, Chu HM: Molecular cloning and analysis of *Schizosaccharomyces pombe rad* 9, a gene involved in DNA repair and mutagenesis. Mol Gen Genet 232:367–376, 1992

Morstyn G, Hsu HS-M, Kinsella T, Gratzner H, Russo A, Mitchell J: Bromodeoxyuridine in tumors and chromosomes detected with a monoclonal antibody. J Clin Invest 72:1844–1850, 1983

Sinclair WK: Radiation survival in synchronous and asynchronous Chinese hamster cells in vitro. In Biophysical Aspects of Radiation Quality: Proceedings of the Second IAEA Panel, pp 39–54. Vienna, IAEA, 1968

Sinclair WK: Dependence of radiosensitivity upon cell age. In Proceedings of the Carmel Conference on Time and Dose Relationships in Radiation Biology as Applied to Radiotherapy, pp 97–107. Upton, NY, BNL Report 50203 (C-57), 1969

Sinclair WK, Morton RA: X-ray sensitivity during the cell generation cycle of cultured Chinese hamster cells. Radiat Res 29:450–474, 1966

Steel G, Hanes S: The technique labeled mitoses: Analysis by automatic curve fitting. Cell Tissue Kinet 4:93–105, 1971

Terasima R, Tolmach LJ: X-ray sensitivity and DNA synthesis in synchronous populations of HeLa cells. Science 140:490–492, 1963

Withers HR, Mason K, Reid BO, Dubraysky N, Barkley HT, Brown BW, Smathers JB: Response of mouse intestine to neutrons and gamma rays in relation to dose fractionation and division cycle. Cancer 34:39–47, 1974

*Radiobiology for the Radiologist, Fourth Edition*, by Eric J. Hall
J. B. Lippincott Company, Philadelphia © 1994.

# 7

# *Repair of Radiation Damage and the Dose-Rate Effect*

Diagnostic Radiology
Nuclear Medicine
Radiation Therapy

# CLASSIFICATION
# OF RADIATION DAMAGE

Radiation damage to mammalian cells can be divided into three categories: (1) **lethal damage,** which is irreversible, is irreparable, and, by definition, leads irrevocably to cell death; (2) **sublethal damage,** which under normal circumstances can be repaired in hours unless additional sublethal damage is added (eg, from a second dose of radiation) with which it can interact to form lethal damage (sublethal damage repair, therefore, is manifest by the increase in survival observed when a dose of radiation is split into two fractions separated by a time interval); and (3) **potentially lethal damage** (PLD), the component of radiation damage that can be modified by postirradiation environmental conditions. All three are simply operational terms, since in mammalian cells the mechanisms of repair and radioresistance are not fully understood at the molecular level.

In several species of yeast, mutants have been isolated that are very sensitive to killing by x-rays (or by ultraviolet light). Many of the wild-type versions of the defective genes have been isolated, and in some cases their DNA sequence has been determined. The gene products appear to be involved directly in the repair process, and/or in functioning as molecular checkpoint controlling elements (molecular checkpoint genes are described in Chapter 6).

In mammalian cells, the first repair gene to be isolated was associated with correcting DNA damage produced by mitomycin C. This gene is located on human chromosome 18, and it has been characterized and its DNA sequence has been determined. The situation is much more difficult in the case of x-rays, since mutant mammalian cell lines that are very radiosensitive compared with the wild type are simply not available. For example, in the case of mitomycin C, the mutant and wild-type cells differed in sensitivity to the drug by a factor of about 500, whereas the most radiosensitive mammalian mutants differ from normal cells by a factor of only 2 or 3. This makes the isolation of normal x-ray repair genes technically difficult. A human gene capable of correcting the x-ray sensitivity of a mutant Chinese hamster cell line has, however, been isolated and localized to chromosome 19, and its DNA sequence has also been ascertained. Unfortunately, the defective gene in the human genetic disorder ataxia-telangiectasia, which is associated with sensitivity to x-ray cell killing, as well as a predisposition to cancer, has not been identified. The isolation of this gene would be of enormous practical importance.

# POTENTIALLY LETHAL
# DAMAGE

Varying environmental conditions after exposure to x-rays can influence the proportion of cells that survive a given dose because of the expression or repair of PLD. This damage is potentially lethal because under ordinary circumstances it causes cell death, but if survival is increased as a result of the manipulation of the postirradiation environment, PLD is considered to have been repaired. PLD is repaired if cells are incubated in balanced salt solution instead of full growth medium for several hours after irradiation. This is a drastic treatment, however, and does not mimic a physiological condition that is ever likely to occur in vivo. Little and his colleagues chose to study PLD repair in density-inhibited stationary-phase cell cultures, which are considered to be a better in vitro model for tumor cells in vivo (Fig. 7-1). Cell survival was enhanced considerably if the cells were allowed to remain in the density-inhibited state for 6 to 12 hours after irradiation before being subcultured and assayed for colony-forming ability.

The relevance of PLD to radiotherapy became much more obvious when it was shown that repair, comparable in magnitude and kinetics to that found in vitro, also occurred in vivo in experimental tumors. In this case, repair took the form of significantly enhanced cell survival if several hours were allowed to elapse between irradi-

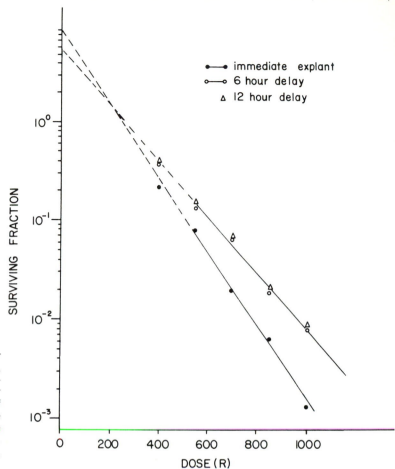

**Figure 7-1.** X-ray survival curves for density-inhibited stationary-phase cells, subcultured (trypsinized and plated) either immediately or 6 to 12 hours after irradiation. Cell survival is *enhanced* if cells are left in the stationary phase after irradiation, allowing time for the repair of potentially lethal damage. (From Little JB: Radiat Res 56:320–333, 1973)

ation of the tumor in situ and removal of the cells from the host to assess their reproductive integrity (Fig. 7-2).

To summarize the available experimental data, there is general agreement that PLD is repaired and the fraction of cells surviving a given dose of x-rays is enhanced if postirradiation conditions are suboptimal for growth, so that cells do not have to attempt the complex process of mitosis while their chromosomes are damaged. If mitosis is delayed by suboptimal growth conditions, DNA damage can be repaired.

The importance of PLD repair to clinical radiotherapy is a matter of debate. That it occurs in transplantable animal tumors has been documented beyond question, and there is no reason to suppose that it does not occur in human tumors. It has been suggested that the radioresistance of certain types of human tumors is linked to their ability to repair PLD; that is, radio-

sensitive tumors repair PLD inefficiently while radioresistant tumors have efficient mechanisms to repair PLD. This is an attractive hypothesis, but it has not stood the test of time!

## POTENTIALLY LETHAL DAMAGE AND HIGH LINEAR ENERGY TRANSFER RADIATIONS

Experiments with cells in culture and animal tumors indicate that there is *no PLD repair* following exposure to high linear energy transfer radiations. Figure 7-3 shows the data for Lewis lung carcinoma cells irradiated in situ with neutrons or cobalt-60 γ-rays. After irradiation the tumor was removed and the proportion of surviving cells assayed by their ability to form colonies, either in vitro or in the lungs of recipient animals

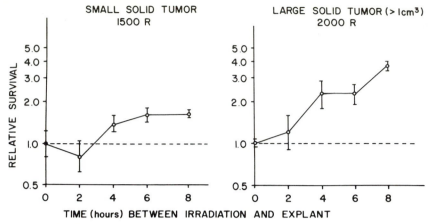

Figure 7-2.   Repair of potentially lethal damage in mouse fibrosarcomas. The tumors were irradiated in situ, then removed and prepared into single cell suspensions. The number of survivors was determined by their ability to form colonies in vitro. The fraction of cells surviving a given dose *increases* if a time interval is allowed between irradiation and removal of the tumor, because during this interval, potentially lethal damage is repaired. (From Little JB, Hahn GM, Frindel E, Tubiana M: Radiology 106:689–694, 1973)

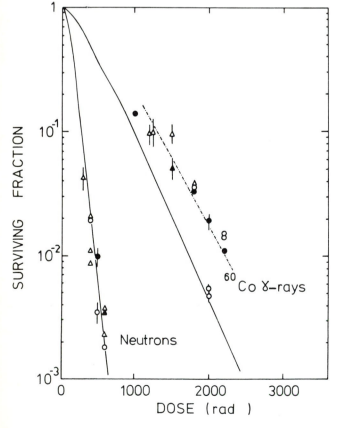

Figure 7-3.   Survival of Lewis lung carcinoma cells irradiated in situ with cobalt-60 γ-rays or neutrons (16-MeV d⁺ →Be). After irradiation, the colony-forming ability of the cells is assessed either by plating in vitro into medium containing soft agar, a technique that yields tight spherical colonies, or by injecting cells into recipient animals and counting the number of lung colonies produced. The solid lines are survival curves for cells from tumors removed *immediately* after irradiation and assayed for colony-forming ability. Closed and open symbols refer to cells from tumors removed 4 to 8 hours or 18 to 24 hours after irradiation, respectively. The circles represent data from the soft agar technique, while triangles refer to in vivo lung colonies. Note that, in the case of γ-rays, survival is enhanced if the cells are left in situ for some hours after irradiation before the assay for colony-forming ability, indicating repair of potentially lethal damage. No such repair is seen after neutron irradiation. (From Shipley WU, Stanley JA, Courtenay VC, Field SB: treatment with fast neutrons and gamma rays. Cancer Res 35:932–938, 1975)

into which they were injected. After exposure to γ-rays, survival was enhanced if the cells were left in situ for 4 to 24 hours, indicating the repair of PLD. After irradiation with neutrons, cell survival was the *same* whether tumors were removed and assayed immediately or left in situ for up to 24 hours. This was interpreted to mean that no PLD repair took place. PLD repair represents one more difference in the properties of neutrons compared with x-rays, but it is not clear whether this is an advantage or disadvantage of densely ionizing radiation in terms of their use for radiotherapy.

## SUBLETHAL DAMAGE REPAIR

*Sublethal damage repair* is the operational term for the increase in cell survival that is observed when a given radiation dose is split into two fractions separated by a time interval.

Figure 7-4 shows data obtained in a split-dose experiment with cultured Chinese hamster cells. A single dose of 15.58 Gy (1558 rads) leads to a surviving fraction of 0.005. When the dose is divided into two equal fractions, separated by 30 minutes, the surviving fraction is already appreciably higher than for a single dose. As the time interval is extended, the surviving fraction increases until a plateau is reached at about 2 hours, corresponding to a surviving fraction of 0.02. This represents about four times as many surviving cells as for the dose given in a single exposure. A further increase in the time interval between the dose fractions is not accompanied by any additional increment in survival. The increase in survival in a split-dose experiment is due to the repair of sublethal radiation damage.

The data shown in Figure 7-4 were obtained with cultured mammalian cells maintained at room temperature (24°C) between the dose fractions to prevent the cells from moving through the cell cycle during this interval. This rather special experiment was described first because it illustrates the phenomenon of the repair of sublethal radiation damage, uncomplicated by the movement of cells through the cell cycle.

Figure 7-5 shows the results of the parallel experiment in which cells were exposed to split doses while being maintained at their normal growing temperature of 37°C. The pattern of repair seen in this case differs from that observed for cells kept at room temperature. In the first few hours prompt repair of sublethal damage is again evident, but at longer intervals between the two split doses the surviving fraction of cells decreases again.

An understanding of this phenomenon is based on the age–response function described in Chapter 6. When an asynchronous population of cells is exposed to a large dose of radiation, more cells are killed in the sensitive than in the resistant phases of the cell cycle. The surviving population of cells, therefore, tends to be partly synchronized.

In Chinese hamster cells most of the survivors from a first dose are located in the S phase of the cell cycle. If about 6 hours are allowed to elapse before a second dose of radiation is given, this cohort of cells will progress around the cell cycle and will be in $G_2$ or M, a sensitive period of the cell cycle, at the time of the second dose. If the increase in radiosensitivity in moving from late S to the $G_{2-M}$ period exceeds the effect of repair of sublethal damage, the surviving fraction will fall.

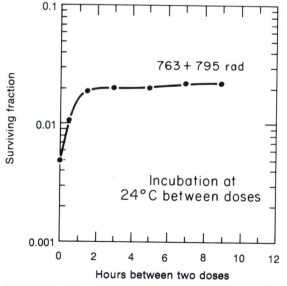

**Figure 7-4.** Survival of Chinese hamster cells exposed to two fractions of x-rays and incubated at room temperature for various time intervals between the two exposures. (From Elkind MM, Sutton-Gilbert H, Moses WB, Alescio T, Swain RW: Radiat Res 25:359, 1965)

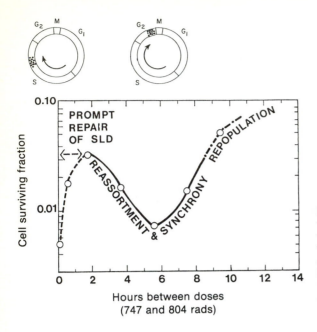

**Figure 7-5.** Survival of Chinese hamster cells exposed to two fractions of x-rays and incubated at 37°C for various time intervals between the two doses. The survivors of the first dose are predominantly in a resistant phase of the cycle (late S). When the interval between doses is about 6 hours, these resistant cells will have moved to the $G_2$–M phase, which is sensitive. (Redrawn from Elkind MM, Sutton-Gilbert H, Moses WB, Alescio T, Swain RW: Radiat Res 25:359, 1965)

The pattern of repair shown in Figure 7-5 is, therefore, a combination of three processes occurring simultaneously. First, there is the prompt repair of sublethal radiation damage. Second, there is progression of cells through the cell cycle during the interval between the split doses, which has been termed *reassortment*. Third, there is an increase of surviving fraction due to cell division, or repopulation, when the interval between the split doses is 10 to 12 hours because this exceeds the length of the cell cycle of these rapidly growing cells.

This simple experiment, performed in vitro, illustrates the three "Rs" of radiobiology: **repair, reassortment,** and **repopulation**. There is a fourth "R," **reoxygenation,** which is discussed in Chapter 8. It should be emphasized that the dramatic dip in the split-dose curve at 6 hours, caused by reassortment, and the increase in survival by 12 hours, because of repopulation, is seen only for rapidly growing cells. Hamster cells in culture have a cycle time of only 9 or 10 hours. The time sequence of these events would be longer in more slowly proliferating normal tissues in vivo.

Repair of sublethal radiation damage has been demonstrated in just about every biological test system for which a quantitative endpoint is avail-able. Figure 7-6 illustrates the pattern for repair of sublethal radiation damage in two in vivo systems in mice, P388 lymphocytic leukemia and skin cells. In neither case is there a dramatic dip in the curve at 6 hours due to movement of cells through the cycle because the cell cycle is long. In resting skin, for example, the cell cycle of stem cells may be as long as 10 days rather than the 9 hours of the rapidly growing cells in Figure 7-5. The mouse tumor data show more repair in small 1-day tumors than in large hypoxic 6-day tumors; this important point illustrates that repair is an active process requiring oxygen and nutrients.

The various factors involved in the repair of sublethal damage are summarized in Figure 7-7. Figure 7-7A shows that when a dose is split into two fractions separated by a time interval more cells survive than for the same total dose given in a single fraction because the shoulder of the curve must be repeated with each fraction. In general, there is a good correlation between the extent of repair of sublethal damage and the size of the shoulder of the survival curve. This is not surprising, since both are manifestations of the same basic phenomenon: the accumulation and repair of sublethal damage. Some mammalian cells are characterized by a survival curve with a

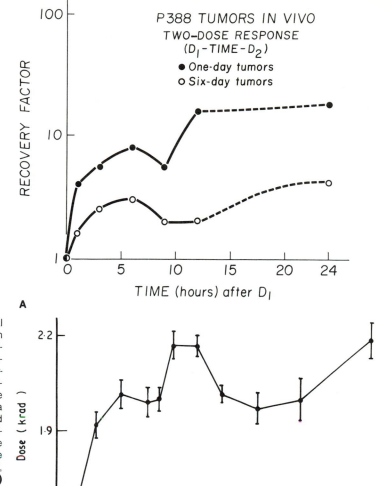

Figure 7-6. Repair of sublethal damage in two in vivo mammalian cell systems. **(A)** Split-dose experiments with P388 lymphocytic leukemia cells in the mouse. The *recovery factor* is the ratio of the surviving fraction resulting from two-dose fractionation to the survival from a single equivalent dose. One-day-old tumors are composed predominantly of oxygenated cells, while the cells in 6-day-old tumors are hypoxic. (From Belli JA, Dicus GJ, Bonte FJ: JNCI 38:673, 1967) **(B)** Split-dose experiments with skin epithelial cells in the mouse. The total x-ray dose, given as two fractions, required to result in one surviving epithelial cell per square millimeter is plotted against the time interval between the two doses. (From Emery EW, Denekamp J, Ball MM: Radiat Res 41:450, 1970)

broad shoulder, and split-dose experiments then indicate a substantial amount of sublethal damage repair. Other types of cells show survival curves with a minimal shoulder, and this is reflected in more limited repair of sublethal damage. In the terminology of the linear-quadratic $(\alpha/\beta)$ description of the survival curve, it is the quadratic component $(\beta)$ that causes the curve to bend and results in the sparing effect of a split dose. A large shoulder corresponds to a small $\alpha/\beta$ ratio.

The time course of the increase in cell survival that results from the repair of sublethal damage is charted in Figure 7-7B. As the time interval between the two dose fractions is increased there is a rapid increase in the fraction of cells surviving owing to the prompt repair of sublethal damage. This repair is complete by 1 or 2 hours for cells in culture but may take longer for late responding tissues in vivo (see Chapter 13). As the time interval between the two dose fractions is increased there will be a dip in the curve owing to

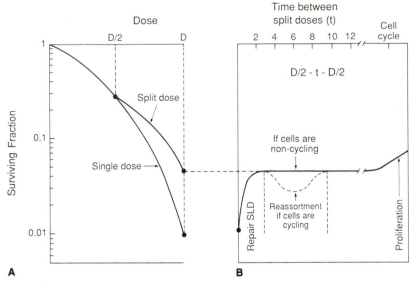

**Figure 7-7.** Diagram summarizing the repair of sublethal damage as evidenced by a split-dose experiment. **(A)** When the dose is delivered in two fractions separated by a time interval, there is an increase in cell survival because the shoulder of the curve must be expressed each time. **(B)** The fraction of cells surviving a split dose increases as the time interval between the two dose fractions increases. As the time interval increases from zero to 2 hours, the increase in survival is due to the repair of sublethal damage. In cells with a long cell cycle, or that are out of cycle, there is no further increase in cell survival by separating the dose by more than 2 or 3 hours. However, in a rapidly dividing cell population there is a dip in cell survival caused by reassortment, as explained in Figure 7-5. When the time interval between the split doses exceeds the cell cycle, there will be an increase in cell survival owing to proliferation or repopulation between the doses.

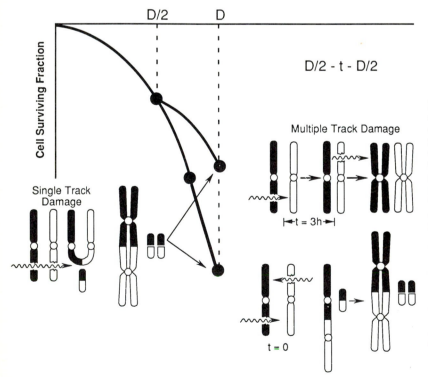

**Figure 7-8.** Repair of sublethal damage. When a dose D is delivered as two fractions of D/2 separated by several hours, the fraction of cells surviving is greater than if the dose is given in a single exposure. The fraction of cells killed by single-track damage is the same whether the dose is given in two fractions or as a single exposure. It is the multiple-track damage that is affected by fractionation. If the two chromosome breaks that must interact to form a lethal lesion (such as a dicentric) occur hours apart, then the first break may be repaired before the second occurs. On the other hand, if the two chromosome breaks are open at the same time, they may interact to form a lethal lesion such as a dicentric.

the movement of surviving cells through the cell cycle, as explained in Figure 7-6. This will only occur in a population of fast-cycling cells. In cells that are noncycling there can be no dip. When the time interval between the two dose fractions exceeds the cell cycle, there will be an increase in the number of cells surviving due to cell proliferation; that is, cells can double in number between the dose fractions.

## MECHANISM OF SUBLETHAL DAMAGE REPAIR

In Chapter 3, evidence was summarized of the correlation between cell killing and the production of asymmetrical chromosomal aberrations, such as dicentrics and rings. This in turn is a consequence of an interaction between two (or more) double-strand breaks in the DNA. On this interpretation the repair of sublethal damage is simply the repair of double-strand breaks. When a dose is split into two parts separated by a time interval, some of the double-strand breaks produced by the first dose are rejoined and repaired before the second dose. The situation is illustrated in Figure 7-8. Here it is assumed that dicentric chromosomes are the cause of cell lethality, but the argument would be the same for rings or anaphase bridges, that is, for any aberration that involves the interaction of two double-strand breaks. The breaks in two chromosomes that must interact to form a dicentric may be formed by (1) a single track breaking both chromosomes (labeled single-track damage) or (2) separate tracks breaking the two chromosomes (labeled multiple-track damage).

The component of cell killing that results from single-track damage will be the same whether the dose is given in a single exposure or fractionated. The same is not true of multiple-track damage. If the dose is given in a single exposure (ie, two fractions with t = 0 between them) all breaks produced by separate electrons can interact to form dicentrics. On the other hand, if the two dose fractions, D/2, are separated by (for example) 3 hours, breaks produced by the first dose may be repaired before the second dose is given. Consequently, there will be fewer interactions between broken chromosomes to form dicentrics and more cells will survive. On this

simple interpretation, the repair of sublethal damage reflects the repair and rejoining of double-strand breaks before they can interact to form lethal lesions. This may not be the whole story, but it is a useful picture to keep in mind.

## REPAIR AND RADIATION QUALITY

For a given biological test system the shoulder on the acute survival curve and, therefore, the amount of sublethal damage repair indicated by a split-dose experiment varies with the type of radiation used. The effect of dose fractionation with x-rays and neutrons is compared in Figure 7-9. For x-rays, dividing the total dose into two equal fractions, separated by 1 to 4 hours, results in a marked increase of cell survival because of the prompt repair of sublethal damage. By contrast, dividing the dose into two fractions has little effect on cell survival when neutrons are used, indicating little repair of sublethal damage.

## THE DOSE-RATE EFFECT

For x- or $\gamma$-rays dose rate is one of the principal factors that determines the biological consequences of a given absorbed dose. As the dose rate is lowered and the exposure time extended, the biological effect of a given dose is generally reduced.

The classic dose-rate effect, which is very important in radiotherapy, results from the repair of sublethal damage that occurs during a long radiation exposure. To illustrate this principle, Figure 7-10 shows an idealized experiment in which each dose ($D_2$, $D_3$, $D_4$, and so on) is delivered in a number of equal fractions of size D, with a time interval between fractions that is sufficient for repair of sublethal damage to be complete. The shoulder of the survival curve is repeated with each fraction. The broken line, F, shows the overall survival curve that would be observed if only single points were determined, corresponding to equal dose increments. This survival curve has no shoulder. Since continuous low dose-rate irradiation may be considered to be an infinite number of infinitely small fractions, the survival curve

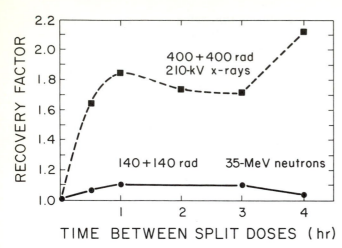

Figure 7-9. Split-dose experiments with Chinese hamster cells. For 210-kV x-rays, two 4-Gy (400-rad) doses, separated by a variable interval, were compared with a single dose of 8 Gy (800 rads). For neutrons (35-MeV d⁺ →Be), two 1.4 Gy (140-rads) doses were compared with a single exposure of 2.8 Gy (280 rads). The data are plotted in terms of the recovery factor, defined as the ratio of surviving fractions for a given dose delivered as two fractions compared with a single exposure. It is evident that repair of sublethal damage during the interval between split doses is virtually nonexistent for neutrons but is a significant factor for x-rays. (From Hall EJ, Roizin-Towle L, Theus RB, August RS: Radiology 117:173–178, 1975)

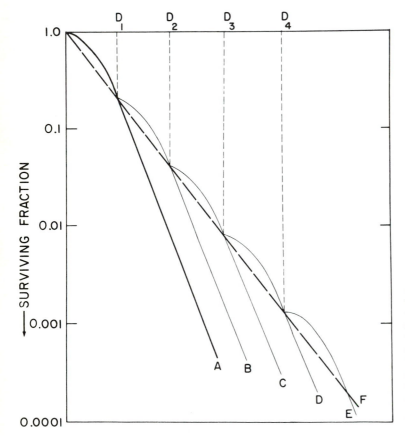

Figure 7-10. Idealized fractionation experiment. Curve A is the survival curve for single acute exposures of x-rays. Curve F is obtained if each dose is given as a series of small fractions of size $D_1$ with an interval between fractions sufficient for repair of sublethal damage to take place. Multiple small fractions approximate to a continuous exposure to a low dose rate. (From Elkind MM, Whitmore GF: Radiobiology of Cultured Mammalian Cells. New York, Gordon and Breach, 1967)

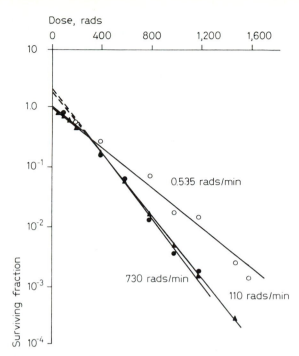

**Figure 7-11.** Survival curves for HeLa cells exposed to γ-rays at high and low dose rates.

under these conditions would also be expected to have no shoulder and to be shallower than for single acute exposures.

## EXAMPLES OF THE DOSE-RATE EFFECT IN VITRO AND IN VIVO

Survival curves for HeLa cells cultured in vitro over a wide range of dose rates, from 7.3 Gy/min to 0.535 cGy/min, are summarized in Figure 7-11. As the dose rate is reduced, the survival curve becomes shallower and the shoulder tends to disappear (ie, the survival curve becomes an exponential function of dose). The dose-rate effect caused by repair of sublethal damage is most dramatic between 0.01 and 1 Gy/min (1 and 100 rads/min). Above and below this dose-rate range, the survival curve changes little, if at all, with dose rate.

The magnitude of the dose-rate effect from the repair of sublethal damage varies enormously between different types of cells. HeLa cells are characterized by a survival curve for acute expo-

sures that has a small initial shoulder, which goes hand in hand with a modest dose-rate effect. This is to be expected, since both are expressions of the cell's capacity to accumulate and repair sublethal radiation damage. By contrast, Chinese hamster cells have a broad shoulder to their acute x-ray survival curve and show a correspondingly large dose-rate effect. This is evident in Figure 7-12; there is a clear-cut difference in biological effect, at least at high doses, between dose rates of 1.07, 0.3, and 0.16 Gy/min (107, 30, and 16 rads/min).

Figure 7-13 shows survival curves for 40 different cell lines of human origin, cultured in vitro and irradiated at high dose rate (HDR) and low dose rate (LDR). At low dose rate the survival curves "fan out" and show a greater variation in slope because in addition to the variation of inherent radiosensitivity evident at high dose rate, there is a range of repair times of sublethal damage. Some cell lines repair sublethal damage rapidly, some more slowly, and this is reflected in the survival curves at low dose rate.

Survival curves for crypt cells in the mouse jejunum irradiated with γ-rays at various dose rates are shown in Figure 7-14. There is a dramatic dose-rate effect owing to the repair of sublethal radiation damage from an acute exposure at 2.74 Gy/min (274 rads/min) to a protracted exposure at 0.92 cGy/min (0.92 rad/min). As the dose rate is lowered further, cell division begins to dominate the picture because the exposure time is longer than the cell cycle. At 0.54 cGy/min (0.54 rad/min) there is little reduction in the number of surviving crypts, even for very large doses, because cellular proliferation occurs during the long exposure and balances cell killing by the radiation.

## THE INVERSE DOSE-RATE EFFECT

There is at least one example of an inverse dose-rate effect, in which decreasing the dose rate results in increased cell killing. This is illustrated in Figure 7-15. Decreasing the dose rate for this cell line from 1.54 to 0.37 Gy/h (154 to 37 rads/h) increases the efficiency of cell killing, so that this low dose rate is almost as effective as an acute

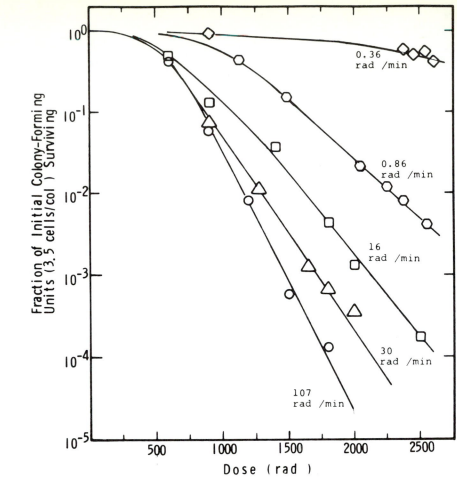

Figure 7-12. Dose–response curves for Chinese hamster cells (CHL-F line) grown in vitro and exposed to cobalt-60 γ-rays at various dose rates. At high doses a substantial dose rate effect is evident even between 1.07, 0.3, and 0.16 Gy (107, 30, and 16 rads/min). The decrease in cell killing becomes even more dramatic as the dose rate is further reduced. (From Bedford JS, Mitchell JB: Dose rate effects in synchronous mammalian cells in culture. Radiat Res 54:316–327, 1973)

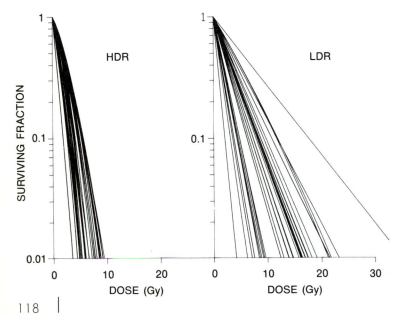

Figure 7-13. Dose survival curves at high dose rate (HDR) and low dose rate (LDR) for a large number of cells of human origin cultured in vitro. Note that the survival curves fan out at low dose rate because in addition to a range of inherent radiosensitivities (evident at HDR) there is also a range of repair times of sublethal damage.

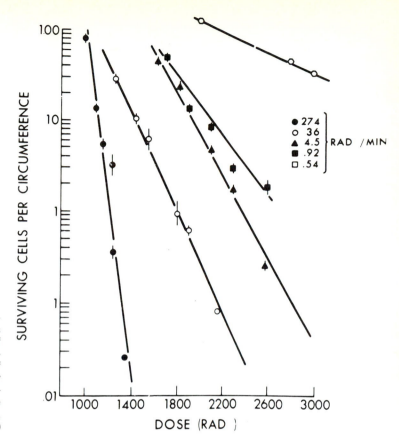

**Figure 7-14.** Response of mouse jejunal crypt cells irradiated with γ-rays from cesium-137 over a wide range of dose rates. The mice were given total-body irradiation, and the proportion of surviving crypt cells was determined by the appearance of regenerating microcolonies in the crypts $3\frac{1}{2}$ days later. Note the large dose-rate effect. (From Fu K, Phillips TL: Radiology 114:709–716, 1975)

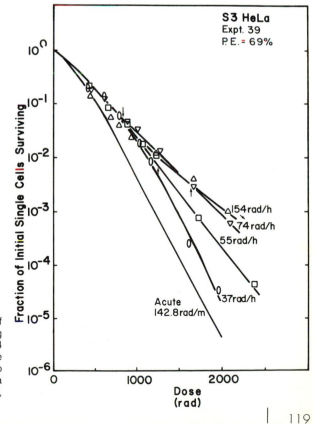

**Figure 7-15.** The inverse dose rate effect. A range of dose rates can be found for HeLa cells such that lowering the dose rate leads to *more* cell killing. At 1.54 Gy/h (154 rads/h) cells are "frozen" in the various phases of the cycle and do not progress. As the dose rate is dropped to 0.37 Gy/h (37 rads/h), cells progress to a block in $G_2$, a radiosensitive phase of the cycle. (From Mitchell JB, Bedford JS, Bailey SM: Radiat Res 79:520–536, 1979)

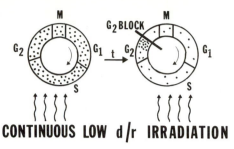

CONTINUOUS LOW d/r IRRADIATION

**Figure 7-16.** The inverse dose rate effect. A range of dose rates can be found, at least for HeLa cells, that allows cells to progress through the cycle to a block in late $G_2$. Under continuous low dose rate irradiation, an asynchronous population becomes a population of radiosensitive $G_2$ cells. (From Hall EJ: Endocurie Hypertherm Oncol 1:141–151, 1985)

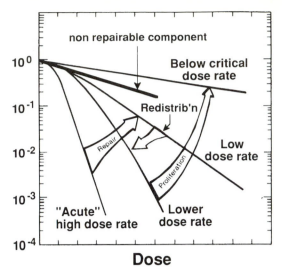

**Dose**

**Figure 7-17.** The dose rate effect due to repair of sublethal damage, redistribution in the cycle, and cell proliferation. The dose–response curve for acute exposures is characterized by a broad initial shoulder. As the dose rate is reduced, the survival curve becomes progressively shallower as more and more sublethal damage is repaired but cells are "frozen" in their positions in the cycle and do not progress. As the dose rate is lowered further and for a limited range of dose rates, the survival curve *steepens* again because cells can progress through the cycle to pile up at a block in $G_2$, a radiosensitive phase but still cannot divide. A further lowering of dose rate allows cells to escape the $G_2$ block and divide; cell proliferation may then occur during the protracted exposure, and survival curves become shallower as cell birth from mitosis offsets cell killing from the irradiation. (Based on the ideas of Dr. Joel Bedford)

exposure. The explanation of this is illustrated in Figure 7-16. At about 0.3 Gy/h (30 rads/h) cells tend to progress through the cycle and become arrested in $G_2$, a radiosensitive phase of the cycle. At higher dose rates they are "frozen" in the phase of the cycle they are in at the start of the irradiation; at lower dose rates they continue to cycle during irradiation.

## THE DOSE-RATE EFFECT SUMMARIZED

Figure 7-17 summarizes the entire dose-rate effect. For acute exposures at high dose rate the survival curve has a significant initial shoulder. As the dose rate is lowered and the treatment time protracted, more and more sublethal damage can be repaired during the exposure. Consequently, the survival curve becomes progressively shallower ($D_0$ increases), and the shoulder tends to disappear. A point is reached at which *all* sublethal damage is repaired, resulting in a limiting slope. In at least some cell lines a further lowering of the dose rate allows cells to progress through the cycle and accumulate in $G_2$. This is a radiosensitive phase, and so the survival curve becomes steeper again. This is the inverse dose-rate effect. A further reduction in dose rate will allow cells to pass through the $G_2$ block and divide. Proliferation may then occur during the radiation exposure if the dose rate is low enough and the exposure time is long compared with the length of the mitotic cycle. This may lead to a further reduction in biological effect as the dose rate is progressively lowered, because cell birth will tend to balance cell death. A dose-rate effect from cell proliferation was evident in studies with mouse jejunal crypt cells (see Fig. 7-14).

## VERY LOW DOSE RATES: CONTINUOUS EXPOSURES

The effects of very low dose rates have been investigated principally by observing renewal tissues of small animals. A steady-state cell population can be maintained under continuous irradiation as long as cell death per generation is less than cell birth. The dose rate that can be tolerated varies with the species and tissue type. The testis is most sensitive: male rats can reproduce for 10 generations or more under continuous exposure at 2 cGy/d, but a slight increase in dose rate above this level results in a depletion of the testis cell population. At the other extreme, the small intestine in the rat has been shown to maintain cell division and a steady-state population at dose rates as high as 4 Gy/d (400 rads/d). The blood-forming tissues are intermediate between these two extremes; red blood cell production in the rat can be maintained at close to normal levels for months during exposure to 0.5 Gy/d (50 rads/d).

Lamerton and Courtenay drew attention to three principal factors that determine the response of renewal tissues to continuous irradiation:

1. The cellular sensitivity of the stem cells involved. Cells that exhibit an acute exposure survival curve with a broad shoulder would be expected to be less susceptible to low dose-rate irradiation, since the shoulder is continuously reconstructed during a protracted exposure.
2. The duration of the cell cycle. The accumulated dose over the cell cycle is a more appropriate indicator of cell lethality than the dose rate. Thus a given dose rate of continuous irradiation will be more damaging to cells with a long cell cycle than to cells with a short cycle, since a larger dose will be absorbed per cell cycle.
3. The ability of some tissues to adapt to the new trauma of continuous irradiation. The red blood cell is one example. At 0.45 Gy/d (45 rads/d) a normal rate of red cell production is resumed after an initial period of adaptation and is then maintained for months. The compensation for cell killing appears to be achieved in the sequence of recognizable red blood cell precursors by lengthening of transit time and shortening of cell cycle, allowing extra divisions to be inserted. The small intestine of the rat adapts rapidly to a continuous exposure of 3.5 Gy/d (350 rads/d). The cell cycle is lengthened within 6 hours of the start of irradiation, but this trend is reversed after 24 hours, and the cell cycle rapidly becomes shorter than normal.

# BRACHYTHERAPY OR ENDOCURIETHERAPY

Implanting radioactive sources directly into a tumor was a strategy first suggested by Alexander Graham Bell soon after the turn of the century. Over the years, various groups in different countries coined various names for this type of therapy, using the prefix *brachy* from the Greek for "short range," or *endo* from the Greek for "within." There are two distinct forms of brachytherapy: (1) intracavitary irradiation using radioactive sources that are placed in body cavities in close proximity to the tumor and (2) interstitial brachytherapy using radioactive seeds implanted directly into the tumor volume.

Both interstitial and intracavitary techniques were developed to an advanced stage at an early date because the technology was readily available. Radium in sufficient quantities was extracted and purified in the early 1900s, whereas radioactive sources of sufficient activity for teletherapy sources of adequate dose rate only came as a spin-off of World War II nuclear technology.

## Intracavitary Therapy

Intracavitary radiotherapy at low dose rate is always temporary and usually takes 1 to 4 days (dose rate about 50 cGy/h). It can be used for a number of anatomical sites, but by far the most common is the uterine cervix. There has been a continual evolution in the radionuclide used; in the early days radium was used, but this went out of favor because of the safety aspects of using an encapsulated source that can leak radioactivity. As an interim measure cesium-137 was introduced, but nowadays most centers use iridium-192; its shorter half-life and lower energy make for ease of radiation protection, especially in conjunction with a remote afterloader.

To an increasing extent, low dose-rate intracavitary therapy is being replaced by high dose-rate intracavitary therapy, delivered in 3 to 12 dose fractions. Replacing continuous low dose-rate therapy with a few large-dose fractions must give up much of the radiobiological advantage, and lose the sparing of late responding normal tissues, as described in Chapter 13. It is only possible because the treatment of carcinoma of the cervix is a special case in which the dose-limiting normal tissues (eg, bladder, rectum) receive a lower dose than the prescribed dose to the tumor (or to point A). For high dose-rate treatments lasting a few minutes it is possible to use retractors that result in even lower doses to the critical normal tissues than are possible with an insertion that lasts 24 hours or more. These physical advantages offset the radiobiological disadvantages so that the general principle that a few large fractions at high dose rate give poorer results than at low dose rate does not apply to this special case.

## Interstitial Therapy

Interstitial brachytherapy can be either temporary or permanent. Permanent implants in earlier times utilized radium, but the most widely used radionuclide at the present time is iridium-192. Implants at low dose rate are considered by many radiotherapists to be the treatment of choice for the 5% or so of human cancers that are accessible to such techniques.

The dose-rate range used in these treatments is in the region of the dose-rate spectrum, in which the biological effect varies rapidly with dose rate. The maximum dose that can be delivered without unacceptable damage to the surrounding normal tissue depends on the volume of tissue irradiated and on the dose rate, which is in turn a function of the number of radioactive sources used and their geometric distribution. To achieve a consistent biological response, the total dose used should be varied according to the dose rate employed.

Ellis and Paterson independently published curves to relate total dose to result in normal tissue tolerance to dose rate (Fig. 7-18); there is remarkable agreement between the two sets of data based on clinical judgment.

Quoting Paterson:

> The graph for radium implants is an attempt to set out the doses in five to ten days which are equivalent to any desired seven-day dose. In its original form it perhaps owed more to inspiration than to science but it has gradually been corrected to match actual experience.

Both Paterson and Ellis regarded a dose of 60 Gy (6000 rads) in 7 days as the standard treatment, corresponding to a dose rate of 0.357 Gy/h (35.7 rads/h). If the sources are of higher activity and the treatment dose rate is higher, then a lower total dose should be used. For example, a dose

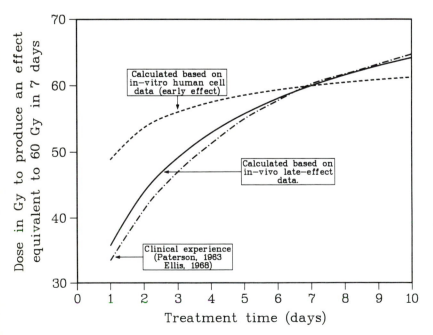

**Figure 7-18.** Dose equivalent to 60 Gy (6000 rads) in 7 days as proposed by Paterson (1963) and by Ellis (1968) based on clinical observation of normal tissue tolerance or calculated from radiobiological principles. The $\alpha/\beta$ ratios and the T1/2 for repair of sublethal damage were chosen for early or for late responding tissues (see Chapter 13).

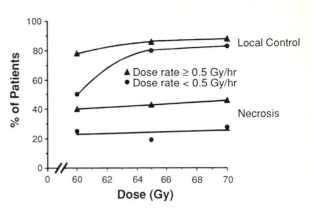

**Figure 7-19.** Local tumor control and necrosis rate at 5 years as a function of dose in patients treated for T1–2 squamous cell carcinomas of the mobile tongue and the floor of the mouth with interstitial iridium-192 implants. The patients were grouped according to whether the implant was characterized by a high dose rate (above 0.5 Gy/h) or low dose rate (below 0.5 Gy/h). The necrosis rate is higher for the higher dose rate at all dose levels. Local tumor control did not depend on dose rate provided the total dose was sufficiently large. (Redrawn from the data of Mazeron JJ, Simon JM, Le Pechoux C et al: Radiother Oncol 21:39–47, 1991)

rate of 0.64 Gy/h (64 rads/h) would produce an equivalent biological effect with a total dose of only 46 Gy (4600 rads) in a treatment time of 3 days.

Also shown in Figure 7-18 are isoeffect curves, matched to 60 Gy in 7 days, based on radiobiological data for early and late responding tissues. The variation of total dose with dose rate is much larger for late than for early responding tissues because of the lower $\alpha/\beta$ characteristic of such tissues. It is interesting to note that the curve for late responding tissues calculated from radiobiological data agrees closely with the clinical estimates of Ellis and of Paterson, as it should since their judgment was stated unequivocally to be based on late equalizing effects. In recent years, Mazeron and his colleagues in Paris have published two papers that show clearly that a dose-rate effect is important in interstitial implants. They have, perhaps, the largest experience in the world of the use of iridium-192 wire implants.

The first describes the analysis of local tumor control and the incidence of necrosis in a large cohort of patients with T1–2 squamous cell carcinoma of the mobile tongue and the floor of the mouth who were treated with interstitial iridium-192. The data are shown in Figure 7-19. Patients were grouped according to dose rate, either more or less than 0.5 Gy/h. It is evident that there is a substantially higher incidence of necrosis in patients treated at the higher dose rate. By contrast, dose rate makes little or no difference to local control provided the total dose is high enough, namely, 65 to 70 Gy, but there is a clear separation at lower doses (60 Gy), with the lower dose rate being less effective. These results are in good accord with the radiobiological predictions.

The second paper analyzes data from a large group of patients with carcinoma of the breast who received an iridium-192 implant as a boost to external-beam radiotherapy. These results allow an assessment of the effect of dose rate on tumor control but provide no information on the effect of dose rate on late effects, since there was only one case that involved necrosis. The interstitial implant comprised only part of the radiotherapy, and a fixed standard dose was used, so only limited conclusions can be drawn from these data. The results (Fig. 7-20), however, show a correlation between the proportion of recurrent tumors and the dose rate. For a given total dose, there were markedly fewer recurrences when the radiation was delivered at a higher dose rate rather than a lower dose rate.

The relatively short half-life of iridium (70 days) means that a range of dose rates will be inevitable because the activity of the sources will decay during the months that they are in use. It is important, therefore, to correct the total dose for the dose rate because of the experience of Mazeron and his colleagues in Paris described earlier. Iridium-192 has two advantages: (1) the source size can be small and (2) its lower photon energy makes protection easier than with radium or cesium-137. Sources of this radionuclide are ideal for use with a computer-controlled afterloader (Fig. 7-21). Catheters can be implanted into the patient inactive, and then the sources transferred from the safe by remote control after the patient has returned to his own room. The sources can be returned to the safe when the patient needs nursing care.

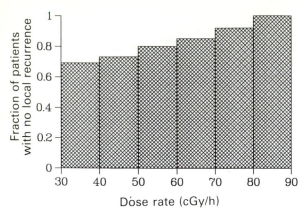

**Figure 7-20.** Percentage of patients who showed no local recurrence as a function of dose rate in patients treated for breast carcinoma by a combination of external-beam irradiation plus iridium-192 interstitial implant. The implant was used to deliver a dose of 37 Gy (3700 rads); the dose rate varied by a factor of 3 owing to different linear activities of the iridium-192 wire and to different size volumes implanted. (Drawn from the data of Mazeron JJ, Simon JM, Crook J et al: Int J Radiat Oncol Biol Phys 21:1173–1177, 1991)

## Permanent Interstitial Implants

Encapsulated sources with a relatively short half-life can be left in place permanently. There are two advantages for the patient: (1) an operation to remove the implant is not needed and (2) the patient can go home with the implant in place. On the other hand, it does involve additional expense, since the sources are not reused. The initial dose rate is high and falls off as the implanted sources decay. Iodine-125 has been most widely used to date for permanent implants. The total prescribed dose is usually about 160 Gy (16,000 rads) at the periphery of the implanted volume, with 80 Gy (8000 rads) delivered in the first half-life of 60 days. The soft emission from iodine has a relative biological effectiveness of about 1.5; this corresponds to 80 × 1.5, or 120 Gy (12,000 rads) of high-energy γ-rays. This is a big dose, even at low dose rate, and corresponds to a good level of cell kill. It is, however, spread over 60 days, and consequently the success of the implant in sterilizing the tumor depends critically on the cell cycle of the clono-

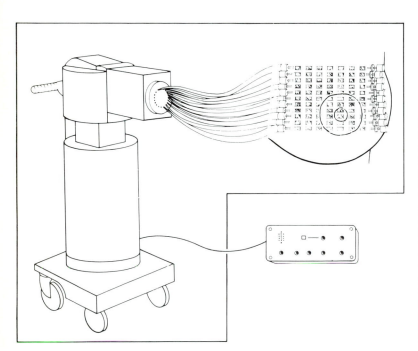

**Figure 7-21.** Diagram illustrating the use of a computer-controlled remote afterloader to minimize radiation exposure of personnel during brachytherapy. Catheters are implanted into the tumor and radiographs are taken to check the validity of the implant using "dummy" nonradioactive sources. The catheters are then connected to a shielded safe containing the radioactive (iridium-192) sources, which are transferred by remote control to the implant in the patient. The control panel is located outside a lightly shielded room. The sources can be retracted temporarily to the safe so that personnel can care for the patient, thus effectively eliminating radiation exposure to personnel.

Table 7-1.
## Characteristics of Radionuclides for Intracavitary or Interstitial Brachytherapy

| RADIONUCLIDE | PHOTON ENERGY | | HALF-LIFE | HVL (mm LEAD) |
| --- | --- | --- | --- | --- |
| | Average (keV) | Range (keV) | | |
| **Conventional** | | | | |
| Cesium-137 | 662 | — | 30 years | 5.5 |
| Iridium-192 | 380 | 136–1060 | 74.2 days | 2.5 |
| | | | | |
| **New** | | | | |
| Iodine-125 | 28 | 3–35 | 60.2 days | 0.025 |
| Gold-198 | 412 | — | 2.7 days | 2.5 |
| Americium-241 | 60 | — | 432 years | 0.125 |
| Palladium-103 | 21 | 20–23 | 17 days | 0.008 |
| Samarium-145 | 41 | 38–61 | 340 days | 0.06 |
| Ytterbium-169 | 100 | 10–308 | 32 days | 0.1 |

*(Data computed by Dr. Ravinder Nath, Yale University)*

genic cells. In a rapidly growing tumor, cell birth by mitosis will compensate for cell killing by the radiation during the prolonged exposure time. This will be much less of a problem with slowly growing tumors, such as carcinoma of the prostate, and it is in such sites that permanent implants with iodine-125 have found a place.

A major advantage of a radionuclide such as iodine-125 is the low energy of the photons emitted (about 30 keV). This makes little difference to the dose distribution in an implanted tumor but greatly simplifies radiation protection problems, since medical and nursing staff are easily shielded. In addition, dose falls off rapidly outside the treatment volume, so that doses to areas of the patient remote from the implant are greatly reduced.

A number of other new radionuclides are under consideration as sources for brachytherapy that share with iodine-125 the properties of a relatively short half-life and a low-energy photon emission to reduce problems of radiation protection. By contrast, americium-241 emits a low-energy photon but has a long half-life of hundreds of years. Table 7-1 summarizes some of the physical characteristics of the newly developed sources and contrasts them to the characteristics of radionuclides more commonly used for brachytherapy.

## RADIOLABELED IMMUNOGLOBULIN THERAPY FOR HUMAN CANCER

Radiolabeled immunoglobulin therapy is the radiotherapy for cancer using an antibody to deliver a radioactive isotope to the tumor. Much of the pioneering work in this field has been done by Stanley Order and his colleagues. They have focused on antiferritin labeled with radioactive iodine or yttrium.

Ferritin is an iron storage protein that is synthesized and secreted by a broad range of malignancies, including hepatomas, lung cancer, neuroblastoma, acute myelogenous leukemia, cancer of the breast and pancreas, and Hodgkin's disease. It is not known why ferritin is produced preferentially in tumors. It has been suggested that messenger RNA for ferritin may resemble that for many viruses. This suggestion is highly speculative but is consistent with the observation that ferritin is present in tumors that are suspected of having a viral etiology. This connection is strongly suspected for hepatomas, which have been associated with hepatitis B virus, and probably exists for Hodgkin's disease, too.

Although ferritin is also present in normal tissues, selective tumor targeting has been demonstrated in animal models and in clinical scanning, historically performed first for Hodgkin's disease. This differential is the basis of the potential therapeutic gain and, therefore, the clinical usefulness of radiolabeled immunoglobulin therapy.

In the early years of radiolabeled immunoglobulin therapy, radiolabeled polyclonal antibodies were used. These were replaced with murine monoclonal antibodies carrying iodine-131, which could be used for both diagnosis and therapy. More recently, chimeric mouse–human antibodies, which are human antibodies derived by tissue culture or produced in genetically altered mice, and synthetically derived antibodies have become available. These developments have progressively reduced the possibility of inducing an immune response, lengthened the effective half-life, and hence increased the tumor dose.

### Radionuclides

Early studies utilized iodine-131, which is easily linked to antibodies. The disadvantage of using iodine-131 is that it requires large doses (about 30 mCi); as a consequence of this, patients must be hospitalized, self-care is needed, and pediatric patients are excluded. In addition, the dose and dose rate to the tumor are limited by the relatively weak $\beta$ emission (0.3 MeV) and by the total-body dose resulting from the $\gamma$ emission, which causes systemic hematopoietic toxicity.

In more recent developments iodine-131 has been replaced by yttrium-90, which is characterized by a pure $\beta$ emission of relatively high energy (0.9 MeV). This allows a higher tumor dose and dose rate and enables the applications to be administered on an outpatient basis. More recently, rhenium-188, rhenium-186, and phosphorus-32 have all been used. New chemical linkages, including a variety of chelates, have been used, all seeking to firmly bind the isotope to the antibody.

### Tumor Target Visualization

When iodine-131 was used, the $\gamma$-ray emission allowed tumor localization as well as providing the bulk of the therapeutic dose. When pure $\beta$-emitters such as yttrium-90 were first introduced, it

was necessary to add a $\gamma$-emitter such as indium-111 to allow visualization. Nowadays, it is no longer acceptable to scan with a conventional gamma-camera since single photon emission computed tomography (SPECT) provides a clearer picture. The "bremstralung" from $\beta$-emitters can be scanned by this means, so that radionuclides such as yttrium-90 can be used without the need to add a $\gamma$-emitter for visualization.

### Targeting

The ability to target tumors with antiferritin mirrors the vascularity of the tumor nodules. In general, tumors with a high degree of vascularity are better targeted with antiferritin than less vascularized tumors. The presence of ferritin per se is not enough to ensure targeting. The need for neovasculature means that uptake tends to be greater in smaller tumors. Uptake can also be affected by radiation or hyperthermia. A dose of external radiation can act as an initiator. This was first observed empirically but is now used routinely to enhance the targeting of the radiolabeled antiferritin. This is probably a consequence of damage to tumor vasculature, which allows antiferritin to leak out of vessels and into tumor cells. The targeting ratio of a tumor to the average for normal tissues is about 2.9 for iodine-131–labeled antiferritin; the corresponding ratio is 1.2 for bone and gastrointestinal tract and 0.8 for lung.

### Clinical Results

The most promising results have been in the treatment of unresectable primary hepatoma, for which 48% partial remission and 7% complete remission rates have been reported by the Johns Hopkins group for patients receiving iodine-131–labeled antiferritin in combination with low doses of doxorubicin (Adriamycin) and 5-fluorouracil. Some success has also been reported by other groups using similar techniques in the treatment of metastatic neuroblastoma, relapsed grade IV gliomas after radiotherapy and chemotherapy, metastatic ovarian cancer resistant to prior radiotherapy, and malignant pleural and pericardial effusions of diverse etiology.

Iodine-131–labeled antiferritin led to partial remissions in patients with Hodgkin's disease, while yttrium-90 antiferritin produced *complete* remissions, indicating the increased effectiveness of the larger doses possible with pure β-ray emitting radionuclides. Radiolabeled immunoglobulin therapy has been used with varying success for a wide range of other malignancies, including hepatoma, ovarian cancer, gliomas, and leukemia. Although a variety of radiolabeled antibodies have been shown to achieve remissions in lymphoma, the question of the effect of the total-body exposure versus tumor targeting is still open.

## Dosimetry

For iodine-131–labeled antiferritin treatment of primary hepatoma, 30 mCi is administered on day 0, followed by 20 mCi on day 5. Escalation of dose beyond these levels is not helpful, since the deposition of labeled antiferritin becomes saturated. This translates into a peak dose rate of 45 to 50 mGy/h (4.5 to 5 rads/h) on days 1 and 5 and a total accumulated dose of 10 to 12 Gy (1000 to 1200 rads) by about 15 days. The corresponding dose rate to normal liver is 10 mGy/h (1 rad/h), and the total-body dose is 2 to 3 mGy/h (0.2 to 0.3 rad/h), which results in limiting hematologic toxicity. It is remarkable that such a small dose at such a low dose rate can produce remissions in patients with tumors of 1 kg or more. This response is difficult to explain on the basis of conventional radiobiological data, but the clinical results are exciting.

For yttrium-90–labeled antiferritin treatment, a single application of 20 mCi results in a peak dose of about 0.16 Gy/h (16 rads/h), which decays with a tumor-effective half-life of 2 days and results in a total dose of about 20 to 35 Gy (2000 to 3500 rads).

► ## Summary of Pertinent Conclusions

### Potentially Lethal Damage

- The component of radiation damage that can be modified by manipulation of the postirradiation conditions is known as potentially lethal damage (PLD).
- Potentially lethal damage repair can occur if cells are prevented from dividing for 6 hours or more after irradiation; this is manifest as an increase in survival. This repair can be demonstrated in vitro by keeping cells in saline or plateau phase for 6 hours after irradiation and in vivo by delayed removal and assay of animal tumors or cells of normal tissues.
- Potentially lethal damage repair is significant for x-rays but does not occur after neutron irradiation.
- It has been suggested that resistant human tumors (eg, melanoma) owe their resistance to large amounts of potentially lethal damage repair. This is still controversial.

### Sublethal Damage

- *Sublethal damage repair* is an operational term that describes the increase in survival when a dose of radiation is split into two fractions separated in time.
- The half-time of sublethal damage repair in mammalian cells is about 1 hour, but it may be longer in late responding normal tissues in vivo.

*(continued)*

► *Summary of Pertinent Conclusions* *(Continued)*

- Sublethal damage repair occurs in tumors and normal tissues in vivo as well as in cells cultured in vitro.
- The repair of sublethal damage reflects the repair of DNA breaks before they can interact to form lethal chromosomal aberrations.
- Sublethal damage repair is significant for x-rays but almost nonexistent for neutrons.

### Dose-Rate Effect

- When the radiation dose rate is reduced from about 1 Gy/min to 0.3 Gy/h (100 rads/min to 30 rads/h) there is a reduction in the cell killing from a given dose because sublethal damage repair occurs during the protracted exposure.
- As the dose rate is reduced, the slope of the survival curve becomes shallower ($D_0$ increases), and the shoulder tends to disappear.
- In some cell lines an *inverse* dose-rate effect is evident (ie, reducing the dose rate increases the proportion of cells killed) owing to the accumulation of cells in $G_2$, which is a sensitive phase of the cycle.

### Brachytherapy

- Implanting sources into or close to a tumor is known as brachytherapy (Gk., *brachy* meaning "short") or endocurietherapy (Gk., *endo* meaning "within").
- Intracavitary radiotherapy involves placing radioactive sources into a body cavity close to a tumor. The most common example is the treatment of carcinoma of the uterine cervix.
- Interstitial therapy involves implanting radioactive sources directly into the tumor and adjacent normal tissue.
- Temporary implants, which formerly utilized radium needles, are now performed most often with iridium-192 wires or seeds.
- When the implant is used as a sole treatment, a commonly used dose is 50 to 70 Gy (5000 to 7000 rads) in 5 to 9 days. Total dose should be adjusted for dose rate. Clinical studies show that both tumor control and late effects vary with dose rate for a given total dose. Often the implant is used as a boost to external-beam therapy and only half the treatment is given with the implant.
- Because of the small size and low photon energy, iridium-192 seeds are suitable for use with computer-controlled remote afterloaders.
- Permanent implants can be performed with radionuclides (such as iodine-125), which have a relatively short half-life.
- A number of novel radionuclides are being considered as sources for brachytherapy. Most emit low-energy photons, which simplifies the problems of radiation protection.

### Radiolabeled Immunoglobulin Therapy

- In the early days of radiolabeled immunoglobulin therapy, radiolabeled polyclonal antibodies were used. These were replaced with murine monoclonal antibodies. More recently, chimeric mouse–human antibodies,

*(continued)*

► **Summary of Pertinent Conclusions** *(Continued)*

> which are human antibodies derived by tissue culture or produced in genetically altered mice, have become available. Finally, synthetically derived antibodies have been produced.
>
> - Iodine-131 has been largely replaced by pure β-ray emitters such as yttrium-90, resulting in an increased tumor dose and decreased total-body toxicity.
> - Single photon emission computed tomography (SPECT) can be used to visualize the tumor, using the "bremstralung" from the β-rays.
> - Radiolabeled immunoglobulin therapy has produced promising results in unresectable primary hepatoma and in patients with Hodgkin's lymphoma. It has been used with varying success for a wide range of other malignancies. These results have been obtained with total tumor doses of 20 to 35 Gy (2000 to 3500 rads) delivered at very low dose rates.

# BIBLIOGRAPHY

Ang KK, Thames HD, van der Vogel AG et al: Is the rate of repair of radiation induced sublethal damage in rat spinal cord dependent on the size of dose per fraction? Int J Radiat Oncol Biol Phys 13:557–562, 1987

Bedford JS, Hall EJ: Survival of HeLa cells cultured in vitro and exposed to protracted gamma irradiation. Int J Radiat Biol 7:377–383, 1963

Bedford JS, Mitchell JB: Dose-rate effects in synchronous mammalian cells in culture. Radiat Res 54:316–327, 1973

Bell AG: The uses of radium. Am Med 6:261, 1903

Belli JA, Bonte FJ, Rose MS: Radiation recovery response of mammalian tumor cells in vivo. Nature 211:662–663, 1966

Belli JA, Dicus GJ, Bonte FJ: Radiation response of mammalian tumor cells: I. Repair of sublethal damage in vivo. JNCI 38:673–682, 1967

Belli JA, Shelton M: Potentially lethal radiation damage: Repair by mammalian cells in culture. Science 165:490–492, 1969

Berry RJ, Cohen AB: Some observations on the reproductive capacity of mammalian tumor cells exposed in vivo to gamma radiation at low dose rates. Br J Radiol 35:489–491, 1962

Bryant PE: Survival after fractionated doses of radiation: Modification by anoxia of the response of *Chlamydomonas*. Nature 219:75–77, 1968

Dale RG: The use of small fraction numbers in high dose-rate gynaecological afterloading: Some radiobiological considerations. Br J Radiol 63:290–294, 1990

Denekamp J, Fowler JF: Further investigations of the response of irradiated mouse skin. Int J Radiat Biol 10:435–441, 1966

Elkind MM, Sutton H: Radiation response of mammalian cells grown in culture: I. Repair of x-ray damage in surviving Chinese hamster Cells. Radiat Res 13:556–593, 1960

Elkind MM, Sutton-Gilbert H, Moses WB, Alescio T, Swain RB: Radiation response of mammalian cells in culture: V. Temperature dependence of the repair of x-ray damage in surviving cells (aerobic and hypoxic). Radiat Res 25:359–376, 1965

Ellis F: Dose time and fractionation in radiotherapy. In Elbert M, Howard A (eds): Current Topics in Radiation Research, vol 4, pp 359–397. Amsterdam, North-Holland, 1968

Hahn GM, Bagshaw MA, Evans RG, Gordon LF: Repair of potentially lethal lesions in x-irradiated, density-inhibited Chinese hamster cells: Metabolic effects and hypoxia. Radiat Res 55:280–290, 1973

Hahn GM, Little JB: Plateau-phase cultures of mammalian cells: An in vitro model for human cancer. Curr Top Radiat Res 8:39–83, 1972

Hall EJ: Radiation dose rate: A factor of importance in radiobiology and radiotherapy. Br J Radiol 45:81–97, 1972

Hall EJ: The biological basis of endocurietherapy: The Henschke Memorial Lecture 1984. Endocurie Hypertherm Oncol 1:141–151, 1985

Hall EJ, Bedford JS: Dose rate: Its effect on the survival of HeLa cells irradiated with gamma rays. Radiat Res 22:305–315, 1964

Hall EJ, Brenner DJ: The dose-rate effect revisited: Radiobiological considerations of importance in radiotherapy. Int J Radiat Oncol Biol Phys 21:1403–1414, 1991

Hall EJ, Brenner DJ: The 1991 George Edelstyn Memorial Lecture: Needles, wires and chips—advances in brachytherapy. Clin Oncol 4:249–256, 1992

Hall EJ, Cavanagh J: The effect of hypoxia on the recovery of sublethal radiation damage in *Vicia* seedlings. Br J Radiol 42:270–277, 1969

Hall EJ, Fairchild RG: Radiobiological measures with californium-252. Br J Radiol 42:263–266, 1970

Hall EJ, Kraljevic U: Repair of potentially lethal radiation damage: Comparison of neutron and x-ray RBE and implications for radiation therapy. Radiology 121:731–735, 1976

Hall EJ, Rossi HH, Roizin LA: Low dose-rate irradiation of mammalian cells with radium and californium-252: A comparison of effects on an actively proliferating cell population. Radiology 99:445–451, 1971

Henschke UK, Hilaris BS, Mahan GD: Afterloading in interstitial and intracavitary radiation therapy. AJR 386:95, 1963

Hornsey S: The recovery process in organized tissue. In Silini G (ed): Radiation Research, pp 587–603. Amsterdam, North-Holland, 1967

Hornsey S: The radiosensitivity of melanoma cells in culture. Br J Radiol 45:158, 1972

Howard A: The role of oxygen in the repair process. In Bond VP (ed): Proceedings of the Carmel Conference on Time and Dose Relationships in Radiation Biology as Applied to Radiotherapy, pp 70–81. Upton, NY, BNL Report 50203 (C-57), 1969

Jeggo PA, Hafezparast M, Thompson AF, Broughton BC, Kaur GP, Zdzienicka MZ, Athwal RS: Localization of a DNA repair gene (XRCC5) involved in double-strand-break rejoining to human chromosome 2. Proc Natl Acad Sci USA 89:6423–6427, 1992

Joslin CAF: High-activity source afterloading in gynecological cancer and its future prospects. Endocurie Hypertherm Oncol 5:69-81, 1989

Joslin CAF, Liversage WE, Ramsay NW: High dose-rate treatment moulds by afterloading techniques. Br J Radiol 42:108–112, 1969

Joslin CAF, Smith CW: The use of high activity cobalt-60 sources for intracavitary and surface mould therapy. Proc R Soc Med 63:1029–1034, 1970

Lajtha LG, Oliver R: Some radiobiological considerations in radiotherapy. Br J Radiol 34:252–257, 1961

Lamerton LF: Cell proliferation under continuous irradiation. Radiat Res 27:119–139, 1966

Lamerton LF, Courtenay VD: The steady state under continuous irradiation. In Brown DG, Cragle RG, Noonan JR (eds): Dose Rate in Mammalian Radiation Biology, pp 3-1–3-12. Washington, DC, United States Atomic Energy Commission, Division of Technical Information, Conference 680410, 1968

Lenhard RE Jr, Order SE, Spunberg JJ, Asbell SO, Leibel SA: Isotopic immunoglobulin: A new systemic therapy for advanced Hodgkin's disease. J Clin Oncol 3:1296–1300, 1985

Lieberman HB, Hopkins KM: A single nucleotide base-pair change is responsible for the radiosensitivity exhibited by *S pombe* cells containing the mutant allele RAD-192 (abstr). In Chapman JD, Devey WC, Whitmore GF (eds): Radiation Research: A Twentieth Century Perspective, vol 1, p 333. San Diego, Academic Press, 1991

Lieberman HB, Hopkins, KM, Chu HM, Laverty M: Molecular cloning and analysis of *Schizosaccharomyces pombe rad* 9, a gene involved in DNA repair and mutagenesis. Mol Gen Genet 232:367–376, 1992

Little JB, Hahn GM, Frindel E, Tubiana M: Repair of potentially lethal radiation damage in vitro and in vivo. Radiology 106:689–694, 1973

Mazeron JJ, Simon JM, Crook J et al: Influence of dose rate on local control of breast carcinoma treated by external beam irradiation plus iridium-192 implant. Int J Radiat Oncol Biol Phys 21:1173–1177, 1991

Mazeron JJ, Simon JM, Le Pechoux C et al: Effect of dose rate on local control and complications in definitive irradiation of $T_{1-2}$ squamous cell carcinomas of mobile tongue and floor of mouth with interstitial iridium-192. Radiother Oncol 21:39–47, 1991

Mitchell JB, Bedford JS, Bailey SM: Dose-rate effects on the cell cycle and survival of S3 HeLa and V79 cells. Radiat Res 79:520–536, 1979

Order SE: Monoclonal antibodies: Potential in radiation therapy and oncology. Int J Radiat Oncol Biol Phys 8:1193–1201, 1982

Order SE, Klein JL, Ettinger D et al: Use of isotopic immunoglobulin in therapy. Cancer Res 40:3001–3007, 1980

Order SE, Porter M, Hellman S: Hodgkin's disease: Evidence for a tumor-associated antigen. N Engl J Med 285:471–474, 1971

Order SE, Stillwagon GB, Klein JL, Leichner PK, Siegelman SS, Fishman EK, Ettinger DS, Haulk T, Kupher K, Finney K, Surdyke M, Self S, Leibel S: Iodine-131 antiferritin: A new treatment modality in hepatoma—a Radiation Therapy Oncology Group study. J Clin Oncol 3:1573–1582, 1985

Orton CG: What minimum number of fractions is required with high dose-rate afterloading? Br J Radiol 60:300–302, 1987

Paterson R: Treatment of Malignant Disease by Radiotherapy. Baltimore, Williams & Wilkins, 1963

Phillips RA, Tolmach LJ: Repair of potentially lethal damage in x-irradiated HeLa cells. Radiat Res 29:413–432, 1966

Phillips TL, Ainsworth EJ: Altered split-dose recovery in mice irradiated under hypoxic conditions. Radiat Res 39:317–331, 1969

Phillips TL, Hanks GE: Apparent absence of recovery in endogenous colony-forming cells after irradiation under hypoxic conditions. Radiat Res 33:517–532, 1968

Pierquin B: L'effet différentiel de l'irradiation continué (ou semi-continué) à faible debit des carcinoms épidermoides. J Radiol Electrol 51:533–536, 1970

Pierquin B, Chassagne D, Baillet F et al: Clinical observations on the time factor in interstitial radiotherapy using iridium-192. Clin Radiol 24:506–509, 1973

Shipley WU, Stanley JA, Courtenay VC, Field SB: Repair of radiation damage in Lewis lung carcinoma cells following in situ treatment with fast neutrons and gamma rays. Cancer Res 35:932–938, 1975

Shuttleworth E, Fowler JF: Nomograms for radiobiologically equivalent fractionated x-ray doses. Br J Radiol 39:154–155, 1966

Stout R, Hunter RD: Clinical trials of changing dose rate in intracavitary low dose-rate therapy. In Mould RF (ed): Brachytherapy. Amsterdam, Nucletron, 1985

Suit H, Urano M: Repair of sublethal radiation injury in hypoxic cells of a $C_3H$ mouse mammary carcinoma. Radiat Res 37:423–434, 1969

Thompson LH, Brookman KW, Jones NJ, Allen A, Carrano V: Molecular cloning of the human XRCC1 gene, which corrects defective DNA strand break repair and sister chromatid exchange. Mol Cell Biol 20:6160–6271, 1990

Travis EJ, Thames HD, Watkins TL et al: The kinetics of repair in mouse lung after fractionated irradiation. Int J Radiat Biol 52:903–19, 1987

Tubiana N, Malaise E: Growth rate and cell kinetics in human tumors: Some prognostic and therapeutic implications. In Symington T, Carter RL (eds): Scientific Foundations of Oncology, pp 126–136. Chicago, Year Book Medical Publishers, 1976

Turesson I, Thames HD: Repair capacity and kinetics of human skin during fractionated radiotherapy: Erythema, desquamation, and telangiectasia after 3 and 5 years' follow-up. Radiother Oncol 15:169–188, 1989

Van't Hooft E: The selection HDR: Philosophy and design. In: Mould RF: Selectron Brachytherapy Journal. Amsterdam, Nucletron, 1985

Weichselbaum RR, Little JB, Nove J: Response of human osteosarcoma in vitro to irradiation: Evidence for unusual cellular repair activity. Int J Radiat Biol 31:295–299, 1977

Weichselbaum RR, Nove J, Little JB: Deficient recovery from potentially lethal radiation damage in ataxia-telangiectasia and xeroderma pigmentosum. Nature 271:261–262, 1978

Weichselbaum RR, Schmitt A, Little JB: Cellular repair factors influencing radiocurability of human malignant tumors. Br J Cancer 45:10–16, 1982

Weichselbaum RR, Withers HR, Tomkinson K, Little JB: Potentially lethal damage repair (PLDR) in x-irradiated cultures of a normal human diploid fibroblast cell strain. Int J Radiat Biol 43:313–319, 1983

Wells RL, Bedford JS: Dose-rate effects in mammalian cells: IV. Repairable and non-repairable damage in noncycling $C_3H$ 10T1/2 cells. Radiat Res 94:105–134, 1983

Whitmore GF, Gulyas S: Studies on recovery processes in mouse L cells. NCI Monogr 24:141–156, 1967

Winans LF, Dewey WC, Dettor CM: Repair of sublethal and potentially lethal x-ray damage in synchronous Chinese hamster cells. Radiat Res 52:333–351, 1972

Withers HR: Capacity for repair in cells of normal and malignant tissues. In Bond VP (ed): Proceedings of the Carmel Conference on Time and Dose Relationships in Radiation Biology as Applied to Radiotherapy, pp 54–69. Upton, NY, BNL Report 50203 (C-57), 1969

*Radiobiology for the Radiologist, Fourth Edition*, by Eric J. Hall
J. B. Lippincott Company, Philadelphia © 1994.

# 8

# *The Oxygen Effect and Reoxygenation*

Diagnostic Radiology
Nuclear Medicine
Radiation Therapy

A host of chemical and pharmacologic agents that modify the biological effect of ionizing radiations have been discovered. None is simpler than oxygen, none produces such a dramatic effect, and, as it turns out, no other agent has such obvious practical implications.

The oxygen effect was observed as early as 1912 by Swartz in Germany, who noted that the skin reaction produced on his forearm by a radium applicator was reduced if the applicator was pressed hard onto the skin. He attributed this to the interruption in blood flow. By 1921 it had been noted by Holthusen that *Ascaris* eggs were relatively resistant to radiation in the absence of oxygen, a result wrongly attributed to the absence of cell division under these conditions. The correlation between radiosensitivity and the presence of oxygen was made by Petry in 1923 from a study of the effects of radiation on vegetable seeds. All of these results were published in the German literature but were apparently little known in the English-speaking world.

In England in the 1930s Mottram explored the question of oxygen in detail, basing his investigations on some work of Crabtree and Cramer on the survival of tumor slices irradiated in the presence or absence of oxygen. He also discussed the importance of these findings to radiotherapy. Mottram began a series of experiments that culminated in a quantitative measurement of the oxygen effect by his colleagues Gray and Read, using as a biological test system the growth inhibition of the primary root of the broad bean *Vicia faba*.

## THE NATURE OF THE OXYGEN EFFECT

Survival curves for mammalian cells exposed to x-rays in the presence and absence of oxygen are illustrated in Figure 8-1. The ratio of hypoxic to aerated doses needed to achieve the same biological effect is called the **oxygen enhancement ratio** (OER). For sparsely ionizing radiations, such as x- and $\gamma$-rays, the OER at high doses has a value of between 2.5 and 3. The

OER has been determined for a wide variety of chemical and biological systems with different end points, and its value for x-rays always tends to fall in this range. There is some evidence that for rapidly growing cells cultured in vitro the OER has a smaller value of about 2 at lower doses, of the order of the daily dose per fraction in radiotherapy. This is believed to be due to the variation of OER with the phase of the cell cycle; cells in $G_1$ have a lower OER than those in S, and since $G_1$ cells are more radiosensitive they dominate the low-dose region of the survival curve. For this reason the OER of an asynchronous population is slightly smaller at low doses than at high doses. This result has been demonstrated for a fast-growing cell cultured in vitro when precise survival measurements are possible but would be difficult to show in a tissue. It is of little, if any, clinical importance.

Figure 8-2 illustrates the oxygen effect for other types of ionizing radiations. For a densely ionizing radiation, such as low-energy $\alpha$-particles, the survival curve does not have an initial shoulder. In this case, survival estimates made in the presence or absence of oxygen fall along a common line; the OER is unity—in other words, there is no oxygen effect. For radiations of intermediate ionizing density, such as neutrons, the survival curves have a much reduced shoulder. In this case the oxygen effect is apparent, but it is much smaller than is the case for x-rays. In the example shown in Figure 8-2 the OER for neutrons is about 1.6.

In summary, the oxygen effect is large and important in the case of sparsely ionizing radiations, such as x-rays, is absent for densely ionizing radiations, such as $\alpha$-particles, and has an intermediate value for fast neutrons.

## THE TIME AT WHICH OXYGEN ACTS AND THE MECHANISM OF THE OXYGEN EFFECT

For the oxygen effect to be observed, oxygen must be present *during* the radiation exposure or, to be precise, during or within microseconds

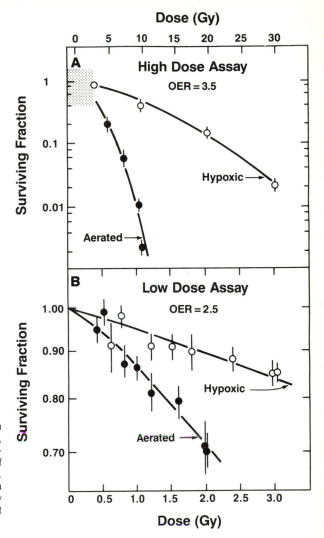

**Figure 8-1.** Cells are much more sensitive to x-rays in the presence of molecular oxygen than in its absence (ie, under hypoxia). The ratio of doses under hypoxia to aerated conditions necessary to produce the same level of cell killing is called the oxygen enhancement ratio (OER). It has a value close to 3 at high doses but may have a lower value of about 2 at x-ray doses below about 2 Gy (200 rads). (Redrawn from Palcic B, Skarsgard LD: Radiat Res 100:328–339, 1984)

after the radiation exposure. Sophisticated experiments have been performed in which oxygen, contained in a chamber at high pressure, was allowed to "explode" onto a single layer of bacteria (and later mammalian cells) at various times before or after irradiation with a 2-microsecond electron pulse from a linear accelerator. It was found that oxygen need not be present *during* the irradiation to sensitize but could be added *afterward*, provided the delay was not too long. Some sensitization occurred with oxygen added as late as 5 milliseconds after irradiation.

Experiments such as these shed some light on the mechanism of the oxygen effect. It is still not fully understood, however. There is general agreement that oxygen acts at the level of the free radicals. The chain of events from the ab-

sorption of radiation to the final expression of biological damage has been summarized as follows. The absorption of radiation leads to the production of fast charged particles. The charged particles, in passing through the biological material, produce a number of ion pairs. These ion pairs have a very short lifetime (about $10^{-10}$ second) and produce free radicals, which are highly reactive molecules because they have an unpaired valence electron. They are important because, although their lifetime is only $10^{-5}$ second, it is appreciably longer than that of the ion pairs.

To a large extent, it is these free radicals that break chemical bonds, produce chemical changes, and initiate the chain of events that results in the final expression of biological damage.

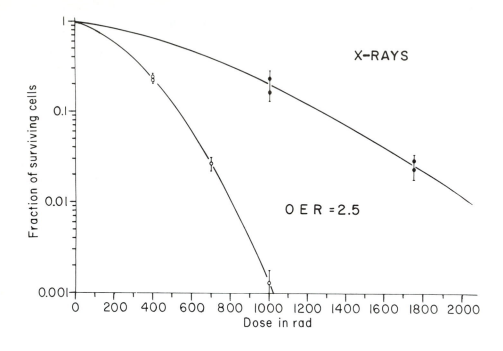

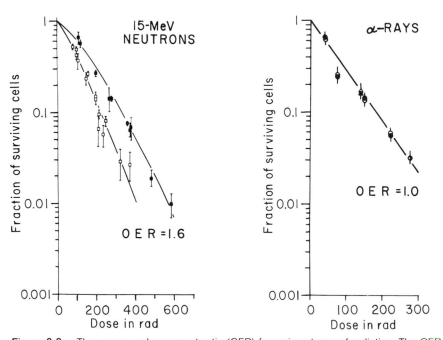

**Figure 8-2.** The oxygen enhancement ratio (OER) for various types of radiation. The OER for α-particles is unity. X-rays exhibit a larger OER of 2.5. Neutrons (15-MeV d⁺ →T) are between these extremes, with an OER of 1.6. (Redrawn from Barendsen GW, Koot CJ, van Kersen GR, Bewley DK, Field SW, Parnell CJ: Int J Radiat Biol 10:317, 1966; and Broerse JJ, Barendsen GW, van Kersen GR: Int J Radiat Biol 13:559, 1967)

If oxygen is present, it reacts with the free radical R·. This reaction produces $RO_2$, an organic peroxide that is a nonrestorable form of the target material; that is, the reaction results in a change in the chemical composition of the material exposed to the radiation. This reaction cannot take place in the absence of oxygen and if oxygen were not present many of the ionized target molecules could repair themselves and recover the ability to function normally. In a sense, then, oxygen may be said to "fix" the radiation lesion. This is known as the *oxygen fixation hypothesis* (Fig. 8-3). The word "fix" is used in the European sense of making something permanent, not in the American sense of repairing.

# THE CONCENTRATION OF OXYGEN REQUIRED

A question of obvious basic importance is the *concentration* of oxygen required to potentiate the effect of radiation. Is the amount required small or large? Many investigations have been performed using bacteria or mammalian cells, and the similarities are striking.

The simple way to visualize the effect of oxygen is by considering the change of slope of the mammalian cell survival curve. Figure 8-4 is a dramatic representation of what happens to the survival curve when oxygen is gradually introduced into the biological system. Curve A is characteristic of the response under conditions of equilibration with air. Curve B is a survival curve for irradiation in as low a level of hypoxia as can usually be obtained under experimental conditions (10 ppm of oxygen in the gas phase). The introduction of a very small quantity of oxygen, 100 ppm, is readily noticeable in a change in the slope of the survival curves. A concentration of 2200 ppm, which is about 0.25% oxygen, moves the survival curve halfway toward the fully aerated condition.

Other experiments have shown that by the time a concentration of oxygen corresponding to 2% has been reached, the survival curve is virtually indistinguishable from that obtained under conditions of normal aeration. Furthermore, increasing the amount of oxygen present from that characteristic of air to 100% oxygen does not further affect the slope of the curve.

The more usual textbook representation of the variation of radiosensitivity with oxygen concentration is shown in Figure 8-5. The term used here to represent radiosensitivity is proportional to the reciprocal of the $D_0$ of the survival curve. It is arbitrarily assigned a value of unity for anoxic conditions. As the oxygen concentration increases, the material becomes progressively more sensitive to radiation, until, in the presence of 100% oxygen, it is about three times as sensitive as under complete anoxia. Note that the rapid change of radiosensitivity occurs as the partial pressure of oxygen is increased from zero to about 30 mm Hg. A further increase in oxygen tension to an atmosphere of pure oxygen has lit-

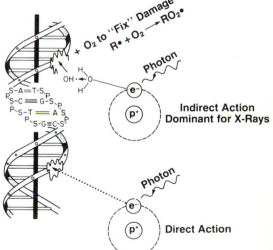

**Figure 8-3.** The oxygen fixation hypothesis. About two thirds of the biological damage produced by x-rays is by indirect action, mediated by free radicals. The damage produced by free radicals in DNA can be repaired under hypoxia but may be "fixed" (made permanent and irreparable) if molecular oxygen is available.

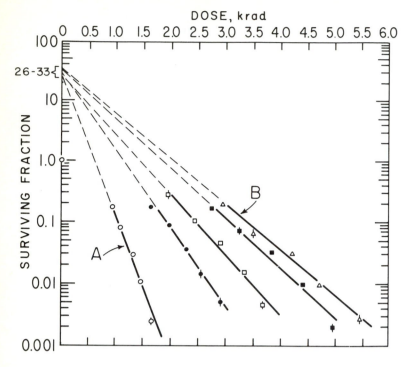

**Figure 8-4.** Survival curves for Chinese hamster cells exposed to x-rays in the presence of various oxygen concentrations. (Open circles, air; closed circles, 2200 ppm of oxygen or PO₂ of 1.7 mm Hg; open squares, 355 ppm of oxygen or PO₂ of 0.25 mm Hg; closed squares, 100 ppm of oxygen or PO₂ of 0.075 mm Hg; open triangles, 10 ppm of oxygen or PO₂ of 0.0076 mm Hg, which corresponded to the lowest level of hypoxia that could be obtained) (From Elkind MM, Swain RW, Alescio T, Sutton H, Moses WB: Cellular Radiation Biology, pp 442–461. Baltimore, Williams & Wilkins, 1965)

tle, if any, further effect. An oxygen concentration of 0.5% (or 3 mm Hg) results in a radiosensitivity halfway between the characteristic of hypoxia and that of fully oxygenated conditions.

It is evident, then, that very small amounts of oxygen are necessary to produce the dramatic and important oxygen effect observed with x-rays. Although it is usually considered that the oxygen tension of most normal tissues is similar to that of venous blood or lymph (20 to 40 mm Hg), in fact, oxygen probe measurements indicate that the oxygen tension between different tissues may vary over a wide range from 1 to 100 mm Hg. Many tissues are borderline hypoxic and contain a small proportion of cells that are radiobiologically hypoxic. This is particularly true of, for example, the liver and skeletal muscles. Even mouse skin has a small proportion of hypoxic cells that show up as a change of slope when the survival curve is pushed to low survival levels.

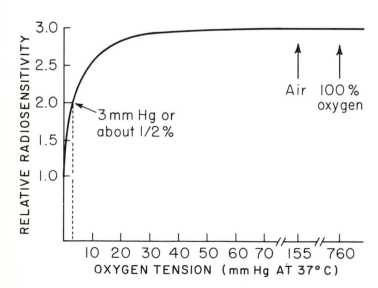

**Figure 8-5.** The dependence of radiosensitivity on oxygen concentration. If the radiosensitivity under anoxic conditions is arbitrarily assigned a value of unity, the radiosensitivity is about 3 under well-oxygenated conditions. Most of this change of sensitivity occurs as the oxygen concentration increases from 0 to 30 mm Hg. A further increase of oxygen content to that characteristic of air or even pure oxygen at high pressure has little further effect. A sensitivity halfway between anoxia and full oxygenation occurs for a PO₂ of about 3 mm Hg, which corresponds to about 0.5%. This illustration is idealized and does not represent any specific experimental data. Experiments have been performed with yeast, bacteria, and mammalian cells in culture; the results conform to the general conclusions summarized here.

# CHRONIC AND ACUTE HYPOXIA

It is important to recognize that hypoxia in tumors can result from two quite different mechanisms. *Chronic* hypoxia results from the limited diffusion distance of oxygen through tissue that is respiring. Cells may remain hypoxic for long periods of time. *Acute* hypoxia is a result of the temporary closing of a tumor blood vessel and is therefore transient.

## Chronic Hypoxia

Radiotherapists began to suspect that oxygen influenced the radiosensitivity of tumors in the 1930s. It was, however, the paper by Thomlinson and Gray in 1955 that triggered the tremendous interest in oxygen as a factor in radiotherapy when they described the phenomenon of chronic hypoxia. Thomlinson and Gray reported a histologic study of fresh specimens of bronchial carcinoma. Cells of the stratified squamous epithelium, normal or malignant, generally remain in contact with one another; the vascular stroma on which their nutrition depends lies in contact with the epithelium, but capillaries do not penetrate between the cells. Tumors that arise in this type of tissue often grow in solid rods that, seen in section, appear to be circular areas surrounded by stroma. The centers of large tumor areas are necrotic and are surrounded by intact tumor cells, which consequently appear as rings. Figure 8-6*A*, reproduced from Thomlinson and Gray, shows a transverse section of tumor cord and is typical of areas of a tumor in which necrosis is not far advanced. Figure 8-6*B* shows large areas of necrosis separated from stroma by a narrow band of tumor cells about 100 µm wide.

By viewing a large number of these samples of human bronchial carcinomas, Thomlinson and Gray recognized that as the tumor cord grew larger, the necrotic center enlarged too, so that the thickness of sheath of viable tumor cells remained essentially constant. This is illustrated in Figure 8-7.

The obvious conclusion was that tumor cells could proliferate and grow actively only if they were close to a supply of oxygen or nutrients from the stroma. They then went on to calculate the distance to which oxygen could diffuse in respiring tissue and come up with a distance of about 150 µm. This was close enough to the thickness of viable tumor cords on their histologic sections for them to conclude that oxygen depletion was the principal factor leading to the development of necrotic areas in tumors. Using more appropriate values of oxygen diffusion coefficients and consumption values, a better estimate of the distance oxygen can diffuse in respiring tissue is about 70 µm. This will of course vary from the arterial to the venous end of a capillary, as illustrated in Figure 8-8.

By histologic examination of sections, it is possible to distinguish only two classes of cells: (1) those that appear to be proliferating well and (2) those that are dead or dying. Between these two extremes, and assuming a steadily decreasing oxygen concentration, one would expect a region in which cells would be at an oxygen tension high enough for cells to be clonogenic but low enough to render the cells protected from the effect of ionizing radiation. Cells in this region would be relatively protected from a treatment with x-rays because of their low oxygen tension and could provide a focus for the subsequent regrowth of the tumor (see Fig. 8-8). On the basis of these ideas it was postulated that the presence of a relatively small proportion of hypoxic cells in tumors could limit the success of radiotherapy in some clinical situations.

These ideas about the role of oxygen in cell killing dominated the thinking of radiobiologists and radiotherapists in the late 1950s and early 1960s. A great deal of thought and effort was directed toward solving this problem. The solutions proposed included the use of high-pressure oxygen chambers and the development of novel radiation modalities, such as neutrons, negative π-mesons, and heavy charged ions.

## Acute Hypoxia

Regions of acute hypoxia develop in tumors as a result of the temporary closing or blockage of a particular blood vessel. If this blockage were permanent, the cells downstream would, of course, eventually die and would be of no further consequence. There is, however, good evi-

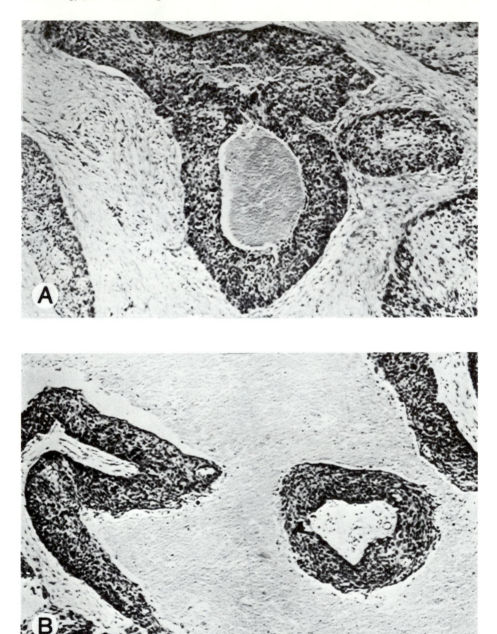

**Figure 8-6.** Transverse sections of tumor cords surrounded by stroma from human carcinoma of the bronchus. **(A)** A typical tumor area in which necrosis is not far advanced. **(B)** Large areas of necrosis separated from the stroma by bands of tumor cells about 100 µm wide. (From Thomlinson RH, Gray LH: Br J Cancer 9:539–549, 1955)

dence that tumor blood vessels open and close in a random fashion so that different regions of the tumor become hypoxic intermittently. At the moment when a dose of radiation is delivered, a proportion of the tumor cells may be hypoxic, but if the radiation were delayed until a later time, a different group of cells may be hypoxic.

The occurrence of acute hypoxia was postulated in the early 1980s by Brown and later demonstrated unequivocally in rodent tumors by Chaplin and his colleagues. Figure 8-9 is an attempt to illustrate the way in which acute hypoxia occurs to explain the difference between acute and chronic hypoxia.

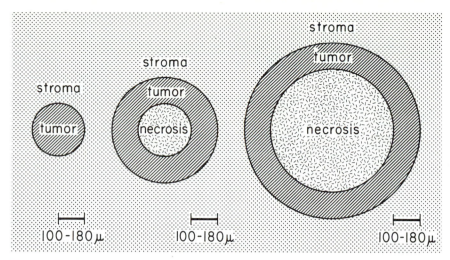

**Figure 8-7.** The conclusions reached by Thomlinson and Gray from a study of histologic sections of human bronchial carcinoma. No necrosis was seen in small tumor cords with a radius of less than about 160 μm. No tumor cord with a radius exceeding 200 μm was without a necrotic center. As the diameter of the necrotic area increased, the thickness of the sheath of viable tumor cells remained essentially constant at 100 to 180 μm.

## THE FIRST EXPERIMENTAL DEMONSTRATION OF HYPOXIC CELLS IN A TUMOR

The dilution assay technique, described in Chapter 5, was used by Powers and Tolmach to investigate the radiation response of a solid subcutaneous lymphosarcoma in the mouse. Survival estimates were made for doses between 2 and 20 Gy (200 and 2000 rads). The results are shown in Figure 8-10, in which the dose on a linear scale is plotted against the fraction of surviving cells on a logarithmic scale.

The survival curve for this solid tumor clearly consists of two separate components. The first, up to a dose of about 9 Gy (900 rads), has a slope ($D_0$) of 1.1 Gy (110 rads). The second has a shallower slope ($D_0$ = 2.6 Gy, or 260 rads). This biphasic survival curve has a final slope about two and one-half times shallower than the initial portion, which strongly suggests that the tumor consists of two separate groups of cells,

**Figure 8-8.** The diffusion of oxygen from a capillary through tumor tissue. The distance to which oxygen can diffuse is limited largely by the rapid rate at which it is metabolized by respiring tumor cells. For some distance from a capillary, cells are well oxygenated (*white*). At greater distances oxygen is depleted, and tumor cells become necrotic (*black*). Hypoxic tumor cells form a layer, perhaps one or two cells thick, in between (*gray*). In this region the oxygen concentration is high enough for the cells to be viable but low enough for them to be relatively protected from the effects of x-rays. These cells may limit the radiocurability of the tumor. The distance to which oxygen can diffuse is about 70 μm at the arterial end of a capillary and less at the venous end.

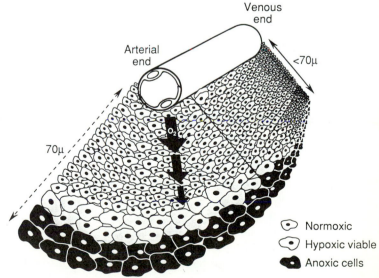

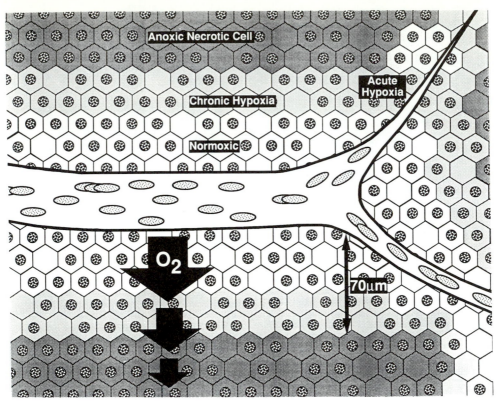

**Figure 8-9.** Diagram illustrating the difference between *chronic* and *acute* hypoxia. *Chronic hypoxia* results from the limited diffusion distance of oxygen in respiring tissue that is actively using up oxygen. Cells that become hypoxic in this way remain hypoxic for long periods of time until they die and become necrotic. *Acute hypoxia* results from the temporary closing of tumor blood vessels. The cells are intermittently hypoxic since normoxia is restored each time the blood vessel opens up again. (Redrawn from Brown JM: JNCI 82, 1990)

one oxygenated and the other hypoxic. If the shallow component of the curve is extrapolated backward to cut the surviving-fraction axis, it does so at a survival level of about 1%. From this it may be inferred that about 1% of the clonogenic cells in the tumor were deficient in oxygen.

The response of this tumor to single doses of radiation of various sizes is readily explained on this basis. If 99% of the cells are well oxygenated and 1% are hypoxic, the response to lower doses is dominated by the killing of the well-oxygenated cells. For these doses the hypoxic cells are depopulated to a negligibly small extent. Once a dose of about 9 Gy (900 rads) is exceeded, however, the oxygenated compartment of the tumor has been severely depopulated, and the response of the tumor is characteristic of the response of hypoxic cells. This was the first unequivocal demonstration that a solid tumor could contain cells sufficiently hypoxic to be protected from cell kill-

ing by x-rays but still clonogenic and capable of providing a focus for tumor regrowth.

## PROPORTION OF HYPOXIC CELLS IN VARIOUS ANIMAL TUMORS

Over the years many investigators have determined the fraction of hypoxic cells in a wide variety of tumors in experimental animals. The most satisfactory and most widely used method is to obtain paired survival curves (Fig. 8-11*A*). The steepest curve relates to a fully oxygenated population of cells; the uppermost curve, to a population made up entirely of hypoxic cells. The intermediate curves refer to mixed populations of hypoxic and oxygenated cells. At low doses the survival curve for a mixed population closely follows that for the oxygenated population. At higher doses the number of surviving oxygenated cells is negligible compared with the number of anoxic cells, and consequently the curve representing the mixed population is parallel to (ie, has the same slope as) the curve for the hypoxic population. The fraction of hypoxic cells in the tumor determines the distance between the parallel terminal slopes of the dose-response curves as shown in Figure 8-11A. This fraction is identical to the ratio of the surviving cells from the partially hypoxic tumor to those of the entirely hypoxic tumor.

In practice the procedure is as follows. Survival measurements are made at several dose levels, under two different conditions:

1. The animal (eg, a mouse) is asphyxiated several minutes before irradiation by breathing nitrogen. Under these conditions, *all* of the tumor cells are hypoxic and the data points obtained define a line comparable to the upper curve in Figure 8-11A.

2. The animal is alive and breathing air, so that the proportion of hypoxic cells in the tumor is at its normal level. The data points obtained define a lower line typical of a mixed population of hypoxic and oxygenated cells. The vertical separation between the two lines gives the proportion of hypoxic cells characteristic of that particular type of tumor.

An example of experimental data for a determination of the hypoxic fraction in a mouse tumor is shown in Figure 8-11B. Hypoxic fractions can also be calculated from a comparison of the $TCD_{50}$ values for clamped and unclamped tumors or from a comparison of growth delays from tumors irradiated under these two conditions. Any of these methods involves several assumptions, notably that cells made hypoxic artificially have the same sensitivity as those that have respired to this condition in the tumor naturally and that the tumor is composed of two distinct populations, one aerated and the other

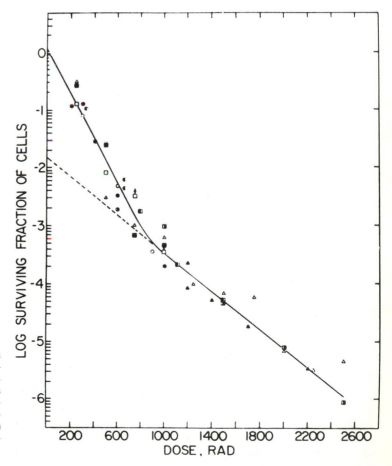

Figure 8-10. Fraction of surviving cells as a function of dose for a solid subcutaneous lymphosarcoma in the mouse irradiated in vivo. The first part of the curve has a slope ($D_0$) of 1.1 Gy (110 rads); the second component of the curve has a shallower slope of 2.6 Gy (260 rads). (From Powers WE, Tolmach LJ: Nature 197:710–711, 1963)

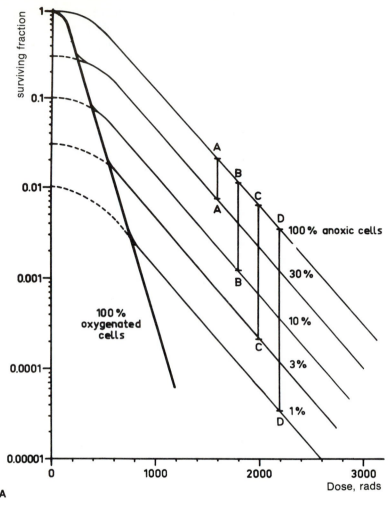

**A**

Figure 8-11. **(A)** Theoretical survival curves for cell populations containing different fractions of hypoxic cells. The fraction of hypoxic cells in each population determines the distance between its survival curve and the curve for the completely hypoxic population. From the relative radiosensitivity at any dose level at which the survival curves are approximated by parallel lines, the fraction of hypoxic cells can be determined from the ratio of survival of the completely and partially hypoxic populations, as indicated by the vertical lines A-A, B-B, and so on. This illustration is based on the model proposed by Hewitt and Wilson. (From van Putten LM, Kallman RF: Oxygenation status of a transplantable tumor during fractionated radiotherapy. JNCI 40:411–451, 1968) **(B)** The proportion of hypoxic cells in a mouse tumor. The biphasic curve labeled air curve represents data for cells from tumors irradiated in mice breathing air, which are therefore a mixture of aerated and hypoxic cells. The hypoxic curve is for cells irradiated in mice asphyxiated by nitrogen breathing or for cells irradiated in vitro in nitrogen, so that they are all hypoxic. The air curve is for cells irradiated in vitro in air. The proportion of hypoxic cells is the ratio of the air to hypoxic curves, or the vertical separation between the curves, since surviving fraction is on a logarithmic scale. (Courtesy of Dr. Sara Rockwell; based on data by Moulder and Rockwell and by Rockwell and Kallman)

hypoxic, with nothing falling in between. Consequently, measured values for hypoxic fractions can only serve as a guide and must not be taken too seriously.

Moulder and Rockwell published a survey of all published data in hypoxic fractions and reported that of 42 tumor types studied, 37 were

found to contain hypoxic cells in at least one study. Hypoxic fractions range from 0% to 50%, with a tendency for many results to average about 15%.

Comparable measurements cannot, of course, be made in human tumors to determine precisely the proportion of hypoxic cells. By irradiating pa-

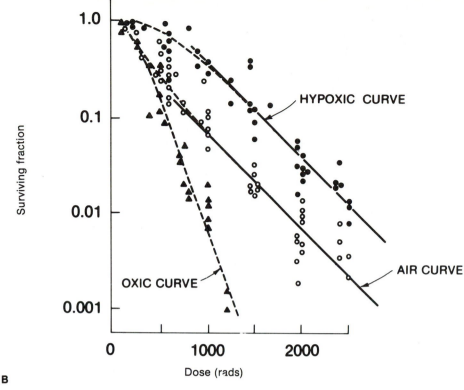

**B**

Figure 8-11. *(Continued)*

tients with multiple skin nodules with and without large doses of the hypoxic cell sensitizer misonidazole, Dische and Denekamp were able to estimate that the proportion of hypoxic cells was consistent with the 10% to 15% characteristic of many animal tumors.

## EVIDENCE FOR HYPOXIA IN HUMAN TUMORS

Although it is not possible to perform experiments in humans to unequivocally demonstrate that at least some tumors contain hypoxic cells, the circumstantial evidence is compelling.

- Analogy can be made with mouse tumors in which hypoxia can be demonstrated unequivocally.
- Histologic appearance suggests the possibility of hypoxia.
- Binding of radioactive-labeled nitroimidazoles occurs.
- Oxygen probe measurements are predictive.

- Pretreatment hemoglobin levels are a powerful prognostic factor in squamous carcinoma of the head and neck, carcinoma of the cervix, carcinoma of the bronchus, and transitional cell carcinoma of the bladder.

## OXYGEN PROBE MEASUREMENTS AS A PREDICTIVE ASSAY

Oxygen probes, that is, electrodes to implant directly into a tumor to measure oxygen concentration by a polarographic technique, have a long and chequered history. Technical developments have, however, resulted in the Eppendorf probe, which has a very fast response time and can be moved quickly through a tumor under computer control to produce an oxygen profile.

Oxygen probes may be used in individual patients before treatment as a predictive assay to sort out those with tumors that are significantly hypoxic. A preliminary clinical trial in Germany suggests that local control in advanced carcinoma of the cervix, treated by radiotherapy, correlated with oxygen probe measurements. This topic is discussed in more detail in Chapter 15.

## REOXYGENATION

Van Putten and Kallman determined the proportion of hypoxic cells in a transplantable sarcoma in the mouse. This tumor, which was of spontaneous origin, was transplanted from one generation of animals to the next by inoculating a known number of tumor cells subcutaneously. The tumor was allowed to grow for 2 weeks, by which time it had reached a size suitable for the experiment. The tumor was irradiated in vivo, then excised and made into a suspension of cells. The proportion of hypoxic cells was determined by the method described in Figure 8-11.

They found that for this mouse sarcoma the proportion of hypoxic cells in the untreated tumor was about 14%. The vital contribution made by van Putten and Kallman involved a determination of the proportion of hypoxic cells in this tumor *after* various fractionated radiation treatments. Groups of tumors were exposed to five daily doses of 1.9 Gy (190 rads), delivered from Monday to Friday, and the proportion of hypoxic cells was determined on the following Monday. The result was 18% hypoxic cells. In another experiment, four daily fractions were given, Monday to Thursday, and the proportion of hypoxic cells was measured on the following day, Friday. In this experiment the proportion of hypoxic cells was found to be 14%.

These experiments have far-reaching implications in radiotherapy. The fact that the proportion of hypoxic cells in the tumor is about the same at the end of a fractionated radiotherapy regimen as in the untreated tumor demonstrates that during the course of the treatment, cells moved from the hypoxic to the well-oxygenated compartment of the tumor. If this were not the case, then the *proportion* of hypoxic cells would increase during the course of the fractionated treatment because the radiation depopulates the aerated cell compartment more than the hypoxic cell compartment. This phenomenon, by which hypoxic cells become oxygenated after a dose of radiation, is termed **reoxygenation.** The oxygen status of cells in a tumor is not static; it is dynamic and constantly changing.

The process of reoxygenation is illustrated in Figure 8-12. A modest dose of x-rays to a mixed

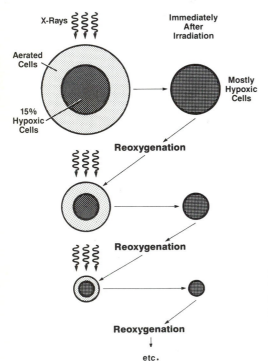

**Figure 8-12.** The process of reoxygenation. Tumors contain a mixture of aerated and hypoxic cells. A dose of x-rays kills a greater proportion of aerated than hypoxic cells because they are more radiosensitive. Immediately after irradiation, most cells in the tumor are hypoxic. But the preirradiation pattern tends to return because of reoxygenation. If the radiation is given in a series of fractions separated in time sufficiently for reoxygenation to occur, the presence of hypoxic cells does not greatly influence the response of the tumor.

population of aerated and hypoxic cells results in significant killing of aerated cells but little killing of those that are hypoxic. Consequently, the viable cell population immediately after irradiation is dominated by hypoxic cells. If a sufficient time is allowed before the next radiation dose, the process of reoxygenation will restore the proportion of hypoxic cells to about 15%. If this process is repeated many times, the tumor cell population will be depleted, despite the intransigence to killing by x-rays of the cells deficient in oxygen. In other words, if reoxygenation is efficient between dose fractions, the presence of hypoxic cells will not have a significant effect on the outcome of a multifraction regimen.

## TIME SEQUENCE
## OF REOXYGENATION

The work of van Putten and Kallman indicated that, in their particular tumor system, the proportion of hypoxic cells had returned to its original pretreatment level by 24 hours after the delivery of a fractionated dosage schedule. Kallman and Bleehen reported experiments in which the proportion of hypoxic cells in the same transplantable mouse sarcoma was determined at various times after the delivery of a single dose of 10 Gy (1000 rads). Their results are shown in Figure 8-13; the shape of the curve indicates that in this particular tumor the process of reoxygenation is very rapid indeed.

Similar results have subsequently been reported by a number of researchers using a variety of tumor systems. The patterns of reoxygenation observed in several different animal tumor systems are summarized in Figure 8-14. Two of the three animal tumors show efficient and rapid reoxygenation, with the proportion of hypoxic cells returning to or even falling below the pretreatment level.

The time sequence, however, is not the same for the three types of tumors. In particular, the mammary carcinoma investigated by Howes shows a minimum in the proportion of hypoxic cells that is very much lower than that characteristic of the unirradiated tumor. This occurs 3 days

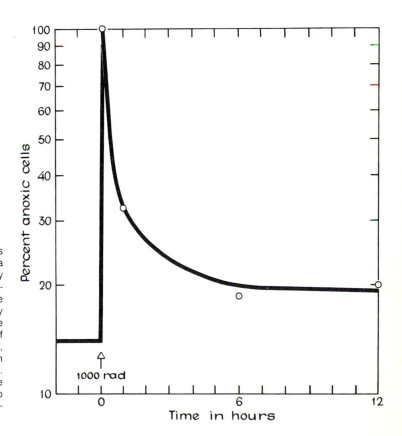

**Figure 8-13.** Percentage of hypoxic cells in a transplantable mouse sarcoma as a function of time after a dose of 10 Gy (1000 rads) of x-rays. Immediately after irradiation, essentially 100% of the viable cells are hypoxic because a dose of 10 Gy (1000 rads) kills a large proportion of the aerated cells. In this tumor the process of reoxygenation is very rapid. By 6 hours, the percentage of hypoxic cells has fallen to a value close to the preirradiation level. (From Kallman RF, Bleehen NM: In: Dose Rate in Mammalian Radiation Biology, pp 20.1–20.23. USAEC Publ CONF-680410, Biology and Medicine [Tid-4500], 1968)

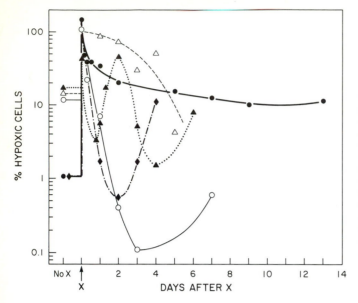

**Figure 8-14.** The proportion of hypoxic cells as a function of time after irradiation with a large dose for five transplanted tumors in experimental animals. Open circles indicate mouse mammary carcinoma that reoxygenates rapidly and well (data from Howes). Closed triangles indicate rat sarcoma that shows two waves of reoxygenation (data from Thomlinson). Open triangles show that mouse osteosarcoma that does not reoxygenate at all for several days and then but slowly (data from van Putten). Closed circles indicate mouse fibrosarcoma that reoxygenates quickly but not as completely as the mammary carcinoma (data from Dorie and Kallman). Closed diamonds indicate mouse fibrosarcoma that reoxygenates quickly and well (data from Kummermehr, Preuss-Bayer, and Trott). The extent and rapidity of reoxygenation is extremely variable and impossible to predict. (Courtesy of Dr. Sara Rockwell)

after the delivery of a single large dose of radiation. The only experimental tumor investigated so far that does not show any significant rapid reoxygenation is the osteosarcoma studied by van Putten, also illustrated in Figure 8-14.

## MECHANISM OF REOXYGENATION

In experimental animals, some tumors take several days to reoxygenate, while in others the process appears to be complete within an hour or so. In a few tumors both fast and slow components to reoxygenation are evident. The differences of time scale reflect the different types of hypoxia that are being reversed, namely, acute or chronic. In the long term, a restructuring or a revascularization of the tumor might be expected as the cells killed by the radiation are broken down and removed from the population. As the tumor shrinks in size, surviving cells that previously were beyond the range of oxygen diffusion find themselves closer to a blood supply and so reoxygenate. This slow component of reoxygenation, taking place over a period of days as the tumor shrinks, involves reoxygenation of cells that were *chronically* hypoxic.

By contrast, the first component of reoxygenation, that is complete within hours, is due to the reoxygenation of *acutely* hypoxic cells. Those cells that are hypoxic at the time of irradiation because they are in a region where a blood vessel is temporarily closed will quickly reoxygenate when that vessel reopens.

## THE IMPORTANCE OF REOXYGENATION IN RADIOTHERAPY

The process of reoxygenation has important implications in practical radiotherapy. If human tumors do in fact reoxygenate as rapidly and as efficiently as most of the animal tumors studied, then the use of a multifraction course of radiotherapy, extending over a long period of time, may well be all that is required to deal effectively with any hypoxic cells in human tumors.

Hypoxia confers an impressive measure of protection to x-rays, and also to many chemotherapeutic agents, at least those such as bleomycin for which free radicals are involved in the mechanism of cell killing.

The reoxygenation studies with $C_3H$ mouse mammary carcinoma, included in Figure 8-14, indicate that by 2 to 3 days after a dose of radiation, the proportion of hypoxic cells is actually *lower* than in untreated tumors. Consequently, it was predicted that several large doses of x-rays given at 48-hour intervals would virtually eliminate the problem of hypoxic cells in this tumor.

Fowler and his colleagues showed that, for the cure of this tumor, the preferred x-ray schedule was five large doses in 9 days. These results suggest that x-irradiation can be an extremely effective form of therapy but ideally requires a sharply optimal choice of fractionation pattern. Making this choice, however, demands a detailed knowledge of the time course of reoxygenation in the particular tumor to be irradiated. This information is available for only a few animal tumors and is impossible to obtain at present for the human. Indeed, in the human it is not known whether any or all tumors reoxygenate. Although the evidence from the radiotherapy clinic that many tumors are eradicated with doses on the order of 60 Gy (6000 rads) given in 30 treatments argues strongly in favor of reoxygenation, since the presence of a very small proportion of hypoxic cells would make "cures" unlikely at these dose levels. It is an attractive hypothesis that some of the human tumors that do not respond to conventional radiotherapy are those that do not reoxygenate quickly and efficiently.

## ► Summary of Pertinent Conclusions

- The presence or absence of molecular oxygen dramatically influences the biological effect of x-rays.
- The oxygen enhancement ratio (OER) is the ratio of doses without and with oxygen to produce the same biological effect.
- The OER for x-rays is about 3 at high doses and is possibly lower (about 2) at doses below about 2 Gy (200 rads).
- OER decreases as linear energy transfer (LET) increases. The OER approaches unity (ie, no oxygen effect) at an LET of about 160 keV/μm. For neutrons, the OER has an intermediate value of about 1.6.
- To produce its effect, oxygen must be present during the radiation exposure or at least during the lifetime of the free radicals ($10^{-5}$ second).
- Oxygen "fixes" (ie, makes permanent) the damage produced by free radicals. In the absence of oxygen, damage produced by the indirect action may be repaired. Oxygen modifies the indirect but not the direct action of radiation.
- Only a small quantity of oxygen is required for radiosensitization; 0.5% oxygen results in a sensitivity halfway between hypoxia and full oxygenation.
- There are two forms of hypoxia that are the consequence of different mechanisms: **chronic** hypoxia and **acute** hypoxia.
- Chronic hypoxia results from the limited diffusion range of oxygen through respiring tissue.
- Acute hypoxia is a result of the temporary closing of tumor blood vessels and is therefore transient.
- In either case there may be cells present during irradiation that are at a sufficiently low oxygen tension to be intransigent to killing by x-rays but high enough to be viable.
- Most transplantable tumors in animals have been shown to contain hypoxic cells that limit curability by single doses of x-rays. Hypoxic fractions vary from 0% to 50% but are frequently about 10% to 15%. Studies of hypoxic cell sensitizers indicate similar proportions in human tumor nodules.
- There is good evidence that human tumors contain hypoxic cells, too. This evidence includes histologic appearance, oxygen probe measurements, the binding of radioactive nitroimidazoles, and the importance of

*(continued)*

▶ **Summary of Pertinent Conclusions**   *(Continued)*

pretreatment hemoglobin levels as a prognostic factor for several types of malignancies.

- Oxygen probes with a fast response time, implanted in a tumor and moving quickly under computer control, may be used to obtain the oxygen profile of a tumor. One clinical trial suggests a correlation between median $PO_2$ values and local control in advanced carcinoma of the cervix treated by radiotherapy. This is discussed further in the Chapter 15.
- Reoxygenation is the process by which cells that are hypoxic at the time of irradiation become oxygenated afterward.
- The extent of reoxygenation and the rapidity with which it occurs varies widely for different experimental animal tumors.
- If reoxygenation is rapid and complete, hypoxic cells have little influence on the outcome of a fractionated radiation schedule.
- The "fast" component of reoxygenation is due to the reoxygenation of *acutely* hypoxic cells; as tumor blood vessels open and close, the slow component is due to the reoxygenation of *chronically* hypoxic cells as the tumor shrinks.
- Reoxygenation cannot be measured in human tumors, but presumably it occurs, at least in those tumors controlled by conventional fractionated radiotherapy.

- ***Evidence for Hypoxia in Human Tumors***

This topic is really outside the scope of a book on radiobiology, but for completeness, the reasons for thinking that some human tumors contain a significant proportion of hypoxic cells are listed below:

1. Local control by radiotherapy, but not survival due to distant metastasis, correlates closely with hemoglobin levels. This has been shown to be true for squamous cell carcinoma of the head and neck, cervix, and bronchus as well as transitional cell carcinoma of the bladder.
2. The histologic appearance of many human tumors suggests regions of hypoxia by analogy with animal tumors where the proportion of hypoxic cells can be measured.
3. Measurements with oxygen probes indicate regions of hypoxia in some human tumors; local control correlates with $PO_2$ levels.
4. Labeled nitroimidazoles are deposited near necrotic areas in some human tumors. This requires bioreduction and therefore implies hypoxia (see Chapter 10).
5. Hyperbaric oxygen and radiosensitizers such as misonidazole improve the results of radiotherapy in a few cases, particularly when a limited (suboptimal) number of dose fractions were used.

The evidence listed in the previous list shows with certainty that hypoxia is a factor in some human tumors. The urgent need is to discover the circumstances in which the presence of hypoxic cells limits tumor control in a full fractionated course of radiotherapy.

# BIBLIOGRAPHY

Brown JM: Evidence for acutely hypoxic cells in mouse tumours, and a possible mechanism of reoxygenation. Br J Radiol 52:650–656, 1979

Chaplin DJ, Durand RE, Olive PL: Acute hypoxia in tumors: Implications for modifiers of radiation effects. Int J Radiat Oncol Biol Phys 12:1279–1282, 1986

Chaplin DJ, Olive PL, Durand RE: Intermittent blood flow in a murine tumor: Radiobiological effects. Cancer Res 47:597–601, 1987

Crabtree HG, Cramer W: Action of radium on cancer cells: Some factors affecting susceptibility of cancer cells to radium. Proc R Soc Long [Biol] 113:238, 1933

Crabtree HG, Cramer W: The action of radium on cancer cells: I. Effects of hydrocyanic acid, iodoacetic acid, and sodium fluoride on the metabolism and transplantability of cancer cells. Sci Rep Imp Cancer Res Fund 11:75, 1934

Denekamp J: Cytoxicity and radiosensitization in mouse and man. Br J Radiol 51:636–637, 1978

Denekamp J, Fowler JF, Dische S: The proportion of hypoxic cells in a human tumor. Int J Radiat Oncol Biol Phys 2:1227–1228, 1977

Deschner EE, Gray LH: Influence of oxygen tension on x-ray–induced chromosomal damage in Ehrlich ascites tumor cells irradiated in vitro and in vivo. Radiat Res 11:115–146, 1959

Elkind MM, Swain RW, Alescio T, Sutton H, Moses WB: Oxygen, nitrogen, recovery, and radiation therapy. In Cellular Radiation Biology, pp 442–461. Baltimore, Williams & Wilkins, 1965

Gray LH, Conger AD, Ebert M, Hornsey S, Scott OCA: The concentraiton of oxygen dissolved in tissues at the time of irradiation as as factor in radiotherapy. Br J Radiol 26:628–6548, 1953

Groebe K, Vaupel P: Evaluation of oxygen diffusion distances in human breast cancer xenografts using tumor-specific in vivo data: Role of various mechanisms in the development of tumor hypoxia. Int J Radiat Oncol Biol Phys 15:691–697, 1988

Hill RP. Bush RS, Yeung P: The effect of anemia on the fraction of hypoxic cells in experimental tumor. Br J Radiol 44:299–304, 1971

Holthusen H; Beitrage zur Biologie der Strahlenwirkung. Pflugers Arch Gesamte Physiol 187:1–24, 1921

Howard-Flanders P, Alper T: The sensitivity of microorganisms to irradiation under controlled gas conditions. Radiat Res 7:518–540, 1957

Howard-Flanders P, Moore D: The time interval after pulsed irradiation within which injury in bacteria can be modified by dissolved oxygen: I. A search for an effect of oxygen 0.02 second after pulsed irradiation. Radiat Res 9:422–437, 1958

Howes AE: An estimation of changes in the proportion and absolute numbers of hypoxic cells after irradiation of transplanted $C_3H$ mouse mammary tumors. Br J Radiol 42:441–447, 1969

Kallman RF, Bleehen NM: Post-irradiation cyclic radiosensitity changes in tumors and normal tissues. In Brown DG, Cragle RG, Noonan JR (eds): Proceedings of the Symposium on Dose Rate in Mammalian Radiobiology, Oak Ridge, TN, 1968, pp 20.1–20.23. Springfield, VA, CONF-680410, 1968

Kallman RF, Jardine LJ, Johnson CW: Effects of different schedules of dose fractionation on the oxygenation status of a transplantable mouse sarcoma. JNCI 44:369–377, 1970

Michael BD, Adams GE, Hewitt HB, Jones WBG, Watts ME: A posteffect of oxygen in irradiated bacteria: A submillisecond fast mixing study. Radiat Res 54:239–251, 1973

Mottram JC: On the action of beta and gamma rays of radium on the cell in different states of nuclear division. Rep Cancer Labs (Middlesex Hospital, London) 30:98, 1913

Mottram JC: Factor of importance in radiosensitivity of tumours. Br J Radiol 9:606–614, 1936

Moulder JE, Rockwell S: Hypoxic fractions of solid tumors: Experimental techniques, methods of analysis and a survey of existing data. Int J Radiat Oncol Biol Phys 10:695–712, 1984

Palcic B, Skarsgard LD: Reduced oxygen enhancement ratio at low doses of ionizing radiation. Radiat Res 100:328–339, 1984

Petry E: Zur Kenntnis der Bedingungen der biologischen Wirkung der Röntgenstrahlen. Biochem Zeitschr 135:353, 1923

Powers WE, Tolmach LJ: A multicomponent x-ray survival curve for mouse lymphosarcoma cells irradiated in vivo. Nature 197:710–711, 1963

Read J: The effect of ionizing radiations on the broad bean root: I. The dependence of the alpha ray sensitivity on dissolved oxygen. Br J Radiol 25:651–661, 1952

Read J: The effect of ionizing radiations on the broad bean root: X. The dependence of the x-ray sensitivity of dissolved oxygen. Br J Radiol 25:89–99, 1952

Read J: Mode of action of x-ray doses given with different oxygen concentrations. Br J Radiol 25:336–338, 1952

Reinhold HS: The post-irradiation behaviour of transplantable solid tumors in relation to the regional oxygenation. In Turano L, Ratti A, Biagini C (eds): Progress in Radiology, vol 2, pp 1482–1486. Amsterdam, Excerpta Medica, 1967

Rockwell S, Moulder JE: Biological factors of importance in split-course radiotherapy. In Paliwal BR, Herbert DE, Orton CG (eds): Optimization of Cancer Radiotherapy, pp 171–182. New York, American Institute of Physics, 1985

Thomlinson RH: Changes of oxygenation in tumors in relation to irradiation. Front Radiat Ther Oncol 3:109–121, 1968

Thomlinson RH: Reoxygenation as a function of tumor size and histopathological type. In Proceedings of the Carmel Conference on Time and Dose Relationships in Radiation Biology as Applied to Radiotherapy, pp 242–254. Upton, NY, BNL Report 50203 (C-57), 1969

van Putten LM: Oxygenation and cell kinetics after irradiation in a transplantable osteosarcoma. In: Effects on Cellular Proliferation and Differentiation, pp 493–505. Vienna, IAEA, 1968

van Putten LM: Tumour reoxygenation during fractionated radiotherapy: Studies with a transplantable osteosarcoma. Eur J Cancer 4:173–182, 1968

van Putten LM, Kallman RF: Oxygenation status of a transplantable tumor during fractionated radiotherapy. JNCI 40:441–451, 1968

Vaupel P, Kallinowski F, Okunieff P: Blood flow, oxygen and nutrient supply, and metabolic microenvironment of human tumors: A review. Cancer Res 49:6449–6465, 1989

Wright EA, Howard-Flanders P: The influence of oxygen on the radiosensitivity of mammalian tissues. Acta Radiol 48:26–32, 1957

*Radiobiology for the Radiologist, Fourth Edition*, by Eric J. Hall
J. B. Lippincott Company, Philadelphia © 1994.

# 9

# Linear Energy Transfer and Relative Biological Effectiveness

THE DEPOSITION OF RADIANT ENERGY
LINEAR ENERGY TRANSFER (LET)
RELATIVE BIOLOGICAL EFFECTIVENESS
RBE AND FRACTIONATED DOSES
RBE FOR DIFFERENT CELLS AND TISSUES
RBE AS A FUNCTION OF LET
THE OPTIMAL LET
FACTORS THAT DETERMINE RBE
THE OXYGEN EFFECT AND LET
RADIATION WEIGHTING FACTOR
SUMMARY OF PERTINENT CONCLUSIONS

Radiation Therapy

153

# THE DEPOSITION OF RADIANT ENERGY

When radiation is absorbed in biological material, ionizations and excitations occur that are not distributed at random but tend to be localized along the tracks of individual charged particles in a pattern that depends on the type of radiation involved. For example, photons of x-rays give rise to fast electrons, particles carrying unit electric charge and having very small mass; neutrons, on the other hand, give rise to recoil protons, particles again carrying unit electric charge but having a mass nearly 2000 times greater than that of the electron. α-Particles carry two electric charges on a particle four times as heavy as a proton. The charge-to-mass ratio for α-particles therefore differs from that for electrons by a factor of about 8000.

As a result, the spatial distribution of the ionizing events produced by different particles varies enormously. This is illustrated in Figure 9-1. The background is an electron micrograph of a human liver cell. The white dots generated by a computer simulate ionizing events. The lowest track represents a low-energy electron, such as might be set in motion by a photon of diagnostic x-rays. The primary events are well separated in space, and for this reason x-rays are said to be **sparsely ionizing.** The second track from the bottom represents an electron set in motion by a photon of cobalt-60 γ-rays, which is even more

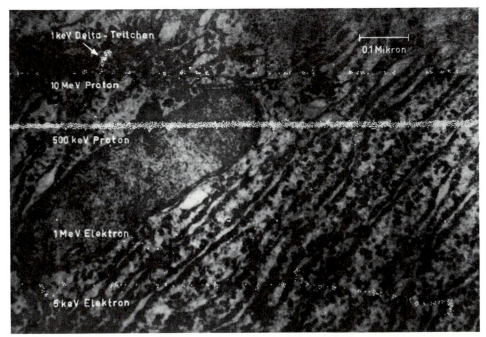

**Figure 9-1.** Variation of ionization density associated with different types of radiation. The background is an electron micrograph of a human cell. The white dots represent ionizations. (*Top to bottom*) *10-MeV proton*, typical of the recoil protons produced by high-energy neutrons used for radiotherapy. The track is intermediate in ionization density. Also shown is a secondary 1-keV δ-ray, an electron set in motion by the proton. *500-keV proton*, produced by lower energy neutrons (eg, from fission spectrum) or by higher energy neutrons after multiple collisions. The ionizations form a dense column along the track of the particle. *I-MeV electron*, produced, for example, by photons of cobalt-60 γ-rays. This particle is very sparsely ionizing. *5-keV electron*, typical of secondary electrons produced by x-rays of diagnostic quality. This particle is also sparsely ionizing but a little denser than the higher energy electron. (Courtesy of Dr. Albrecht Kellerer)

sparsely ionizing. For a given particle the density of ionization decreases as the energy goes up. The third track from the bottom represents a proton that might be set in motion by a fission spectrum neutron from a reactor; a dense column of ionization is produced, so the radiation is referred to as **densely ionizing.** The uppermost track refers to a 10-MeV proton, such as may be set in motion by a high-energy neutron used for radiotherapy. The track is intermediate in ionization density.

## LINEAR ENERGY TRANSFER

**Linear energy transfer** (LET), a term introduced by Zirkle, is the energy transferred per unit length of the track. The special unit usually used for this quantity is kiloelectron volt per micron (KeV/μm) of unit density material. The International Commission of Radiological Units in 1962 defined this quantity as follows:

> The linear energy transfer ($L$) of charged particles in medium is the quotient of $dE/dl$, where $dE$ is the average energy locally imparted to the medium by a charged particle of specified energy in traversing a distance of $dl$.

That is,

$$L = dE/dl$$

If it were possible to deal with monoenergetic particles—particles that all have the same energy—then their tracks would be similar, and LET would be meaningful. In practice, most radiations consist of a wide spectrum. For example, a 250-kV x-ray beam consists of photons with energies from a maximum of 250 keV down to the lowest energy that can escape through the tube casing and added filters. The tracks produced by such a conglomerate beam vary enormously.

As a result, LET can only be an average quantity. Furthermore, at the microscopic level, the energy per unit length of track varies over such a wide range that the average has very little meaning. This can be illustrated by the story of the Martian visitor to Earth who arrives knowing that Earth is inhabited by living creatures with an average mass of 1 g. Not only is this information of very little use, but it may also be positively misleading, particularly if the first animal that the

Martian encounters is an elephant. An average has little meaning when individual variation is great.

The situation for LET is further complicated by the fact that it is possible to calculate an average in many different ways. The most commonly used method is to calculate the **track average,** which is obtained by dividing the track into equal lengths, calculating the energy deposited in each length, and finding the mean. This is illustrated in Figure 9-2. The **energy average** is obtained by dividing the track into equal energy increments and averaging the lengths of track over which these energy increments are deposited.

In the case of either x-rays, or monoenergetic charged particles, the two methods of averaging yield similar results. In the case of 14-MeV neutrons, by contrast, the track average LET is about 12 keV/μm while the energy average LET is about 75 keV/μm. The biological properties of neutrons tend to correlate with the energy average.

As a result of these considerations, LET is a quantity condemned by the purists as worse than useless, since it can in some circumstances be very misleading. It is, however, useful as a simple and naive way to indicate the quality of different types of radiation. Typical LET values for commonly used radiations are listed in Table 9-1. Note that for a given type of charged particle, the higher the energy, the *lower* the LET and therefore the lower its biological effectiveness. For example, γ-rays and x-rays both give rise to fast secondary electrons; therefore 1.1 MV cobalt-60 γ-rays have a lower LET than 250 kV x-rays and are less effective biologically by about 10%. By

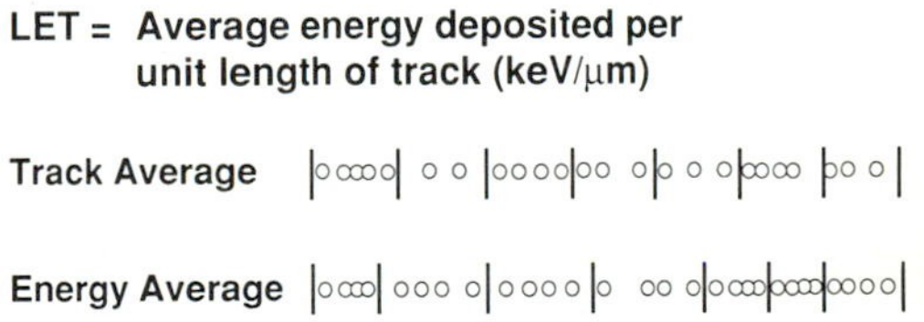

LET = **Average energy deposited per unit length of track (keV/μm)**

**Figure 9-2.** Linear energy transfer (LET) is the average energy deposited per unit length of track. The *track average* is calculated by dividing the track into equal lengths and averaging the energy deposited in each length. The *energy average* is calculated by dividing the track into equal energy intervals and averaging the lengths of the tracks that contain this amount of energy. The method of averaging makes little difference for x-rays or for monoenergetic charged particles, but the track average and energy average are different for neutrons.

Table 9-1.
Typical LET Values

| RADIATION | | LET (keV/μm) | |
|---|---|---|---|
| Cobalt-60 γ-rays | | 0.2 | |
| 250-kV x-rays | | 2.0 | |
| 10-MeV protons | | 4.7 | |
| 150-MeV protons | | 0.5 | |
| | Track Avg. | | Energy Avg. |
| 14-MeV neutrons | 12 | | 100 |
| 2.5-MeV α-particles | | 166 | |
| 2-GeV Fe ions | | 1000 | |

the same token, 150-MeV protons have a lower LET than 10-MeV protons, and therefore are slightly less effective biologically.

## RELATIVE BIOLOGICAL EFFECTIVENESS

The amount or quantity of radiation is expressed in terms of the **dose,** a physical quantity with the units of gray or rad. Dose is a measure of the energy absorbed per unit mass of tissue. Equal doses of different types of radiation do not, however, produce *equal* biological effects. One gray of neutrons produces a greater biological effect than 1 Gy of x-rays. The key to the difference lies in the pattern of energy deposition at the microscopic level.

In comparing different radiations it is customary to use x-rays as the standard. The formal definition of **relative biological effectiveness** (RBE) is as follows:

The RBE of some test radiation (r) compared with x-rays is defined by the ratio $D_{250}/D_r$, where $D_{250}$ and $D_r$ are, respectively, the doses of x-rays and the test radiation required for equal biological effect.

To measure the RBE of some test radiation, one first chooses a biological system in which the effect of radiations may be scored quantitatively. To illustrate the process involved, we will discuss a specific example. Suppose we are measuring the RBE of fast neutrons compared with 250-kV x-rays, using the lethality of plant seedlings as a test system. Groups of plants are exposed to various doses of x-rays, while parallel groups are ex-

posed to a range of neutron doses. At the end of the period of observation, it is possible to calculate the dose of x-rays and then of neutrons, which results in the death of half of the plants in a group. This quantity is known as the $LD_{50}$, the mean lethal dose. Suppose that for x-rays the $LD_{50}$ turns out to be 6 Gy (600 rads) and that for neutrons the corresponding quantity is 4 Gy (400 rads). The RBE of neutrons compared with x-rays is then simply the ratio 6/4, or 1.5.

The study of RBE is relatively straightforward so long as a test system with a single, unequivocal end point is used. It becomes more complicated if, instead, a test system such as the response of mammalian cells in culture is chosen. Figure 9-3*A* shows survival curves obtained when mammalian cells in cultures are exposed to a range of doses of, on the one hand, fast neutrons and, on the other hand, 250-kV x-rays. The RBE may now be calculated from these survival curves as the ratio of doses that produce the same biological effect. If the endpoint chosen for comparison is the dose required to produce a surviving fraction of 0.01, then the dose of neutrons necessary is 6.6 Gy (660 rads), while the corresponding dose of x-rays is 10 Gy (1000 rads). The RBE, then, is the quotient of 10/6.6, or 1.5. If the comparison is made at a surviving fraction of 0.6, however, the neutron dose required is only 1 Gy (100 rads) and the corresponding x-ray dose is 3 Gy (300 rads). The resultant RBE is 3/1, or 3.0. Because the x-ray and neutron survival curves have different *shapes*, the x-ray survival curve having an initial shoulder while the neutron curve is an exponential function of dose, the resultant RBE will depend on the level of biological damage (and therefore the dose) chosen.

## RBE AND FRACTIONATED DOSES

Because the RBE of more densely ionizing radiations, such as neutrons, varies with the dose per fraction, the RBE for a fractionated regimen with neutrons will be greater than for a single exposure, because a fractionated schedule consists of a number of small doses and the RBE is large for small doses.

Figure 9-3*B* illustrates a hypothetical treatment with neutrons consisting of four fractions. For a

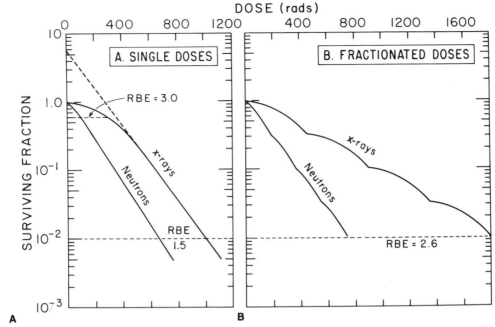

**Figure 9-3.** Typical survival curves for mammalian cells exposed to x-rays and fast neutrons. **(A)** Single doses. The survival curve for x-rays has a large initial shoulder; for fast neutrons the initial shoulder is smaller and the final slope steeper. Because the survival curves have different shapes, the relative biological effectiveness (RBE) does not have a unique value but varies with dose, getting larger as the size of the dose is reduced. **(B)** Fractionated doses. The effect of giving doses of x-rays or fast neutrons in four equal fractions to produce the same level of survival as in *A*. The shoulder of the survival curves is re-expressed after each dose fraction; since the shoulder is larger for x-rays than for neutrons, this results in an enlarged RBE for fractionated treatments.

surviving fraction of 0.01 the RBE for neutrons relative to x-rays is about 2.6. The RBE for the same radiations in Figure 9-3*A* at the same level of survival was 1.5 because only single exposures were involved. This is a direct consequence of the larger shoulder that is characteristic of the x-ray curve, which must be repeated for each fraction. The width of the shoulder represents a part of the dose that is wasted; the larger the number of fractions, the greater the extent of the wastage. By contrast, the neutron survival curve has little or no shoulder, so there is correspondingly less wastage of dose from fractionation. The net result is that neutrons become progressively more efficient than x-rays as the dose per fraction is reduced and the number of fractions is increased. The same is true, of course, for exposure to continuous low dose-rate irradiation. The neutron RBE will be larger at low dose rate than for an acute exposure, since the effectiveness of neutrons decreases with dose rate to a much smaller extent than is the case for x or γ-

rays. Indeed, for low-energy neutrons there is no loss of effectiveness.

## RBE FOR DIFFERENT CELLS AND TISSUES

Even for a given total dose or dose per fraction, the RBE varies greatly according to the tissue or endpoint studied. Broerse and Barendsen and their colleagues in the Netherlands have obtained survival curves for a number of different cell lines exposed to either neutrons or x-rays. A summary of their data is shown in Figure 9-4, which illustrates the differences in intrinsic radiosensitivity among the various types of cells. In this figure survival curves are presented for mouse bone marrow stem cells, mouse lymphocytic leukemia cells, cultured cells of human kidney origin, rat rhabdomyosarcoma cells, and mouse intestinal crypt cells. These curves demonstrate clearly that different cells exhibit a considerable spectrum of

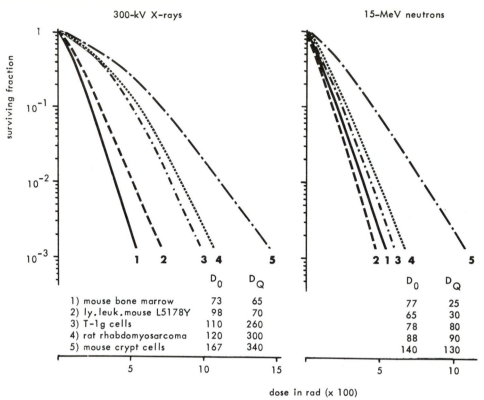

Figure 9-4. Survival curves for various types of clonogenic mammalian cells irradiated with 300-kV x-rays or 15-MeV d⁺→T neutrons: curve 1, mouse hematopoietic stem cells; curve 2, mouse lymphocytic leukemia cells L5178Y; curve 3, Tl cultured cells of human kidney origin; curve 4, rat rhabdomyosarcoma cells; curve 5, mouse intestinal crypt stem cells. Note that the variation in radiosensitivity among different cell lines is markedly less for neutrons than for x-rays. (Broerse JJ, Barendsen GW: Curr Top Radiat Res Q 8:305–350, 1973)

radiosensitivities for x-rays. Of the cells tested, bone marrow stem cells are the most sensitive, while intestinal crypt cells are the most resistant.

There is still a range of radiosensitivities for irradiation with neutrons, but the differences between the various cell types is now much smaller. The principal difference is that the x-ray survival curves have large and variable initial shoulders; the shoulder region for neutrons is smaller and less variable. As a consequence, the RBE will be different for each cell line. In general, cells characterized by an x-ray survival curve with a *large shoulder,* indicating that they can accumulate and repair a large amount of sublethal radiation damage, will show a large RBE for neutrons. Conversely, cells for which the x-ray survival curve has *little if any shoulder* will exhibit small neutron RBE values.

In Figure 9-4 the crypt cells of the mouse jejunum have the largest shoulder to their x-ray sur-

vival curve; they also result in the highest neutron RBE. At the other end of the scale, colony-forming units in the bone marrow are characterized by a survival curve that is close to an exponential function of dose, with little if any shoulder. The RBE for neutrons is likewise smallest for this biological system.

## RBE AS A FUNCTION OF LET

Figure 9-5 illustrates the survival curves obtained for x-rays, 15-MeV neutrons, and α-particles. As the LET increases from about 2 keV/μm for x-rays up to 150 keV/μm for α-particles, the survival curve changes in two important respects. First, the survival curve becomes steeper. Second, the extrapolation number tends toward unity; that is, the shoulder of the curve becomes

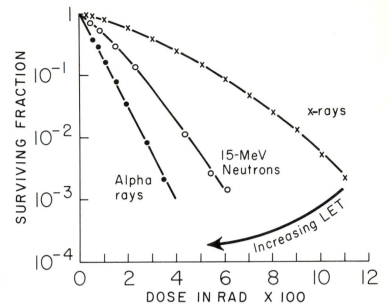

**Figure 9-5.** Survival curves for cultured cells of human origin exposed to 250-kVp x-rays, 15-MeV neutrons, and 4-MeV α-particles. As the LET of the radiation increases, the slope of the survival curves gets steeper and the size of the initial shoulder gets smaller. (Redrawn from Broerse JJ, Barensen GW, van Kersen, GR: Int J Radiat Biol 13:559–572, 1967; Barendsen GW: Curr Top Radiat Res Q 4:293–356, 1968)

progressively smaller as the LET increases. A more common way to represent these data is to plot the RBE as a function of LET (Fig. 9-6). As the LET increases, the RBE increases slowly at first, and then more rapidly as the LET increases beyond 10 keV/μm. Between 10 and 100 keV/μm, the RBE increases rapidly with increasing LET and in fact reaches a maximum at about 100 keV/μm. Beyond this value for the LET, the RBE again falls to lower values. This is an important effect and is explained in more detail in the next section.

The LET at which the RBE reaches a peak is much the same (about 100 keV/μm) for a wide range of mammalian cells, from mouse to human, and is the same for mutation as an endpoint as for cell killing. It probably reflects the "target" size and is related to the DNA content, which is similar for all mammalian cells.

## THE OPTIMAL LET

It is of interest to inquire why radiation with a LET of about 100 keV/μm is optimal in terms of producing a biological effect. At this density of ionization, the *average* separation between ionizing events just about coincides with the diameter of the DNA double helix (20 Å or 2 nm).

Radiation with this density of ionization is most likely to cause a double-strand break by the passage of a single charged particle, and double-strand breaks are the basis of most biological effects, as discussed in Chapter 2. This is illustrated in Figure 9-7. In the case of x-rays, which are more sparsely ionizing, the probability of a single track causing a double-strand break is low, and in general more than one track will be required. As a consequence, x-rays have a low biological effectiveness. At the other extreme, much more densely ionizing radiations (with a LET of 200 keV/μm, for example) will readily produce double-strand breaks, but energy will be "wasted" because the ionizing events are too close together. Since RBE is the ratio of *doses* to produce equal biological effect, this more densely ionizing radiation will have a lower RBE than the optimal LET radiation. The more densely ionizing radiation will be just as effective *per track*, but less effective per unit dose. It is possible, therefore, to understand why RBE reaches a maximum value in terms of the production of double-strand breaks, since the interaction of two double-strand breaks to form an exchange type aberration is the basis of most biological effects. Radiations having this optimal LET include neutrons of a few hundred kiloelectron volts, as well as low energy protons and α-particles.

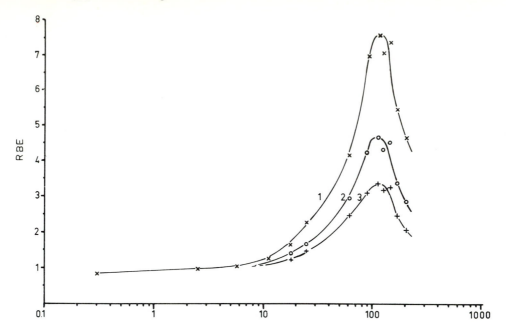

**Figure 9-6.** Variation of RBE with LET for survival of mammalian cells of human origin. The RBE rises to a maximum at an LET of about 100 keV/μm and subsequently falls for higher values of LET. Curves 1, 2, and 3 refer to cell survival levels of 0.8, 0.1, and 0.01, respectively, illustrating that the absolute value of the RBE is not unique but depends on the level of biological damage and, therefore, on the dose level. (From Barendsen GW: Curr Top Radiat Res Q 4:293–356, 1968)

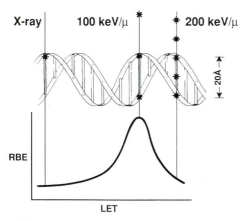

**Figure 9-7.** Diagram illustrating why radiation with an LET of 100 keV/μm has the greatest RBE for cell killing, mutagenesis, or oncogenic transformation. For this LET, the average separation between ionizing events coincides with the diameter of the DNA double helix (ie, about 20 Å [2 nm]). Radiation of this quality is most likely to produce a double-strand break from one track for a given absorbed dose.

## FACTORS THAT DETERMINE RBE

The earlier discussion of RBE began with a simple illustration of how this ratio may be determined for neutrons compared with x-rays, using a simple biological test system with a single, unequivocal endpoint, such as the $LD_{50}$ for plant seedlings. Under these circumstances, RBE is conceptually very simple. In the years immediately after World War II it was commonplace to see references to *the* RBE for neutrons, as if it were a single, unique quantity.

Now that more information is available from different biological systems, many of which allow the researcher to investigate the relationship between biological response and radiation dose rather than observing one endpoint at a single dose, it is apparent that RBE is a very complex quantity. RBE depends on the following:

Radiation quality (LET)
Radiation dose
Number of dose fractions
Dose rate
Biological system or endpoint

In this context, radiation quality means the type of radiation and its energy, whether electromagnetic or particulate and whether charged or un-charged. To a first approximation, the RBE varies with the LET, which for charged particles is about proportional to $Q^2/V$, where $Q$ is the charge carried by the particle and $V$ is its velocity.

RBE depends on the dose level and the number of dose fractions (or alternatively, the dose per fraction) because, in general, the shape of the dose–response relationship varies for radiations that differ substantially in their LET.

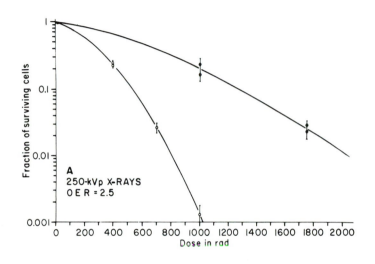

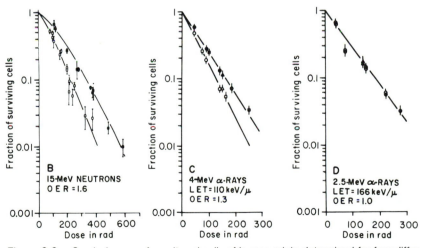

**Figure 9-8.** Survival curves for cultured cells of human origin determined for four different types of radiation. Open circles refer to aerated and closed circles to hypoxic conditions. **(A)** 250-kVp x-rays; OER = 2.5. **(B)** 15-MeV d⁺ →T neutrons; OER = 1.6. **(C)** 4-MeV α-particles; LET, 110 KeV/μm; OER = 1.3. **(D)** 2.5-MeV α-particles; LET, 166 keV/μm; OER = 1. (Redrawn from Broerse JJ, Barendsen GW: Int J Radiat Biol 13:559, 1967; and Barendsen GW, Koot CJ, van Kersen GR, Bewley DK, Field SB, Parnell CJ: Int J Radiat Biol 10:317–327, 1966)

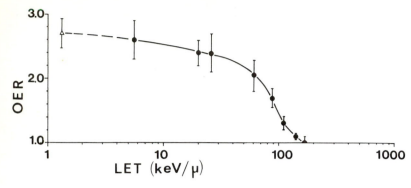

**Figure 9-9.** OER as a function of LET. Measurements of OER were made with cultured cells of human origin. Closed circles refer to monoenergetic charged particles, the open triangle to 250-kVp x-rays with an assumed track average LET of 1.3 keV/μ. (From Barendsen GW, Koot CJ, van Kersen GR, Bewley DK, Field SB, Parnell CJ: Int J Radiat Biol 10:317–327, 1966)

RBE can vary with the dose rate because the slope of the dose–response curve for sparsely ionizing radiations, such as x- or γ-rays, varies critically with a changing dose rate. By contrast, the biological response to densely ionizing radiations depends little on the rate at which the radiation is delivered.

The biological system or endpoint that is chosen has a marked influence on the RBE values obtained. In general, RBE values are high for tissues that accumulate and repair a great deal of sublethal damage and low for those that do not.

## THE OXYGEN EFFECT AND LET

A most important relationship exists between LET and the oxygen enhancement ratio (OER). Figure 9-8 shows mammalian cell survival curves for various types of radiation that have very different LETs and that exhibit very different OERs. Figure 9-8*A* refers to x-rays, which are sparsely ionizing, have a low LET, and consequently exhibit a large OER of about 2.5. Figure 9-8*B* refers to neutrons, which are intermediate in ionizing density and characteristically show an OER of 1.6. Figure 9-8*D* refers to 2.5-MeV α-particles, which have densely ionizing high-LET radiation; survival estimates, whether in the presence or absence of oxygen, fall along a common line, and so the OER is unity. Figure 9-8*C* contains data for 4-MeV α-particles, which are slightly less densely ionizing; in this case the OER is about 1.3.

Barendsen and his colleagues have used mammalian cells cultured in vitro to investigate the OER for a wide range of radiation types. Their results are summarized in Figure 9-9, in which OER is plotted as a function of LET. At low LET, corresponding to x- or γ-rays, the OER is between 2.5 and 3; as the LET increases, the OER falls slowly at first, until the LET exceeds about 60 keV/μm, after which the OER falls rapidly and reaches unity by the time the LET has reached about 200 keV/μm.

Both OER and RBE are plotted as a function of LET in Figure 9-10. (The curves are taken from the more complete plots in Figures 9-6 and 9-9.) Interestingly, the two curves are virtually mirror

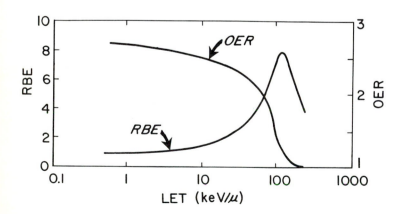

**Figure 9-10.** Variation of the oxygen enhancement ratio (OER) and the relative biological effectiveness (RBE) as a function of the LET of the radiation involved. The data were obtained by using T1 kidney cells of human origin, irradiated with various naturally occurring α-particles or with deuterons accelerated in the Hammersmith cyclotron. Note that the rapid increase of RBE and the rapid fall of OER occur at about the same LET, 100 keV/μm. (Redrawn from Barendsen GW: In: Proceedings of the Conference on Particle Accelerators in Radiation Therapy, pp 120–125. US Atomic Energy Commission, Technical Information Center, LA-5180-C, October 1972)

images of one another. The optimal RBE and the rapid fall of OER occur at about the same LET value, namely 100 keV/μm.

# RADIATION WEIGHTING FACTOR

Radiations differ in their biological effectiveness per unit of absorbed dose, as discussed earlier. The complexities of RBE are too difficult to apply in specifying dose limits in radiation protection; it is necessary to have a simpler way to consider differences in biological effectiveness of different radiations. One rad of neutrons, for example, is more hazardous than 1 rad of x-rays. The term **radiation weighting factor** ($W_R$) has been introduced for this purpose. The quantity produced by multiplying the absorbed dose by the weighting factor is called the *equivalent dose*. When dose is expressed in gray, (Gy), the equivalent dose is in sieverts (Sv); when dose is in rads, the equivalent dose is in rems. Radiation weighting factors are chosen by the International Commission on Radiological Protection (ICRP), based on a consideration of experimental RBE values, biased for biological endpoints relevant to radiation protection at low dose and low dose rate. There is a considerable element of judgment involved. The $W_R$ is set at unity for all low LET radiations (x-rays, γ-rays, and electrons), with a value of 20 for maximally effective neutrons and α-particles. Detailed values recommended by the ICRP are discussed in more detail in Chapter 25. Thus, using this system, an absorbed dose of 0.1 Gy (10 rads) of radiation with a radiation weighting factor of 20 would result in an equivalent dose of 2 Sv (200 rem).

► *Summary of Pertinent Conclusions*

- X- and γ-rays are called sparsely ionizing because along the tracks of the electrons set in motion, primary ionizing events are well separated in space.
- α-Particles and neutrons are densely ionizing because the tracks consist of dense columns of ionization.
- Linear energy transfer (LET) is the energy transferred per unit length of track. Typical values are 0.3 keV/μm for cobalt-60 γ-rays, 2 keV/μm for 250-kV x-rays, and 100 to 2000 keV/μm for heavy charged particles.
- Relative biological effectiveness (RBE) of some test radiation (r) is the ratio $D_x/D_r$, where $D_x$ and $D_r$ are the doses of 250-kV x-rays and the test radiation, respectively, required to produce equal biological effect.
- RBE increases with LET to a maximum at about 100 keV/μm, thereafter decreasing with higher LET.
- For radiation with the optimal LET of 100 keV/μm, the average separation between ionizing events is similar to the diameter of the DNA double helix (2 nm). It can most efficiently produce a double-strand break by a single track.
- The RBE of high-LET radiations compared with low-LET radiations increases as the dose per fraction decreases. This is a direct consequence of the fact that the dose–response curve for low-LET radiations has a broader shoulder than for high-LET radiations.
- RBE varies according to the tissue or endpoint studied. In general, RBE values are high for cells or tissues that accumulate and repair a great deal of sublethal damage, so that their dose–response curves for x-rays have a broad initial shoulder.
- RBE depends on the following:

*(continued)*

▶ *Summary of Pertinent Conclusions* *(Continued)*

> Radiation quality (LET)
> Radiation dose
> Number of fractions
> Dose rate
> Biological system or endpoint
>
> - The oxygen enhancement ratio (OER) has a value of about 3 for low-LET radiations, falls when the LET rises above about 30 keV/µm, and reaches unity by an LET of about 200 keV/µm.
> - The radiation weighting factor ($W_R$) depends on LET and is specified by the International Commission on Radiological Protection as a representative RBE at low dose and low dose rate for biological effects relevant to radiation protection such as cancer induction and heritable effects. It is used in radiological protection to reduce radiations of different biological effectiveness to a common scale.
> - Equivalent dose is the product of absorbed dose and the radiation weighting factor ($W_R$). If absorbed dose is expressed in gray (Gy), equivalent dose is in sieverts (Sv). If absorbed dose is in rads, equivalent dose is in rems.

# BIBLIOGRAPHY

Barendsen GW: Impairment of the proliferative capacity of human cells in culture by alpha particles with differing linear energy transfer. Int J Radiat Biol 8:453–466, 1964

Barendsen GW, Beusker TLJ, Vergroesen AJ, Budke L: Effects of different ionizing radiations on human cells in tissue culture: II. Biological experiments. Radiat Res 13:841–849, 1960

Barendsen GW, Walter HMD: Effects of different ionizing radiations on human cells in tissue culture: IV. Modification of radiation damage. Radiat Res 18:106–119, 1963

Berry RJ, Bewley DK, Parnell CJ: Reproductive capacity of mammalian tumor cells irradiated in vivo with cyclotron-produced fast neutrons. Br J Radiol 38:613–617, 1965

Bewley DK: Radiobiological research with fast neutrons and the implications for radiotherapy. Radiology 86:251–257, 1966

Bewley DK, Field SB, Morgan RL, Page BC, Parnell CJ: The response of pig skin to fractionated treatments with fast neutrons and x-rays. Br J Radiol 40:765–770, 1967

Broerse JJ, Barendsen GW: Relative biological effectiveness of fast neutrons for effects on normal tissues. Curr Top Radiat Res Q 8:305–350, 1973

Field SB: The relative biological effectiveness of fast neutrons for mammalian tissues. Radiology 93:915–920, 1969

Field SB, Jones T, Thomlinson RH: The relative effect of fast neutrons and x-rays on tumor and normal tissue in the rat: II. Fractionation recovery and reoxygenation. Br J Radiol 41:597–607, 1968

Fowler JF, Morgan RL: Pretherapeutic experiments with the fast neutron beam from the Medical Research Council Cyclotron: VIII. General review. Br J Radiol 36:115–121, 1963

International Commission on Radiation Units and Measurements: The quality factor in radiation protection. Report 40. Bethesda, MD, ICRU, 1986

ICRP: Recommendations of the International Commission on Radiological Protection: International Commission on Radiological Protection publication 26. New York, Pergamon Press, 1977

ICRP: Recommendations of the International Commission on Radiological Protection. Oxford, Pergamon Press, 1990

ICRP/ICRU: Report of the RBE Committee to the International Commissions on Radiological Protection and on Radiological Units and Measurements. Health Phys 9:357, 1963

ICRU: Radiation Quantities and Units. Report 33. Washington, DC, International Commission on Radiation Units and Measurements, 1980

*Radiobiology for the Radiologist, Fourth Edition,* by Eric J. Hall
J. B. Lippincott Company, Philadelphia © 1994.

*10*

# Radiosensitizers and Bioreductive Drugs

Radiation Therapy

Radiosensitizers are chemical or pharmacologic agents that increase the lethal effects of radiation when administered in conjunction with it. Many compounds that modify the radiation response of mammalian cells have been discovered over the years, but most offer no practical gain in radiotherapy because they do not show a **differential effect** between tumors and normal tissues. There is no point in employing a drug that increases the sensitivity of tumor and normal cells to the same extent.

When this all-important criterion of a differential effect is applied, only two types of sensitizers have found practical use in clinical radiotherapy:

1. The halogenated pyrimidines, which sensitize cells to a degree dependent on the amount of the analogue incorporated. In this case a differential effect is based on the premise that tumor cells cycle faster and, therefore, incorporate more of the drug than the surrounding normal tissues.
2. Hypoxic cell sensitizers, which increase the radiosensitivity of cells deficient in molecular oxygen but have no effect on normally aerated cells. In this case a differential effect is based on the premise that hypoxic cells occur only in tumors and not in normal tissues.

These two classes of sensitizers are discussed in turn. The basic strategy of all radiosensitizers is illustrated in Figure 10-1. The aim is to move the tumor control curve to lower doses by sensitizing tumor cells while not affecting the normal tissue complication curve, or at least not altering it as much. The outcome would be to increase the tumor control probability that would be achieved for a given level of normal tissue complications.

## THE HALOGENATED PYRIMIDINES

The combining size (the van der Waal radius) of an atom of chlorine, bromine, or iodine is very similar to that of the methyl group $CH_3$. The halogenated pyrimidines, 5-iododeoxyuridine and 5-bromodeoxyuridine, are consequently very similar indeed to the normal DNA precursor thymidine, having a halogen substituted in place of the methyl group.

The similarity is so close that they are incorporated into the DNA chain in place of thymidine. This substitution "weakens" the DNA chain, and consequently the cells are more susceptible to damage by $\gamma$-rays or ultraviolet light. These substances are effective as sensitizers only if they are made available to cells for several cell generations, so that an appreciable quantity of the analogue may be actually incorporated into the DNA. As the percentage of thymidine bases replaced increases, so does the extent of radiosensitization.

The effectiveness of the halogenated pyrimidines as sensitizers was first shown in bacteria,

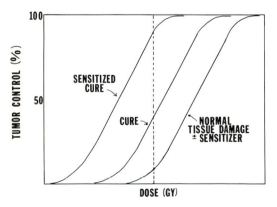

**Figure 10-1.** The basic strategy of all radiosensitizers. The addition of the drug is expected to move the tumor control curve to the left, while not affecting the normal tissue complication curve, or at least not altering it as much. For halogenated pyrimidines this expectation is based on the premise that tumor cells are cycling more rapidly than cells of the dose-limiting normal tissues so that they incorporate more sensitizer. For hypoxic cell radiosensitizers this expectation is based on the premise that hypoxic cells are present only in tumors, not in normal tissues, and these drugs preferentially sensitize hypoxic cells. (Based on an idea by Dr. Ged Adams)

but a similar effect has been amply demonstrated in mammalian cells both in vitro and in vivo. Figure 10-2 shows the sensitization of hamster cells to x-rays and to fluorescent light by the incorporation of bromodeoxyuridine and iododeoxyuridine. Although there is little to choose between the bromine or the iodine analogues as far as sensitization to x-rays is concerned, bromodeoxyuridine is a much more efficient sensitizer for fluorescent light. This turns out to be an important difference in the clinical application of these drugs. One of the unpleasant side effects of bromodeoxyuridine in some patients is a rash, caused by phototoxicity from the interaction of light with the drug. This is much less of a problem with the iodine analogue, as might be predicted from Figure 10-2.

The use of halogenated pyrimidines as an adjunct to radiotherapy began in the 1970s. The rationale was that tumor cells may be cycling more rapidly than the normal cells in surrounding tissues, so that more drug could be replaced in the tumor cell DNA, resulting in "selective" radiosensitization. It was perhaps unfortunate that head

and neck tumors were among those treated in this early study at Stanford University, since they are surrounded by actively proliferating normal tissues. The choice of tumors in the head and neck was determined partly by the need to deliver the analogue by an intraarterial infusion into the main vessel supplying the neoplasm to be treated, because the liver tends to dehalogenate the circulating drug. Tumor responses were reported to be good, but normal tissue damage was unacceptable.

Consequently, these sensitizers were not used for a number of years, until several centers began an evaluation in more suitable tumor sites, where the proximity of actively proliferating normal tissues is not such a problem. Among the tumors evaluated were high-grade glioblastomas and large unresectable sarcomas.

Since the all-important differential effect between tumor and normal tissues is based on the greater uptake of the halogenated pyrimidines in the malignant cells, the most appropriate tumors are those characterized by a high growth fraction and high labeling index, both indicators of cell

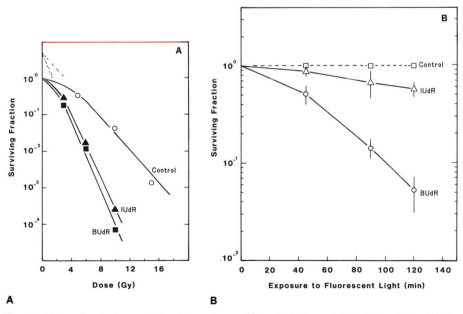

**Figure 10-2.** Survival curves for bromodeoxyuridine (BUdR)- and iododeoxyuridine (IUdR)-substituted cells exposed to x-rays **(A)** and fluorescent light **(B)**. Both halogenated pyrimidines sensitize equally to x-rays, and there is little to choose between them on this count. However, iododeoxyuridine has little effect with fluorescent light; thus it is preferred clinically because it avoids the light-induced rash produced by bromodeoxyuridine. (From Mitchell JB, Morstyn G, Russo A, Kinsella TJ, Fornace A, McPherson S. Gladstein E: Int J Radiat Oncol Biol Phys 10:1447–1451, 1984)

division. In the future, measurements of these quantities in individual patients may be used as a basis for choosing suitable cases.

## SENSITIZERS OF HYPOXIC CELLS

As described in Chapter 8, a great deal of experimental work through the years had established that, at least in transplanted tumors in animals, tumor control by x-rays is frequently limited by the presence of foci of hypoxic cells that are intransigent to killing by x-rays, which may result in tumor regrowth. Among the methods suggested to overcome this problem are treatment in hyperbaric oxygen chambers and the introduction of high linear energy transfer radiations, such as neutrons and heavy ions. Chemical sensitizers address the same problem.

Spurred largely by the efforts of radiation chemists (most notably Adams), a search was under way in the early 1960s for compounds that mimic oxygen in their ability to sensitize biological materials to the effects of x-rays. Instead of trying to "force" oxygen into tissues by the use of high-pressure tanks, the emphasis of this approach shifted to oxygen substitutes that diffuse into poorly vascularized areas of tumors and achieve the desired effect by chemical means. The vital difference between these drugs and oxygen, on which their success depends, is that the sensitizers are not rapidly metabolized by the cells in the tumor through which they diffuse. Because of this, they can penetrate further than oxygen and reach *all* of the hypoxic cells in the tumor, including those most remote from a blood supply. In the early 1960s many simple chemical compounds were found to have the ability to sensitize hypoxic microorganisms. These studies were guided by the hypothesis, now known to be correct, that sensitizing efficiency is related directly to the electron affinity of the compounds. A number of sensitizers were studied, notably TAN, PNAP, and a group of substances known as the nitrofurans. Although these compounds were highly effective as sensitizers of microorganisms in the petri dish, their application to mammalian cells in vivo was limited by their toxicity and their chemical and pharmacologic instability.

Adams and his colleagues listed properties that would be essential for a clinically useful hypoxic cell sensitizer. First, it had to selectively sensitize hypoxic cells at a concentration that would result in acceptable toxicity to normal tissues. Second, it should be chemically stable and not subject to rapid metabolic breakdown. Third, it must be highly soluble in water or lipids and must be capable of diffusing a considerable distance through a nonvascularized cell mass to reach the hypoxic cells, which in a tumor may be located as far as 200 μm from the nearest capillary. Fourth, it must be effective throughout most of the cell cycle, certainly in the early part, since it is likely that hypoxic cells in the tumor will be arrested in the $G_1$ phase of the cell cycle. Fifth, it should be effective at the relatively low daily doses of a few Gy (a few hundred rads) used in conventional fractionated radiotherapy.

## MISONIDAZOLE

Figure 10-3 illustrates the numbering of the basic ring structure of the nitroimidazoles. The side chain determines position 1, and the position of the nitro group ($NO_2$) leads to the classification of the drug as a 2-nitroimidazole, 4-nitro-

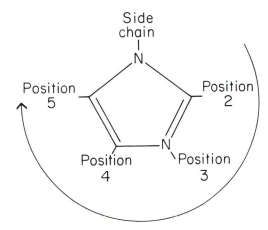

**Figure 10-3.** Method of numbering the basic ring structure of the nitroimidazoles. The side chain determines position 1. If the nitro group ($NO_2$) is in the second position, the drug is a 2-nitroimidazole. If the $NO_2$ group is in the fifth position, the drug is a 5-nitroimidazole. In general, 2-nitroimidazoles are more efficient radiosensitizers of hypoxic cells.

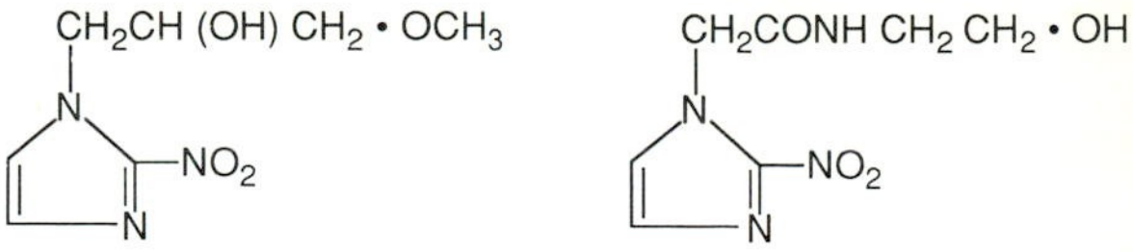

**Figure 10-4.** The structure of misonidazole compared with that of etanidazole. Both are 2-nitroimidazoles. Etanidazole is hydrophilic because of the composition of the side chain. Consequently, it does not cross the blood–brain barrier and is less neurotoxic.

$CH_2CH(OH)CH_2 \cdot OCH_3$

—$NO_2$

**Misonidazole**

$CH_2CONH\,CH_2\,CH_2 \cdot OH$

—$NO_2$

**Etanidazole**

imidazole, and so on. In general, 2-nitro-imidazoles have a higher electron affinity than 5-nitroimidazoles, the class that includes metronidazole which was briefly tried as a radiosensitizer. Several 2-nitroimidazoles had been synthesized as possible new trichomonacides, and one of these, produced by Roche Products, proved to be a very potent radiosensitizer. This compound, misonidazole, has been the subject of intensive investigation in the petri dish, experimental animals, and the clinic. The structure of misonidazole is shown in Figure 10-4.

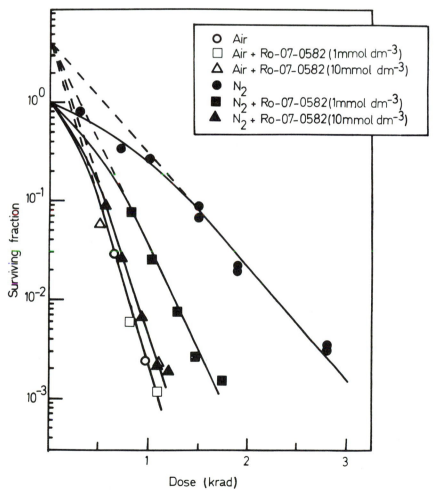

| | |
|---|---|
| ○ | Air |
| □ | Air + Ro-07-0582 (1mmol dm$^{-3}$) |
| △ | Air + Ro-07-0582 (10mmol dm$^{-3}$) |
| ● | N$_2$ |
| ■ | N$_2$ + Ro-07-0582 (1mmol dm$^{-3}$) |
| ▲ | N$_2$ + Ro-07-0582 (10mmol dm$^{-3}$) |

**Figure 10-5.** Survival data for aerated and hypoxic Chinese hamster cells x-irradiated in the presence of various concentrations of misonidazole (Ro-07-0582). At a concentration of 10 mM of this drug the radiosensitivity of hypoxic cells approaches that of aerated cells. The response of aerated cells is not affected by the drug at all. (From Adams GE, Flockhart IR, Smithen CE, Stratford IJ, Wardman P, Watts ME: Radiat Res 67:9–20, 1976)

## Fast Sensitization

That misonidazole produces appreciable sensitization can be demonstrated with cells in culture (Fig. 10-5). Hypoxic cells in the presence of 10 mM of misonidazole have a radiosensitivity approaching that of aerated cells. Because of its greater effectiveness at lower concentrations, misonidazole also has a dramatic effect on tumors in experimental animals. This is illustrated in Figure 10-6, which shows the proportion of mouse mammary tumors controlled as a function of x-ray dose delivered in a single fraction. If x-rays are used alone, the dose required to control half of the tumors is 43.8 Gy (4380 rads). This falls to 24.1 Gy (2410 rads) if the radiation is delivered 30 minutes after the administration of misonidazole (1 mg/g body weight). This corresponds to an enhancement ratio (ER) of 1.8. Dramatic results, such as those shown in Figure 10-6, in which an ER of 1.8 was obtained, are rather misleading; they represent single-dose treatments in contrast to the multifraction regimens common in conventional radiotherapy. Most animal tumors reoxygenate to some extent between irradiations, so that in a multifraction regimen the ER for a hypoxic sensitizer is usually much less than for a single-dose treatment.

## Cytotoxicity

In addition to radiosensitizing hypoxic cells, several of the nitroimidazoles have also been shown to be preferentially cytotoxic to cells that are deficient in oxygen (Fig. 10-7). Cells deficient in oxygen are readily killed in a period of several hours at concentrations of 5 mM of misonidazole, whereas much longer times are required for cells that are aerated. This cytotoxicity is also strongly dependent on temperature. Figure 10-7 shows a family of survival curves exposed to misonidazole at a concentration of 1 mM for various periods of time at several differ-

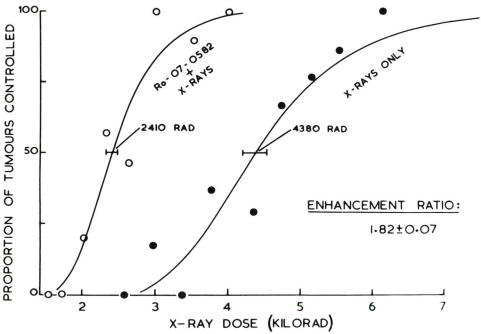

**Figure 10-6.** Proportion of mouse mammary tumors controlled at 150 days as a function of x-ray dose for a single treatment. The right curve represents x-rays only; the left curve refers to x-rays delivered after the administration of 1 mg/g body weight of misonidazole (Ro-07-0582). The enhancement ratio is the ratio of x-ray doses in the absence or presence of the drug that result in the control of 50% of the tumors; it has a value of 1.8. (From Sheldon PW, Foster JL, Fowler JF: Br J Cancer 30:560–565, 1974)

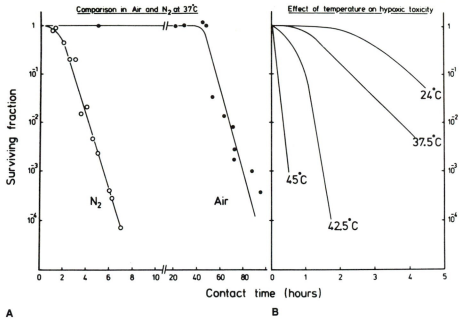

**Figure 10-7.** **(A)** Misonidazole is preferentially cytotoxic to hypoxic cells. Much larger concentrations or much larger exposure times are necessary to kill cells in air compared with cells in $N_2$. (Courtesy of Dr. Ged Adams) **(B)** The cytotoxicity of misonidazole strongly depends on temperature. Elevation of temperature by a few degrees causes many more cells to be killed by a given exposure. (From Hall EJ, Astor M, Geard C, Bigalow J: Br J Cancer 35:809, 1977)

ent temperatures. The cell-killing potential of the drug is greatly enhanced when the temperature is elevated by a few degrees.

## Thiol Depletion

The radiosensitization produced by a given concentration of misonidazole is significantly enhanced if the cells are incubated for a time in the presence of the drug *before* the irradiation is delivered. This supersensitization, or "slow" sensitization, is due to the reduction of the levels of natural radioprotectors, such as glutathione, in the cell, resulting from a prolonged exposure to compounds such as misonidazole.

## Clinical Use

After encouraging results in laboratory studies, misonidazole was introduced into a large number of clinical trials, involving many different types of human tumors in Europe and the United States.

In general, the results have been disappointing. Of the 20 or so randomized prospective controlled clinical trials performed in the United States by the Radiation Therapy Oncology Group, none yielded a statistically significant advantage for misonidazole, although a number indicated a slight benefit. The only trial that shows a clear advantage for misonidazole was the head and neck trial performed in Denmark, the largest single trial performed with the sensitizer. When patients of all categories are compared in this trial, the addition of misonidazole to the radiotherapy schedule conferred no significant advantage. When the patients are categorized into a number of subgroups, however, males with high hemoglobin levels and cancer of the pharynx showed a great benefit from the addition of misonidazole. Tumor control at 3 years was about double in the group receiving the drug compared with those patients receiving radiotherapy alone. This interesting result is shown in Figure 10-8. Other subgroups, including patients with cancer of the larynx, showed no benefit from the addition of the sensitizer.

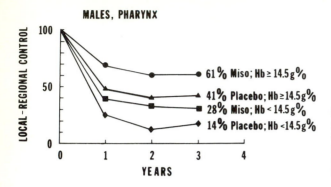

**MALES, PHARYNX**

LOCAL–REGIONAL CONTROL

61% Miso; Hb ≥ 14.5 g%
41% Placebo; Hb ≥ 14.5 g%
28% Miso; Hb < 14.5 g%
14% Placebo; Hb < 14.5 g%

YEARS

**Figure 10-8.** Some results from the Danish head and neck (DAHANCA) trial of misonidazole. Misonidazole produced a significant improvement of tumor control by radiotherapy only for males with tumors of the pharynx and depended on hemoglobin (Hb) status. (Data from Dr. Jens Overgaard)

When misonidazole was used in the clinic, the dose-limiting toxicity was found to be peripheral neuropathy that progressed to central nervous system toxicity if drug administration was not stopped. This toxicity prevented use of the drug at adequate dose levels throughout multifraction regimens. The disappointing results obtained with misonidazole in the clinic must be attributed largely to the fact that doses were limited to inadequate levels because of this toxicity.

## ETANIDAZOLE

Spurred by the success of misonidazole in the laboratory compared with its relative failure in the clinic, researchers began to search for a better drug. The result was etanidazole, synthesized by Stanford Research International. It was the drug chosen for the next series of randomized prospective clinical trials in the United States, which are nearing completion. The structure of etanidazole is shown in Figure 10-4. Its development represents a logical and elegant piece of research. Figure 10-9 illustrates the rationale for the development of this class of drugs. The position of the nitro group largely determines the electron affinity and therefore the radiosensitizing properties. The side chain determines the pharmacokinetics and hence the toxicity of the

drug. By varying the side chain, a whole family of drugs was synthesized that have similar radiosensitizing properties in vitro. Although they all have the nitro group in the 2 position, they have a wide range of partition coefficients and therefore pharmacologic properties.

There are two reasons for the superiority of etanidazole over misonidazole. First, etanidazole has a shorter half-life in vivo. Figure 10-10*A* shows the concentration versus time curves for two drugs, such as etanidazole and misonidazole, that have different half-lives in vivo. If the peak concentrations are the same and the drugs have equal electron affinities and sensitizing properties, then their efficiency as radiosensitizers should be indistinguishable. On the other hand, the drug with the shorter half-life results in a smaller area under the curve and might therefore be expected to show less toxicity. The second advantage of etanidazole is a function of its partition coefficient. Figure 10-10*C* shows the ratio of tumor concentration to serum concentration and of brain concentration to serum concentration for the range of compounds synthesized in the Stanford series. These ratios are plotted against the partition coefficient, which is a measure of the solubility of the drugs in water and lipids. Misonidazole has a partition coefficient of about 0.4, which means that it is widely distributed in all tissues because it is soluble in water or lipids.

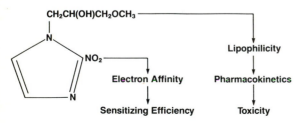

CH₂CH(OH)CH₂OCH₃

N

NO₂ → Electron Affinity → Sensitizing Efficiency

Lipophilicity → Pharmacokinetics → Toxicity

**Figure 10-9.** The guiding principles for the design of new radiosensitizers that led to the synthesis of etanidazole. The nitro group in the 2 position of the nitroimidazole ring largely determines the electron affinity and therefore the radiosensitizing properties. The side chain determines the solubility in water and lipids and therefore the pharmacokinetics. (Based on an idea from Dr. Martin Brown)

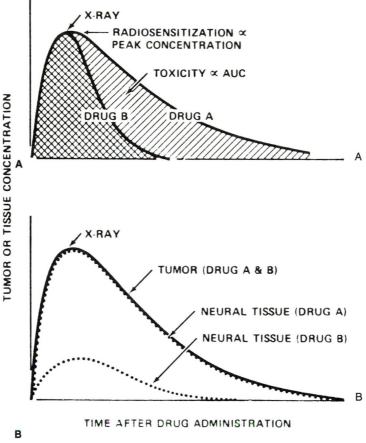

**Figure 10-10.** The reasons for expecting etanidazole (SR 2508) to be a superior radiosensitizer to misonidazole. **(A)** Relationships between concentration and time for two drugs with different half-lives in vivo. If the two drugs are equal as sensitizers in vitro and the x-ray dose is delivered when tumor concentration peaks, then the effectiveness of the two drugs as sensitizers will be the same in vivo. However, toxicity is related to the area under the curve, which is smaller for drug B (etanidazole) than for drug A (misonidazole:). **(B)** If drug B is able to penetrate into tumors as well as drug A but is unable to cross the blood–brain barrier or penetrate neural tissue, then less neurotoxicity would be expected for a given level of sensitization with drug B than with drug A. (Courtesy of Dr. Martin Brown) **(C)** The tumor to plasma ratio of drug concentrations and the brain to plasma ratio for ten 2-nitroimidazole radiosensitizers as a function of their octanol-water partition coefficient. Misonidazole has a partition coefficient of 0.4 (ie, it dissolves well in water or lipids). It is distributed in all tissues of the body. The tumor-to-plasma and brain-to-plasma ratios are both close to 1. As the partition coefficient decreases, the drug becomes more hydrophilic (ie, it dissolves in water better than lipids). The tumor-to-plasma ratio then falls because the drug does not cross the blood–brain barrier. The etanidazole tumor-to-plasma ratio is still close to 1, so the drug penetrates the tumor well. The brain-to-plasma ratio is only 0.1 because the drug does not readily cross the blood–brain barrier. Drugs with partition coefficients much smaller than that of etanidazole are not useful because they do not penetrate tumors effectively, so that the tumor-to-plasma and brain-to-plasma ratios begin to fall. (From Brown JM: In: Modification of Radiosensitivity in Cancer Treatment, pp 139–176. Tokyo, Academic Press, 1984)

*(continued)*

Consequently, the tumor-to-serum and the brain-to-serum ratios are close to unity for misonidazole; in other words, the drug is widely distributed through essentially all tissues of the body. When the partition coefficient is reduced, the tumor-to-serum ratio begins to drop because the drug is hydrophilic rather than lipophilic and does not cross the blood–brain barrier. For etanidazole, with a partition coefficient 0.04, the tumor-to-serum ratio is still close to unity, whereas the brain-to-serum ratio is 10 times smaller. It was reasoned that if the drug was poorly penetrating into the nervous system tissues and did not cross the blood–brain barrier,

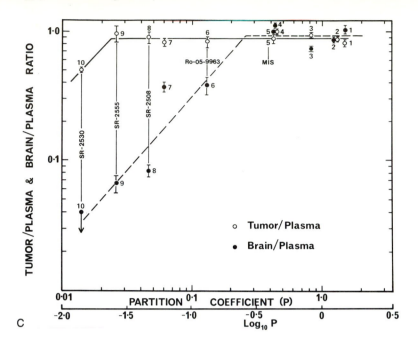

Figure 10-10. *(Continued)*

then it should produce less neurotoxicity than misonidazole. It can also be seen from Figure 10-10*C* that if the partition coefficient is further reduced and the drug is made even more hydrophilic, it does not penetrate into the tumor either.

On the basis of these considerations, etanidazole was chosen as having about the optimal partition coefficient. Phase 1 and 2 clinical trials have been performed with this drug, and it turns out that doses with etanidazole can be increased by a factor of about 3 compared with misonidazole. The dose-limiting toxicity is also a peripheral neuropathy, but at a much higher drug concentration. Phase 3 controlled randomized prospective clinical trials are in progress and nearing completion.

## CHEMOPOTENTIATION

Although the nitroimidazoles were developed principally as radiosensitizers, they have also proved to be effective chemosensitizers. In vitro they have been shown to potentiate the cell killing of a range of chemotherapeutic agents, including melphalan, bleomycin, and cisplatin. In vivo the effectiveness of the nitroimidazoles as chemopotentiators is most dramatic with the alkylating agents, such as cyclophosphamide, melphalan, and the nitrosoureas.

In vitro, hypoxia is an absolute prerequisite for chemopotentiation. Furthermore, it has been shown that levels of oxygen required for chemopotentiation are even lower than those required for hypoxic radioprotection. Nevertheless, the levels of chemopotentiation observed in animal tumors is greater than can be accounted for in terms of the proportion of cells known to be radiobiologically hypoxic. For whatever reason, misonidazole and etanidazole appear to be potent potentiators of chemotherapy agents, and a number of clinical trials are in progress combining a radiosensitizer with alkylating agents.

The mechanism of chemopotentiation by the nitroimidazoles is not clear. In fact, it is likely that more than one mechanism is involved. Part of the effect almost certainly results from the reduction of the thiol levels in the cell. An additional factor for some chemotherapeutic agents may be an increase in DNA interstrand cross-link formation as a result of treatment with the nitroimidazole. A further possible development in chemopotentiation is the use of compounds specifically and primarily designed to deplete cells of glutathione (eg, buthionine sulfoximine).

## BIOREDUCTIVE DRUGS

Bioreductive drugs are compounds that are reduced intracellularly to form active cytotoxic agents. The term **bioreductive drug** was first used by Sartorelli in the context of the development of mitomycin C. Usually, bioreduction is favored under hypoxic conditions, so that these compounds display differential cytotoxicity to hypoxic cells. This is one of the rationales for selectivity in solid tumors.

The development of some major classes of bioreductive drugs grew out of the field of hypoxic cell radiosensitizers when it was observed that misonidazole was preferentially cytotoxic to hypoxic cells. This was discussed earlier in this chapter.

There are several main classes of bioreductive drugs. The principal ones are listed below:

1. Fused-ring benzoquinones, some of which are related to mitomycin C
2. Organic N-oxides of different structures
3. Dual-function nitroheterocyclic compounds

### Mitomycin C

Mitomycin C is a natural product and has been shown to be active in a wide range of tumors in experimental animals as well as in some human malignancies. The drug is activated by biore-

duction to form products that cross link intracellular DNA. The cytotoxicity is greater under hypoxic than aerated conditions, but only by a small factor. This prompted the search for related compounds with less toxicity to aerated normal tissues. One such compound is porfiromycin, which shows a larger hypoxic differential than mitomycin C, principally because of a reduced cytotoxic effect on aerobic cells. The reductases DT diaphorase and cytochrome P450 have both been implicated in the bioactivation of these drugs. Mitomycin C is discussed in more detail in Chapter 17.

### Organic Nitroxides (SR 4233)

Organic nitroxides show considerable promise as antitumor agents. These agents are activated by metabolic chemical reduction and are highly potent against hypoxic cells, showing large hypoxic/oxic cytotoxicity ratios. The lead compound is a triazene-di-N-oxide, SR 4233, synthesized by Stanford Research International, now known as Tirapazamine. Figure 10-11 shows survival curves for Chinese hamster cells treated with graded concentrations of Tirapazamine. Note the hypoxic/oxic toxicity ratio of about 100. This compound is believed to be activated by the enzyme cytochrome P450. The hypoxic/oxic toxicity ratio is not as large (about 20) in cell lines of human origin, presumably reflecting a different spectrum, or different levels, of enzymes. Tirapazamine has been shown to be active in several experimental tumors and is, at present, entering phase I clinical trials. These compounds are not radiosensitizers because they do not modify the

Figure 10-11. Dose–response curves for Chinese hamster cells exposed for $1\frac{1}{2}$ hours to graded concentrations of SR 4233 (Tirapazamine) under aerated and hypoxic conditions. Cells deficient in oxygen are preferentially killed. The hypoxic cytoxicity ratio (defined as the ratio of drug concentrations under aerated and hypoxic conditions required to produce the same cell survival) is variable between different cell lines. For Chinese hamster cells shown, the ratio is about 100; for cells of human origin the ratio is somewhat smaller, closer to 20. Tirapazamine is an organic nitroxide synthesized by Stanford Research International. Its structure is shown in the inset. (Courtesy of Dr. J. Martin Brown)

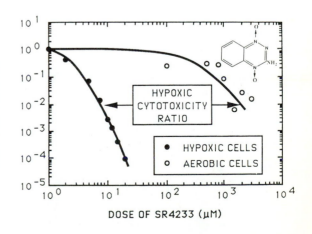

radiation response. They are, however, designed to be adjuncts to radiation, with the radiation killing the aerated cells and the drug killing the hypoxic cells.

## Dual-Function Nitroheterocyclic Compounds (RB 6145)

These compounds consist of a 2-nitroimidazole ring that can act as a hypoxic cell radiosensitizer in much the same way as misonidazole or etanidazole but with an aziridine ring at the terminal end of the side chain that confers on the molecule much more potency as a hypoxic cytotoxin. The lead compound is RSU 1069. This compound shows high activity in vitro and in experimental animals, but preliminary results from a phase I clinical trial revealed dose-limiting gastrointestinal toxicity. Toxicity can be avoided by using the compound RB 6145, a compound containing the bromoethyl chain (Fig. 10-12). In vivo, the bromoethyl group cyclises with the loss of HBr, so that RB 6145 is reduced to RSU 1069. Figure 10-12 shows the results of an experiment with a murine tumor treated with x-rays and with RB 6145. A single dose of 10 Gy (1000 rads) alone results in about 1½ logs of cell kill; the addition of the drug produces a further 1½ logs of cell kill, whether the drug is used before or after the radiation exposure, indicating that the drug is

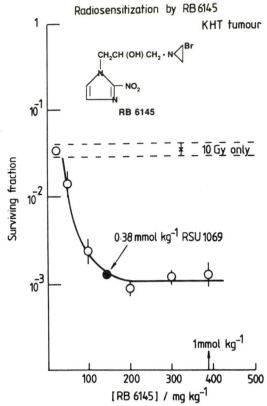

**Figure 10-12.**    Effect on the survival of KHT tumor cells produced by various doses of RB 6145 administered 45 minutes before a dose of 10 Gy (1000 rads) of x-rays. The effect of x-rays alone is shown between the dotted lines. The structure of RB 6145 is shown in the insert. (Courtesy of Dr. Ged Adams)

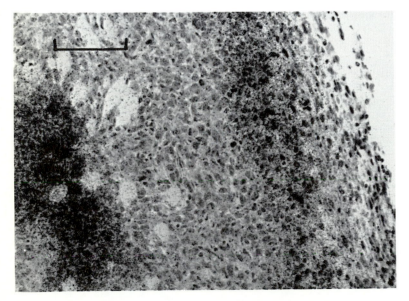

**Figure 10-13.**    Autoradiograph of a section of a human small cell lung carcinoma from a patient who received radioactive-labeled misonidazole the previous day. There are areas of intense labeling (many grains in the emulsion), suggesting the presence of hypoxic regions in the tumor. In areas deficient in oxygen the misonidazole undergoes anaerobic metabolism and is broken down, and the radioactive label is deposited. (Courtesy of Drs. J.D. Chapman and R. Urtasun)

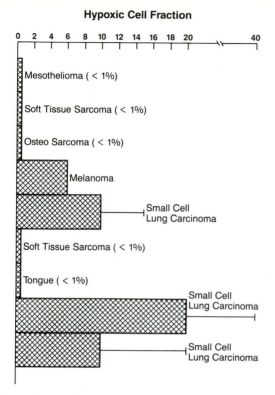

**Hypoxic Cell Fraction**

**Figure 10-14.** Summary of the labeling levels found in the first eight patients to be administered radioactive-labeled misonidazole. Only four of the eight patients show levels of labeling commensurate with the presence of hypoxic cells. (Courtesy of Drs. J.D. Chapman and R. Urtasun)

acting as a potent hypoxic cytotoxin, not as a radiosensitizer. RB 6145 can be administered orally and is already in phase I clinical trials.

## MARKERS OF HYPOXIC CELLS

A major development in the past decade has been the synthesis of radioactive-labeled nitro-imidazoles for use as markers of hypoxic cells. The technique is as follows. A dose of misonidazole, or one of its analogues, carrying a radioactive label is administered. The drug is quickly excreted without being broken down from tissues that are well aerated, but under conditions of reduced oxygen tension, the drug is metabolized, and broken down. Chapman and Urtusan in Edmonton, Canada, performed a study in which patients were given a nitro-imidazole labeled with tritiated thymidine 22 hours before the tumor was surgically removed. Figure 10-13 is a section of a melanoma showing the density of grains over a region of the tumor, indicating the presence of hypoxic cells. The interesting result of the study is that only four of nine patients had tumors with a significant proportion of hypoxic cells (Fig. 10-14). In this small group of patients, biased inasmuch as only accessible tumors could be studied, only melanoma and small cell lung cancer appeared to contain a proportion of hypoxic cells that would prejudice the outcome of radiotherapy. Until recently it was only possible to use β-emitting isotopes as labels, which can only be detected by autoradiography when the tumor is removed and sectioned. More recently, Chapman has successfully labeled a nitroimidazole by attaching a positron emitting radionuclide (iodine-123) using a sugar molecule. The presence of hypoxia may then be detected by SPECT (single photon emission computed tomography) imaging, which of course is noninvasive. This exciting development opens up the possibility of screening patients prospectively to select those in which hypoxia is a problem for inclusion in protocols involving hypoxic cell sensitizers or bioreductive drugs. This topic is discussed further in Chapter 15.

▶ *Summary of Pertinent Conclusions*

*Nonhypoxic Sensitizers*
- If the methyl group in thymidine is replaced by a halogen and incorporated into DNA, it results in radiosensitization.
- The halogenated pyrimidine must be incorporated into DNA for sensitization to occur. Consequently, cells must be grown in the presence of the analogue for several cell cycles. The extent of radiosensitization increases with the amount incorporated.

*(continued)*

► *Summary of Pertinent Conclusions* (Continued)

- For a sensitizer to be useful there must be a differential effect between tumors and normal tissues. The halogenated pyrimidines require the tumor to be cycling faster than the dose-limiting normal tissues.
- Iododeoxyuridine is preferred to bromodeoxyuridine because it is an equally effective radiosensitizer but a less effective photosensitizer. Rash is therefore reduced in patients.
- Gliomas may be a suitable tumor for clinical studies because they are rapidly growing and surrounded by slowly growing or nongrowing normal tissue.

### Hypoxic Cell Sensitizers

- Hypoxic cell sensitizers increase the radiosensitivity of hypoxic cells but not aerated cells. The differential effect on tumors is based on the presence of hypoxic cells in tumors but not in normal tissues.
- Fast sensitization is a free-radical process. The sensitizer mimics oxygen by "fixing" damage produced by free radicals.
- Slow sensitization refers to the extra sensitization that occurs if the sensitizer is incubated with cells for a prolonged period, resulting in thiol depletion.
- Misonidazole, the first compound used widely, sensitizes cells in culture and animal tumors.
- Doses of misonidazole that can be used clinically are limited to suboptimal levels by peripheral neuropathy. Only 1 of 30 or so clinical trials shows a clear advantage for misonidazole.
- Etanidazole has a shorter half-life in vivo than misonidazole. It does not cross the blood–brain barrier because it is more hydrophilic. Neurotoxicity is dose limiting, but about three times larger doses can be given than with misonidazole. Phase III clinical trials are in progress.
- Nitroimidazoles sensitize cells to chemotherapy drugs, especially alkylating agents. This is called chemopotentiation.

### Hypoxic Cytotoxins

- Bioreductive drugs are compounds that are reduced intracellularly to form cytotoxic agents.
- Usually bioreduction is favored under hypoxia; this is a rationale for selectivity in solid tumors.
- Mitomycin C is active in a wide range of tumors. The hypoxic/oxic cytotoxicity ratio is quite small.
- SR 4233 is an organic nitroxide. It shows a large hypoxic/oxic toxicity ratio. The compound is active in many animal tumors and has entered phase I clinical trials.
- RB 6145 is a dual-function nitroheterocylic compound. The nitroimidazole ring functions as a hypoxic cell radiosensitizer, while the aziridine ring at the end of the side chain functions as an alkylating agent. It is a potent hypoxic cytotoxin.

*(continued)*

▶ **Summary of Pertinent Conclusions** *(Continued)*

- Both SR 4233 and RB 6145 are designed to be used as adjuncts to irradiation, with the radiation killing the aerobic cells and the drug targeted to kill the hypoxic cells.

### Markers of Hypoxic Cells

- Nitroimidazoles labeled with a radionuclide can be used as markers of hypoxic cells. The drug is quickly excreted from aerobic tissues without breaking down. In areas of hypoxia, the drug undergoes bioreduction and the radionuclide is deposited.
- Nitroimidazoles labeled with a β-emitter have been available for some time. By autoradiography on sections of a tumor surgically removed about a day after administration of a labeled drug, hypoxic areas can be identified. Only a minority of human tumors (notably melanomas and small cell lung carcinomas) showed an appreciable proportion of hypoxic cells.
- Nitroimidazoles can now be labeled with iodine-123. Hypoxic regions of a tumor can be visualized by single-photon emission computed tomography (SPECT). This is a noninvasive procedure that can be used as a predictive assay in individual patients. In the few patients, about 40% show the presence of hypoxic areas.
- The availability of methods to detect significant areas of hypoxia will allow **selection** of patients who may benefit from methods to overcome hypoxia (eg, radiosensitizers, hypoxic cytotoxins, neutrons).

## BIBLIOGRAPHY

Adams GE: Chemical radiosensitization of hypoxic cells. Br Med Bull 29:48–53, 1973

Adams GE: Redox, radiation and reductive bioactivation. Radiat Res, 132:129–139, 1992

Adams GE, Clarke ED, Flockhart IR, Jacobs RS, Sehmi DS, Stratford IJ, Wardman P, Watts ME, Parrick J, Wallace RG, Smithen CE: Structure–activity relationships in the development of hypoxic cell radiosensitizers: I. Sensitization efficiency. Int J Radiat Biol 35:133–150, 1979

Adams Ge, Clarke ED, Gray P, Jacobs RS, Stratford IJ, Wardman P, Watts ME, Parrick J, Wallace RG, Smithen CE: Structure–activity relationships in the development of hypoxic cell radiosensitizers: II. Cytotoxicity and therapeutic ratio. Int J Radiat Biol 35:151–160, 1979

Alper T: The modification of damage caused by primary ionization of biological targets. Radiat Res 5:573–585, 1956

Ash DV, Peckham MJ, Steel GG: The quantitative response of human tumours to radiation and misonidazole. Br J Cancer 40:883–889. 1979

Bagshaw MA, Doggett RL, Smith KC: Intra-arterial 5-bromodeoxyuridine and x-ray therapy. AJR 99:889–894, 1967

Baker MA, Zeman EM, Hirst VK, Brown JM: Metabolism of SR 4233 by Chinese hamster ovary cells: Basis for selective hypoxic toxicity. Cancer Res 48:5947–5952, 1988

Brown JM, Goffinet DR, Cleaber JE, Kallman RF: Preferential radiosensitization of mouse sarcoma relative to normal skin by chronic intra-arterial infusion of halogenated pyrimidine analogs. JNCI 47:75–89, 1971

Chapman JD, Urtasun RC, Franko AJ, Raleigh JA, Meeker BE, McKinnon SA: The measurement of oxygenation status of individual tumors. In: Prediction of Response in Radiation Therapy: The Physical and Biological Basis. Proceedings of the American Association of Physical Medicine Symposium, No. 7, pp 49–60, 1989

Chapman JD, Whitmore GF (eds): Chemical modifiers of cancer treatment. Int J Radiat Oncol Biol Phys 10:1161–1813, 1984

Cole S, Stratford IJ, Bowler J, Nolan J, Wright EG, Horwich A, Holliday SB, Deacon JM, Peckham MJ: A toxicity and pharmacokinetic study in man of the hypoxic cell radiosensitizer RSU 1069. Br J Radiol 59:1238–1240, 1986

Coleman CN: Hypoxic cell radiosensitizers: Expectations and progress in drug development. Int J Radiat Oncol Biol Phys 11:323–329, 1985

Dische S, Gray AJ, Zanelli GD: Clinical testing of the radiosensitizer Ro-07-0582: II. Radiosensitization of normal and hypoxic skin. Clin Radiol 27:159–166, 1976

Foster JL, Conroy PM, Searle AJ, Willson RL: Metronidazole (Flagyl): Characterization as a cytotoxic drug specific for hypoxic tumor cells. Br J Cancer 33:485–490, 1976

Gray AJ, Dische S, Adams GE, Flockhart IR, Foster JL: Clinical testing of the radiosensitizer Ro-07-0582: I. Dose, tolerance, serum and tumor concentrations. Clin Radiol 27:151–157, 1976

Hall EJ, Astor M, Geard C, Bigalow J: Cytotoxicity of Ro-07-0582: Enhancement by hyperthermia and protection by cysteamine. Br J Cancer 35:809–815, 1977

Hall EJ, Roizin-Towle L: Hypoxic sensitizers: Radiobiological studies at the cellular level. Radiology 117:453–457, 1975

Jenkins TC, Naylor MA, O'Neill P, Threadgill MD, Cole S, Stratford IJ, Adams GE, Fielden EM, Suto MJ, Stier MA: Synthesis and evaluation of 1-(3-[2-haloethylamino]propyl)-2-nitroimidazoles as pro-drugs of RSU 1069 and its analogues, which are radiosensitizers and bioreductively activated cytotoxins. J Med Chem 33:2603–2610, 1990

Jette DC, Wiebe LI, Flanagan RJ, Lee J, Chapman JD: Iodoazomycin riboside (1-[5′-iodo-5′-deoxyribofuranosyl]-2-nitroimidazole): A hypoxic cell marker: I. Synthesis and in vitro characterization. Radiat Res 105:169, 1986

Kinsella T, Mitchell J, Russo A, Aiken M, Morstyn G, Hsu S, Rowland J, Glatstein E: Continuous intravenous infusions of bromodeoxyuridine as a clinical radiosensitizer. J Clin Oncol 2:1144–1150, 1984

Kinsella T, Mitchell J, Russo A, Morstyn G, Glatstein E: The use of halogenated thymidine analogs as clinical radiosensitizers: Rationale, current status, and future prospects—non-hypoxic cell sensitizers. Int J Radiat Oncol Biol Phys 10:139–1406, 1984

Kinsella T, Russo A, Mitchell J, Collins J, Rowland J, Wright D, Glatstein E: A phase I study of intravenous iododeoxyuridine as a clinical radiosensitizer. Int J Radiat Oncol Biol Phys 11:1941–1946, 1985

Laderoute K, Wardman P, Rauth AM: Molecular mechanisms for the hypoxia-dependent activation of 3-amino-1,2,4-benzotriazine-1, 4-dioxide (SR 4233). Biochem Pharmacol 37:1487–1495, 1988

Lin AJ, Cosby LA, Shansky CW, Sartorelli AC: Potential bioreductive alkylating agents: I. Benzoquinone derivatives. J Med Chem 15:1247–1252, 1972

Lorimore SA, Adams GE: Oral (PO) dosing with RS 1069 or RB 6145 maintains their potency as hypoxic cell radiosensitizers and cytotoxins but reduces systemic toxicity compared with parenteral (IP) administration in mice. Int J Radiat Oncol Biol Phys 21:387–395, 1991

Mitchell J, Kinsella T, Russo A, McPherson S, Rowland J, Smith B, Kornblith P, Glatstein E: Radiosensitization of hematopoietic precursor cells (CFUc) in glioblastoma patients receiving intermittent intravenous infusions of bromodeoxyuridine (BUdR). Int J Radiat Oncol Biol Phys 9:457–463, 1983

Mitchell J, Morstyn G, Russo A, Kinsella T, Fornace A, McPherson S, Glatstein E: Differing sensitivity to fluorescent light in Chinese hamster cells containing equally incorporated quantities of BUdR versus IUdR. Int J Radiat Oncol Biol Phys 10:1447–1451, 1984

Mitchell J, Russo A, Kinsella T, Glatstein E: The use of non-hypoxic cell sensitizers in radiobiology and radiotherapy. Int J Radiat Oncol Biol Phys 12:1513–1518, 1986

Mohindra JK, Rauth A: Increased cell killing by metronidazole and nitrofurazone of hypoxic compared to aerobic mammalian cells. Cancer Res 36:930, 1976

Morstyn G, Hsu S, Kinsellas T, Gratzner H, Russo A, Mitchell J: Bromodeoxyuridine in tumors and chromosomes detected with a monoclonal antibody. J Clin Invest 72:1644–1850, 1983

Parliament MB, Chapman JD, Urtasun RC, McEwan AJ, Golberg L, Mercer JR, Mannan RH, Wiebe LI: Noninvasive assessment of human tumor hypoxia with [123]I-iodoazomycin arabinoside: Preliminary report of a clinical study. Br J Cancer 65:90–95, 1992

Rasey JS, Koh W, Grierson JR, Granbaum Z, Krohn KA: Radiolabelled fluoromisonidazole as an imaging agent for tumor hypoxia. Int J Radiat Oncol Biol Phys 17:985, 1989

Roizin-Towle LA, Hall EJ, Flynn M, Bigalow JE, Varnes ME: Enhanced cytotoxicity of melphalan by prolonged exposure to nitroimidazoles: The role of endogenous thiols. Int J Radiat Oncol Biol Phys 8:757–760, 1982

Rose CM, Millar JL, Peacock JH, Phelps TA, Stephens TC: Differential enhancement of melphalan cytotoxicity in tumour and normal tissue by misonidazole. In Brady LW (ed): Radiation Sensitizers, pp 250–257. New York, Masson, 1980

Stratford IJ, Adams GE: Effect of hyperthermia on differential cytotoxicity of a hypoxic cell radiosensitizer, Ro-07-0582, on mammalian cells in vitro. Br J Cancer 35:309, 1977

Sutherland RM: Selective chemotherapy of non-cycling cells in an in vitro tumour model. Cancer Res 34:3501–3503, 1974

Thomlinson RH, Dische S, Gray AJ, Errington LM: Clinical testing of the radiosensitizer Ro-07-0582: III. Response of tumors. Clin Radiol 27:167–174, 1976

Urtasun RC, Band P, Chapman JD, Feldstein ML, Mielke B, Fryer C: Radiation and high dose metronidazole (Flagyl) in supratentorial glioblastomas. N Engl J Med 294:1364–1367, 1976

Urtasun RC, Band P, Chapman JD, Rabin HR, Wilson

AF, Fryer CG: Clinical phase 1 study of the hypoxic cell radiosensitizer Ro-07-0582, a 2-nitroimidazole derivative. Radiology 122:801–804, 1977

Urtasun RC, Chapman JD, Raleigh JA, Franko AJ, Koch CJ: Binding of $^3$H-misonidazole to solid human tumors as a measure of tumor hypoxia. Int J Radiat Oncol Biol Phys 12:1263–1267, 1986

Wong TW, Whitmore GF, Gulyas S: Studies on the toxicity and radiosensitizing ability of misonidazole under conditions of prolonged incubation. Radiat Res 75:541–555, 1978

Zeman EM, Brown JM, Lemmon MJ, Hirst VK, Lee WW: SR 4233: A new bioreductive agent with high selective toxicity for hypoxic mammalian cells. Int J Radiat Oncol Biol Phys 12:1239–1242, 1986

Zeman EM, Hirst VK, Lemmon MJ, Brown JM: Enhancement of radiation induced tumour cell killing by the hypoxic cell toxin SR 4233. Radiother Oncol 12:209–218, 1988

*Radiobiology for the Radiologist, Fourth Edition*, by Eric J. Hall
J. B. Lippincott Company, Philadelphia © 1994.

# 11

# *Radioprotectors*

THE DISCOVERY OF RADIOPROTECTORS
MECHANISM OF ACTION
DEVELOPMENT OF MORE EFFECTIVE COMPOUNDS
AMIFOSTINE (WR-2721) AS A RADIOPROTECTOR
  IN RADIOTHERAPY
RADIOPROTECTORS AND CHEMOTHERAPY
SUMMARY OF PERTINENT CONCLUSIONS

Diagnostic Radiology
Nuclear Medicine
Radiation Therapy

# THE DISCOVERY OF RADIOPROTECTORS

Some substances, while not directly affecting the radiosensitivity of cells, nevertheless may protect whole animals because they cause vasoconstriction or in some way upset normal processes of metabolism to such an extent that the oxygen concentration in critical organs is reduced. Because cells are less sensitive to x-rays under hypoxia, this confers a measure of protection. Examples are sodium cyanide, carbon monoxide, epinephrine, histamine, and serotonin. Such compounds are not really radioprotectors per se and are not discussed further.

The most remarkable group of *true* radioprotectors are the sulfhydryl compounds. The simplest is a **cysteine,** a sulfhydryl compound containing a natural amino acid, the structure of which is

$$SH—CH_2—CH \overset{NH_2}{\underset{COOH}{\diagup \diagdown}}$$

In 1948, Patt discovered that cysteine could protect mice from the effects of total-body x-radiation when the drug was injected or ingested in large amounts before the radiation exposure. At about the same time Bacq and his colleagues in Europe independently discovered that cysteamine could also protect animals from total-body irradiation. This compound has a structure represented by

$$SH—CH_2—CH_2—NH_2.$$

Animals injected with cysteamine to a concentration of about 150 mg/kg require a dose of x-rays 1.8 times larger than control animals to produce the same level of mortality. This factor of 1.8 is called the *dose reduction factor* (DRF), defined as

$$DRF = \frac{\text{Dose of radiation in the presence of the drug}}{\text{Dose of radiation in the absence of the drug}}$$

to produce a given level of lethality.

# MECHANISM OF ACTION

Many similar compounds have been tested and found to be effective as radioprotectors. The most efficient tend to have certain structural features in common: a free SH group (or potential SH group) at one end of the molecule and a strong basic function such as amine or guanidine at the other end, separated by a straight chain of two or three carbon atoms. Sulfhydryl compounds are efficient radioprotectors against sparsely ionizing radiations, such as x- or γ-rays. The mechanism of action involves the scavenging of free radicals. Chapter 1 includes a discussion of the chain of events between the absorption of a photon and the production of biological damage, which may be briefly summarized as follows. The photons give up their energy to fast electrons; these electrons produce ion pairs in the biological materials through which they pass. As an intermediate step between the ion pairs and the breaking of chemical bonds, free radicals are formed. These carry no charge but are highly reactive because of the presence of an unpaired electron in the outer orbit and have a lifetime of about $10^{-5}$ second. In the presence of oxygen the following reaction occurs, where F· represents the free radical:

$$F· + O_2 \rightarrow FO_2·$$

This highly reactive product, $FO_2·$, already constitutes a new changed molecule in the system. Sulfhydryl compounds block this process by reacting with the free radicals in competition with oxygen. Their protective effect, therefore, stems from their ability to scavenge free radicals, facilitating the chemical restitution of the original target molecule. This process is illustrated in Figure 11-1. The protective effect of sulfhydryl compounds tends to parallel the oxygen effect, being maximal for sparsely ionizing radiations (eg, x- or γ-rays) and minimal for densely ionizing radiations (eg, low energy α-particles). It might be predicted that with effective scavenging of all free radicals the largest possible value of DRF would equal the oxygen enhancement ratio, with a value of 2.5 to 3.0.

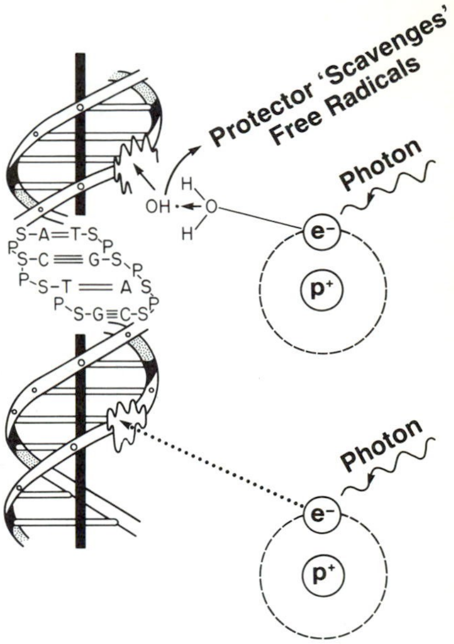

**Figure 11-1.** Radioprotectors containing a sulfhydryl group exert their effect by scavenging free radicals. Therefore they are effective against the indirect action of x-rays and have little effect with high linear energy transfer radiations in which direct action is dominant. Since the indirect action accounts for about two thirds of the biological effect of x-rays, a perfect protector that scavenged all of the free radicals could have a dose reduction factor approaching 3.

This simple description of the mechanism of action of sulfhydryl radioprotectors is intellectually satisfying, but it is clearly not the whole story since radioprotectors of this class have more effect with densely ionizing radiations (such as neutrons) than would be expected. Other factors must be involved that are not fully understood.

## DEVELOPMENT OF MORE EFFECTIVE COMPOUNDS

It is not surprising that the discovery in 1948 of a compound that offered protection against radiation excited the interest of the US Army, since the memory of Nagasaki and Hiroshima was vivid in the years immediately after World War II. Although cysteine is a radioprotector, it is also toxic and induces nausea and vomiting at the dose levels required for radioprotection.

Consequently, the Walter Reed Army Hospital in Washington, DC, synthesized more than 3000 compounds in an attempt to find the perfect radioprotector, one that would protect against radiation without debilitating side effects. At an early stage the important discovery was made that the toxicity of the compound could be greatly reduced if the sulfhydryl group was covered by a phosphate group. This is illustrated in Table 11-1. The $LD_{50}$ of the compound in animals can be doubled and the protective effect in terms of the DRF greatly enhanced if the SH group in cysteamine is covered by a phosphate. This tends to reduce systemic toxicity. Once in the cell, the phosphate group is stripped, and the SH group begins scavenging for free radicals.

The structures of three typical compounds of the more than 3000 synthesized in the Walter Reed series are shown in Table 11-2. The first

Table 11-1.
**Effect of Adding a Phosphate-Covering Function on the Free Sulfhydryl of β-Mercaptoethylamine (MEA)**

| DRUG | FORMULA | $LD_{50}$ IN MICE | DRF |
|------|---------|-------------------|-----|
| MEA | $NH_2$—CH—$CH_2$—SH | 343 (323–364) | 1.6 at 200 mg/kg |
| MEA·$PO_3$ | $NH_2$—$CH_2$—CH—$SH_2PO_3$ | 777 (700–864) | 2.1 at 500 mg/kg |

Table 11-2.
Three Protectors in Practical Use

| COMPOUND | STRUCTURE | USE |
|---|---|---|
| WR-638 | $NH_2CH_2CH_2SPO_3HNa$ | Carried in field pack by Russian army (Cystaphos) |
| WR-2721 | $NH_2(CH_2)_3NHCH_2CH_2SPO_3H_2$ | Protector in radiotherapy and carried by US astronauts on lunar trips (amifostine) |
| WR-1607 | $CH_3(CH_2)_9NHCH_2CH_2SSO_3H$ | Marketed as rat poison (d-CON) |

Comparison of Hematopoietic and Gastrointestinal Dose Reduction Factors in Mice for the Three Compounds Listed Above

| COMPOUND | DRUG DOSE (mg/kg) | DRF (7 DAYS) | DRF (30 DAYS) |
|---|---|---|---|
| WR-638 | 500 | 1.6 | 2.1 |
| WR-2721 | 900 | 1.8 | 2.7 |
| WR-1607 | 10 | — | 2.1 |

compound, WR-638, called Cystaphos, was said to be carried routinely in the field pack of Russian infantry in Europe during the era of the Cold War for use in the event of a nuclear conflict. Its usefulness must be largely psychological, since the compound was carried as a tablet to be administered orally, when in fact these sulfhydryl compounds break down in stomach acid and are only effective when administered intravenously or intraperitoneally. A further factor, of course, is that such compounds will protect only from sparsely ionizing radiation; consequently, they would offer little protection against the prompt release of neutrons produced by the detonation of a nuclear device. They would be effective only against the γ-rays from the resulting fallout.

The second compound, WR-2721, now known as amifostine, is perhaps the most effective of those synthesized in the Walter Reed series. It gives good protection to the blood-forming organs, as can be seen by the DRF for 30-day death in mice, which approaches the theoretical maximum value of 3. It was probably the compound carried by the US astronauts on their trips to the moon to be used if a solar event occurred. On these missions, when the space vehicle left earth's orbit and began coasting toward the moon, the astronauts were committed to a 14-day mission, since they did not have sufficient fuel to turn around without first orbiting the moon and using its gravitational field. If there had been a major solar event in that period, the astronauts would have been exposed to a shower of high-energy protons, resulting in an estimated dose of several hundred Gy (several hundred rads). The availability of a radioprotector with a DRF of between 2 and 3 would have been very important in such a circumstance. As it turned out, no major solar event ever occurred during any manned lunar mission. Amifostine also has a potential in radiotherapy, which is discussed in more detail later.

The third compound, WR-1607, has a structure similar to the other two but is in fact marketed as the rat poison d-CON. It kills by producing cardiac arrest. It is a much more effective radioprotector than either of the others listed in Table 11-2, producing equivalent protection at one hundredth of the dose, but it is not usable because of its toxicity. This compound is included in Table 11-2 because it illustrates how a small change in the structure can result in a dramatic change of properties and because it also points to the potential dose-limiting cytotoxicity of this series of sulfhydryl compounds. For instance, the dose-limiting toxicity of amifostine is hypotension.

# AMIFOSTINE AS A RADIOPROTECTOR IN RADIOTHERAPY

Amifostine (WR-2721), an aminothial, is a prodrug that is dephosphorylated to the active species, which is designated WR-1065. Radioprotectors have a number of potential applications in radiotherapy. For use in total-body irradiation the drug is administered at maximum tolerable concentration immediately before the radiation dose is delivered. Protection of normal tissues versus tumors is achieved through a differential uptake and conversion of amifostine to WR-1065 in tumors. There is evidence of active transport of the drug into normal tissues, with only passive diffusion into tumors; on the other hand the differential effect may be due simply to the better vasculature in normal tissues. Whatever the mechanism, the compound quickly floods normal tissues but penetrates more slowly into the tumor. Consequently, if the radiation dose is given within minutes after the administration of the radioprotector, there is a differential sparing of normal tissue compared with tumor cells. This strategy is effectively illustrated from many experiments with animal tumors, particularly by Yuhas and his colleagues. A typical example is shown in Figure 11-2. Soon after administration of the drug, the concentration of amifostine is found to be high in several normal tissues, while it rises much more slowly in the tumor. Many different tumor types have been studied, and this appears to be a general finding.

There is an interesting variability in the extent to which amifostine protects normal tissues (Table 11-3). In general, there is good protection of the hematopoietic system, the lining of the gut, and particularly the salivary glands. There is no protection of the brain, since the drug dose not cross the blood–brain barrier, and a disappointing level of protection is seen in the lung. The mechanism by which amifostine exerts a differential effect between normal tissues and tumors is not entirely clear. Part of the reason for the slower uptake in tumors may be that they generally have a poorly developed vascular system, but this is clearly not the whole story. An

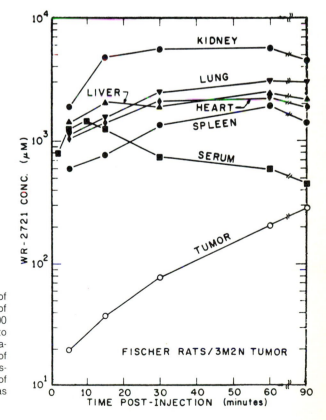

**Figure 11-2.** Serum, tissue, and tumor concentration of the radioprotector Amifostine (WR-2721) as a function of time after intraperitoneal administration of the drug (200 mg/kg). The radioprotector penetrates more slowly into the tumor than into many normal tissues, so that if the radiation dose is delivered soon after the administration of the drug, there is a differential protection of normal tissues. Similar results have been shown in a wide variety of transplantable tumors in laboratory animals. (From Yuhas J: Cancer Res 40:1519–1524, 1980)

Table 11-3.
## Summary of Normal Tissue Responsiveness to Protection by WR-2721

| TISSUES PROTECTED* | TISSUES NOT PROTECTED |
|---|---|
| Bone marrow (2.4–3) | Brain |
| Immune system (1.8–3.4) | Spinal cord |
| Skin (2–2.4) | |
| Small intestine (1.8–2) | |
| Colon (1.8) | |
| Lung (1.2–1.8) | |
| Esophagus (1.4) | |
| Kidney (1.5) | |
| Liver (2.7) | |
| Salivary gland (2.0) | |
| Oral mucosa (>1) | |
| Testes (2.1) | |

*Numbers in parentheses are the dose reduction factors or factor increases in resistance associated with WR-2721 injection. (From Yuhas JM, Spellman JM, Culo F: In Brady L [ed]: Radiation Sensitizers, pp 303–308. New York, Masson, 1980)*

essential feature of the design of successful radioprotectors is that they must be hydrophilic (ie, more soluble in water than in lipids). Lipophilic radioprotectors do not show this differential uptake between normal tissues and tumors. Therefore it may be that the difference in uptake of amifostine between normal tissues and tumors is due in some way to a difference in the membrane structure of the tumor cells, which allows hydrophilic drugs to penetrate only slowly.

Figure 11-3 shows an autoradiograph of an animal given a radioactive-labeled amifostine 20 minutes before sacrifice. A number of features already discussed are illustrated dramatically in this section. First, the tumor (a transplanted EMT6 tumor) is entirely cold—it has not taken up the drug at all. The bone marrow, gut, and salivary glands are very black, indicating a high uptake of the drug. The lungs show an intermediate uptake.

The clinical exploitation of radioprotectors has been slow in coming. Phase 1 toxicity trials of amifostine conducted in humans in the United States have shown that the dose-limiting toxicity is hypotension. Other symptoms include sneezing and somnolence. These undesirable side effects tend to limit the amount of drug given to levels lower than necessary to achieve maximum protection, based on animal experiments. A randomized clinical trial of a radioprotector has been conducted in mainland China. One hundred patients with inoperable unresectable or recurrent adenocarcinoma of the rectum were stratified and randomized to amifostine plus radiotherapy or to radiotherapy alone. The radioprotector was administered 15 minutes before radiotherapy, 4 days a week for 5 weeks. Those patients pretreated with amifostine showed pro-

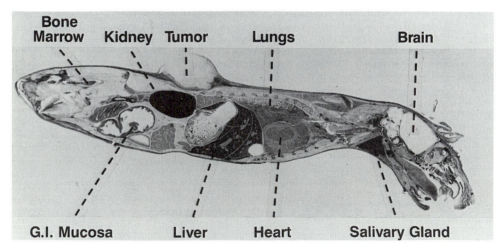

**Figure 11-3.** Autoradiograph of a mouse showing the distribution of amifostine, labeled with radioactive sulfur-35, at 6 minutes after intravenous injection. The greatest densities are seen in the kidney, liver, intestinal mucosa, and submandibular salivary gland. The brain shows little drug concentration because amifostine is hydrophilic and does not cross the blood–brain barrier. The drug has also not concentrated in the tumor (a transplanted EMT6). (From Utley JF, Marlow C, Waddell WJ: Radiat Res 68:284–291, 1976)

tection of the skin, mucous membrane, bladder, and pelvic structures against late moderate and severe reactions. In the radiation-only group, 5 of 37 patients did exhibit such reactions; with none receiving the radioprotector the difference is statistically significant. At the same time there was no apparent protection afforded the tumor.

One of the difficult and worrisome factors in the experimental use of radioprotectors in the clinic is that their use is not fail-safe. To exploit a benefit, radiation doses must be *increased* with the confidence that the normal tissues are protected and that the extra dose will improve tumor response. If radioprotection does not occur, unacceptable normal tissue morbidity results. This requires courage on the part of the investigator.

In addition to whole-body administration, radioprotectors have the tantalizing potential of local topical applications in radiotherapy. Two particular examples have been suggested. First, intrathecal delivery of a drug could be used to protect the spinal cord during radiotherapy. Sec-

ond, a radioprotector could be "sprayed" into the oral cavity just before radiotherapy to minimize mucositis, if a suitable formulation were available.

# RADIOPROTECTORS AND CHEMOTHERAPY

Although sulfhydryl compounds were developed as radioprotectors against ionizing radiation, they also protect against the cytotoxic effects of a number of chemotherapeutic agents, the mode of action of which depends at some stage on the production of free radicals.

The clinical use of amifostine has shown that the compound offers significant protection against nephrotoxicity, ototoxicity, and neuropathy from cisplatin and hematologic toxicity from cyclophosphamide. The same experimental studies indicated no obvious antitumor activity of the radioprotector.

► *Summary of Pertinent Conclusions*

---

- Radioprotectors are chemicals that *reduce* the biological effects of radiation.
- The sulfhydryl compounds cysteine and cysteamine were discovered early but are toxic. If the SH group is covered by a phosphate group, toxicity is reduced.
- The dose reduction factor (DRF) is the ratio of radiation doses required to produce the same biological effect in the absence and presence of the radioprotector.
- The best available radioprotectors can attain DRF values of 2 to 2.7 for bone marrow or gut death in mice irradiated with x-rays.
- The mechanism of action is the scavenging of free radicals and restitution of free radical damage.
- Since radioprotectors modify the indirect action of radiation, DRF values close to the oxygen enhancement ratio are possible for x-rays, but their effectiveness decreases with increasing LET.
- Radioprotectors were carried to the moon by US astronauts to be taken in the event of a solar flare. During the era of the Cold War, it is said that Soviet infantry in Europe carried radioprotectors for use in a possible nuclear war.
- More than 3000 compounds have been synthesized by researchers at the Walter Reed Army Hospital. Amifostine (WR-2721) appears to be the best for radiotherapy.

*(continued)*

▶ *Summary of Pertinent Conclusions*  *(Continued)*

- Bone marrow, the gut, and the salivary glands are well protected by amifostine; the lung is protected poorly and the brain not at all because the drug is hydrophilic and does not cross the blood–brain barrier.
- Amifostine is used in radiotherapy because it floods many normal tissues rapidly after administration but penetrates tumors much more slowly. The strategy is to begin irradiation soon after administration of the drug to exploit a differential effect.
- A clinical trial of amifostine in mainland China has shown protection of normal tissues, with no evidence of protection of the tumor in patients with adenocarcinoma of the rectum treated with radiation.
- Sulfhydryl compounds are useful as protectors for chemotherapy as well as radiotherapy.

# BIBLIOGRAPHY

Kligerman MM, Liu T, Liu Y, Scheffler B, He S, Zhang Z: Interim analysis of a randomized trial of radiation therapy of rectal cancer with/without WR-2721. Int J Radiat Oncol Biol Phys 22:799–802, 1992

Liu T, Liu Y, He S, Zhang Z, Kligerman MM: Use of radiation with or without WR-2721 in advanced rectal cancer. Cancer 69:2820–2825, 1992

Patt HM, Tyree B, Straube RL, Smith DE: Cysteine protection against x-irradiation. Science 110:213–214, 1949

Rasey JS, Nelson NJ, Mahler P, Anderson K, Krohn KA, Menard T: Radioprotection of normal tissues against gamma-rays and cyclotron neutrons with WR2721: $LD_{50}$ studies and $^{35}$S-WR2721 biodistribution. Radiat Res 97:598–607, 1984

Utley JF, Marlowe C, Waddell WJ: Distribution of $^{35}$S-labeled WR-2721 in normal and malignant tissues of the mouse. Radiat Res 68:284–291, 1976

Washburn LC, Carlton JE, Hayes RL: Distribution of WR-2721 in normal and malignant tissues of mice and rats bearing solid tumors: Dependence on tumor type, drug dose, and species. Radiat Res 59:483–575, 1974

Yuhas J: Active versus passive absorption kinetics as the basis for selective protection of normal tissues by S-2-(3-aminopropylamino)-ethyl-phosphorothioic acid. Cancer Res 40:1519–1524, 1980

Yuhas JM, Spellman JM, Culo F: The role of WR2721 in radiotherapy and/or chemotherapy. In Brady L (ed): Radiation Sensitizers, pp 303–308, New York, Masson, 1980

*Radiobiology for the Radiologist, Fourth Edition*, by Eric J. Hall
J. B. Lippincott Company, Philadelphia © 1994.

# 12

# *Cell, Tissue, and Tumor Kinetics*

Radiation Therapy

## THE CELL CYCLE

Mammalian cells replicate and increase in number by mitosis. If growing cells are observed with a conventional light microscope, the only event that can be distinguished is the process of mitosis itself. For most of the cell cycle the chromosomes are diffuse and not clearly seen, but for a short time before mitosis they condense into discrete and recognizable entities. There is a brief flurry of activity as the chromosomes separate into two groups and move to the two poles of the cell; division then occurs to form two daughter cells. The average interval between successive mitoses or divisions is called the **cell cycle** or **mitotic cycle time** ($T_C$).

Howard and Pelc were the first to further subdivide the mitotic cycle by the use of a labeled DNA precursor. This is described in Chapter 6 and is only reviewed briefly here. It is a simple matter to identify the proportion of cells synthesizing DNA (ie, in S phase). The DNA precursor is made available to a growing population of cells, where it is taken up and incorporated into the DNA of cells that are actively synthesizing DNA at that time. Cells that are not making DNA will not take up the label. The cell preparation is then fixed and stained and viewed through a microscope. The DNA precursor may be thymidine labeled with radioactive tritium, which may be identified later by autoradiography, or 5-bromodeoxyuridine, which may be identified later by the use of a specific stain or antibody.

These labeling techniques can be applied to cells growing in vitro in petri dishes or to tissues in vivo, if, after the incorporation of the label, the tissue or tumor of interest is removed and sliced into sections a few microns thick.

By the use of these techniques, the cell cycle in all dividing mammalian cells may be divided as shown in Figure 12-1. After the cells pass through mitosis (M), there is a period of apparent inactivity, termed $G_1$ by Howard and Pelc, simply because it was the first "gap" in activity observed in the cell cycle. After this period of inactivity, the cells actively synthesize DNA during

S phase. Between S phase and the onset of the next division or mitosis, there is another gap in inactivity, termed $G_2$.

## QUANTITATIVE ASSESSMENT OF THE CONSTITUENT PARTS OF THE CELL CYCLE

Two relatively simple measurements can be made on a population of cells. First, it is possible to count the proportion of cells that are seen to be in mitosis; this quantity is called the **mitotic index** (MI). If it is assumed that all of the cells in the population are dividing, that all of the cells have the same mitotic cycle, then,

$$MI = \lambda \, \frac{T_M}{T_C}$$

where $T_M$ is the length of mitosis (ie, the time taken for cells to complete division), and $T_C$ is the total length of the mitotic or cell cycle.

The $\lambda$ is a correction to allow for the fact that cells cannot be distributed uniformly in time around the cycle since they double during mitosis (Fig. 12-2). The simplest assumption is that cells are distributed around the cycle exponen-

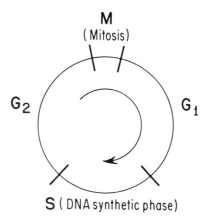

**Figure 12-1.** The phases of the cell cycle. Mitosis (M) is the only event that can be distinguished through the light microscope. The DNA synthetic phase (S) may be identified by the technique of autoradiography (see Chapter 6). The intervals of apparent inactivity are labeled $G_1$ and $G_2$.

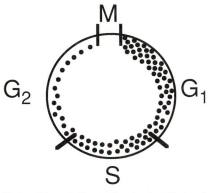

**Figure 12-2.** Diagram illustrating the fact that cells cannot be distributed uniformly in time around the cell cycle because they double in number during mitosis. The simplest assumption is that they are distributed as an exponential function of time.

tially in time, in which case $\lambda$ has a value of 0.69. At all events, the $\lambda$ is a relatively small and unimportant correction factor.

The second relatively simple measurement requires that the cell population be fed for a brief time with a quantity of tritiated thymidine or bromodeoxyuridine. In the jargon of cell kinetics, it is said to be **flash-labeled.** The cell population, whether on a petri dish or in a thin section cut from tissue, is then fixed, stained, and viewed through a microscope. A count is made of the proportion of labeled cells. This quantity is called the **labeling index** (LI).

Given the assumptions that all the cells are dividing with the same cell cycle, then

$$LI = \lambda \frac{T_s}{T_C}$$

where $T_s$ is the duration of the DNA synthetic period, and $T_C$ is the total cell cycle time.

In practice these two quantities—the mitotic index and the labeling index—can be determined from a single specimen by counting the proportion of cells in mitosis and the proportion of cells that are labeled. This is a very important consideration in human studies, in which it is usually not practical to obtain a large number of serial specimens of tumor or normal tissue material. Although these measurements yield *ratios* of the duration of mitosis and DNA synthesis as a fraction of the total cell cycle, they do not give the absolute duration in hours of any part of the cycle.

## THE PERCENT-LABELED-MITOSES TECHNIQUE

A complete analysis of the cell cycle to obtain the length of each phase is only possible by labeling a cohort of cells in one phase of the cycle and observing the progress of this labeled cohort through a "window" in some other readily observable phase of the cycle. In practice the easiest phase to label is S, and the easiest to observe is M.

As stated before, the labeling can be achieved either by using tritiated thymidine, identifiable by autoradiography, or bromodeoxyuridine, identifiable by a specific stain or antibody. The basis of the technique, therefore, is to feed the population of cells a label that is taken up in S, and then to observe the appearance of that label in mitotic cells as they move around the cycle from S to M. To avoid confusion, the technique involving tritiated thymidine will be described in detail, partly because it is the original and classic technique and partly because pictures of autoradiographs show up well in black and white. The technique works equally well if bromodeoxyuridine is used. The bright colors that bromodeoxyuridine-containing DNA can be stained show up well under a microscope but do not reproduce well in black and white.

The percent-labeled-mitoses technique is laborious, is time consuming, and requires a large number of serial samples. It is readily applicable in vitro, for which it is not difficult to obtain a large number of parallel replicate samples. It may also be applied in vivo for determining the cell cycle parameters of normal tissue or tumors, provided a large number of sections from matched animals or tumors can be obtained at accurately timed intervals. The cell population must first be flash-labeled with tritiated thymidine. Theoretically, the labeled DNA precursor should be available to the cells for a negligibly short time; in practice, an exposure time of about 20 minutes is usually used. In vitro the thymidine is added to the growth medium; at the end of the flash-labeling period it is simple to remove the radioactive medium and add fresh medium. In vivo, the tritiated thymidine is injected intraperitoneally; it clearly cannot be removed after 20 minutes, so the exposure time is terminated by the injection of a massive dose of "cold," ie, nonradioactive, thymidine.

During the period when tritiated thymidine is available, cells in S phase take up the radioactive label. After the label is removed, cells will progress through their cell cycle. At regular intervals, usually of 1 hour, a specimen of the cell population must be removed, fixed, and stained and an autoradiograph prepared. This is continued for a total time longer than the cell cycle of the population under study. For each sample the percentage of mitotic cells that carry a radioactive label must then be counted; this is the **percentage of labeled mitoses.** A photomicrograph of a cell preparation is shown in Figure 12-3. An example of a labeled mitosis is marked LM; two unlabeled mitoses are marked UM. This is a particularly laborious process, since only 1% or 2% of the cells are in mitosis in any case and only a fraction of these will be labeled.

The basis for this type of experiment, when applied to an idealized population of cells that all have identical cell cycles, is illustrated in Figure 12-4, a plot of the percentage of labeled mitoses

as a function of time. The cells that are in S while the radioactive thymidine is available take up the label. This labeled cohort of cells then moves through the cell cycle (as indicated by the circles at the top of Figure 12-4) after the pool of radioactive thymidine has been removed. Samples obtained in the first few hours contain no labeled mitotic figures, and the first labeled mitotic figure appears when the leading edge of the cohort of labeled cells reaches M. This point in time is labeled b on the time axis of Figure 12-4; the position of the labeled cohort is indicated above on the circle also marked b.

The percentage of mitotic figures labeled will increase rapidly as the leading edge of the labeled cohort of cells passes through the M phase; when it reaches the end of the M phase, all mitotic figures will be labeled (see position c). For the next few hours all mitotic figures will continue to be labeled until the trailing edge of the labeled cohort of cells reaches the beginning of mitosis (see position d), after which the per-

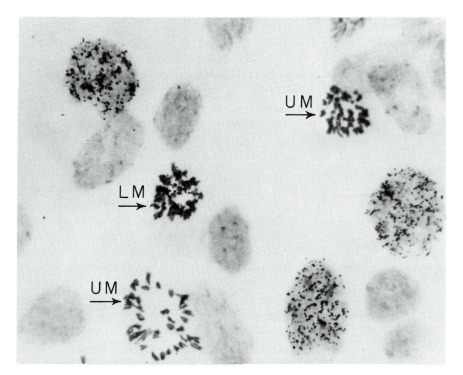

**Figure 12-3.** Photomicrograph of a preparation of mouse corneal cells. The cell preparation was flash-labeled some hours before with tritiated thymidine, which was taken up by cells in S. By the time the autoradiograph was made, the cell marked LM had moved around the cycle into mitosis; it is an example of a labeled mitotic figure. Other cells in mitosis are not labeled (UM). (Courtesy of Dr. M. Fry)

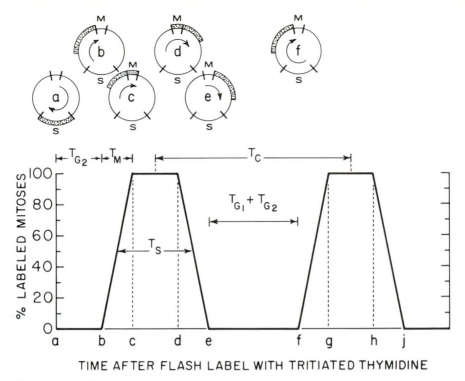

**Figure 12-4.** Percent-labeled-mitoses curve for an idealized cell population in which all of the cells have identical mitotic cycle times. The cell population is flash-labeled with tritiated thymidine, which labels all cells in S. The proportion of labeled mitotic cells is counted as a function of time after labeling. The circles at the top of the figure indicate the position of the labeled cohort of cells as it progresses through the cycle. The length of the various phases (eg, $T_{G2}$, $T_M$) of the cycle ($T_C$) may be determined as indicated.

centage of labeled mitoses will rapidly fall and reach zero when the trailing edge reaches the end of mitosis (see position e).

There will then be a long interval during which no labeled mitotic figures will be seen until the labeled cohort of cells goes around the entire cycle and comes up to mitosis again, after which the whole pattern of events will be repeated.

All of the parameters of the cell cycle may be calculated from Figure 12-4. The time interval before the appearance of the first labeled mitosis, the length ab, is in fact the length of $G_2$ or $T_{G_2}$. The time it takes for the percent-labeled-mitoses curve to rise from 0% to 100% (bc) corresponds to the time necessary for the leading edge of the labeled cohort of cells to proceed through mitosis and is therefore equal to the length of mitosis, $T_M$. The duration of DNA synthesis ($T_S$) is the time taken for the cohort of labeled cells to pass the beginning of mitosis (bd).

Likewise, it is the time required for the labeled cohort to pass the end of mitosis, ce. In practice, $T_S$ is usually taken to be the width of the curve at the 50% level, as marked in Figure 12-5.

The total cycle ($T_C$) is the distance between corresponding points on the first and second wave (bf, cg, dh, or ej) or the distance between the centers of the two peaks as marked on the figure. The remaining quantity, $T_{G_1}$, is usually calculated by subtracting the sum of all the other phases of the cycle from the total cell cycle, or

$$T_{G_1} = T_C - (T_S + T_{G_2} + T_M)$$

Experimental data are never as clear-cut as the idealized picture in Figure 12-4. Points such as b and e, at which the curve begins to rise and reaches zero, are poorly defined. A more typical experimental result is illustrated in Figure 12-5. The only points that can be defined with any certainty are the peaks of the curves and the 50% levels, and these may be used to give a rough es-

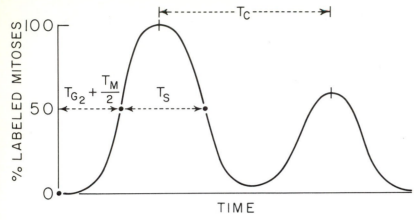

**Figure 12-5.** Typical percent-labeled-mitoses curve obtained in practice for the cells of a tissue or tumor. It differs from the idealized curve in Figure 12-4 in that the only points that can be identified with precision are the peaks of the curve and the 50% levels. The first peak is asymmetrical, and the second peak is lower than the first because the cells of a population have a range of cell cycle times.

timate of the lengths of the various phases of the cycle. The S period is given approximately by the width of the first peak, from the 50% level on the ascending portion of the wave to the corresponding point on the descending curve. The total cell cycle, $T_C$, is readily obtained as the time between successive peaks. In a separate experiment the mitotic index may be counted, which is equal to $T_M/T_C$; since $T_C$ is known, $T_M$ may be calculated. The time from flash-labeling to the point at which the curve passes the 50% level in Figure 12-5 is $T_{G_2} + \frac{1}{2} T_M$; since $T_M$ is already known, $T_{G_2}$ may be calculated. The remaining quantity, $T_{G_1}$, is deduced by subtraction, since the total cycle time and all other phases are known.

A careful examination of an actual set of experimental data makes it plain that the first wave in the percent-labeled-mitoses curve is not symmetrical; the downswing is shallower than the upswing. This observation, coupled with the fact that the second peak is much smaller than the first, indicates that the population is made up of cells with a wide range of cycle times. In many instances, particularly when the population of cells involved is an in vivo specimen of a tumor or a normal tissue, the spread of cell cycle times is so great that a second peak is barely discernible.

In practice, therefore, the constituent parts of the cycle are not simply read off from the percent-labeled-mitoses curve. Instead, a complex computer program is used to try various distributions of cell cycle times and to calculate the curve that best fits the experimental data. In this way an estimate is obtained of the *mean* cell cycle time and also of the *range* of cell cycle times in the population.

## EXPERIMENTAL MEASUREMENTS OF CELL CYCLE TIMES IN VIVO AND IN VITRO

A vast number of cell cycle measurements have been made. Only a few representative results will be reviewed here to highlight the most important points.

Figure 12-6 shows the percent-labeled-mitoses data for two transplantable rat tumors with very different growth rates. The tumor represented in the upper panel has a gross doubling time of 22 hours, which can easily be judged from the separation of the first and second waves of labeled mitotic cells. For the tumor illustrated in the lower panel, there is no discernible second peak in the percent-labeled-mitoses curve because of the large range of cell cycle times among the cells of the population. To obtain an estimate of the average cell cycle in this case, it is necessary to pool information from the percent-labeled-mitoses curve and from a knowledge of the labeling index.

The width of the first wave of the percent-labeled-mitoses curve indicates that the length of the DNA synthetic phase $(T_S)$ is about 10 hours. To obtain the average cell cycle time $(T_C)$, it is essential in this situation to know the labeling index (LI). For this tumor, the labeling index is about 3.6%. The average cell cycle time $(T_C)$

can then be calculated from the following equation:

$$LI = \lambda \frac{T_S}{T_C}$$

Therefore,

$$T_C = \frac{0.693 \times 10}{3.6 / 100}$$
$$= 190 \text{ hours}$$

The absence of a second peak is a clue to the fact that there is a wide range of cell cycle times for the cells of this population, so that 190 hours is very much an *average* value.

A computer analysis makes it possible to estimate the distribution of cell cycle times in a population. For example, Figure 12-7 shows the percent-labeled-mitoses curve for a transplantable mouse tumor, together with an analysis of cell cycle times based on a mathematical model. There is a wide range of cell cycle times, from less than 10 to more than 40 hours,

with a modal value of about 19 hours. This range of cycle times explains the damped-labeled-mitoses curve and the fact that the first peak is not symmetrical.

Table 12-1 is a summary of the cell cycle parameters for cell lines in culture and some of the tissues and tumors for which percent-labeled-mitoses curves have been shown in this chapter. The top line of Table 12-1 shows the data for Chinese hamster cells in culture. These cells are characterized by a short cell cycle of only 10 hours and a minimal $G_1$ period. The second row of the table gives the comparable figures for HeLa cells. From a comparison of these two in vitro cell lines, a very important point emerges. The cell cycles of the two cell lines differ by a factor of more than 2, nearly all of which is due to a difference in the length of $G_1$. The other phases of the cycle are very similar in the two cell lines.

Also included in Table 12-1 are data for the cells of the normal cheek pouch epithelium in

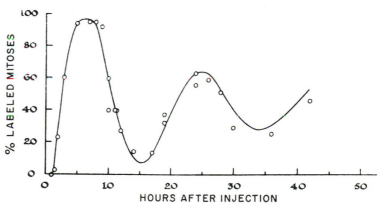

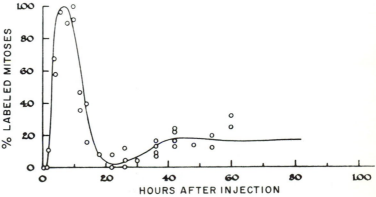

**Figure 12-6.** Percent-labeled-mitoses curve for two transplantable rat sarcomas with widely different growth rates. The tumor in the upper panel has a gross doubling time of 22 hours, compared with 190 hours for the tumor in the lower panel. (From Steel GG, Adams K, B Parratt JC: Br J Cancer 20:784, 1966)

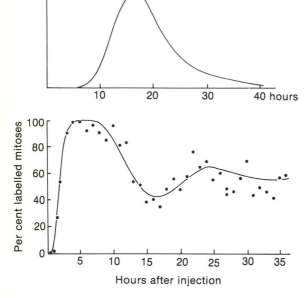

**Figure 12-7.** (*Bottom*) Percent-labeled-mitoses curve for an EMT6 mouse tumor (data from Dr. Sara Rockwell). (*Top*) The distribution of cell cycle times consistent with the damped-labeled-mitoses curve, obtained by computer analysis of the data and a mathematical model. (From Steel GG: Laryngoscope 85:359–370, 1975)

the hamster and a chemically induced carcinoma in the pouch. These are representative of a number of studies in which cells from a solid tumor have been compared with their normal tissue counterpart. In general, it is usually found that the malignant cells have the shorter cycle time.

In reviewing the data summarized in Table 12-1, it is at once evident that while the length of the cell cycle varies enormously between popula-tions, particularly in vivo, the lengths of $G_2$, mito-sis, and S are remarkably constant. The vast bulk of the cell cycle variation is accounted for by dif-ferences in the length of the $G_1$ phase.

## PULSED PHOTO CYTOMETRY

During the past decade or so, classic autoradiog-raphy has been largely replaced by pulsed photo

Table 12-1.
**The Constituent Parts of the Cell Cycle for Some Cells in Culture and Tumors in Experimental Animals**

| AUTHOR(S) | CELL OR TISSUE | HOURS | | | | |
|---|---|---|---|---|---|---|
| | | $T_C$ | $T_S$ | $T_M$ | $T_{G_2}$ | $T_{G_1}$ |
| Bedford | Hamster cells in vitro | 10 | 6 | 1 | 1 | 2 |
| | HeLa cells in vitro | 23 | 8 | 1 | 3 | 11 |
| Steel | Mammary tumors in the rat | | | | | |
| | BICR/M1 | 19 | 8 | ~1 | 2 | 8 |
| | BICR/A2 | 63 | 10 | ~1 | 2 | 50 |
| Quastler and Sherman | Mouse intestinal crypt | 18.75 | 7.5 | 0.5 | 0.5–1 | 9.5 |
| Brown and Berry | Hamster cheek pouch epithelium | 120–152 | 8.6 | 1.0 | 1.9 | 108–140 |
| | Chemically induced carcinoma in pouch | 10.7 | 5.9 | 0.4 | 1.6 | 2.8 |

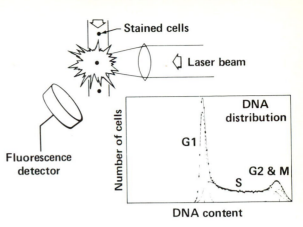

**Figure 12-8.** The principles of DNA distribution analysis of flow cytometry. Suspensions of fluorescent-stained single cells flow one at a time through a light beam with its wavelength adjusted to excite the fluorescent dye. The fluorescence stimulated in each cell is recorded as a measure of that cell's DNA content. Thousands of cells can be measured each second and the results accumulated to form a DNA distribution like that shown for asynchronously growing CHO cells. (From Gray JW, Dolbeare F, Pallavicini MG, Beisker W, Waldman F: Int J Radiat Biol 49:237–255, 1986)

cytometry (Fig. 12-8). The conventional techniques of autoradiography give precise, meaningful answers, but they are laborious and so slow that information is never available quickly enough to act as a predictive assay to influence the treatment options of an individual patient. Techniques based on flow cytometry provide data that are available within a few days. Detailed cell kinetic data can be obtained by such techniques, including an analysis of the distribution of cells in the various phases of the cycle, but in practice the measurement of most immediate relevance to clinical radiotherapy is the estimate of $T_{pot}$, the potential tumor doubling time.

## MEASUREMENT OF POTENTIAL TUMOR DOUBLING TIME ($T_{pot}$)

$T_{pot}$ is a measure of the rate of increase of cells capable of continued proliferation and therefore determines the outcome of a radiotherapy treatment protocol delivered in fractions over an extended period of time.

Tumors with a short $T_{pot}$ may repopulate if fractionation is extended over too long a period. $T_{pot}$ can be calculated from the following:

$$T_{pot} = \frac{\lambda T_S}{LI}$$

where $T_S$ is the length of the DNA synthetic period, LI is the labeling index (ie, the fraction of cells synthesizing DNA at any time) and $\lambda$ is a correction factor to allow for the nonlinear distribution in time of the cells as they pass through the cycle; this factor has a value between 1 and 0.67.

To measure $T_{pot}$ precisely requires a knowledge of $T_S$ and the labeling index. The labeling index can be determined from a single sample, but to measure $T_S$ precisely it is necessary to label the cell population with tritiated thymidine or bromodeoxyuridine, take a sample every hour for a time period about equal to the cell cycle, and count the proportion of labeled mitoses as a function of time as previously described. This is out of the question in a clinical situation but an *estimate* of $T_{pot}$ can be made by flow cytometry from a single biopsy specimen taken 4 to 8 hours after the injection of a tracer amount of a thymidine analogue (bromodeoxyuridine or iododeoxyurine). The biopsy specimen is treated with fluorescent-labeled monoclonal antibody, which detects the incorporation of the thymidine analogue into the DNA.

The specimen is also stained with propidium iodide to determine DNA content. A single cell suspension of the biopsy specimen is then passed through a flow cytometer, which simultaneously measures DNA content (red) and bromodeoxyuridine content (green). This is illustrated in Figure 12-9.

The labeling index is simply the proportion of cells that show significant green fluorescence. $T_S$ can be calculated from the mean red fluorescence of S cells relative to $G_1$ and $G_2$ cells. The DNA content of cells in $G_2$ is double that in $G_1$. The method assumes that the red fluorescence of bromodeoxyuridine-labeled cells (ie, the DNA content of cells in S phase) increases linearly with time (Fig. 12-10). If, for example, the biopsy specimen were obtained 6 hours after administration of bromodeoxyuridine, and the relative

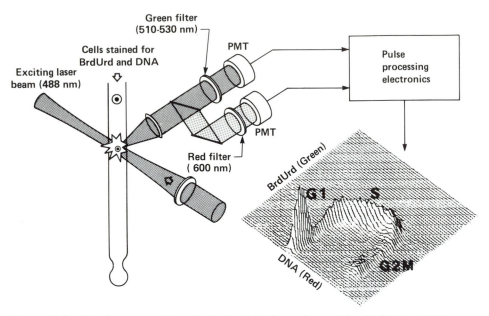

**Figure 12-9.** The flow cytometric analysis of cellular bromodeoxyuridine (BrdUrd) and DNA content for cells stained with fluorescein (linked to BrdUrd) and propidium iodide (linked to DNA). The cells are processed one at a time through a blue (488 nm) laser beam that excites cellular BrdUrd content, and red fluorescence is recorded as a measure of cellular DNA content. The BrdUrd (green fluorescence) axis in the bivariate is logarithmic, with every seven channels representing a doubling of fluorescence intensity. (From Gray JW, Dolbeare F, Pallavicini MG, Beisker W, Waldman F: Int J Radiat Biol 49:237–255, 1986)

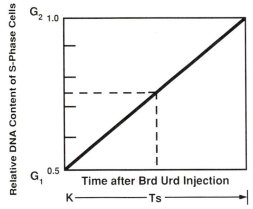

**Figure 12-10.** Graph illustrating the way in which $T_s$ can be estimated by flow cytometry on cells from a single tumor biopsy specimen taken 4 to 8 hours after an injection of a thymidine analogue (bromodeoxyuridine or iododeoxyuridine). Cells in S phase are identified by the *green* fluorescence from an antibody to the thymidine analogue. The relative DNA content is measured by the *red* fluorescence owing to the incorporated propidium iodide. The DNA content in $G_2$ cells is double that in $G_1$. The length of the DNA synthetic phase ($T_s$) can be estimated by the relative DNA content of the S-phase cells in relation to the time between the injection of the thymidine analogue and the biopsy.

DNA content of cells labeled with bromodeoxyuridine (ie, in S phase) was 0.75, midway between that characteristic of $G_1$ and that of $G_2$, the duration of $T_S$ would be simply 12 hours. The method has been validated in a number of in vitro cell lines and also in animal tumor systems, where it can be checked by conventional cell kinetic studies.

This technique gives an *average* value for $T_{pot}$ of the cells in the biopsy specimen since the cells are disaggregated and made into a single cell suspension. There is some evidence from animal experiments that individual cells may have much shorter $T_{pot}$ values.

This technique to measure $T_{pot}$ has proven to be practical as a predictive assay and has been used on a large number of patients entered on a clinical trial of altered fractionation patterns by the European Cooperative Radiotherapy Group (EORTC). This is described in more detail in Chapters 13 and 15. Briefly, estimates of $T_{pot}$ were used to divide patients into those with fast-growing tumors ($T_{pot}$ < 4 days) and those with slow-growing tumors ($T_{pot}$ > 4 days). Patients with fast-growing tumors were found to benefit from an accelerated treatment regimen. This is the first occasion on which a tumor kinetic measurement has been used successfully as a predictive assay. This is a very important development and likely to be widely used.

## THE GROWTH FRACTION

Central to an appreciation of the pattern of growth of solid tumors is the realization that, at any given moment, not all of the tumor cells that are viable and capable of continued growth are actually proceeding through the cell cycle. The population consists of proliferating (P) cells and quiescent (Q) cells. The **growth fraction**, a term introduced by Mendelsohn, is defined as the ratio of the number of proliferating cells (P) to the total number of cells, (P + Q), or

$$GF = \frac{P}{P + Q}$$

There are various ways to estimate GF. One method consists of injecting tritiated thymidine into an animal with a tumor, then, several cell generations later, preparing an autoradiograph from sections of the tumor. The growth fraction is given by the expression

$$GF = \frac{\text{Fraction of cells labeled}}{\text{Fraction of mitoses labeled}}$$

This method assumes that there are two distinct subpopulations, one growing with a uniform cell cycle, the other not growing at all. Continuous labeling is an alternative way to provide an approximate measure of the proportion of proliferating cells. Tritiated thymidine is infused continuously for a time equal to the cell cycle (minus the length of S phase). The fraction of labeled cells then approximates to the growth fraction. Table 12-2 is a summary of growth fractions measured for a variety of solid tumors in experimental animals, which frequently fall between 30% and 50%, even though the tumors vary widely in degree of differentiation, arise in different species, and are of varied histologic types. As a tumor outgrows its blood supply, areas of necrosis often develop that are frequently accom-

**Table 12-2.**
**The Growth Fraction (GF) for Some Tumors in Experimental Animals**

| TUMOR | AUTHOR | GF(%) |
|---|---|---|
| Primary mammary carcinoma in the mouse ($C_3H$) | Mendelsohn | 35–77 |
| Transplantable sarcoma in the rat ($RIB_5$) | Denekamp | 55 |
| Transplantable sarcoma in the rat (SSO) | Denekamp | 47 |
| Transplantable sarcoma in the rat ($SSB_1$) | Denekamp | 39 |
| Mammary carcinoma in the mouse ($C_3H$) | Denekamp | 30 |
| Chemically induced carcinoma in the hamster cheek pouch | Brown | 29 |

panied by the presence of hypoxic cells, the proportion of which for many solid tumors is about 15%. This accounts for part but not all of the quiescent cell population.

## CELL LOSS

The overall growth of a tumor is the result of a balance achieved between cell production from division and various types of **cell loss.** In most cases, tumors grow much more slowly than would be predicted from a knowledge of the cycle time of the individual cells and the growth fraction. The difference is due to cell loss. The extent of the cell loss from a tumor is estimated by comparing the rate of production of new cells with the observed growth rate of the tumor. The discrepancy will provide a measure of the rate of cell loss. Suppose $T_{pot}$ is the *potential* tumor-doubling time (the time during which the tumor volume would be expected to double), calculated from the cell cycle time and the growth fraction. Suppose $T_d$ is the *actual* tumor-doubling time, obtained from simple direct measurements on the diameter of the tumor mass. The **cell loss factor** ($\varphi$) has been defined by Steel to be

$$\Phi = 1 - T_{pot} / T_d$$

The cell loss factor represents the ratio of the *rate of cell loss* to the *rate of new cell produc-*

*tion*. It expresses the loss of growth potential by the tumor. A cell loss factor of 100%, for instance, indicates a steady state of neither growth nor regression.

Cells in tumors can be lost in a number of ways, such as

1. Death from inadequate nutrition. As the tumor outgrows its vascular system, rapid cell proliferation near capillaries will push other cells into regions remote from blood supply, where there is an inadequate concentration of oxygen and other nutrients. These cells will die, giving rise to a progressively enlarging necrotic zone.
2. Apoptosis, or programmed cell death. This form of cell death is manifested by the occurrence of isolated degenerate nuclei remote from regions of overt necrosis.
3. Death from immunologic attack.
4. Metastasis, including all processes by which tumor cells are lost to other parts of the body, such as spread through the bloodstream and lymphatic system.
5. Exfoliation, which would not apply to most model tumors in experimental animals but which could be an important mechanism of cell loss from, for example, carcinoma of the gastrointestinal tract, where the epithelium is renewed at a considerable rate.

There are limited data on the relative importance of these different processes in different tumor types, but it is clear that death from inadequate nutrition—by entry into necrotic areas—is often a major factor. It reflects the latent inability of the vascular system to keep up with the rate of cell production. There is still a great deal to be learned about the occurrence of cell loss from tumors, the mechanisms by which it occurs, and the factors by which it can be controlled. It is clear, however, that any understanding of the growth rate of tumors at the cellular level must include a consideration of this often dominant factor.

## DETERMINATIONS OF CELL LOSS IN EXPERIMENTAL ANIMAL TUMORS

The cell loss factor has been estimated in a considerable number of tumors in experimental animals. Some of the results are listed in Table 12-3. Values for the cell loss factor vary from 0% to more than 90%. In reviewing the literature on this subject, Denekamp pointed out that sarcomas tended to have *low* cell loss factors, while carcinomas tended to have *high* cell loss factors. All of the sarcomas investigated had a cell loss factor of less than 30%, while the carcinomas had a cell loss factor in excess of 70%. Therefore cell loss appears to be a dominant factor in the growth of carcinomas and of considerably less importance for sarcomas.

If this is found to be a general phenomenon, it might be attributed to the origin of carcinomas from continuously renewing epithelial tissues in which the cell loss factor is 100%. This difference between sarcomas and carcinomas may also account for their differing response to radiation. In carcinomas, when the production of new cells is temporarily stopped or reduced by a dose of radiation, cells continue to be removed from the tumor because of the high cell loss factor, and the tumor shrinks. In sarcomas, however, even when a large proportion of the cells are sterilized by a dose of radiation, they do not disappear from the tumor mass as quickly.

It would be simple, then, to explain why two tumors, one a carcinoma and one a sarcoma, containing the same number of cells and exposed to be the same radiation dose, would appear to behave quite differently. The carcinoma might shrink dramatically soon after the radiation dose, while the sarcoma would not appear as affected by the radiation. In the long term, the

Table 12-3.
The Cell Loss Factor ($\Phi$) for Some Tumors in Experimental Animals

| TUMOR | AUTHOR | $\Phi$(%) |
|---|---|---|
| Mouse sarcoma | Frindel | |
|    3-day-old tumor | | 0 |
|    7-day-old tumor | | 10 |
|    20-day-old tumor | | 55 |
| Rat carcinoma | Steel | 9 |
| Rat sarcoma | Steel | 0 |
| Mouse carcinoma | Mendelsohn | 69 |
| Hamster carcinoma | Brown | 75 |
| Rat sarcoma | Hermens | 26 |
| Hamster carcinoma | Reiskin | 81–93 |
| Mouse carcinoma | Tannock | 70–92 |

"cure" rate of both tumors may well be identical, but in the short term the carcinoma would be said to have "responded" to the radiation, whereas the sarcoma might be said to be unresponsive or resistant to radiation.

## THE OVERALL PATTERN OF TUMOR GROWTH

Three factors determine the growth rate of a tumor: (1) the cell cycle of the proliferative cells in the population; (2) the growth factor, that fraction of cells in the population that are proliferating as opposed to those that are quiescent; and (3) the rate of cell loss, either by cell death or loss from the tumor (Fig. 12-11).

The proliferative cells of a tumor, unrestrained as they are by any homeostatic control, divide and proliferate as rapidly as they are able to, limited only by their own inherited characteristics and the availability of an adequate supply of nutrients. Since a tumor is not an organized tissue, it tends to outgrow its blood supply. Areas of necrosis often develop and are frequently accompanied by hypoxic cells, which often constitute about 15% of the total viable cells.

Another manifestation of the overstretched vascular supply is that only a proportion of the viable cells (the growth fraction) are actually proceeding through the cell cycle and multiplying.

The growth fraction is frequently 30% to 50% but tends to be higher in regions close to blood capillaries and lower near necrotic areas.

The potentially explosive growth rate of tumor is seldom realized in practice because of cell loss from metastasis, exfoliation, random cell death, or cell death in the necrotic areas of the tumor. The cell loss factor (the fraction of cells produced by mitosis that are lost) is the most variable factor observed among tumors in experimental animals; values from 0% to more than 90% have been reported.

## GROWTH KINETICS OF HUMAN TUMORS

The first quantitative study of the growth rate of human tumors was done by Collins and his colleagues in 1956. They observed the growth of pulmonary metastases from serial chest radiographs. It is now possible to gather from the literature information on the doubling time of more than 1000 human tumors. Most of the data were obtained either by measurements from radiographs or by direct measurements of skin tumors or metastases in soft tissue. The doubling time of human tumors varies widely from patient to patient and is on the average very long; Tubiana and Malaise have estimated that the median value is about 2 months.

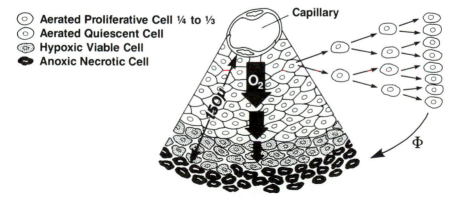

**Aerated Proliferative Cell ¼ to ⅓**
**Aerated Quiescent Cell**
**Hypoxic Viable Cell**
**Anoxic Necrotic Cell**

Capillary

$O_2$

150µ

Φ

**Figure 12-11.** The overall pattern of the growth of a tumor. Clonogenic cells consist of proliferative (P) and quiescent (Q) cells. Quiescent cells can be recruited into the cell cycle as the tumor shrinks after treatment with radiation or a cytotoxic drug. In animal tumors the growth fraction is frequently 30% to 50%. Of the cells produced by division, many are lost, principally into necrotic areas of the tumor remote from the vasculature. The cell loss factor (Φ) varies from 0% to 100% and dominates the pattern of tumor growth. As the tumor outgrows its blood supply, some cells become hypoxic. This accounts for some of the quiescent cells that are out of cycle.

Tumors of the same histologic type arising in different patients differ widely in growth rate. By contrast, metastases arising in the same patient tend to have similar rates of growth. This latter observation is the basis for using patients with multiple skin or pulmonary metastases to test and compare new treatment modalities, such as high linear energy transfer radiations or hyperthermia. There is certainly a correlation between histologic type and growth rate. Tubiana and Malaise have collected values for the doubling time in 389 patients with pulmonary metastases, classified into five histologic categories. They can be arranged in order of doubling time as follows: embryonic tumors, 27 days: malignant lymphomas, 29 days; mesenchymal sarcomas, 41 days; squamous cell carcinomas, 58 days; and adenocarcinomas, 82 days. In addition, the degree of differentiation seems to be related to the doubling time, with poorly differentiated cancers generally progressing more rapidly.

Data have been accumulated comparing the growth rate of primary breast and bronchial cancers to that of metastases in the same person. The primary carcinomas grew significantly more slowly than the metastases (Table 12-4). No entirely satisfactory explanation has been suggested for the more rapid proliferation of metastases. It may be a question of selection or a function of the unusually favorable milieu into which secondary tumors tend to be seeded.

In addition to growth rate measurements, studies of cell population kinetics have also been performed on a limited number of human tumors. Studies of this kind raise practical and ethical problems. The ethical problems stem from the fact that in vivo experiments require an injection of tritiated thymidine or bromodeoxyuridine, which limits such studies to patients who have a short life expectancy and in whom the injection of the label does not raise any problems of possible genetic consequences. The practical problems arise because the percent-labeled-mitoses technique, which is the most satisfactory way to obtain the duration of the various phases of the cell cycle, requires a large number of sequential samples to be taken for several days after the injection of the label. In mice or rats the multiple samples are obtained from a large number of identical animals, bearing transplanted tumors of the same size and type, by sacrificing one or more animals each time. In humans each spontaneous tumor is unique, so the multiple samples must be obtained by repeated biopsies at frequent intervals from the same tumor. This heroic procedure is uncomfortable and inconvenient for the patient and is only practical with large superficial skin tumors, which may not be truly representative of human tumors in general. Nevertheless, a surprisingly large number of human tumors have been studied in this way. The percent-labeled-mitoses curves obtained are similar to those for laboratory animals, although in general the second wave of labeled mitoses is rarely distinct and is usually altogether absent.

Tubiana and Malaise surveyed the field and reported 41 cases in which the cell cycle of solid tumors in humans had been evaluated with the percent-labeled-mitoses technique. The cell cycle obtained was between 15 and 125 hours in 90% of the cases, with a modal value of 48 hours (Table 12-5). The duration of $S(T_s)$ was less variable than the total cell cycle, with 90% of the values falling between 9.5 and 24 hours and a modal value of about 16 hours. As a first approximation, it can be assumed that $T_s$ has a duration of about 16 hours and that the mean duration of the cell cycle is about three times the duration of $T_s$.

Although the percent-labeled-mitoses technique has been used on relatively few human tumors, the labeling index has been measured in many more after in vitro incubation of a fresh piece of excised tumor with tritiated thymidine. The rationale underlying this technique is that

**Table 12-4.**
**Comparison of the Doubling Times of Primary Human Tumors With Metastases in the Same Individuals**

| HISTOLOGIC TYPE | AVERAGE DOUBLING TIME (DAYS)* | |
|---|---|---|
| | Primary Tumors | Lung Metastases |
| Squamous cell carcinomas | 81.8 (97) | 58.0 (51) |
| Adenocarcinomas | 166.3 (34) | 82.7 (134) |

*Number of patients in parentheses.
(From Charbit A, Malaise E, Tubiana M: Eur J Cancer 7:307, 1971)

Table 12-5.
Individual Values for the Duration of the Cell Cycle ($T_C$) in 41 Human and Solid Tumors of Various Histologic Types

| AUTHORS | $T_C$ (HOURS) |
|---|---|
| Frindel et al. (1968) | 97, 51.5, 27.5, 48, 49.8 |
| Bennington (1969) | 15.5, 14.9 |
| Young and de Vita (1970) | 42, 82, 74 |
| Shirakawa et al. (1970) | 120, 144 |
| Weinstein and Frost (1970) | 217 |
| Terz et al. (1971) | 44.5, 31, 14, 25.5, 26, 42 |
| Peckham and Steel (1973) | 59 |
| Estevez et al. (1972) | 37, 30, 48, 30, 38, 96, 48 |
| Terz and Curutchet* (1974) | 18, 19, 19.2, 120 |
| Malaise et al.* (unpublished data) | 24, 33, 48, 42 |
| Muggia et al. (1972) | 64 |
| Bresciani et al. (1974) | 82, 50, 67, 53, 58 |

*Measured by the mean grain count halving time. (From Tubiana M, Malaise E: In Symington T, Carter RL [eds]: Scientific Foundations of Oncology, pp 126–136. Chicago, Year Book Medical Publishers, 1976)

cells already synthesizing DNA in vivo are able to continue synthesis of DNA in vitro, while no new cells will enter synthesis under the incubation conditions that are normally used.

The growth fraction, too, has been measured in only a limited number of human tumors by the method of continuous labeling. If a population of cells is labeled continuously during a period corresponding to the duration of the cell cycle less the duration of the DNA synthetic phase (ie, $T_C - T_S$), all the actively proliferating cells should be labeled. This method of continuous labeling can only be performed with a small number of patients, who are in no way representative. An alternative procedure is to estimate the growth fraction by assuming that the proportion of cells in cycle is about equal to three times the labeling index, an assumption based on the notion that the cell cycle is three times the length of the S phase. The growth fraction calculated in this way correlates well with the tumor-doubling time: it is 0.9 in malignant lymphomas and embryonic tumors and less than 0.06 in adenocarcinomas. The relation between the growth rate and growth fraction appears to be much closer in human tumors than in animal tumors.

Of the various parameters that characterize tumor kinetics, the cell loss factor is, in general, the most difficult to evaluate. The cell loss factor for human tumors has generally been calculated by comparing the *observed tumor volume doubling time* to the *potential doubling time*, which is the time required for the population of cells to double, assuming that all the cells produced are retained in the tumor. Tubiana and Malaise calculated a mean value of the cell loss factor for five histologic groups of human tumors, assuming the duration of S to be 16 hours. Their results suggest that, in general, the mean cell loss factor exceeds 50%. Furthermore, it appeared to be higher when the tumor was growing quickly and when its growth fraction was high. In humans, the smallest cell loss factors seem to be associated with those histologic types of tumors that have the slowest rate of growth. The cell loss factor, therefore, tends to reduce the spread of growth rates that results from the differences in growth fraction of the various types of tumors.

Steel has independently estimated the extent of cell loss in human tumors by comparing the potential doubling time with observed tumor growth rates. The relevant data on the volume-doubling time for six groups of human tumors are shown in Table 12-6. They consist mostly of measurements on primary and secondary tumors of the lung. There are differences between individual series, which may indeed reflect significant differences in the growth rates of the various types of tumors, but if the results are all pooled, they yield an average median doubling time of 66 days, with 80% of the values falling in the range of 18 to 200 days. Taking the median values for the labeling index, doubling time, and S phase as suggested by Steel, the median cell loss factor in all human tumors studied is 77%. It would thus appear that for human tumors cell loss is generally the most important factor determining the pattern of tumor growth.

The high cell loss in human tumors largely accounts for the great disparity between the cell cycle time of the individual dividing cells and the overall doubling time of the tumor. Although the tumor-doubling time is characteristically 40 to 100 days, the cell cycle time is relatively short, 1 to 5 days. This has important implications, which are often overlooked, in the use of cycle-specific chemotherapeutic agents or radiosensitizing drugs, for which it is the cell cycle time that is relevant.

Table 12-6.
Volume-Doubling Times of Human Tumors

| AUTHOR(S) | SITE | VOLUME-DOUBLING TIME (DAYS) | RANGE (DAYS) |
|---|---|---|---|
| Breuer | Lung metastases | 40 | 4–745 |
| Collins et al. | Lung metastases | 40 | 11–164 |
| Collins | Lung metastases from colon or rectum | 96 | 34–210 |
| Garland | Primary bronchial carcinoma | 105 | 27–480 |
| Schwartz | Primary bronchial carcinomas | 62 | 17–200 |
| Spratt | Primary skeletal sarcomas | 75 | 21–366 |

*(Based on data from Steel GG: Cell Tissue Kinet 1:193–207, 1968)*

Since Bergonie and Tribondeau established a relation between the rate of cell proliferation and the response to irradiation in normal tissues, it might be supposed that this would be the same for tumors. It is of interest to note that the histologic groups of human tumors that have the most rapid mean growth rate and the highest growth fraction and cell turnover rate are indeed those that are the most radiosensitive. There is also a correlation between, on the one hand, the growth rate and the labeling index or the cell loss and, on the other hand, the reaction to chemotherapy. This is not surprising, since the majority of drugs act essentially on cells in S phase. It is remarkable, however, that the only human tumors in which it is possible to achieve cures by chemotherapy are the histologic types with a high labeling index. Furthermore, a high level of cell loss appears to favor the response to chemotherapy, and in humans this occurs especially in tumors with a high labeling index.

## A COMPARISON OF THE CELL CYCLE TIMES OF THE CELLS OF SOLID TUMORS AND THEIR NORMAL COUNTERPARTS

A number of authors have attempted to compare the cell cycle times of normal and malignant tissues. Despite the paucity of data available, it is fair to draw the general conclusion that the cell cycle time of the malignant cells is appreciably *less* than that of their normal counterparts. An exception to this generalization would be tumors arising from rapidly proliferating normal tissues, such as leukemias and tumors of the gastrointes-

tinal tract. In these cases it is unlikely that the tumor cells would have a shortened cell cycle *compared with the comparable normal tissue.*

It is generally found that irradiation causes an *elongation* of the generation cycle of tumor cells, while a corresponding *shortening* of the cell cycle of normal cells is frequently reported. There are exceptions to this rule, but it is often found to be true.

From investigations of the morphologic and proliferative changes produced by radiation in the epidermis of hairless mice, Devik showed that the cell cycle time of the basal cells of this epidermis was dramatically reduced compared with unirradiated cells and that this reduction occurred in regions showing a gross hyperplastic reaction after irradiation. A similar dramatic shortening of the cell cycle of irradiated epidermal cells is suggested by data reported by Breuer from patients who had just completed a course of radiotherapy, after which the skin overlying the treated region had undergone moist desquamation.

It would seem, therefore, that the cycle time of cells with a long generation time can be substantially shortened by irradiation. Such results would, however, appear to depend on a gross tissue response. When the turnover time, or the cell cycle time, of a tissue is very long, the tissue will take a long time to recognize the fact that most of its cells have been sterilized by a dose of radiation, since cells only die when attempting a subsequent mitosis.

The probable consequence of this is that normal tissues will not respond by speeding up the progress of cells through their cell cycle for some time after the delivery of the dose of radiation. If this time is comparable to the overall time of a fractionated course of radiotherapy, then the preirradiation values of the cell cycle times of the normal and malignant tissues will be relevant to a discussion of dose–time relationships in radiotherapy or to the use of cycle-specific chemotherapeutic or radiosensitizing drugs in combination with radiotherapy.

## GLOSSARY OF TERMS

| Symbol | Meaning |
|---|---|
| $T_C$ | Average cell cycle of the dividing cells of a population |
| $T_M$ | Duration of mitosis (M) |
| $T_{G_1}$ | Duration of G1 period |
| $T_{G_2}$ | Duration of G2 period |
| $T_S$ | Duration of DNA synthetic period (S) |
| GF | Growth fraction; proportion of viable cells in active cell division |
| $T_d$ | Observed volume-doubling time of a tumor or tissue |
| $T_{pot}$ | Potential doubling time of a tumor: theoretical doubling time calculated from the cell cycle and growth fraction, assuming no cell loss |
| $\Phi$ | Cell loss factor; rate of loss of cells is a fraction of the rate of new cell production $$\Phi = 1 - T_{pot}/T_d$$ |
| MI | Mitotic index; proportion of cells in mitosis at any time |
| LI | Labeling index; proportion of cells in the population that take up tritiated thymidine |
| RCS | Radioactivity per cell in S phase |
| PLM | Percent-labeled-mitoses |

## ► Summary of Pertinent Conclusions

- Mammalian cells proliferate by mitosis (M). The interval between successive mitoses is the cell cycle time ($T_C$).
- In mitosis the chromosomes condense and are visible. The DNA synthetic (S) phase can be identified by autoradiography. The first gap ($G_1$) separates mitosis from S phase. The second gap ($G_2$) separates S phase from the subsequent mitosis.
- Fast-growing cells in culture and some cells in self-renewal tissues in vivo have a $T_C$ of 10 hours; stem cells in a resting normal tissue, such as the skin, have a cell cycle time of 10 days.
- Most of the difference in cell cycle between fast- and slow-growing cells is a result of differences in $G_1$, which varies from less than 1 hour to more than a week.
- The mitotic index (MI) is the fraction of cells in mitosis.

$$MI = \lambda T_M / T_C.$$

- The labeling index (LI) is the fraction of cells that take up tritiated thymidine (ie, the fraction of cells in S).

$$LI = \lambda T_S / T_C.$$

- The percent-labeled-mitoses (PLM) technique allows an estimate to be made of the lengths of the constituent phases of the cell cycle. The basis of the technique is to label cells with tritiated thymidine or bromodeoxyuridine in S phase and time their arrival in mitosis.
- Flow cytometry allows a rapid analysis of the distribution of cells in the cycle. Cells are stained with a DNA-specific dye and sorted on the basis of DNA content.
- The bromodeoxyuridine-DNA assay in flow cytometry allows cells to be stained simultaneously with two dyes that fluoresce at different wave-

*(continued)*

► *Summary of Pertinent Conclusions* (Continued)

lengths: one that binds in proportion to DNA content to indicate the phase of the cell cycle and the other that binds in proportion to bromo-deoxyuridine incorporation to show if cells are synthesizing DNA.

- $T_{pot}$, the potential doubling time of a tumor, reflects the cell cycle of individual cells and the growth fraction but ignores cell loss.
- $T_{pot}$ is the relevant parameter for estimating the effect of cell proliferation on a protracted radiotherapy protocol.
- $T_{pot}$ can be estimated by means of flow cytometric analysis on cells from a single biopsy specimen taken 4 to 8 hours after an intravenous administration of bromodeoxyuridine.
- $T_{pot}$ has been shown to be a useful predictive assay for selecting patients that might benefit from accelerated treatment.
- The growth fraction (GF) is the fraction of cells in active cell cycle (ie, the fraction of proliferative cells).
- In animal tumors, the growth fraction frequently ranges from 30% to 50%.
- The cell loss factor ($\Phi$) is the fraction of cells produced by cell division lost from the tumor.
- In animal tumors, $\Phi$ varies from 0% to more than 90%, tending to be small in small tumors and to increase with tumor size.
- The $\Phi$ tends to be large for carcinomas and small for sarcomas.
- Volume-doubling time of a tumor is the gross time for it to double overall in size as measured, for example, in serial radiographs.
- Potential doubling time $T_{pot}$ of a tumor is the calculated time for a tumor to double in size, allowing for the growth fraction but assuming that all cells produced are retained in the tumor.
- Tumors grow much more slowly than would be predicted from the cycle time of individual cells. One reason is the growth fraction, but the principal reason is the cell loss factor.
- The overall pattern of tumor growth may be summarized as follows. A minority of cells (the GF) are proliferating rapidly, while most are quiescent. The majority of the new cells produced by mitosis are lost from the tumor.
- In general, the cell cycle time of malignant cells is appreciably *shorter* than that of their normal tissue counterparts.
- In general, irradiation causes an *elongation* of the cell cycle time in tumor cells and a *shortening* of the cell cycle in normal tissues.

### Human Tumors

- In 90% of human tumors the cell cycle time is between 15 and 125 hours (modal value, 48 hours).
- In human tumors, $T_s$ has a modal value of about 16 hours (a range of 9.5 to 24 hours).
- As a first approximation, the mean duration of the cell cycle is about three times the duration of the S phase.
- Growth fraction is more variable in human tumors than in rodent tumors and correlates better with gross volume-doubling time.
- Cell loss factor for human tumors has been estimated by Tubiana and Malaise to have an average value for a range of tumors in excess of 50%. Steel's estimate for a median value for all human tumors studied is 77%.

# BIBLIOGRAPHY

Begg AC, Hofland I, Van Glabekke M, Bartlelink H, Horiot JC: Predictive value of potential doubling time for radiotherapy of head and neck tumor patients: Results from the EORTC Cooperative Trial 22851. Semin Radiat Oncol 2:22–25, 1992

Begg AC, McNally NJ, Shrieve D et al: A method to measure the duration of DNA synthesis and the potential doubling time from a single sample. Cytometry 6:620–625, 1985

Begg AC, Moonen I, Hofland I et al: Human tumor cell kinetics using a monoclonal antibody against iododeoxyuridine: Intratumoral sampling variations. Radiother Oncol 11:337–347, 1988

Bergonie J, Tribondeau L (trans): Interpretation of some results of radiotherapy in an attempt at determining a logical technique of treatment. Radiat Res 11:587, 1959

Bresciani F: A comparison of the generative cycle in normal hyperplastic and neoplastic mammary gland of the C3H mouse. In Cellular Radiation Biology, pp 547–557. Baltimore, Williams & Wilkins, 1965

Breuer K: Growth rate and radiosensitivity of human tumours: I. Growth rate of human tumours. Eur J Cancer 2:157–171, 1966

Brown JM: The effect of acute x-irradiation on the cell proliferation kinetics of induced carcinomas and their normal counterpart. Radiat Res 43:627–653, 1970

Brown JM, Berry RJ: Effects of x-irradiation on the cell population kinetics in a model tumor and normal tissue system: Implication for the treatment of human malignancies. Br J Radiol 42:372–377, 1969

Collins VP, Loeffer K, Tivey J: Observation on growth rates of human tumors. AJR 6:988, 1956

Denekamp J: The cellular proliferation kinetics of animal tumors. Cancer Res 30:393–400, 1970

Denekamp J: The relationship between the "cell loss factor" and the immediate response to radiation in animal tumours. Eur J Cancer 8:335, 1972

Dolbeare F, Beisker W, Pallavicini MG, Vanderlaan M, Gary JW: cytochemistry for BrDUrd/DNA analysis: Stoichiometry and sensitivity. Cytometry 6:521–530, 1985

Dolbeare F, Gratzner H, Pallavicini M, Gray JW: Flow cytometric measurement of total DNA content and incorporated bromodeoxyuridine. Proc Natl Acad Sci USA 80:5573–5577, 1983

Frankfurt OS: Mitotic cycle and cell differentiation in squamous cell carcinomas. Int J Cancer 2:304–310, 1967

Frindel E, Malaise EP, Alpen E, Tubiana M: Kinetics of cell proliferation of an experimental tumor. Cancer Res 27:1122–1131, 1967

Frindel E, Malaise EP, Tubiana M: Cell proliferation kinetics in five human solid tumors. Cancer 22:611–620, 1968

Frindel E, Valleron AJ, Vassort F, Tubiana M: Proliferation kinetics of an experimental ascites tumor of the mouse. Cell Tissue Kinet 2:51–65, 1969

Gray JW: Cell-cycle analysis of perturbed cell populations: Computer simulation of sequential DNA distributions. Cell Tissue Kinet 9:499–516, 1976

Gray JW, Carver JH, George YS, Mendelsohn ML: Rapid cell cycle analysis by measurement of the radioactivity per cell in a narrow window in S-phase (RCSi). Cell Tissue Kinet 10:97–104, 1977

Gray JW, Dolbeare F, Pallavicini MG, Beisker W, Waldman F: Cell cycle analysis using flow cytometry. Int J Radiat Biol 49:237–255, 1986

Hermens AF, Barendsen GW: Cellular proliferation patterns in an experimental rhabdomyosarcoma in the rat. Eur J Cancer 3:361–369, 1967

Hoshima T, Yagashima T, Morovic J, Livin E, Livin V: Cell kinetic studies of in situ human brain tumors with bromodeoxyuridine. Cytometry 6:627–632, 1985

Howard A, Pelc SR: Synthesis of deoxyribonucleic acid in normal and irradiated cells and its relation to chromosome breakage. Heredity (Suppl) 6:261, 1952

Lesher S: Compensatory reactions in intestinal crypt cells after 300 roentgens of cobalt-60 gamma irradiation. Radiat Res 32:510–519, 1967

Mendelsohn ML: The growth fraction: A new concept applied to tumors. Science 132:1496, 1960

Mendelsohn ML: Autoradiography analysis of cell proliferation in spontaneous breast cancer of the $C_3H$ mouse: III. The growth fraction. JNCI 28:1015–1029, 1962

Mendelsohn ML: Principles, relative merits, and limitations of current cytokinetic methods. In Drewinko B, Humphrey RM (eds): Growth Kinetics and Biochemical Regulation of Normal and Malignant Cells, pp 101–112. Baltimore, Williams & Wilkins, 1977

Morstyn G, Hsu S-M, Kinsella T, Gratzuer H, Russo A, Mitchell J: Bromodeoxyuridine in tumors and chromosomes detected with a monoclonal antibody. J Clin Invest 72:1844–1850, 1983

Palekar SK, Sirsat SM: Replication time pattern of transplanted fibrosarcoma in the mouse. Indian J Exp Biol 5:173–175, 1967

Post J, Hoffman J: The replication time and pattern of carcinogen-induced hepatoma cells. J Cell Biol 22:341–350, 1964

Quastler H, Sherman FG: Cell population kinetics in the intestinal epithelium of the mouse. Exp Cell Res 17:420–4389, 1959

Raashad AL, Evans CA: Radioautographic study of epidermal cell proliferation and migration in normal and neoplastic tissues of rabbits. JNCI 41:845–853, 1968

Refsum SB, Berdal P: Cell loss in malignant tumours in man. Eur J Cancer 3:235–236, 1967

Reiskin AB, Berry RJ: Cell proliferation and carcinogenesis in the hamster cheek pouch. Cancer Res 28:898–905, 1968

Reiskin AB, Mendelsohn ML: A comparison of the cell cycle in induced carcinomas and their normal counterpart. Cancer Res 24:1131–1136, 1964

Simpson-Herren L, Blow JG, Brown PH: The mitotic cycle of sarcome 180. Cancer Res 28:724–726, 1968

Steel GG: Cell loss as a factor in the growth rate of human tumours. Eur J Cancer 3:381–387, 1967

Steel GG: Cell loss from experimental tumors. Cell Tissue Kinet 1:193–207, 1968

Steel GG: The kinetics of cell proliferation in tumors. In Bond VP (ed): Proceedings of the Carmel Conference on Time and Dose Relationships in Radiation Biology as Applied to Radiotherapy, pp 130–149. Upton, NY, BNL Report 50203 (C-57), 1969

Steel GG: Autoradiographic analysis of the cell cycle: Howard and Pelc to the present day. Int J Radiat Biol 49:227–235, 1986

Steel GG, Adams K, Barratt JC: Analysis of the cell population kinetics of transplanted tumours of widely differing growth rate. Br J Cancer 20:784–800, 1966

Steel GG, Haynes S: The technique labeled mitoses: Analyses by automatic curve fitting. Cell Tissue Kinet 4:93–105, 1971

Tubiana M, Malaise EB: Growth rate and cell kinetics in human tumors: Some prognostic and therapeutic implications. In Symington T, Carter R (eds): Scientific Foundations of Oncology, pp 126–136. Chicago, Year Book Medical Publishers, 1976

*Radiobiology for the Radiologist, Fourth Edition*, by Eric J. Hall
J. B. Lippincott Company, Philadelphia © 1994.

# 13

# *Time, Dose, and Fractionation in Radiotherapy*

Radiation Therapy

## THE INTRODUCTION
## OF FRACTIONATION

The multifraction regimens commonly used in conventional radiation therapy are a consequence largely of radiobiological experiments performed in France in the 1920s and 1930s. It was found that a ram could not be sterilized by exposing its testes to a single dose of radiation without extensive skin damage to the scrotum, whereas if the radiation was spread out over a period of weeks in a series of daily fractions, sterilization was possible without producing unacceptable skin damage (Fig. 13-1). It was postulated that the testes were a model of a growing tumor, whereas the skin of the scrotum represented a dose-limiting normal tissue. The reasoning may be flawed, but the conclusion proved to be valid; fractionation of the radiation dose produces, in most cases, better tumor control for a given level of normal tissue toxicity than a single large dose.

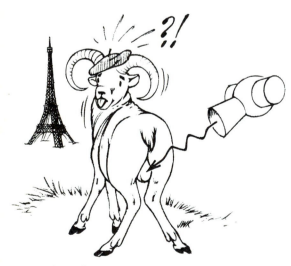

**Figure 13-1.** Conventional multifraction radiotherapy was based on experiments performed in Paris in the 1920s and 1930s. Rams could not be sterilized with a single dose of x-rays without extensive skin damage, whereas if the radiation were delivered in daily fractions over a period of time, sterilization was possible without skin damage. The testes were regarded as a model of a growing tumor and skin as dose-limiting normal tissue.

## THE FOUR *R*s
## OF RADIOBIOLOGY

Now, more than 60 years later, we can account for the efficacy of fractionation based on more relevant radiobiological experiments. We can appeal to the four *R*s of radiobiology:

Repair of sublethal damage
Reassortment of cells within the cell cycle
Repopulation
Reoxygenation

The basis of fractionation in radiotherapy can be understood in simple terms. Dividing a dose into a number of fractions *spares* normal tissues because of repair of sublethal damage between dose fractions and repopulation of cells if the overall time is sufficiently long. At the same time dividing a dose into a number of fractions *increases* damage to the tumor because of reoxygenation and reassortment of cells into radiosensitive phases of the cycle.

The advantages of prolongation of treatment are to spare early reactions and to allow adequate reoxygenation in tumors. Excessive prolongation, however, will allow surviving tumor cells to proliferate during treatment.

## THE STRANDQUIST PLOT
## AND THE ELLIS NSD SYSTEM

Early attempts to understand and account for fractionation gave rise to the well-known Strandquist plot, in which effective single dose was plotted as a function of the overall treatment time (Fig. 13-2). Since all treatments were given as three or five fractions per week, overall time in this plot contains by implication the number of fractions as well. It was commonly found in these plots that the slope of the isoeffect curve for skin was about 0.33; that is, the total dose for an isoeffect was proportional to $T^{0.33}$.

The most important contribution in this area, made by Ellis and his colleagues with the introduction of the nominal standard dose (NSD) system, was the recognition of the importance of

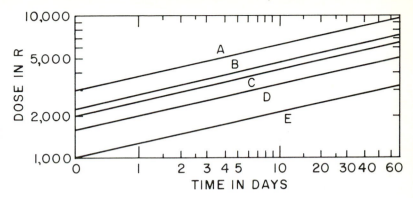

**Figure 13-2.** Isoeffect curves relating the total dose to the overall treatment time for A, skin necrosis; B, cure of skin carcinoma; C, moist desquamation of skin; D, dry desquamation of skin; and E, skin erythema. (Redrawn from Strandquist M: Acta Radiol (Suppl) 55:1–300, 1944)

separating overall time from the number of fractions. According to this hypothesis, total dose for the tolerance of connective tissue is related to the number of fractions (N) and the overall time (T) by the relation

$$\text{Total dose} = (\text{NSD})T^{0.11}N^{0.24}$$

The NSD system has been discussed extensively. It does enable predictions to be made of equivalent dose regimens, provided that the range of time and number of fractions is not too great and does not exceed the range over which the data were available. For example, in changing a treatment protocol from five fractions per week to four fractions per week, the formula can be used to calculate the size of dose fractions needed to result in the same normal tissue tolerance with the two different protocols. Of course, since the system is based ultimately on skin-reaction data, it does *not* in any way predict **late effects.** An obvious weakness of the NSD system is that time is allowed for in terms of a single power function, where the nominal single dose is proportional to $T^{0.11}$. In fact, biological experiments with small animals have shown that this relationship is far from accurate. Proliferation does not affect the total dose required to produce a given biological reaction at all until some time after the start of irradiation, but then the dependence in time is much greater than allowed for by the Ellis formula.

## PROLIFERATION AS A FACTOR IN NORMAL TISSUES

Experimental evidence indicates that the total dose required to produce a given biological effect is not a power function of time, as postulated by the Ellis NSD system, but turns out to be more complex. The extra dose required to counter proliferation and result in a given level of skin damage in mice, does not increase at all until about 12 days into a fractionated regimen, but then increases very rapidly as a function of time. The shape of the curve is roughly sigmoidal (Fig. 13-3). If similar data were available for humans, the effects of proliferation would not be seen until a longer period into a fractionation regimen because of the slower response of the human skin and the longer cell cycle of the individual cells. Figure 13-3 is not meant to be quantitative but to indicate that the *shape* of the curve relating extra dose to proliferation is sigmoidal. This illustrates immediately that the method of allowing for overall time in the NSD system is incorrect or at best a very crude approximation.

A further consideration is that all normal tissues are not the same. In particular, there is a clear distinction between tissues that are **early responding,** such as the skin, mucosa, and intestinal epithelium, and those that are **late responding,** such as the spinal cord. Figure 13-4 shows the extra dose required to produce a given level of damage for a fractionated protracted regimen in the case of representative tissues from the early- and late-responding groups. This diagram compares mouse skin, representative of early-responding tissues, and rat spinal cord, representative of late-responding tissues. It is recognized that these may not be ideal examples, but suitable data for more relevant systems are simply not available; comparable quantitative data are certainly not available for humans. The point made by this figure is that the time after the start of a fractionated regimen at which extra

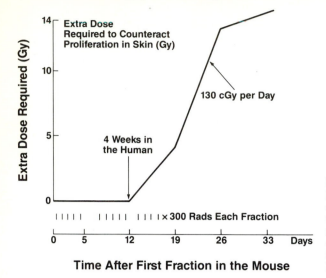

**Time After First Fraction in the Mouse**

Figure 13-3. The extra dose required to counteract proliferation in the skin of mice as a function of time after starting daily irradiation with 300 cGy per fraction. A delay followed by a rapid rise is typical of time factors in proliferating normal tissues. In mouse skin the delay is about 2 weeks; in humans it is about 4 weeks. (Modified from Fowler JF: Acta Radiol 23:209–216, 1984; data from Denekamp J: Br J Radiol 46:381, 1973)

dose is required to compensate for cellular proliferation is quite different for late-, as opposed to early-, responding tissues. The other point made, of course, is that these are data from rodents and that in the case of humans the time scales (although they are not known with any precision) are likely to be very much longer. In particular, the time at which extra dose is required to compensate for proliferation in late-responding tissues in humans is far beyond the overall time of any normal radiotherapy regimen.

Figure 13-5 is an attempt to convert the experimental laboratory data contained in Figure 13-4 into a general principle that can be applied to clinical practice. Early-responding tissues are triggered to proliferate within a few weeks of the start of a fractionated regimen so that the "extra dose to counter proliferation" increases with

time, certainly during conventional radiotherapeutic protocols. By contrast, conventional radiotherapy extending to 6 or 8 weeks is **never** long enough to allow the triggering of proliferation in late-responding tissues. These considerations lead to the important axiom that

> Prolonging overall time within the normal radiotherapy range has little sparing effect on late reactions but a large sparing effect on early reactions.

This has far-reaching consequences in radiotherapy. Early reactions, such as reactions of the skin or of the mucosa, can be dealt with easily by the simple expedient of prolonging the overall time. Although such a strategy overcomes the problem of the early reactions, it has no effect whatsoever on the late reactions.

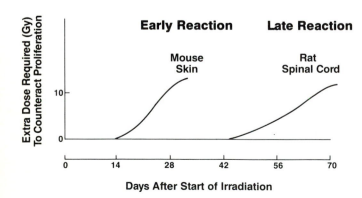

**Days After Start of Irradiation**

Figure 13-4. The extra dose required to counteract proliferation only as a function of time after starting daily irradiation in rodents. The left curve represents a typical early reaction; the right curve represents a typical late reaction. The delays are much longer in humans. (Modified from Fowler JF: Radiother Oncol 1:1–22, 1983)

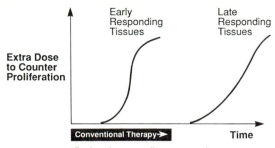

"Prolonging overall treatment time spares **Early** but not **Late** responding tissues"

**Figure 13-5.** Highly speculative illustration attempting to extrapolate the experimental data for early- and late-responding tissue in rats and mice to principles that can be applied in clinical radiotherapy. The extra dose required to counter proliferation in early responding tissues begins to increase after a few weeks into a fractionated regimen, certainly during the time course of conventional therapy. By contrast, conventional protocols are never sufficiently long to include the proliferation of late-responding tissues.

## THE SHAPE OF THE DOSE–RESPONSE RELATIONSHIP FOR EARLY- AND LATE-RESPONDING TISSUES

Clinical and laboratory data suggest that there is a consistent difference between early- and late-responding tissues in their response to changing fractionation patterns. When fewer and larger dose fractions are given, late reactions are more severe, even though early reactions are matched by an appropriate adjustment in total dose. This dissociation can be interpreted as differences in repair capacity or shoulder shape of the underlying dose–response curves. The dose–response relationship for late-responding tissues is *more curved* than that for early-responding tissues. In terms of the linear-quadratic relationship between effect and dose this translates into a larger $\alpha/\beta$-ratio for *early* than *late* effects. The difference in the shapes of the dose–response relationships is illustrated in Figure 13-6. The $\alpha/\beta$ ratio is the dose at which cell killing by the linear ($\alpha$) and quadratic ($\beta$) components are equal.

For early effects $\alpha/\beta$ is large; as a consequence, $\alpha$ dominates at low doses, so that the dose-response curve has a marked initial slope and does not bend until higher doses. The linear and quadratic components of cell killing are not equal until about 10 Gy (1000 rads). For late effects $\alpha/\beta$ is small, so that the $\beta$ term has an influence at low doses. The dose-response curve bends at lower doses to appear more curvy; the linear and quadratic components of cell killing are equal by about 2 Gy (200 rads).

Dose–response curves for organ function must be distinguished clearly from those for clonogenic cell survival. The distinction is not a trivial one. Organ function is obviously related more to the proportion of functional cells remaining in an irradiated organ at a particular time than to the proportion of clonogenic (stem) cells. The dose-effect curves for clonogenic cells tend to be straight, with a relatively small shoulder, whereas dose-effect relations for organ function tend to be more curved with a larger shoulder. It is, of course, the dose–response curves for organ function that are more relevant to the tolerance of normal tissues.

There are four different pieces of information, some from clinical experience and some from animal studies, that represent circumstantial evidence for the conclusion that the shape of the dose–response relationship differs for early- and late-responding tissues. First, when a fractionation scheme is changed in clinical practice from many small doses to a few large fractions and the total dose is titrated to produce equal early effects, the treatment protocol involving a few large fractions results in *more severe late effects*.

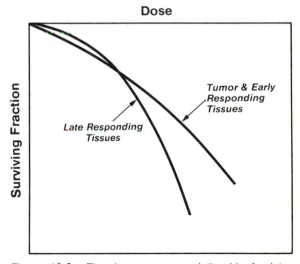

**Figure 13-6.** The dose–response relationship for late-responding tissues is more curved than for early-responding tissues. In the linear-quadratic formulation this translates into a larger $\alpha/\beta$ for early than for late effects. The ratio $\alpha/\beta$ is the dose at which the linear ($\alpha$) and the quadratic ($\beta$) components of cell killing are equal: that is, $\alpha D = \beta D^2$. (Redrawn from the concepts of Dr. H. R. Withers)

There is an abundance of clinical evidence for the truth of this statement.

Second, the relative biological effectiveness (RBE) for neutrons compared with x-rays is *larger* for late effects than for early effects, at least in treatment schedules involving many fractions. There is good evidence from the early neutron trials, especially from Edinburgh, that this statement is valid. The clinical data are illustrated in Figure 13-7, which shows a patient treated for ankylosing spondylitis in which the top half of the field was treated with x-rays and the bottom half of the field was treated with neutrons. At the end of treatment the early response of the two areas is about equal, but by 2 years after treatment there is clearly a more severe late reaction in the neutron-treated than in the x-ray treated field. This observation is compatible with the concept that the dose–response relationship for late-responding tissues is more curved than for early-responding tissues, as illustrated in Figure 13-8. In the case of both early- and late-responding tissues the dose–response relationship for neutrons is an exponential function of dose (at least up to the daily doses used clinically), and so there is no effect of fractionation. For x-rays, late-responding tissues have a more curved dose–response relationship and consequently show a bigger fractionation effect than early-responding tissues. Therefore, if total doses are matched to produce equivalent early effects of neutrons and x-rays, then the late effects will be more severe for neutrons. This would be expected to be true, at least for multifraction regi-

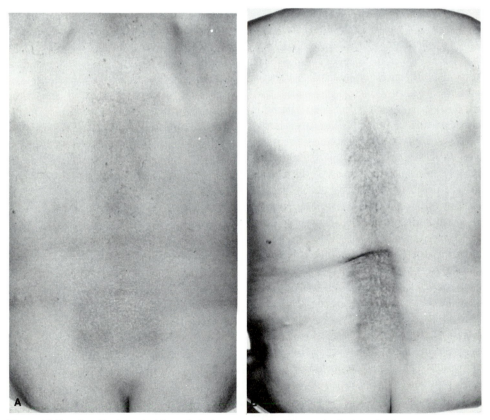

**Figure 13-7.** A patient treated for ankylosing spondylitis. The top half of the field was treated with x-rays, the bottom half with neutrons. Doses were matched in a 20-fraction regimen so that the early responses to x-rays and neutrons at the end of treatment were equivalent **(A)**. Two years later **(B)**, the neutron-treated area shows a much more severe late response than the area treated with x-rays. This demonstrates clearly that the neutron relative biological effectiveness (RBE) is greater for late- than for early-responding tissues, at least in multifraction regimens. (Courtesy of Prof. William Duncan, Edinburgh University)

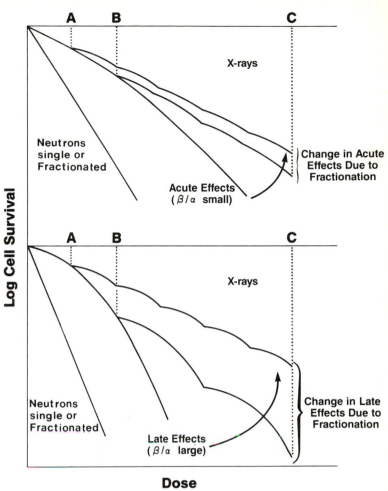

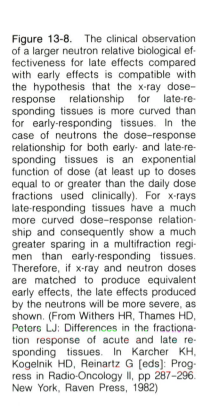

**Figure 13-8.** The clinical observation of a larger neutron relative biological effectiveness for late effects compared with early effects is compatible with the hypothesis that the x-ray dose–response relationship for late-responding tissues is more curved than for early-responding tissues. In the case of neutrons the dose–response relationship for both early- and late-responding tissues is an exponential function of dose (at least up to doses equal to or greater than the daily dose fractions used clinically). For x-rays late-responding tissues have a much more curved dose–response relationship and consequently show a much greater sparing in a multifraction regimen than early-responding tissues. Therefore, if x-ray and neutron doses are matched to produce equivalent early effects, the late effects produced by the neutrons will be more severe, as shown. (From Withers HR, Thames HD, Peters LJ: Differences in the fractionation response of acute and late responding tissues. In Karcher KH, Kogelnik HD, Reinartz G [eds]: Progress in Radio-Oncology II, pp 287–296. New York, Raven Press, 1982)

mens, with enough fractions for the difference in shape of the dose–response curves for early- and late-responding tissues to become evident.

Third, clinical trials of hyperfractionation, in which two doses are delivered per day for 6 to 7 weeks, appear to result in greatly reduced late effects if the total dose is titrated to produce equal or possibly slightly more severe acute effects. Tumor control is the same or slightly improved. This important clinical observation has been made in a number of centers and again is compatible with the same difference of shape of dose–response curves between early- and late-responding tissues. Late-effect tissues are more sensitive to changes in fractionation patterns than early-responding tissues.

Fourth, in experiments with laboratory animals the isoeffect curves (ie, dose versus number of fractions to produce an equal biological effect)

are *steeper* for a range of late effects than for a variety of acute effects. The data are shown in Figure 13-9, in which early effects are represented by, for example, skin desquamation or jejunal crypt colonies, while late effects are represented by, for example, the lung or spinal cord injury. Table 13-1 is a summary of the values of $\alpha/\beta$ for a number of early- and late-responding tissues. The important result is that for early-responding tissues $\alpha/\beta$ (ie, the dose at which the single and multiple event cell killing are about equal) occurs at the dose of about 10 Gy (1000 rads). By contrast, $\alpha/\beta$ for late-responding tissues is about 2 Gy (200 rads). These results come from experiments in small laboratory animals. The values of $\alpha/\beta$ shown in Table 13-1 come from experiments in which the reciprocal of the total dose is plotted against the quadratic relationship in biological systems in which it is possi-

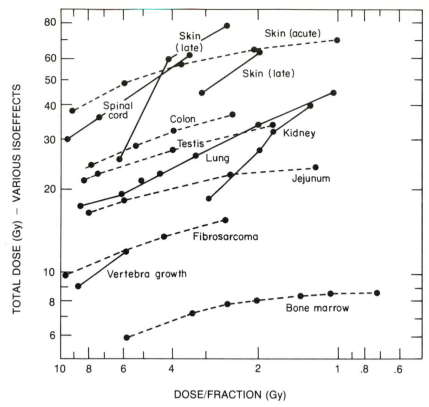

**Figure 13-9.** Isoeffect curves in which the total dose necessary for a certain effect in various tissues is plotted as a function of dose per fraction. Late effects are plotted with solid lines, acute effects with dashed lines. The data were selected to exclude an influence on the total dose of regeneration during the multifraction experiments. The main point of the data is that the isodoses for late effects increase more rapidly with decrease in dose per fraction than is the case for acute effects. (From Withers HR: Cancer 55:2086, 1985)

Table 13-1.
### Ratio of Linear to Quadratic Terms From Multifraction Experiments

| REACTIONS | α/β (Gy) |
|---|---|
| **Early** | |
| Skin | 9 –12 |
| Jejunum | 6 –10 |
| Colon | 10 –11 |
| Testis | 12 –13 |
| Callus | 9 –10 |
| **Late** | |
| Spinal cord | 1.7–4.9 |
| Kidney | 1 –2.4 |
| Lung | 2 –6.3 |
| Bladder | 3.1–7 |

ble to observe equal effects from various fractionation regimens, even though single-cell dose-survival curves cannot be generated (see Fig. 4-24).

The parameters derived from curves reconstructed from multifraction experiments are specifically relevant to the multifraction end point measured in each experiment, whether it is a proportion of clonogenic cells or a stated reduction in organ function. The dose–response curve that is constructed from multifraction experimental data by making simple assumptions is a functional dose–response curve, deduced from data in which repair after each fractional dose is basically the quantity being measured. It is just such functional dose–response curves that are required to elucidate the relationship between tolerance dose in radiotherapy and size of dose per fraction, with overall time considered separately.

# POSSIBLE EXPLANATIONS FOR THE DIFFERENCE IN SHAPE OF DOSE–RESPONSE RELATIONSHIPS FOR EARLY- AND LATE-RESPONDING TISSUES

The radiosensitivity of a population of cells varies with the distribution of cells through the cycle. In general, cells are most resistant in late S phase; slowly growing cells with a long cycle may, however, have a second resistant phase in late $G_1$ phase, which may be termed $G_0$ if the cells are out of cycle. Thus, two quite different cell populations may be radioresistant:

1. A population proliferating so fast that S phase occupies a major portion of the cycle
2. A population proliferating so slowly that many cells are in late $G_1$ or not proliferating at all, so that many resting cells are in $G_0$

It is thought that many *late-responding normal tissues* are resistant owing to the presence of many resting cells. This type of resistance applies particularly to small doses per fraction and disappears at larger doses per fraction.

If resistance is due to the presence of many cells in S phase in a rapidly proliferating population, redistribution occurs through all the phases of the cell cycle, which can be considered a "self-sensitizing" activity. The fast proliferation itself is a form of resistance, since the new cells produced by division offset those killed by the dose fractions. This applies to *acutely responding tissues* and also to *tumors*. Proliferation occurring during a protracted, fractionated regimen helps to spare normal tissues but, of course is a potential danger as far as the tumor is concerned.

# FRACTION SIZE AND OVERALL TREATMENT TIME: INFLUENCE ON EARLY- AND LATE-RESPONDING TISSUES

The difference in shape of the dose–response relationship for early- and late-responding tissues leads to an important axiom:

Fraction size is the dominant factor in determining late effects, while overall treatment time has little influence. By contrast, fraction size and overall treatment time both determine the response of acutely responding tissues.

It is remarkable that both clinical radiation therapists and experimental radiobiologists did not come to recognize this simple fact until the mid 1980s.

# ACCELERATED REPOPULATION

Treatment with any cytotoxic agent, including radiation, can trigger surviving cells (clonogens) in a tumor to divide faster than before. This is known as **accelerated repopulation.**

Figure 13-10 illustrates this phenomenon in a transplanted rat tumor. Part *A* of this figure shows the overall growth curve for this tumor, together with the shrinkage and regrowth that occurs after a single dose of 20 Gy (2000 rads) of x-rays. Part *B* shows the proliferation of individual surviving cells (ie, clonogenic cells) that, after treatment, are dividing with a cycle time of 12 hours. The important point to note is that during the time that the tumor is overtly shrinking and regressing the surviving clonogens are dividing and increasing in number more rapidly than ever.

There is evidence for a similar phenomenon in human tumors. Withers and his colleagues surveyed the literature on radiotherapy for head and neck cancer and estimated the dose to achieve local control in 50% of cases ($TCD_{50}$) as a function of the overall duration of fractionated treatment. The results are summarized in Figure 13-11. The analysis suggests that clonogen repopulation in this human cancer accelerates at about 28 days after the initiation of radiotherapy in a fractionated regimen. A dose increment of about 0.6 Gy (60 rads) per day is required to compensate for this repopulation. Such a dose increment is consistent with a 4-day clonogen doubling rate, compared with a median of about 60 days for unperturbed growth.

The conclusion to be drawn from this is that radiotherapy, at least for head and neck cancer, and probably in other instances, too, should be completed as soon after it has begun as is practicable. It may be better to delay initiation of treat-

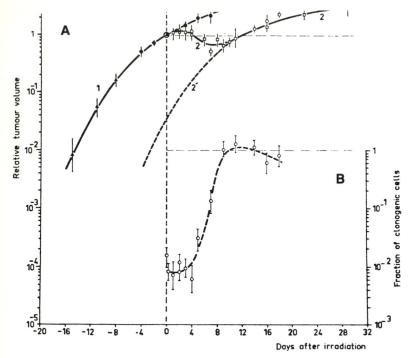

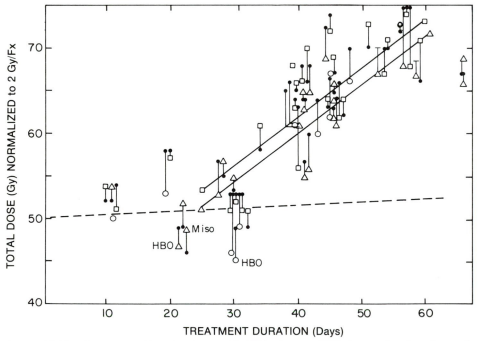

Figure 13-10. Illustrating Accelerated Repopulation. Growth curves of a rat rhabdomyosarcoma showing the shrinkage, growth delay, and subsequent recurrence following treatment with a single dose of 20 Gy (2000 rads) of x-rays. **(A)** Curve 1: Growth curve of unirradiated control tumors. Curve 2: Growth curve of tumors irradiated at time t = 0, showing tumor shrinkage and recurrence. **(B)** Variation of the fraction of clonogenic cells as a function of time after irradiation, obtained by removing cells from the tumor and assaying for colony formation in vitro. (From Hermens AF, Barendsen GW: Eur J Cancer 5:173–189, 1969)

Figure 13-11. Doses to achieve local control in 50% of cases (TCD$_{50}$), as a function of overall treatment time, for squamous cell tumors of the head and neck. The data points include many published results from the literature, including high-pressure oxygen trials (HBO), and the trial of misonidazole (Miso). The dashed line shows the rate of increase in TCD$_{50}$ predicted from a 2-month clonogen doubling rate. (From Withers HR, Taylor JMG, Maciejewski B: Acta Oncol 27:131–146, 1988)

ment than to introduce delays during treatment. If overall treatment time is too long, the effectiveness of later dose fractions will be prejudiced because the surviving clonogens in the tumor have been triggered into rapid repopulation.

The experimental data referred to above all relate to radiotherapy. It might, however, be anticipated that similar considerations would apply to chemotherapy, or to a combination of radiotherapy and chemotherapy. There is evidence in some human malignancies that radiotherapy produces poorer results if preceded by a course of chemotherapy. It may be that accelerated repopulation, triggered by the chemotherapy, is the explanation.

## MULTIPLE FRACTIONS PER DAY

We are now in a position to sum up the pros and cons of fractionation and prolongation of treatment in a much more sophisticated way than would have been possible at the beginning of this chapter. The advantages of prolongation of treatment are to spare early reactions and to allow adequate reoxygenation in tumors. Excessive prolongation, however, has two disadvantages: (1) it can decrease deceptively the acute reactions without sparing late injury, and (2) it will allow the surviving tumor cells to proliferate during treatment. There are two separate strategies that use multiple treatments per day:

1. Hyperfractionation
2. Accelerated treatment

The aims and objectives of these strategies are quite different.

### Hyperfractionation

The basic aim of hyperfractionation is to further separate early and late effects. The overall treatment time remains conventional at 6 to 8 weeks, but since two fractions per day are used, the number of fractions is doubled to between 60 and 80. The dose must be increased since the dose per fraction has been decreased. The intent is to further reduce late effects while achieving the same or better tumor control and the same or slightly increased early effects.

Two fractions per day may not be the limit of hyperfractionation; a further sparing of late effects by splitting the dose into more and more fractions of smaller and smaller size would occur as long as the dose fraction is still on the curved portion of the dose–response curve.

Withers introduced the concept of *"flexure" dose* ($D_f$), defined as the point at which the dose–response curve starts to bend significantly, and suggested that in practice this occurs at a dose of 0.1 $\alpha/\beta$; that is, the curve bends at a dose one tenth of that at which the linear and quadratic components are equal. Values of the $\alpha/\beta$ are 6 to 12 Gy (600 to 1200 rads) for early-responding tissues and 1 to 5 Gy (100 to 500 rads) for late-responding tissues. The flexure dose, therefore, with a value of 0.1 $\alpha/\beta$, is remarkably small: 0.6 to 1.2 Gy (60 to 120 rads) for early-responding tissues and 0.1 to 0.5 Gy (10 to 50 rads) for late-responding tissues, such as the spinal cord, kidney, lung, or late contraction in skin.

The important conclusion is that to exploit fully the sparing of late damage, doses per fraction as low as this should be used. It should be emphasized that there would not be further sparing of early-reacting tissues or, indeed, of tumors by such low doses per fraction. To not prolong overall treatment time too much, these small doses per fraction would necessitate three or even four fractions per day. Prospective controlled clinical trials have shown that hyperfractionation can improve local control in head and neck cancer by 15%.

### Accelerated Treatment

The alternative strategy of *accelerated treatment* involves an approximately conventional total dose with a conventional fraction number, but since two fractions a day are given, the overall time is approximately halved. In practice, it is never possible to quite achieve this, since the early effects become limiting. It is usually necessary either to interpose a rest period in the middle of the treatment or to slightly reduce the dose with early effects as the limiting factor. The intent of this strategy is to reduce repopulation in rapidly proliferating tumors. There is little or no change in the late effects, since the number of fractions and the dose per fraction are unaltered.

Accelerated treatment is claimed to improve local control in head and neck cancer.

## THE TIME INTERVAL BETWEEN TWO FRACTIONS WHEN TOTAL DOSE IS GIVEN TWICE DAILY (BID)

One thing the two strategies of hyperfraction and accelerated treatment have in common is that both involve multiple fractions per day, and in this context it is important to ensure that the two fractions are separated by a sufficient time interval for the effects of the two doses to be independent: that is, for the repair of sublethal damage from the first dose to be complete before the second dose is delivered. With cells cultured in vitro, the half-time of repair is usually about 1 hour. Although there is evidence that for cells of human origin cultured in vitro, it may vary widely from a few minutes to several hours. For normal tissues in vivo it is more difficult to make precise estimates, but it has been inferred from fractionation experiments that the repair of sublethal damage may be very much slower in late-responding tissues. The most pertinent and remarkable evidence comes from twice-a-day trials by the Radiation Therapy Oncology Group (RTOG) that indicate that, for a given total dose delivered in a given number of fractions, the incidence of late effect was *worse* for interfraction intervals less than 4 hours compared with interfraction intervals longer than 6 hours. These data imply that the repair of sublethal damage in late-responding tissues is slow and so current wisdom dictates an interfraction interval of 6 hours or more when multiple fractions per day are used. This is radiobiology learned from the clinic!

## THE CHOICE BETWEEN ACCELERATED TREATMENT AND HYPERFRACTIONATION

There is clearly a trade-off between the relative benefits of hyperfractionation to reduce late effects and accelerated treatment to improve tumor control by avoiding tumor cell proliferation during an elongated course of treatment.

In 1982, Thames and his colleagues calculated that if conventional overall times of 6 or 7 weeks are shortened to one half or one third by using either two or three fractions per day, then this procedure will give bigger gains in local control than the hyperfractionation procedure if the doubling time of clonogenic cells in the tumor is 5 days or shorter. This could correspond to labeling indices of 10% to 15% or greater, which are not uncommon in human tumors.

Almost everything, therefore, depends on the *clonogenic cell number doubling time.* Some authors have equated this with the *potential doubling time* ($T_{pot}$). Recent data justify this view with the possibility of a predictive assay applicable to the individual patient.

## $T_{pot}$ AND ACCELERATED TREATMENT

A study of the European Cooperative Radiotherapy Group (EORTC) has demonstrated in a dramatic way the usefulness of measuring cell kinetic parameters as a predictive assay in patients receiving radiotherapy for head and neck cancer. In a comparison of accelerated to conventional radiotherapy, each patient was given intravenously a tracer dose of the thymidine analogue iododeoxyuridine.

A tumor biopsy was performed between 4 to 8 hours after administration of the iododeoxyuridine and a specimen was sent for flow cytometric analysis to estimate $T_{pot}$ as described in Chapter 12 on cell, tissue, and tumor kinetics. The conventional radiotherapy arm consisted of daily 2-Gy fractions, whereas the accelerated radiotherapy arm consisted of 1.6-Gy fractions given *three* times per day with 4 hours between fractions. In the accelerated radiotherapy arm, a gap of 2 weeks followed the first week of treatment to allow for normal tissue recovery, followed by a further 2 weeks of treatment. Patients in the two protocol arms received a similar total dose but given in different overall times: 70 Gy in 7 weeks for the conventional and 72 Gy in 5 weeks for the accelerated treatment.

The results of the randomized prospective controlled clinical trials are shown in Figure 13-12. Patients were divided retrospectively into those with *"fast"*-growing tumors (ie, $T_{pot} < 4$ days) or *"slow"*-growing tumors (ie, $T_{pot} > 4$

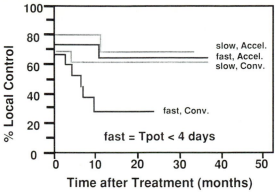

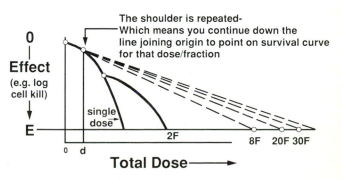

Figure 13-12. Graph illustrating the results of the EORTC Cooperative Trial to compare conventional fractionation (200 cGy once per day for 7000 cGy in 7 weeks) with accelerated treatment (160 cGy three times daily for 7200 cGy in 5 weeks). In the figure, Conv. represents conventional and Accel. represents the accelerated protocol. "Fast"-growing tumors were those with a $T_{pot}$ less than 4 days. Slow-growing tumors had a measured $T_{pot}$ greater than 4 days. (Redrawn from Begg AC, Hofland I, Van Glabekke M, Bartlelink H, Horiot JC: Semin Radiat Oncol 2:22–25, 1992)

days). For the slow- growing tumors, there was no detectable difference between the results of conventional and accelerated treatment. For fast-growing tumors, however, the accelerated treatment resulted in substantially better local control than the conventional protocol and indeed produced results comparable to those obtained for slow-growing tumors. It is remarkable that such a dramatic difference could be achieved by reducing overall treatment time by only 2½ weeks.

If all patients were pooled, there was no significant difference between conventional and accelerated regimens. Only when a small minority of patients with fast-growing tumors were considered did the superiority of the accelerated treatment become evident. This illustrates the dramatic use of a predictive assay to *select* a subgroup of patients who would benefit from a new treatment modality.

# USING THE LINEAR-QUADRATIC CONCEPT TO CALCULATE EFFECTIVE DOSES IN RADIOTHERAPY

It is often useful in practice to have a simple way to compare different fractionation regimens and to assign them a numerical score. For many years the nominal standard dose (NSD) system, developed by Ellis and colleagues, was widely used. It proved useful for assessing modest changes in fractionation but fell into dispute when extrapolated beyond the data range on which it was based. The linear-quadratic model is now more widely used and has received greater acceptance. The following section was suggested by Dr. Jack Fowler; the format is based on tutorials that he has given at ASTRO (American Society of Therapeutic Radiology and Oncology) and at ESTRO (European Society of Therapeutic Radiology and Oncology).

Use of the Linear Quadratic (LQ) model, with appropriate values for the parameters, $\alpha$ and $\beta$, emphasizes the difference between early- and late-responding tissues and the fact that it is never possible to match two different fractionation regimens to be equivalent for both. Calculations of this sort, although a useful guide for residents in training or for research purposes, are not to be considered a substitute for clinical judgment and experience. They are presented only as examples.

Figure 13-13 illustrates the familiar way in which biological effect as a function of dose varies with the number of fractions into which the radiation is delivered—always assuming that the fractions are spaced sufficiently to allow full repair of sublethal radiation damage. For a multifraction regimen, the shoulder of the curve has to be repeated many times, and as a consequence

Figure 13-13. Graph illustrating that, if the dose–response relationship is linear quadratic in form for graded single doses, the *effective* dose–response curve for a multifraction regimen approaches an exponential function of dose for many doses. The effective dose–response relationship is a straight line from the origin through the point on the single dose survival curve corresponding to the daily dose fraction (typically 2 Gy). (Drawn from the concepts of Dr. J. Fowler)

the effective dose–response relationship is a straight line from the origin through the point on the single-dose survival curve for that dose fraction (typically 2 Gy). This was previously discussed in Chapter 3. For the linear portion of the curve, $\alpha$ represents the $\log_e$ of the cells killed per gray. As the curve bends, the quadratic component of cell killing is represented by $\beta$, which is the $\log_e$ of the cells killed per $(gray)^2$. This is illustrated in Figure 13-14. The ratio $\alpha/\beta$ has the dimensions of dose, and is the dose at which the linear and quadratic components of cell killing are equal.

For a single acute dose D, the biological effect is given by

$$E = \alpha D + \beta D^2 \qquad (1)$$

For n well separated fractions of dose d, the biological effect is given by

$$E = n(\alpha d + \beta d^2) \qquad (2)$$

As suggested some years ago by Barendsen, this equation may be rewritten as

$$E = (nd)(\alpha + \beta d)$$
$$= (\alpha)(nd)(1 + \frac{d}{\alpha/\beta}) \qquad (3)$$

but nd = D, the total dose, so

$$E = \alpha \text{ (total dose) (relative effectiveness)}$$

where the quantity $1 + [d/(\alpha/\beta)]$ will be called relative effectiveness. If this equation is divided through by $\alpha$, we have

$$\frac{E}{\alpha} = \text{(Total dose)} \times \text{(Relative effectiveness)}$$
$$= nd \times (1 + \frac{d}{\alpha/\beta}) \qquad (4)$$

The quantity $E/\alpha$ is the **biologically effective dose** and is the quantity by which different fractionation regimens are intercompared. In words, the final equation is

Biologically effective dose = (Total dose) × (Relative effectiveness)

$$\frac{E}{\alpha} = nd \times (1 + \frac{d}{\alpha/\beta}) \qquad (5)$$

## Choice of $\alpha/\beta$

For calculating the examples that follow, $\alpha/\beta$ is assumed to be 3 Gy for late-responding tissues and 10 Gy for early-responding tissue. The reader may, of course, substitute other values if they seem to be more appropriate. It should be noted that parts of schedules can be added, that is, (partial effect)$_1$ and (partial effect)$_2$, as in the concomitant boost. It should also be noted that while it is permissible to compare biologically effective doses for late effects (in Gy$_3$) of one schedule with another and permissible to compare biologically effective doses for early effects (in Gy$_{10}$) of one schedule with another, it is clearly **not** permissible or meaningful to compare early with late effects!

## Model Calculations

1. Conventional treatment, 30 fractions of 2 Gy given one fraction per day, 5 days per week, for an overall treatment time of 6 weeks. This will be written as 30F × 2 Gy/6 weeks.

Early effects: $\frac{E}{\alpha} = (nd)(1 + \frac{d}{\alpha/\beta}) = 60(1 + \frac{2}{10})$
$$= 72 \text{ Gy}_{10}$$

Late effects: $\frac{E}{\alpha} = 60(1 + \frac{2}{3})$
$$= 100 \text{ Gy}_3$$

*Comment:* The subscripts to the biologically effective dose are a reminder that this figure is

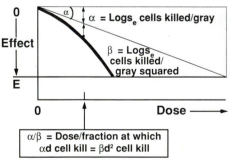

**Figure 13-14.** Graph illustrating the linear-quadratic nature of the radiation cell survival curve, $S = e^{-\alpha D - \beta D^2}$ where S is the fraction of cells surviving a dose D, $\alpha$ is the number of logs of cell kill per gray from the linear portion of the curve, and $\beta$ is the number of logs of cell kill per $(gray)^2$ from the quadratic component. The linear and quadratic components of cell kill are equal at a dose D = $\alpha/\beta$.

**not** in grays and a reminder of the particular values of $\alpha/\beta$ used in the calculation.

2. Hyperfractionation, 70 fractions of 1.15 Gy given twice daily (BID), 6 hours apart, 5 days per week, for an overall treatment time of 7 weeks, that is, 70F $\times$ 1.15 BID/7 weeks

$$\text{Early effects: } \frac{E}{\alpha} = (nd)\ (1 + \frac{d}{\alpha/\beta})$$
$$= 80.5\ (1 + \frac{1.15}{10})$$
$$= 89.8\ Gy_{10}$$
$$\text{Late effects: } \frac{E}{\alpha} = 80.5\ (1 + \frac{1.15}{3})$$
$$= 111.4\ Gy_3$$

*Comment:* This treatment is much "hotter," ie, more effective than the conventional for both early and late effects.

3. A one-fraction-a-day control schedule frequently used to compare with hyperfractionation is 35 fractions of 2 Gy given once a day for 5 days a week, for an overall treatment time of 7 weeks, that is, 35F $\times$ 2 Gy/7 weeks

$$\text{Early effects: } \frac{E}{\alpha} = (nd)\ (1 + \frac{d}{\alpha/\beta})$$
$$= 70\ (1 + \frac{2}{10})$$
$$= 84\ Gy_{10}$$
$$\text{Late effects: } \frac{E}{\alpha} = 70\ (1 + \frac{2}{3})$$
$$= 116.7\ Gy_3$$

*Comment:* This "control" schedule is **not** comparable to the hyperfractionation since it is less effective by 7% for early effects, which includes tumor control (84 vs 89.8 $Gy_{10}$) but hotter for late effects by 5% (116.7 vs 111.4 $Gy_3$).

4. Concomitant boost 30 fractions of 1.8 Gy given once a day, 5 days a week and at the same time (concomitant) a boost to a smaller field of 12 fractions of 1.5 Gy once a day. Overall treatment time is 6 weeks, that is, {(30F $\times$ 1.8 Gy) + (12F $\times$ 1.5 Gy)}/6 weeks. This protocol is much favored at the MD Anderson Hospital. By giving the boost concomitantly, a prolongation of overall time is avoided.

$$\text{Early effects: } \frac{E}{\alpha} = (nd)\ (1 + \frac{d}{\alpha/\beta})$$
$$= 54\ (1 + \frac{1.8}{10}) + 18(1 + \frac{1.5}{10})$$
$$= 84.4\ Gy_{10}$$
$$\text{Late effects: } \frac{E}{\alpha} = 54\ (1 + \frac{1.8}{3}) + 18(1 + \frac{1.5}{3})$$
$$= 113.4\ Gy_3$$

*Comment:* The $Gy_{10}$ and $Gy_3$ values should be compared with the comparable figures for the previous schedules given earlier. The concomitant boost is hotter than the conventional schedule for both early and late effects. Compared with hyperfractionation, however, this concomitant boost is almost the same for late effects but less effective for early effects, including tumor control.

5. Continuous Hyperfractionated Accelerated Radiotherapy (CHART) of 36 fractions of 1.5 Gy given three fractions a day, 6 hours apart, for 12 consecutive days with overall treatment time, 12 days, that is, 36F $\times$ 1.5 Gy (3F/day) /12 days.

$$\text{Early effects including tumor: } \frac{E}{\alpha} = (nd)\ (1 + \frac{d}{\alpha/\beta})$$
$$= 54\ (1 + \frac{1.5}{10})$$
$$= 62.1\ Gy_{10.}$$
$$\text{Late effects: } \frac{E}{\alpha} = 54\ (1 + \frac{1.5}{3})$$
$$= 81.0\ Gy_3$$

*Comment:* Direct comparison of CHART with the previous examples 1 through 4 in terms of $Gy_{10}$ and $Gy_3$ is meaningless since CHART has an overall time of only 12 days compared with 6 or 7 weeks for the other schedules.

## Allowance for Tumor Proliferation

The correction proposed here for tumor proliferation is a crude approximation and should not be taken too seriously. It assumes, among other things, that the rate of cellular proliferation remains constant throughout the overall treatment time.

The number of clonogens (N) at time t is related to the initial number of clonogens ($N_0$) by the expression

$$N = N_0 \, e^{\lambda t} \qquad (6)$$

where $\lambda$ is a constant related to the potential doubling time of the tumor, $T_{pot}$, by the expression

$$\lambda = \frac{\log_e 2}{T_{pot}} = \frac{0.693}{T_{pot}} \qquad (7)$$

As the number of clonogens decreases due to cell killing by the fractionated radiation regimen, it will be balanced to some extent by cell division of the surviving clonogens. The biological effect in equation 2 now becomes

$$E = n \, (\alpha d + \beta d^2) - 0.693 \, \frac{t}{T_{pot}} \qquad (8)$$

The biologically effective dose $E/\alpha$ becomes

$$\frac{E}{\alpha} = (nd) \left(1 + \frac{d}{\alpha/\beta}\right) - \frac{0.693}{\alpha} \frac{(t)}{T_{pot}} \qquad (9)$$

or, in words,

$$\begin{array}{l} \text{Biologically} \\ \text{effective dose} \end{array} = \left(\begin{array}{c}\text{Total} \\ \text{dose}\end{array}\right) \times \left(\begin{array}{c}\text{Relative} \\ \text{effectivess}\end{array}\right)$$
$$\qquad\qquad (10)$$
$$- \frac{\log_e 2}{\alpha} \, (\text{No. of cell doublings})$$

It is now necessary to assume a value for $\alpha$, the initial slope of the cell survival curve, as well as for $T_{pot}$, the potential doubling time of the tu-

mor. A reasonable value for $\alpha$ is $0.3 \pm 0.1$/Gy. $T_{pot}$ may have a value of 2 to 25 days with a median value of about 5 days.

For typical 6-week (39-day) schedules referred to earlier, proliferation may reduce the biologically effective dose by

$$\frac{E}{\alpha} = \frac{0.693}{0.3} \times \frac{39}{5} = 18 \; Gy_{10}$$

Note that since we are concerned with tumor proliferation, the reduction in biologically effective dose is in $Gy_{10}$; that is, an early-effect $\alpha/\beta$ value was used. By the same token, proliferation during a 7-week protocol (ie, 46 days) would decrease the biologically effective dose by

$$\frac{E}{\alpha} = \frac{0.693}{0.3} \times \frac{46}{5} = 21.3 \; Gy_{10}$$

CHART calls for three fractions per day over 12 days, and thus proliferation during this time would reduce the biologically effective dose by

$$\frac{E}{\alpha} = \frac{0.693}{0.3} \times \frac{12}{5} = 5.6 \; Gy_{10}$$

Table 13-2 summarizes the effect of tumor proliferation on the biologically effective doses characteristic of the various treatment regimens discussed earlier.

Based on the assumptions made, hyperfractionation results in the largest biologically effective dose and therefore may be expected to result in the best tumor control, followed closely

Table 13-2.
Effect of Tumor Proliferation on Biologically Effective Doses Characteristic of Various Treatment Regimens

| PROTOCOL | $E/\alpha$ EARLY ie, TUMOR $Gy_{10}$ | PROLIFERATION CORRECTION $Gy_{10}$ | CORRECTED FOR TIME $Gy_{10}$ |
|---|---|---|---|
| Conventional protocol 30F × 2 Gy/6 wk (39 d) | 72 | −18.0 | 54 |
| Hyperfractionation 70F × 1.15 Gy/7 wk | 89.8 | −21.3 | 68.5 |
| Concomitant boost (30F × 1.8 Gy) + (12F × 1.5 Gy)/6 wk (39 d) | 84.4 | −18.0 | 66.4 |
| CHART 36F × 1.5 Gy/12 d | 62.1 | −5.6 | 56.5 |

by the concomitant boost schedule. CHART is a much less effective schedule based on a $T_{pot}$ of 5 days. It is necessary to assume a very fast growing tumor, with a $T_{pot}$ of 3 days or less, for CHART to become the most effective schedule.

It must be emphasized again that calculations of this sort should be used only as a guide for residents in training, since they do not in any way replace clinical judgment. It is useful, however, to have a yardstick by which new fractionation schemes may be judged. A number of software packages are being developed to perform on a personal computer calculations of the type described earlier.

► ## Summary of Pertinent Conclusions

- The four *R*s of radiobiology are

  Repair of sublethal damage
  Reassortment of cells within the cell cycle
  Repopulation
  Reoxygenation
- The basis of conventional fractionation may be explained as follows. Dividing a dose into a number of fractions *spares* normal tissues because of the repair of sublethal damage between dose fractions and cellular repopulation. At the same time, fractionation *increases* tumor damage because of reoxygenation and reassortment.
- The Strandquist plot is the relation between total dose and overall treatment time. In this context "time" includes the number of fractions. On a double log plot the slope of the line for normal tissues is often close to 0.33.
- The Ellis NSD system made the important contribution of separating the effects of a number of fractions and overall time. The time correction was a power function ($T^{0.11}$) that is far from accurate.
- The extra dose required to counteract proliferation in a normal tissue irradiated in a fractionated regimen is a sigmoidal function of time. No extra dose is required until some weeks into a fractionated schedule.
- The delay before an extra dose is required to counteract the effects of proliferation is much longer for late-responding tissues and is beyond the overall time for conventional radiotherapy schedules.
- Prolonging overall time within the normal radiotherapy range has little sparing effect on *late reactions* but a large sparing effect on *early reactions*.
- The dose–response relationship for late effects is more curvy than for early effects. The ratio $\alpha/\beta$ is about 10 Gy (1000 rads) for early effects and about 2 Gy (200 rads) for late-responding tissues. Consequently, late-responding tissues are more sensitive to changes in fractionation pattern.
- Fraction size is the dominant factor in determining *late effects*, while overall treatment time has little influence. By contrast, fraction size and overall treatment time both determine the response of *acutely responding* tissues.
- Accelerated repopulation refers to the triggering of surviving cells (clonogens) to divide more rapidly as the tumor shrinks after irradiation or treatment with any cytotoxic agent.
- Accelerated repopulation starts in head and neck cancer in the human about 4 weeks after initiation of fractionated radiotherapy. About 0.6 Gy (60 rads) per day is needed to compensate for this repopulation.

*(continued)*

► **Summary of Pertinent Conclusions** *(Continued)*

- This phenomenon mandates that treatment should be completed as soon as practical once it has started; it may be better to delay the start than to introduce interruptions during treatment.
- The basic aim of hyperfractionation is to further separate early and late effects. The overall treatment time remains conventional at 6 to 8 weeks, but since two fractions per day are used, the total number of fractions is 60 to 80. The dose must be increased, since the dose per fraction is decreased. Early reactions may be slightly increased, tumor control improved, and late effects greatly reduced.
- In accelerated treatment, to reduce repopulation in rapidly proliferating tumors, approximately conventional doses and number of fractions are used; but since two doses per day are given, the overall treatment time is halved.
- **Hyperfractionation** improves local control in head and neck cancer by about 15%; this has been demonstrated in prospective controlled randomized clinical trials in the United States and by the European Cooperative Group.
- **Accelerated treatment** has been shown to improve local control in patients with "fast" growing tumors, that is, those with a $T_{pot} < 4$ days as measured by flow cytometry after administration of iododeoxyuridine.
- The linear-quadratic concept may be used to calculate the biological effectiveness of various radiotherapy protocols.
- The useful formula is

(Biological Effective Dose) = (Total Dose) × (Relative Effectiveness)

$$E/\alpha = nd \times (1 + \frac{d}{\alpha/\beta})$$

- An approximate allowance can be made for tumor proliferation during an extended radiotherapy course by assuming a value for $T_{pot}$.

# BIBLIOGRAPHY

Begg AC, Hofland I, Van Glabekke M, Bartlelink H, Horiot JC: Predictive value of potential doubling time for radiotherapy of head and neck tumor patients: Results from the EORTC Cooperative Trial 22851. Semin Radiat Oncol 2:22–25, 1992

Begg AC, McNally NJ, Shrieve D et al: A method to measure the duration of DNA synthesis and the potential doubling time from a single sample. Cytometry 6:620–625, 1985

Begg AC, Moonen I, Hofland I et al: Human tumor cell kinetics using a monoclonal antibody against iododeoxyuridine: Intratumoral sampling variations. Radiother Oncol 11:337–347, 1988

Douglas BG, Fowler JF: The effect of multiple small doses of x-rays on skin reactions in the mouse and a basic interpretation. Radiat Res 66:401–426, 1976

Ellis F: Dose time and fractionation: A Clinical Hypothesis. Clin Radiol 20:1–7, 1969

Ellis F: Nominal standard dose and the ret. Br J Radiol 44:101–108, 1971

Fowler JF: Dose–response curves for organ function in cell survival. Br J Radiol 56:497–500, 1983

Fowler JF: 40 years of radiobiology: Its impact on radiotherapy. Phys Med Biol 29:97–113, 1984

Fowler JF: What next in fractionated radiotherapy? Br J Cancer (Suppl VI) 49:285S–300S, 1984

Fowler JF: Potential for increasing the differential response between tumors and normal tissues: Can proliferation rate be used? Int J Radiat Oncol Biol Phys 12:641–646, 1986

Fowler JF: The linear-quadratic formula and progress in fractionated radiotherapy. Br J Radiol 62:679–694, 1989

Parsons JT, Bova FJ, Million RR: A reevaluation of split-course technique for squamous cell carcinoma of the head and neck. Int J Radiat Oncol Biol Phys 6:1645–1652, 1980

Peters LJ, Withers HR, Thames HD: Radiobiological bases for multiple daily fractionation. In Kaercher KH, Kogelnik HD, Reinartz G (eds): Progress in Radio-Oncology II, pp 317–323. New York, Raven Press, 1982

Ronde LA: Radiation sciences and medical radiology. Radiother Oncol 1:1–22, 1983

Thames HD, Peters LJ, Withers HR, Fletcher GH: Accelerated fractionation vs. hyperfractionation: Rationales for several treatments per day. Int J Radiat Oncol Biol Phys 9:127–138, 1983

Thames HD Jr, Withers HR: Test of equal effect per fraction and estimation of initial clongen number in microcolony assays of survival after fractionated irradiation. Br J Radiol 53:1071–1077, 1980

Thames HD, Wither HR, Peters LJ, Fletcher GH: Changes in early and late radiation responses with altered dose fractionation: Implications for dose–survival relationships. Int J Radiat Oncol Biol Phys 8:219–226, 1982

Withers HR: Cell cycle redistribution as a factor in multifraction irradiation. Radiology 114:199–202, 1975

Withers HR: Response of tissues to multiple small dose fractions. Radiat Res 71:24–33, 1977

Withers HR, Peters LJ, Kogelnik HD: The pathobiology of late effects of irradiation. In Meyn RE, Withers HR (eds): Radiation Biology in Cancer Research, pp 439–448. New York, Raven Press, 1980

Withers HR, Taylor JMG, Maciejewski B: The hazard of accelerated tumor clonogen repopulation during radiotherapy. Acta Oncol 27:131, 1988

Withers HR, Thames HE Jr, Flow BL, Mason HA, Hussey DH: The relationship of acute to late skin injury in 2 and 5 fraction/week gamma-ray therapy. Int J Radiat Oncol Biol Phys 4:595–601, 1978

Withers HR, Thames HD, Peters LJ, Fletcher GH: Normal tissue radioresistance in clinical radiotherapy. In Fletcher GH, Nervi C, Withers HR (eds): Biological Bases and Clinical Implications of Tumor Radioresistance, pp 139–152. New York, Masson, 1983

*Radiobiology for the Radiologist, Fourth Edition,* by Eric J. Hall
J. B. Lippincott Company, Philadelphia © 1994.

# 14

# *New Radiation Modalities*

Radiation Therapy

The early recognition that x-rays could produce local tumor control in some patients and not in others led to the notion that other forms of ionizing radiations might be superior.

Neutrons were first introduced in a speculative way, not based on any particular hypothesis. The later use of neutrons, as well as the introduction of protons, negative π-mesons, and heavy ions were all based clearly on a putative advantage, either of physical dose distribution or radiobiological properties.

The use of neutrons following World War II was based squarely on the premise that the presence of hypoxic cells limits the curability of human tumors by x-ray therapy, so that the lower oxygen enhancement ratio (OER) characteristic of neutrons might confer an advantage. An alternative rationale for neutrons, proposed at a later date, was that their relative biological effectiveness (RBE) is larger for slow-growing tumors, so that they may have an advantage in a limited number of specific human tumors.

Protons have radiobiological properties similar to x-rays, and their introduction into radiotherapy was based entirely on the superiority of the physical dose distribution possible with charged particles. Negative π-mesons and heavy ions were introduced with the hope of combining the radiobiological advantages attributed to neutrons, with the dose distribution advantage characteristic of protons.

Neutrons have been shown to be superior to x-rays in a limited number of situations, specifically for the treatment of prostatic cancer and salivary gland tumors. A number of controlled clinical trials have been performed for a wide variety of cancer sites, but a gain was only apparent in these few circumstances. Protons have found a small, but important niche for the treatment of uveal melanoma and tumors such as chordomas that are located close to the spinal cord and so benefit greatly from the localized dose distribution. The wider use of protons for broad-beam radiotherapy is being tested but no advantage has yet been proven. Negative π-mesons and heavy ions have been used to treat hundreds of patients, but prospective randomized trials have never been completed to prove their superiority over conventional x-rays. Their enormous cost may be justified by a significant gain.

The casual reader may be content with this summary of new radiation modalities and may not wish to proceed farther in this chapter. Interest in high linear energy transfer (LET) radiations for radiotherapy has largely waned, but protons are very much in vogue. In this chapter neutrons and protons are considered in turn.

## FAST NEUTRONS

### Rationale

Neutrons were first used for cancer therapy at the Lawrence Berkeley Laboratory in California in the 1930s. Their use was not based on any biological or physical rationale; they were used only because they represented a new modality that might be useful in hopeless cancer cases, for which conventional radiations were known to be ineffective.

After World War II, interest in neutrons for cancer treatment was renewed at the Hammersmith Hospital in London as a result of studies that implied that tumors contain hypoxic cells and that cells deficient in oxygen are resistant to killing by x-rays. The rationale for neutrons at this stage, therefore, was their lower dependence on oxygen for cell killing, together with the premise that viable hypoxic cells limit curability by x-rays.

Clinical trials to date have clearly shown that neutrons do *not* offer an advantage over x-rays across the board for a broad spectrum of tumor types. Nevertheless, there is tantalizing evidence that they give better results for certain types of tumors. This, together with other evidence, has resulted in a rethinking of the role of hypoxic cells and the admission that they are probably not as important as previously thought, at least in multifraction regimens in which reoxygenation can be effective. The revised rationale for neutrons, therefore, is that RBE varies for different tumor types, being high for some that are slowly proliferating. On this basis they would be expected to offer an advantage only in a few selected types of cases. The idea is that slowly growing, well-differentiated tumors may be analogous to the slowly proliferating tissues responsible for late effects, and it is well documented that neutron RBEs are higher for late than for early effects, at least for treatment schedules involving many fractions.

The rationale for the use of neutrons has undergone a considerable evolution over the years. The biological properties of neutrons differ from those of x-rays in a number of respects, and it is not clear which is the most important in a clinical situation.

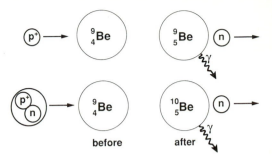

**Figure 14-1.** Diagram illustrating the two neutron production processes in common usage. (*Top*) The d⁺→Be stripping process. Deuterons are accelerated to high energy in the cyclotron and are then made to impinge on a beryllium target. When incident on the target, the proton is "stripped" from the deuteron, leaving a neutron that retains part of the incident kinetic energy of the accelerated deuteron. For each neutron produced, one atom of beryllium is converted to boron. (*Bottom*) The p⁺→Be process. Protons are accelerated to high energy in a cyclotron and made to impinge on a target of beryllium where they "knock out" neutrons.

## Practical Sources

The only practical source of neutrons for clinical radiotherapy is a cyclotron. A **cyclotron** is an electrical device capable of accelerating positively charged particles, such as protons or deuterons, to an energy of millions of volts. The particle is accelerated by being made to pass repeatedly through an electrical gradient while being held in a circular orbit by a magnetic field produced by a huge magnet. The path of the particle, as it accelerates, is a spiral, until it is extracted from the machine. The principle of the cyclotron was conceived by Ernest Lawrence at the University of California at Berkeley in 1931 when he realized that the time taken for a charged particle to complete a circular orbit in magnetic field was independent of the radius of the orbit.

Neutrons can be produced in a cyclotron by accelerating deuterons or protons and making them impinge on a beryllium target (Fig. 14-1). Using the d⁺ → Be process, a high yield of neutrons is readily achievable; the disadvantage is that the cyclotrons needed are relatively massive. Early on, a few low-energy machines, of 15 MeV or less, were built specially for medical use and installed in hospitals, with their time divided between neutron cancer therapy and the production of short-lived positron-emitting radionuclides. This was the policy in Great Britain, with neutron therapy being administered with small cyclotrons using the d⁺ → Be process at

Hammersmith and Edinburgh. Unfortunately, the limited energy from this process results in poor percentage depth doses, and only relatively superficial tumors in the head and neck region could be treated adequately. To obtain penetration comparable to megavoltage x-rays using neutrons produced by the d⁺ → Be process requires an accelerating energy of about 50 MeV, and that means a massive cyclotron, much too big to be accommodated in a hospital. In the United States several high-energy machines (22 to 50 MeV), initially designed and built at enormous cost for high-energy physics research, were modified and used to generate neutron beams for cancer therapy on a part-time basis.

More recently, cyclotrons to produce neutrons have been built using the p⁺ → Be reaction. Since a proton has half the mass of a deuteron, the cyclotron can be sufficiently small to be installed in a hospital, particularly in the case of cyclotrons based on superconducting technology.

Neutron spectra produced by the two processes are shown in Figure 14-2. When a beam of deuterons impinges on a beryllium target, the proton is stripped from the deuteron and carries with it some of the kinetic energy of the deuterons, a process illustrated in Figure 14-1. The neutron spectrum consists of a single peak, with a modal value about 40% of the accelerated energy of the incident deuterons. Thus, 50-MeV deu-

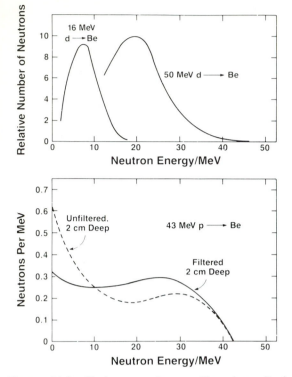

Figure 14-2. Neutron spectra resulting from (*top*) cyclotron-produced neutrons by the d⁺→Be process for the highest and lowest energies used clinically and (*bottom*) cyclotron-produced neutrons by the p⁺→Be process, with and without a hydrogenous filter to remove the "soft" low-energy neutrons. (Compiled from published data by Dr. Paul Kliauga)

terons would produce a neutron beam with a modal energy of about 20 MeV. When accelerated protons impinge on a beryllium target, neutrons are produced by a knock-on process, and the neutron spectrum spans a wide range (see Fig. 14-1). Many low-energy neutrons are produced, as well as neutrons up to energies close to the accelerating energy of the incident protons. In many cases it is necessary to use a filter of some hydrogenous material, such as polyethylene, to preferentially filter out some of the low-energy neutrons that would "spoil" the depth-dose curves because they are absorbed at superficial depths (see Fig. 14-2). A 50-MeV proton cyclotron produces neutrons with depth doses similar to a deuteron cyclotron of the same or slightly higher energy, while being a fraction of the size. Dedicated hospital-based

cyclotrons in the 50- to 70-MeV range using the p⁺ → Be reaction are used in neutron cancer therapy in a number of countries. Such machines can be built with an isocentric mount and adjustable collimators. The resultant depth doses are comparable to a 6-MV x-ray Linac. Controlled clinical trials to compare neutrons with x-rays can now be performed without the neutrons being at a disadvantage because of poor physical characteristics.

## Percentage Depth Doses for Neutron Beams

An essential factor in the choice of a neutron beam for clinical use is its ability to penetrate to a sufficient depth. Figure 14-3 is a comparison of the percentage depth doses for various photon beams with those for neutrons produced by cyclotrons using the d⁺ → Be or p⁺ → Be processes. The lower energy Hammersmith cyclotron, used in the early trials, gave appreciably poorer depth-dose characteristics and is in fact comparable to a cesium-137 unit. The higher-energy cyclotrons show considerably better penetration. The depth doses associated with a 50-MeV cyclotron using the d⁺ → Be process or high-energy cyclotrons using the p⁺ → Be process rival those of linear accelerator in the 4- to 6-MeV range. The acceptable depth doses associated with neutron machines are to some extent a function of the long treatment distances used, which are usually 100 to 140 cm. This distance is necessitated by the collimator, which must be thick because it is made of a hydrogenous material to absorb the neutrons and a metal such as lead to remove the γ-ray component.

## The First Clinical Use of Neutrons

The first clinical trial of neutrons was not based on any radiobiological rationale but was prompted largely by the availability of a new and unique beam (Fig. 14-4). It is said that it received some impetus when the mother of the Lawrence brothers (E. O. Lawrence was the inventor of the cyclotron and the director of what was to become the Lawrence Berkeley Laboratory) con-

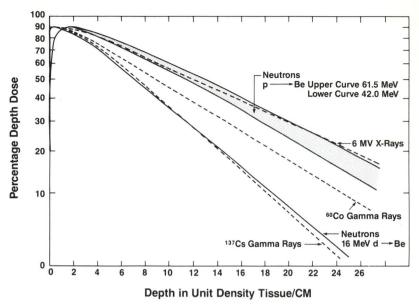

**Figure 14-3.** A comparison of the percentage depth doses for selected neutron beams with x- and γ-rays. Neutrons generated by 16-MeV d⁺→Be have poor depth doses, comparable to a cesium-137 unit with a short source–skin distance. To obtain depth doses comparable to megavoltage photon beams requires about 50 MeV, using either the d⁺→Be or the p⁺→Be reaction. A cyclotron to accelerate protons to this energy is much smaller and can be accommodated in a hospital. (Compiled from published data by Dr. Paul Kliauga)

tracted cancer, which was judged by her physician to be incurable by conventional means. She was treated with neutrons and lived for many years, although from a retrospective review of the case it is probable that she did not have cancer in the first place! This early effort at Berkeley was hampered because the complexities of the relationship between RBE and dose for high LET radiations were not understood at the time. Consequently, a number of patients were seriously overdosed before the trial was terminated by the entry of the United States into World War II. In reviewing their experience many years later, Stone concluded, in his famous Janeway Lecture of 1948, that "neutron therapy as administered by us resulted in such bad late sequelae in proportion to a few good results that it should not be continued."

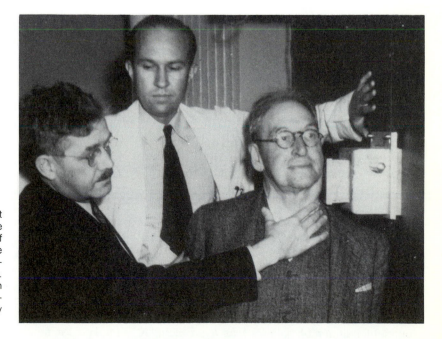

**Figure 14-4.** The first patient treated with neutrons at the Lawrence Berkeley Laboratory of the University of California. On the left is Dr. Robert Stone, the radiotherapist, and in the center is Dr. John Lawrence, the physician brother of the inventor of the cyclotron, E.O. Lawrence (Courtesy of the University of California).

## The Hammersmith Neutron Experience

The renewed interest in neutrons in the postwar years originated at the Hammersmith Hospital in London, where neutrons were generated by the Medical Research Council's 60-inch cyclotron. In this machine 16-MeV deuterons incident on a beryllium target produced neutrons with a modal value of 6 MeV. The Hammersmith cyclotron was suggested and conceived by Gray, based on the notion that a lowered OER would be advantageous to radiotherapy. The machine suffered from the limitations of poor depth doses (equivalent to 250 kVp x-rays) and a fixed horizontal beam.

A prospective randomized clinical trial to compare neutrons with x-rays was started in 1971. Advanced tumors of the head and neck were chosen because the poor depth-dose characteristics made neutrons suitable only for treating relatively superficial lesions. The trial involved patients with tumors of the salivary glands, buccal cavity, hypopharynx, and larynx.

The neutron treatments delivered in only 12 fractions were clearly superior as judged by local control of the primary tumor, but there is some question that the gain was achieved at the expense of a higher complication rate.

## The United States Neutron Experience

Because of the limitations associated with low-energy cyclotrons, interest in a number of centers in the United States turned to the use of large cyclotrons that accelerate deuterons to energies of 22 to 50 MeV. Several such machines were built for high-energy physics research and were converted for part-time neutron therapy. In addition, neutrons were produced at the Fermilab in Batavia, Illinois, by bombarding a beryllium target with 67-MeV protons.

The early US neutron therapy experience was accumulated in these four facilities. All had adequate dose rates and quite good depth doses. Unfortunately, they had disadvantages: all machines had fixed horizontal beams, and all were located in physics installations rather than in large busy hospitals, so that the availability of a sufficient number of patients was a problem. A number of controlled clinical trials were performed for a variety of tumor sites and showed no advantage for neutrons over x-rays. Neutrons, however, appeared to be superior for salivary gland tumors, soft tissue sarcomas, and prostate carcinoma.

## Current Efforts With Neutrons

Enthusiasm for neutron therapy has certainly waned just at a time when technology allows machines to be built that are suitable for clinical use. The new generation of hospital-based cyclotrons, using the $p^+ \rightarrow Be$ reaction have adequate dose rates, good percentage depth doses, and a full isocentric mount, similar to a conventional Linac. A few centers operate such machines in the United States, Europe, and Japan. A fair test should now be possible of neutrons compared with x-rays without the high LET radiation being handicapped from the outset by limitations of access or physical specifications. Emphasis will be placed on two factors. First, subgroups of patients with specific types of tumors that may benefit from neutrons must be found. It is already reasonably clear that there is not an across-the-board benefit from neutrons, which was expected, perhaps naively, in the early days. Second, different fractionation patterns will be tried for neutrons. There is no a priori reason to expect that the best or most effective fractionation pattern and overall time is the same for neutrons as for x-rays. Indeed, the contrary is likely to be the case, and different fractionation regimens will be tried, especially smaller numbers of fractions in a shorter time (ie, accelerated treatment).

Emphasis will be placed on slowly growing tumors in view of the observation of Breuer and Batterman that neutron RBE, measured from pulmonary metastases in patients, increases as tumor volume doubling time increases (Fig. 14-5). This coincides with the clinical experience that neutrons appear to be superior for prostate and salivary gland tumors and soft tissue sarcoma—all relatively slowly growing tumors. The rationale for this decision may be based on the notion that slowly growing tumors have more cells in $G_1$ and the age–response function is less marked for neutrons than x-rays, but the choice

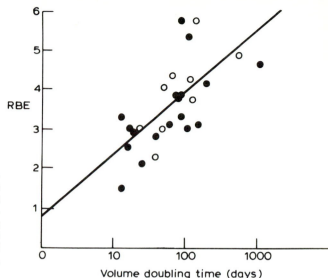

**Figure 14-5.** Values of relative biological effectiveness (RBE) relative to cobalt-60 γ-rays for volume changes of pulmonary metastases in patients as a function of the volume doubling time. The dots indicate the measured RBE values; the open circles are estimated values when only neutron irradiation was given. (From Batterman JJ: Clinical Application of Fast Neutrons: The Amsterdam Experience, p 43, Amsterdam, Rodipi, 1981)

of patients is in fact empirical and based on earlier clinical observations.

## BORON NEUTRON CAPTURE THERAPY

The basic idea behind boron neutron capture therapy (BNCT) is elegant in its simplicity. It has appealed to physicians, and particularly to physicists, for the best part of half a century. The idea is to deliver to the cancer patient a boron-containing drug that is taken up only in tumor cells and then to expose the patient to a beam of low energy (thermal) neutrons that themselves produce little radiobiological effect but that interact with the boron to produce short range, densely ionizing, α-particles. Thus, the tumor is intensely irradiated, while the normal tissues are spared. There are two problems inherent in this idea that have so far proved to be intractable.

1. How do you find a "magic" drug that can distinguish malignant cells from normal cells? (The skeptic might add that searching for such a drug has been the Holy Grail of cancer research and that if one were found, the obvious strategy would be to attach an alkylating agent or an α-emitting radionuclide to it; combining its use with neutrons would be a distant third!)
2. The low-energy neutrons necessary for BNCT

are poorly penetrating in tissue and consequently result in percentage depth doses that are horrible by today's standards.

A number of nuclides have a high propensity for absorbing low energy or thermal neutrons; that is, they have a high neutron capture cross-section. Boron is the most attractive because it is readily available in a nonradioactive form, its chemistry is such that it can be incorporated into a wide variety of compounds, and when it interacts with low-energy neutrons it emits short-range, high LET, α-particles.

For BNCT to be successful, the compounds to be used should have high specificity for malignant cells, with concomitantly low concentrations in adjacent normal tissues and in blood. This, of course, is a tall order.

In the early days, the compounds used were not specially synthesized for BNCT but were already available. In the brain, which is the site for which BNCT has been largely used, some selectivity is obtained because compounds do not penetrate normal brain tissue to the same degree as brain tumors where the blood–brain barrier is absent or severely compromised.

### Boron Compounds

Over the years much effort has been expended in attempts to synthesize compounds specifically for BNCT. Experimental studies as early as 1966 identified a boron compound, $B_{12} H_{11} S H$, which was found to bond to protein molecules, probably due to the sulfhydryl group. These compounds appear to be selectively concentrated in experimentally produced gliomas (as much as seven times higher concentration in tumor compared with normal brain tissue).

Subsequently, a variety of approaches have been adopted in an effort to get boron to concentrate in tumor cells. Boron-containing purines and pyrimidines have been tried, on the premise that they would be incorporated into rapidly dividing tumor cells. Boron has been attached to porphyrins and related phthalocyanines and also to various antibodies. This is an ongoing effort, but the results to date are not particularly impressive.

## Neutron Sources

During fission within the core of a nuclear reactor, neutrons are "born" that have a wide range of energies. Neutron beams can be extracted from the reactor by the application of suitable techniques and the use of appropriate moderators. Thermal neutrons, or room temperature neutrons (0.025 eV), react best with boron to produce densely ionizing α-particles. Unfortunately, thermal neutrons are attenuated rapidly by tissue; the half-value layer is only about 1.5 cm. Consequently, it is not possible to treat to depths of more than a few centimeters without heavily irradiating surface normal tissues. Nevertheless, most clinical trials in Japan have utilized neutrons of this energy.

Current interest in the United States focuses on the use of epithermal neutron beams (1 to 10,000 eV), which have a somewhat greater depth of penetration. These can be obtained by using moderators or filters to slow the fast neutrons into the epithermal range and filtering out the residual thermal neutrons. These epithermal neutrons do not themselves interact with the boron but are degraded at depth in the tissue by collisions with hydrogen atoms. Even so, the peak in dose occurs at a depth of only 2 to 3 cm, with a rapid fall-off beyond this depth. Thus, the very high surface doses are avoided but the depth doses are still poor.

The need for a nuclear reactor as a source of neutrons is a serious limitation and would preclude BNCT facilities in densely populated urban areas. If BNCT were shown to have a clear therapeutic effect, it may be possible to generate appropriate neutron beams by using a proton accelerator or an isotopic source. Little has been done in this area.

## Clinical Trials

A number of clinical trials have been performed over the years, beginning in the 1950s and 1960s. Results are tantalizing but never definitive. The concept of BNCT is as attractive as ever, but it continues to be difficult to convert into a practical treatment modality even for shallow tumors.

# PROTONS

Protons are attractive for radiotherapy because of their physical dose distribution; their radiobiological properties are unremarkable. The RBE of protons is indistinguishable from that of 250-kV x-rays, which means that they are 10% to 15% more effective than cobalt-60 γ-rays or megavoltage x-rays generated by a linear accelerator. The OER for protons is also indistinguishable from that for x-rays, namely 2.5 to 3. These biological properties are consistent with the physical characteristics of high-energy proton beams; they are sparsely ionizing, except for a very short region at the end of the particles' range, just before they stop. In the entrance plateau the average LET is about 0.5 keV/mm, rising to a theoretical maximum of 100 keV/mm over a few microns as the particles come to rest. This high LET component is, however, restricted to such a tiny length of track that for high-energy protons it does not have any significant effect.

The dose deposited by a beam of monoenergetic protons increases slowly with depth but reaches a sharp maximum near the end of the particles' range in the **Bragg peak.** The beam has sharp edges, with little side-scatter, and the dose falls to zero after the Bragg peak, at the end of the particles' range. The possibility of precisely confining the high-dose region to the tumor volume while minimizing the dose to surrounding normal tissue is an obvious attraction to the radio-therapist. Protons and helium ions come closest to realizing this dream at modest cost.

Proton beams ranging in energy from 150 to 200 MeV are of interest in radiotherapy because this corresponds to a range in tissue of 16 to 26 cm. Intense proton beams in this energy range are readily produced by cyclotrons, many of which were built initially for high-energy physics research.

Figure 14-6 shows the depth-dose curve for the 187-MeV proton beam from the synchrocy-clotron at Uppsala, Sweden. The sharply defined Bragg peak occurs at a depth in tissue that depends on the initial energy of the particles.

The early medical use of proton beams involved treatment of the pituitary, first in patients with advanced breast cancer and later in patients with diabetic retinopathy, Cushing's disease, and acromegaly. Protons were used for these applications to exploit their well-defined beam, which made it possible to give a huge dose to the pituitary without causing unacceptable damage to nearby structures. These treatments have been performed at both Berkeley and Harvard, al-

though the two institutions adopted very different strategies. At Harvard, an attempt was made to use a narrow pencil beam of protons of just the right range for the Bragg peak to fall exactly in the pituitary; in this way a huge local dose could be delivered to the gland with minimal irradiation of surrounding tissues. This would appear to be a very elegant approach to the problems, but it is fraught with difficulty because the exact location of the Bragg peak can vary considerably with small inhomogeneities in the tissue traversed. For this reason the Berkeley group favored the use of the plateau portion of a very high-energy beam that passed right through the patient's head; the Bragg peak was not within the patient at all. Multiple beams in a pseudorotation technique were then used, converging on the pituitary, to obtain good dose localization.

The way in which the Bragg peak can be spread out to encompass a tumor of realistic size is illustrated in Figure 14-7. In this figure curve A shows the narrow Bragg peak of the primary beam of the 160-MeV proton beam at the Harvard cyclotron. Beams of lower intensity and

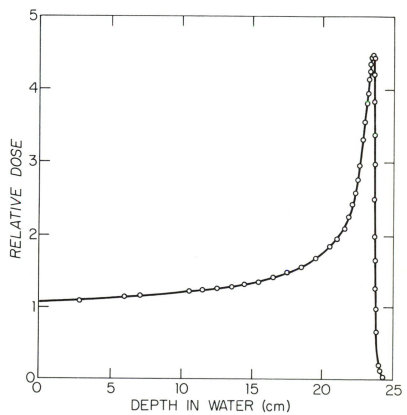

**Figure 14-6.** Depth-dose curve for 187-MeV protons from the Uppsala synchrocyclotron. The dose reaches a sharp peak at a depth of about 23 cm. (Redrawn from Larsson B: Br J Radiol 34:143–151, 1961)

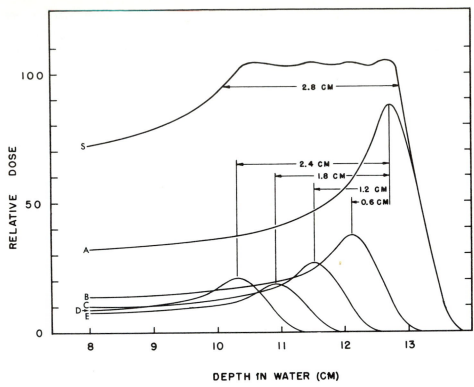

**DEPTH IN WATER (CM)**

Figure 14-7. The way in which the Bragg peak for a proton beam can be spread out. Curve A is the depth-dose distribution for the primary beam of 160-MeV protons at the Harvard cyclotron, which has a half-width of only 0.6 cm. Beams of lower intensity and shorter range, as illustrated by curves B, C, D, and E, can be added to give a composite curve S, which results in a uniform dose over 2.8 cm. The broadening of the peak is achieved by passing the beam through a rotating wheel with sectors of varying thickness. (Redrawn from Koehler AM, Preston WM: Radiology 104:191–195, 1972)

shorter range, shown in curves B, C, D, and E, are readily obtainable by passing the beam through a rotating wheel with plastic sectors of varying thickness. The composite curve, S, which is the sum of all the individual Bragg peaks of the beams of varying range, results in a uniform dose over 2.8 cm. The spread-out Bragg peak can, of course, be made narrower or broader than this, as necessary.

Many researchers consider protons to be the treatment of choice for choroidal melanoma. Figure 14-8 shows the dose distribution that is achieved at the Harvard cyclotron, which allows very high doses to be delivered to small tumors without unacceptable damage to nearby normal tissues. Protons have found a small but important place in the treatment of ocular tumors and also some specialized tumors close to the spinal cord.

Broad-beam radiotherapy, with the Bragg peak spread out to cover a large tumor, has been in progress at Uppsala since 1957, and a comparable US effort has begun at Harvard. Protons are seldom used alone in such applications since there is no skin-sparing effect, but rather they are mixed with high-energy x-rays. This is highly experimental and has shown no obvious advantage, so that the use of protons appears to be limited to those specialized situations in which a sharply defined high-dose region with rapid fall-off of dose is important.

By July 1992, a total of about 10,846 patients had been treated with proton beams, with 5,583 of them treated at the Harvard cyclotron, operated by the Massachusetts General Hospital. Table 14-1 lists the current and planned proton therapy facilities worldwide.

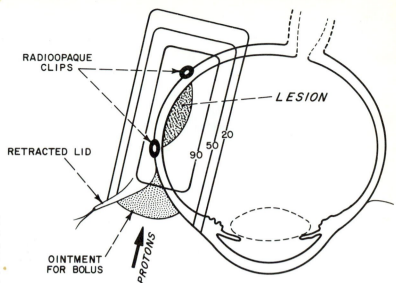

**Figure 14-8.** Dose distribution used for the treatment of choroidal melanoma at the Harvard cyclotron. Note the sharp edges to the beam and rapid fall-off of dose outside the treatment volume. (Courtesy of Dr. Herman Suit)

Table 14-1.
**Proton Facilities and the Number of Patients Treated to July 1992***

| FACILITY | LOCATION | PARTICLE | NO. PATIENTS TREATED |
|---|---|---|---|
| **Existing Facilities** | | | |
| Berkeley 184″ | California, USA | p | 30 |
| Berkeley | California, USA | He | 2054 |
| Uppsala | Sweden | p | 73 |
| Harvard | Massachusetts, USA | p | 5583 |
| Dubna | Russia | p | 84 |
| Moscow | Russia | p | 2200 |
| St. Petersburg | Russia | p | 719 |
| Chiba | Japan | p | 80 |
| Tsukuba | Japan | p | 274 |
| PSI (SIN) | Switzerland | p | 1246 |
| Dubna | Russia | p | 20 |
| Uppsala | Sweden | p | 23 |
| Clatterbridge | England | p | 244 |
| Loma Linda | California, USA | p | 76 |
| Louvain-la-Neuve | Belgium | p | 14 |
| Nice | France | p | 96 |
| Orsay | France | p | 84 |
| **Proposed Facilities** | | | |
| Indiana Cyclotron | Indiana, USA | p | |
| N.A.C. | South Africa | p | |
| PSI | Switzerland | p | |
| A.P.D.C. | Illinois, USA | p | |
| Novosibirsk | Russia | p | |
| ITEP Moscow | Russia | p | |
| NPTC (Harvard) | Massachusetts, USA | p | |
| Sacramento | California, USA | p | |
| Antwerp | Belgium | p | |
| Clatterbridge | England | p | |
| TRIUMF | Canada | p | |
| Tsukuba | Japan | p | |
| Chicago | Illinois, USA | n, p | |
| Julich (KFA) | Germany | p | |

*Based on Particles, a newsletter sponsored by the Proton Therapy Cooperative Group (PTCOG)

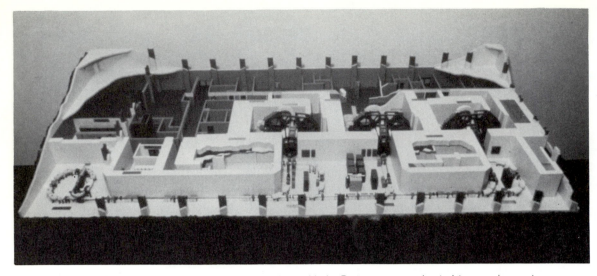

**Figure 14-9.** Model of the proton facility at Loma Linda. Protons are accelerated to energies up to 250 MeV in a large cyclotron. The protons can then be directed into any one of three treatment rooms. This arrangement minimizes "idle" time since while one patient is being treated in one room the next two patients can be set up in adjoining treatment rooms. This sort of facility sets the scene for the future, that is, a large radiation therapy facility with multiple treatment rooms in the context of a cancer center. (Courtesy of Drs. James Slater and John Archambeau, Loma Linda University, Loma Linda, California)

## Hospital-Based Proton Facilities

Many of the proton machines used in the past had been built initially for physics research and were located in physics laboratories. There is much current interest in the development of hospital-based proton facilities producing beams sufficiently penetrating to make possible the treatment of any cancer sites in the human and including a gantry with an isocentric mount. The prototype facility has been built at Loma Linda University in California, where a 250-MeV cyclotron produces a proton beam that can be directed into any one of four treatment rooms. The layout of the facility is shown in Figure 14-9.

The intention is to treat a broad spectrum of human cancers, not just the limited sites for which the dose distributions possible with protons have already proved their worth. Similar facilities are being built or are in the planning stage at several places in the United States, Europe, and Japan. Such facilities set the scene for the future.

## ► *Summary of Pertinent Conclusions*

### *Neutrons*

- Neutrons are indirectly ionizing. In tissue they give up their energy to produce recoil protons, α-particles, and heavier nuclear fragments.
- Biological properties differ from x-rays in several regards; reduced OER, little or no repair of sublethal damage or potentially lethal damage, and less variation of sensitivity through the cell cycle.
- The rationale for the use of neutrons in radiotherapy has changed. The earlier rationale was the reduced OER to overcome the problem of hypoxic cells. The revised rationale is based on a higher neutron RBE for slowly cycling tumors.

*(continued)*

► *Summary of Pertinent Conclusions* (Continued)

- An advantage has been proved clinically for neutrons in the treatment of salivary gland and prostate tumors and soft tissue sarcoma.
- The new generation of hospital-based cyclotrons, generating neutrons by the $p^+ \rightarrow$ Be reaction, will be used for future clinical trials.

### Boron Neutron Capture Therapy

- The principle is to deliver a drug containing boron that localizes only in tumors and then to treat with low-energy thermal neutrons that interact with boron to produce $\alpha$-particles.
- Boron is a suitable substance because it has a large cross-section for thermal neutrons and emits short-range densely ionizing $\alpha$-particles when bombarded by thermal neutrons. Its chemistry is such that it can be incorporated into a wide range of compounds.
- Early boron compounds were selectively localized in brain tumors only to the extent that the blood–brain barrier is absent or compromised.
- Many attempts have been made to synthesize boron-containing compounds that are selectively localized in tumors relative to normal tissues, with marginal success.
- Thermal neutrons are poorly penetrating in tissue with a half value layer of only 1.5 cm.
- Epithermal neutrons are somewhat more penetrating. They are degraded to thermal neutrons by collisions with hydrogen atoms in tissue. The peak dose is at 2 to 3 cm, and the high surface dose is avoided.
- Results of clinical trials are tantalizing but not definitive.
- The concept of BNCT is very attractive, but formidable practical difficulties are involved in making it a practical treatment modality even for relatively shallow tumors.

### Protons

- Protons result in excellent physical dose distributions.
- Protons have biological properties similar to x-rays.
- There is an established place for protons in the treatment of choroidal melanoma or tumors close to the spinal cord, where a sharp cutoff of dose is important.
- Hospital-based high-energy cyclotrons with an isocentric mount are currently being used to treat a broader spectrum of cancer patients with protons. Their efficacy has yet to be proven.

## BIBLIOGRAPHY

Asbury AK, Ojeann RG, Nielsen SL, Sweet WH: Neuropathologic study of fourteen cases of malignant brain tumor treated by boron-10 slow neutron capture radiation. J Neuropathol Exp Neurol 31:278–303, 1972

Barth RF, Soloway AH, Fairchild RG: Boron neutron capture therapy of cancer. Cancer Res 50:1061–1070, 1990

Batterman JJ: Clinical Application of Fast Neutrons: The Amsterdam Experience. Amsterdam, Rodipi, 1981

Broerse JJ, Barendsen GW: Relative biological effectiveness of fast neutrons for effects on normal tissues. Curr Top Radiat Res 8:305–350, 1973

Broerse JJ, Barendsen GW, van Kersen GR: Survival of cultured human cells after irradiation with fast neutrons of different energies in hypoxic and oxygenated conditions. Int J Radiat Biol 13:559, 1967

Catterall M: Results of neutron therapy: Differences, correlations, and improvements. Int J Radiat Oncol Biol Phys 8:2141–2144, 1982

Catterall M, Sutherland I, Bewley DK: First results of a clinical trial of fast neutrons compared with x or gamma rays in treatment of advanced tumors of the head and neck. Br Med J 2:653–656, 1975

Catterall M, Vonberg DD: Treatment of advanced tumors of head and neck with fast neutrons. Br Med J 3:137–143, 1974

D'Angio GJ, Aceto M, Nisce LZ, Kim JH, Jolly R, Buckle D, Holt JG: Preliminary clinical observations after extended Bragg peak helium ion irradiation. Cancer 34:6–11, 1974

Drake CG: Arteriovenous malformations of the brain. N Engl J Med 309:308, 1983

Field, SB, Hornsey S: RBE values for cyclotron neutrons for effects on normal tissues and tumors as a function of dose and dose fractionation. Eur J Cancer 7:151–169, 1971

Fowler JF, Morgan RL, Wood CAP: Pretherapeutic experiments with fast neutron beam from the Medical Research Council Cyclotron: I. The biological and physical advantages and problems of neutron therapy. Br J Radiol 36:77–80, 1963

Hall EJ: Radiobiology of heavy particle radiation therapy: Cellular studies. Radiology 108:119–129, 1973

Hall EJ, Graves RG, Phillips TL, Suit HD (eds): Particle accelerators in radiation therapy. Int J Radiat Oncol Biol Phys 8:2041–2207, 1982

Hatanaka H: A revised boron-neutron capture therapy for malignant brain tumors: II. Interim clinical result with the patients excluding previous treatments. J Neurol 209:81–94, 1975

Hatanaka H, Amano K, Kanemitsu H, Ikeuchi I, Yoshizaki T: Boron uptake by human brain tumors and quality control of boron compounds. In Hatanaka H (ed): Boron Neutron Capture Therapy for Tumors, pp 77–106. Niigata, Japan, Nishimura Co, 1986

Javid M, Brownell GL, Sweet WH: The possible use of neutron-capture isotopes such as boron-10 in the treatment of neoplasms: II. Computation of the radiation energy and estimates of effects in normal and neoplastic brain. J Clin Invest 31:603–610, 1952

Kjellberg RN, Hanamura T, Davis KR, Lyons SL, Adams RD: Bragg-peak proton-beam therapy for arteriovenous malformations of the brain. N Engl J Med 309:269, 1983

Locher GL: Biological effects and therapeutic possibilities of neutrons. AJR 36:1–13, 1936.

Laramore GE, Krall JM, Thomas FJ, Griffin TW, Maor MH, Hendrickson FR: Fast neutron radiotherapy for locally advanced prostate cancer: Results of an RTOG randomized study. Int J Radiat Oncol Biol Phys 11:1621–1627, 1985

Raju MR: Heavy Particle Radiotherapy. New York, Academic Press, 1980

Sweet WH: The use of nuclear disintegration in the diagnosis and treatment of brain tumor. N Engl J Med 245:875–878, 1951

Withers HR, Thames HD, Peters LJ: Biological bases for high RBE values for late effects of neutron irradiation. Int J Radiat Oncol Biol Phys 8:2071–2076, 1982

*Radiobiology for the Radiologist, Fourth Edition*, by Eric J. Hall
J. B. Lippincott Company, Philadelphia © 1994.

# 15

# *Predictive Assays*

Radiation Therapy

In the routine day-to-day practice of radiotherapy, treatment schedules are designed for the "average" patient with a given type of malignancy at a given site. Although much "lip service" is rendered to the subject, in practice little is done to tailor a treatment schedule to the individual case. This chapter was only included after much thought, because the techniques are by no means fully developed or universally accepted. The potential is, however, so great that the resident in training should be aware of the basic ideas.

## RADIOSENSITIVITY OF NORMAL TISSUES

A number of studies have been performed, notably in Japan, to determine in vitro radiation survival curves for skin fibroblasts and peripheral lymphocytes from a large number of persons. In general, it was found that the radiosensitivity of cells of normal tissues vary little from one person to another; indeed, from hundreds of normal persons studied the variation was within the errors of the measurement techniques. There are, of course, some striking exceptions. Persons who are homozygous for *ataxia-telangiectasia* (AT) are exquisitely sensitive to radiation. Cells cultured from such persons have a $D_0$ of only about 0.5 Gy (50 rads), and when these persons receive radiotherapy, both normal tissues and tumors respond to doses only one half to one third of the doses used on the average patient. It is suspected that there may be other groups of persons who are slightly more radiosensitive than average, but this has never been proven and no means of identifying sensitive individuals has been developed. There is, however, the possibility that the doses used in conventional radiotherapy are limited to avoid problems to a radiosensitive minority and that the average patient is, therefore, underdosed.

A few pilot studies with small numbers of patients undergoing radiotherapy have indicated a correlation between the radiosensitivity of fibro-blasts grown from skin biopsy specimens and the score of early or late effects in the same patients. These data, however, are far from convincing and contradict directly the much larger Japanese studies.

In the long run it may turn out that predictive assays for normal tissue radiosensitivity may be the most useful. At the present time, however, when the term *predictive assay* is used, what comes to mind is an assay to determine some property of a tumor.

## PREDICTIVE ASSAYS FOR TUMORS

Assays to predict the radiation characteristics of a tumor fall into three categories:

1. Intrinsic cellular radiosensitivity
2. Oxygen status
3. Proliferative potential

### Intrinsic Cellular Radiosensitivity

Clonogenic cell survival, assessed by the single cell plating techniques described in Chapter 3, has long been considered to be the "gold standard" for judging the cellular response to anticancer agents, including radiation. The formation of a microscopic colony from a single cell requires sustained cell division and is the ultimate proof of reproductive integrity. Cells taken directly from human tumor biopsy specimens, however, do not grow readily and are usually characterized by a poor plating efficiency (often about 1%). It is not easy to obtain a repeatable estimate of the cell surviving fraction to a dose of, say, 2 Gy.

The possibility of a predictive assay for intrinsic cellular radiosensitivity derives from the many attempts that have been made to correlate the in vitro radiosensitivity of **cell lines** derived from human tumors with the clinical responsiveness of tumors of the same histologic group. The most extensive studies are those of Deacon, Peckham, and Steel in the United Kingdom and of Malaise and Fertil in France.

The conclusion from these studies is that the steepness of the initial slope of the survival curve correlates with clinical responsiveness. This initial region of the survival curve is best characterized by the surviving fraction at 2 Gy; or $SF_2$ as it is known. The characteristics of the survival curve at higher doses, designated by the final $D_0$, or $\beta$ in the linear-quadratic formula, did *not* correlate with clinical outcome. Malaise and his colleagues divided tumors into six histologic groups: from the most radioresistant to the most radiosensitive, these are glioblastomas, melanomas, squamous cell carcinomas, adenocarcinomas, lymphomas, and oat cell carcinomas. The order of the $SF_2$s correlates with clinical responsiveness. This is illustrated in Figure 15-1. But most important, Malaise and his colleagues demonstrated widely diverse sensitivities within each histologic group, such that the most-sensitive glioblastoma had a radiosensitivity similar to the most-resistant lymphoma.

These findings are of significant radiobiological interest because they contradict the widely held view that clinical responsiveness is not related to inherent cellular radiosensitivity. To some extent it also weakens the equally widely held view that differences in responsiveness between tumors must be attributable to differences in hypoxic fraction. It is, however, not of much use to the clinical radiotherapist, who does not need in vitro measurements to tell him or her that lymphomas are more radiosensitive than glioblastomas! What the radiotherapist needs is information on the individual patient. These data from Malaise and his colleagues indicate that, since radioresponsiveness may vary with the DNA characteristics of the tumor cells involved, at least between histologic types, then the possibility exists that individual responsiveness may be predicted if a suitable assay were available. The radiobiological experiments with cell lines derived from human tumors laid the groundwork for predictive assays of radiosensitivity of cells from individual patients.

## Growth in Soft Agar—The Courtenay Assay

Although cell lines derived from human tumors can be studied using standard in vitro plating assays (described in Chapter 3), fresh explants from tumor biopsy specimens are much more difficult to grow. Conventional cell culture techniques using cells attached to plastic dishes prove to be unsuitable. Many cells do not grow at all, and those that do have a very low plating efficiency. More success has been achieved by growing fresh explants of tumor biopsy specimens in soft agar, using the so-called Courtenay technique. In this technique, cells do not attach to the surface of the petri dish but grow as spheres or clumps in a semisolid agar gel, supplemented with growth factors. Using this technique, West and her colleagues at the Christie Hospital in Manchester, England, analyzed prospectively for intrinsic radiosensitivity over 50 patients with stage I, II, and III carcinoma of the cervix who were to receive radical radiotherapy. They found that patients with an $SF_2$ of greater than 0.55 had a significantly lower probability of local control than those with an $SF_2$ smaller than 0.55. Their data are shown in Figure 15-2. Stage alone was a poorer prognostic factor for local control than radiosensitivity. These findings suggest that intrinsic radiosensitivity may be a useful predictor of local recurrence after radical radiotherapy.

Malaise and his colleagues in France used a similar technique to culture cells from head and

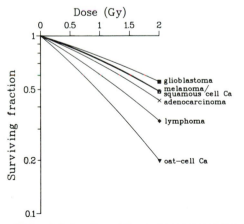

**Figure 15-1.** Initial portion of the mean representative survival curves for cells from each of six histologic groups of human tumors, showing also the surviving fraction at 2 Gy ($SF_2$). (Compiled from the data of Malaise EP, Fertil B, Chavandra N, Guichard M: Int J Radiat Oncol Biol Phys 12:617–624, 1986)

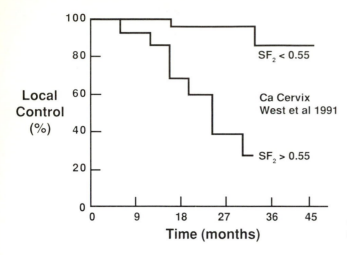

**Figure 15-2.** Local control curves for carcinoma of the cervix (stages I, II, and III) treated by radiotherapy alone. Patients were separated into two groups according to the intrinisic radiosensitivity of the tumor biopsy, measured in vitro by the "Courtenay" assay. The two groups showed a surviving fraction at 2 Gy ($SF_2$) above and below 0.55. (Redrawn from West CML, Davidson SE, Hendry JH, Hunter RD: Lancet 338:818, 1991)

neck tumors and reported a correlation between $\alpha$ (the linear component of the linear-quadratic survival curve) and local control in the patients from whom the biopsy specimens were taken.

Because of the difficulties of performing clonogenic assays on fresh explants of tumor cells, several attempts have been made to develop nonclonogenic assays that depend on growth, are easier to handle, and yield usable results more quickly. Growth rate can be assessed quantitatively by several methods, including exclusion of vital dyes and the incorporation of labeled biochemical precursors. Only two are described here.

### Colorimetric Assays

Cells either from an established cell line or from a tumor biopsy specimen are plated into 96-well plates, treated with graded doses of radiation or of a cytotoxic drug, and allowed to grow for several days. The cells are then stained in one way or another, where quantitation of cell growth is based on the assumption that only *viable* tumor cells are stained. The density of the stain in a given well measured by a spectrophotometer correlates with the number of surviving cells. The technique is much simpler and faster than a clonogenic assay and is amenable to automation.

One of the earliest colorimetric assays was the tetrazolium (MTT) assay. Viable tumor cells reduce a tetrazolium-based compound to a blue formazan product that can be assessed with a spectrophotometer. A stained dish from a typical experiment with the MTT assay is shown in Figure 15-3, together with a typical survival curve. This assay was adopted by the National Cancer Institute to screen large numbers of potential anticancer drugs. It is also useful to identify compounds that are radiosensitizers or radioprotectors.

More recently, the technique has been modified to utilize dyes that can measure the total protein content or total DNA content of a well, rather than using the tetrazolium-based compound, but the principle remains the same. A large proportion of biopsy specimens will grow and give results, but a major drawback of the assay is the possible admixture of normal cells within the sample, since the technique in no way distinguishes between normal and malignant cells.

Assays of this sort are suitable for screening compounds for activity but lack the accuracy to measure $SF_2$, or any other quantity needed in a predictive assay.

### Cell Adhesive Matrix Assay

The basis of the cell adhesive matrix assay is to provide tumor cells from a biopsy specimen with an optimal substrate to facilitate cell attachment and growth. To accomplish this, the surface of plastic dishes is coated with a mixture of fibronectin and fibrinopeptides (CAM) and cells are grown in a special medium supplemented with hormones and growth factors. A cell suspension is prepared from a tumor biopsy specimen and known numbers of cells plated into 24-well microtest plates with a special surface, as described earlier. Control and treated cells are grown for about 2 weeks, after which they are fixed and stained with crystal violet. Growth is quantitated by computerized image analysis of the stained cell monolayer in each well. The staining density of treated is related to untreated wells, and a survival curve is generated. An example of plates used to establish a radiation dose–response relationship is shown in Figure 15-4. Various survival curve parameters can be assessed, notably the surviving fraction at 2 Gy. In common with the colorimetric assays referred to earlier, this is a growth assay, it does not measure reproductive integrity, it is limited to 1 log of killing, and its accuracy at 2 Gy is questionable.

Trials have been performed to evaluate the correlation between the pretreatment CAM assay and clinical responsiveness. Early encouraging results have not been confirmed in later studies,

and the predictive usefulness of the test in individual patients is uncertain.

### Chromosome Aberrations by Premature Chromosome Condensation and Fluorescent in Situ Hybridization

The basic idea of this assay is to take cells from a tumor biopsy *after* the first treatment dose (of, for example, 2 Gy) and then to assess the relative radiosensitivity of the cells by counting the aberration frequency induced in the cells by the treatment dose. This is made possible by combining two relatively recent technical developments, namely, premature chromosome condensation and fluorescent in situ hybridization, described in Chapter 2. The human tumor cells are fused with mitotic hamster cells, which forces their chromosomes to condense prematurely. Symmetrical translocations are readily scorable by using the chromosome painting technique. The beauty of

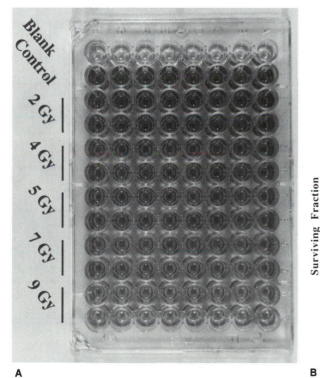

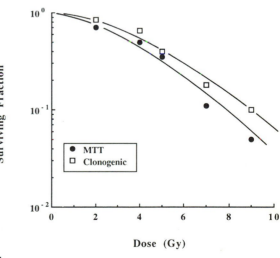

**A**  **B**

Figure 15-3. **(A)** A stained 96-well dish from a typical radiation experiment using the tetrazolium (MTT) assay. The same number of cells were plated into each well, irradiated with graded doses as indicated, and allowed to grow for several days before being stained. The graded density of stain reflects fewer and fewer cells surviving as the dose is increased. **(B)** "Survival curve" based on spectrophotometer measurements of the dishes in *A* compared with a clonogenic survival curve for the same cell. (Courtesy of Dr. James Mitchell)

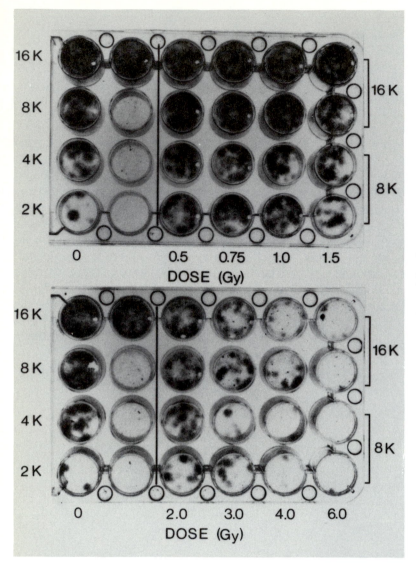

**Figure 15-4.** The adhesive matrix assay. The photograph is of two multiwell culture dishes in which cells from a human melanoma were grown. The two dishes are from the same patient, but different original numbers of cells were used and different radiation doses were applied. The wells on the left (marked 0) are controls with increasing cell numbers. The cultures are stained with crystal violet 2 weeks after plating, and the total amount of stain uptake, expressed as optical density, is measured by a video image analysis system. This measurement of staining density is proportional to the number of cells that have grown in each culture well. It is clear from the figure that increasing doses of radiation result in less and less cell growth. The ratio of the density of cell growth at each radiation dose to the growth of unirradiated controls is used as a surrogate for surviving fraction. (Brock WA, Campbell B, Goepfert H, Peter LJ: Cancer Bull 39:98–102, 1987)

this idea is that the human tumor cells do not have to grow well in culture. The potential problem is that it may be too difficult to score translocations in tumor cells that already have many chromosome changes. As well, the time between in vivo irradiation and biopsy must be standardized to allow for equal DNA repair between different specimens.

## Oxygen Status

### Labeled Nitroimidazoles

New modalities aimed at overcoming the perceived problem of hypoxic cells did not enjoy great success when applied indiscriminately across the board to large groups of patients. This was true for neutrons and hypoxic cell sensitizers, both of which were introduced initially on the premise that the curability of human tumors by x-rays was limited by the presence of hypoxic cells that are resistant to killing with x-rays. It would be desirable to have available an assay that would identify which individual patients have tumors containing hypoxic cells. A successful approach has been based on a nitroimidazole labeled with a radioactive material. In regions of low oxygen tension, the nitroimidazole undergoes bioreduction and radioactive material becomes covalently linked to cellular molecules.

Early studies used misonidazole tagged with a β-emitter radionuclide assayed by autoradiography. This is described in detail in Chapter 10. The test could not be used prospectively as a predictive assay in individual patients, but it was used in a limited number of patients to show that only a minority of tumors contain hypoxic cells. In a more recent development, Chapman and his colleagues have successfully attached radioactive iodine-123 to a nitroimidazole. The radioactive label deposited in the tumor can be detected by single photon emission computed tomography (SPECT). Figure 15-5 shows a SPECT axial section of a patient with a small cell carcinoma of the lung. The patient had received the labeled nitroimidazole 18 hours earlier. The center of the tumor shows up clearly, indicating the presence of hypoxic cells. In practice, the SPECT scan is color-coded and shows up much more clearly than this black and white print. In the preliminary studies conducted so far, about 40% of the patients had tumors containing some fraction of hypoxic cells. This represents a noninvasive test that can be performed on individual patients prospectively. The results could be used to "select" those patients likely to benefit from, for example, a hypoxic cell cytotoxin or radiosensitizer.

## Oxygen Probes

Oxygen probes, that is, electrodes implanted directly into tumors to measure oxygen concentration by a polarographic technique, have a long and chequered history. In the past, they have not been widely used in clinical practice and they have certainly never proved their usefulness. The situation has changed, however, as a consequence of recent technical developments of considerable interest and importance. One of the long-standing problems is that the implantation of a rigid probe crushes tissue, compresses vessels, and causes damage, thereby altering the oxygen tension, the very quantity that is being measured! The recent breakthrough is the development of the Eppendorf probe, a commercially available polarographic electrode that moves quickly through tissue under computer control and has a *very fast* response time of about 1 second. These properties circumvent any significant effect on the recorded local tissue $PO_2$ brought about by the compression of vessels in the vicinity of the electrode and the oxygen consumption of the cathode. The fact that the probe is rigid and not particularly small is then irrelevant. The probe moves under computer control, making a measurement of $PO_2$ every second as it moves along a track through the tumor in steps of about 1 mm.

A prospective clinical trial has been conducted at the University of Mainz in Germany to investigate the usefulness of this new generation of oxygen probes. Patients with locally advanced carcinoma of the uterine cervix were treated with a combination of external-beam radiotherapy

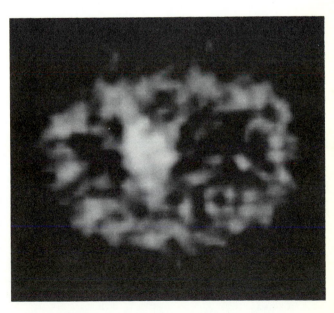

**Figure 15-5.** SPECT axial section through the thorax of a man with limited-stage small cell lung carcinoma. The scan was taken 18 hours after the infusion of $^{123}$I-iodoazomycin arabinoside. The presence of a substantial region of hypoxia is indicated by the binding of the radionuclide. (From Parliament MB, Chapman JD, Urtasun RC, McEwan AJ, Goldberg L, Mercer JR, Mannan RH, Wiebe LI: Br J Cancer 65: 90–95, 1992)

and three high dose-rate brachytherapy insertions. Before treatment, measurements of oxygen concentration were made in each patient, 25 to 30 measurements along each of two tracks through the tumor.

Patients whose tumors exhibited median $PO_2$ values of less than or equal to 10 mm Hg had a significantly lower survival and recurrence-free survival compared with patients with tumors in which the $PO_2$ was greater than 10 mm Hg. Figure 15-6 shows the data for recurrence-free survival. Other factors such as tumor stage, size, histologic grading, and treatment protocol were not significantly different between the two groups. The implication is that tumor descriptors such as size, site, or histologic grade do not predict for the presence of hypoxia. The total number of patients is small, but the results reported are both dramatic and statistically significant. If the results are confirmed in trials involving more patients with longer follow-up, it would appear that oxygen probe measurements represent a practical predictive assay to identify hypoxic tumors that may benefit from alternate treatment strategies. They will be in direct competition with radiolabeled nitroimidazoles detected by SPECT, although they do suffer the disadvantage that an invasive procedure is involved.

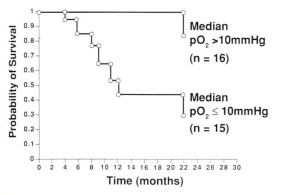

**Figure 15-6.** Recurrence-free survival in patients with advanced carcinoma of the cervix treated by a combination of external-beam radiotherapy and high dose-rate brachytherapy. The patients were divided into two groups on the basis of pretreatment oxygen probe measurements that indicated mean $PO_2$ values of greater than or of less than or equal to 10 mm Hg. (Redrawn from Hoeckel M, Knoop C, Schlenger K, Vomdran B, Baumann E, Mitze M, Knapstein P, Vaupel P: Intratumoral $PO_2$ predicts survival in advanced cancer of the uterine cervix. Radiother Oncol, in press).

# Proliferative Potential

## Potential doubling time (from a single biopsy after Brd Urd)

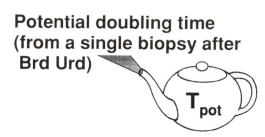

**Figure 15-7.** The potential doubling time ($T_{pot}$) can be measured by flow cytometry on a single tumor biopsy specimen obtained about 8 hours after an injection of bromodeoxyuridine.

## Proliferative Potential

One of the most promising developments in radiotherapy in recent years has been the introduction of altered fractionation patterns—specifically hyperfractionation and accelerated treatment, both of which involve giving two or more radiation treatments per day.

Accelerated treatment is designed to deliver the entire radiotherapy treatment in a time shorter than conventional therapy to minimize the impact of tumor cell proliferation. Two, or in some cases three, radiation treatments are delivered on a given day so that the total number of dose fractions is not reduced even though the overall treatment time is shorter. This is an extremely inconvenient, labor intensive, and expensive form of treatment and should therefore be reserved for patients likely to benefit. The European Cooperative Radiotherapy Group (EORTC) performed a trial to compare an accelerated protocol (72 Gy/5 wk/3 fractions per day) with conventional therapy (70 Gy/7 wk/1 fraction per day) in patients suffering from head and neck cancer. If all patients were considered together, there was no significant difference in local tumor control between the conventional and accelerated protocol. An estimate of the potential tumor doubling time ($T_{pot}$) was, however, made in all the patients in this trial. $T_{pot}$ is estimated from measurements of the labeling index and the length of the DNA synthetic phase ($T_S$), possible by flow cytometry on a single sample of tumor cells taken 4 to 6 hours following an injection of bromodeoxyuridine (Fig. 15-7). The details of the

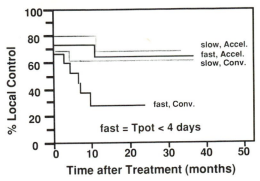

**Figure 15-8.** Graph illustrating the results of the EORTC cooperative trial to compare conventional fractionation (200 cGy once per day for 7000 cGy in 7 weeks) with accelerated treatment (160 cGy three times daily for 7200 cGy in 5 weeks). In the figure, Conv represents conventional and Accel the accelerated protocol. "Fast" growing tumors were those with a $T_{pot}$ less than 4 days. Slow-growing tumors had a measured $T_{pot}$ greater than 4 days. (Redrawn from Begg AC, Horfland I, Van Glabekke M, Bartolink H, Horiot JC: Semin Radiat Oncol 2:22–25, 1992)

method are described in Chapter 12. Tumors with a $T_{pot}$ less than 4 days were described as "fast" growing, and those with a $T_{pot}$ larger than 4 days were regarded as "slow" growing. It was found that local control in patients with slow-growing tumors did not benefit from the accelerated treatment protocol. By contrast, the minority of patients with fast-growing tumors ($T_{pot}$ less than 4 days) showed greatly improved local tumor control on the accelerated protocol. The data are shown in Figure 15-8. In summary, this simple measurement of a parameter of cell population kinetics makes it possible to select out, prospectively and on an individual basis, the minority of patients with head and neck cancer with fast-growing tumors who should benefit substantially from an accelerated treatment protocol.

## CONCLUSION

Predictive assays are in the developmental stage and have not found an accepted place in routine radiotherapy. For the most part they are restricted to a few research-oriented institutions, and then a given laboratory usually specializes in the test that particularly interests it—radiosensitivity, oxygen status, or tumor proliferation—with no one, to my knowledge, measuring them all.

One can easily imagine the day when a battery of predictive assays may be ordered for a radiotherapy patient as routinely as blood chemistry or histologic grading. A knowledge of any unusual normal tissue radiosensitivity, an index of tumor radiosensitivity/radioresistance, the oxygen status of the tumor, and the proliferative potential of the tumor would greatly aid in **selecting** groups of patients who might benefit from accelerated treatment, hyperfractionation, or bioreductive drugs as adjuncts to radiotherapy, or even neutrons. In the past, the trial of new strategies in radiotherapy has been significantly hampered by the heterogeneity of patient populations, as illustrated in some of the examples described in this chapter. Patient selection is likely to be an important issue in the future. Clinical trials require greatly increased numbers of patients in each arm of the protocol if the new agent or technique benefits only a subset of the patients entered on the trial.

► *Summary of Pertinent Conclusions*

- The aim of predictive assays is to identify patients whose tumors (or normal tissues) show unusual intrinsic sensitivity or resistance to radiation or whose tumors are intransigent to conventional treatment due to the presence of hypoxic cells or a rapid proliferative potential.
- It is possible that conventional protocols are designed to avoid problems in the normal tissues of a radiosensitive minority, thus underdosing the average patient.
- Pilot studies with patients on radiotherapy indicate a correlation between the radiosensitivity of normal tissue fibroblasts cultured in vitro and early or late reactions in the same patients from whom the cells were taken.

*(continued)*

► *Summary of Pertinent Conclusions* *(Continued)*

- In the long run, assays for the radiosensitivity of normal tissues may turn out to be most important; at the present time, however, most predictive assays are directed toward the patient's tumor.
- Predictive assays for tumors fall into three categories: intrinsic radiosensitivity, oxygen status, and proliferative potential.

### Intrinsic Radiosensitivity

- Intrinsic cellular radiosensitivity can be measured by clonogenic assays. Cell lines from human tumors can be grown by conventional culture techniques.
- The initial region of the survival curve correlates best: either the $SF_2$, the fraction of cells surviving 2 Gy, or $\alpha$, the linear component or initial slope.
- West and her colleagues found a lower probability of local tumor control in patients with carcinoma of the cervix treated with radiotherapy when the $SF_2$ (measured by the Courtenay assay) was greater than 0.55.
- Tumors have been divided into six histologic groups. From the most radioresistant to the most radiosensitive they are glioblastomas, melanomas, squamous cell carcinomas, adenocarcinomas, lymphomas, and oat cell carcinomas. The order of $SF_2$s correlates with clinical responsiveness, but these data come from cell lines and do not allow predictions of individual patients.
- Nonclonogenic assays have been developed based on cell growth in multi-well dishes. Growth is assessed by density of stain. These assays are rapid, easy, and amenable to automation.
- Cells from biopsy specimens of human tumors do not grow well as attached cells, using conventional techniques, but can be grown in soft agar using the Courtenay assay.
- Colorimetric assays such as the MTT assay, or derivatives of it, are based on the ability of viable cells to reduce a compound that can be visualized by staining or are based on total DNA or RNA content of a colony of cells growing after irradiation. These endpoints are surrogates for reproductive integrity. Such assays are suitable for screening drugs for activity but are not suitable for predictive assays.
- The cell adhesive matrix assay is also based on cell growth, not clonogenicity. It utilizes a specially prepared surface so that cells from a biopsy specimen will attach and grow. Such assays have yet to be proven as predictive assays.
- A new idea, not yet tested, is to measure intrinsic radiosensitivity in cells taken from a tumor biopsy specimen *after* the first treatment of, for example, a 2-Gy dose fraction, by counting chromosome aberrations using the premature chromosome condensation and fluorescent in situ hybridization techniques.

### Oxygen Status

- The oxygen status of a tumor may be assessed by deposited labeled nitroimidazoles in the tumor or by polarographic oxygen probes.
- Nitroimidazoles can now be labeled with the short-lived $\gamma$-emitting isotope iodine-123. In regions of low oxygen tension, the nitroimidazole is

*(continued)*

► **Summary of Pertinent Conclusions**   (Continued)

covalently linked and the isotope deposited. The presence of hypoxia can be visualized by SPECT.

- The recently developed Eppendorf probes have a very fast response and can be moved quickly through a tumor under computer control to obtain an oxygen profile.

- A clinical trial in Germany of patients with advanced carcinoma of the cervix treated with radiotherapy has shown lower survival and recurrence-free survival in patients whose tumors exhibited median $PO_2$ values less than or equal to 10 mm Hg as measured by the Eppendorf probe.

*Proliferative Potential*

- The proliferative potential of a tumor can be expressed in terms of the potential doubling time $(T_{pot})$, which takes into account cell cycle time and growth fraction but not cell loss.

- $T_{pot}$ can be measured in individual patients by flow cytometry on a single tumor biopsy specimen taken some hours after an injection of bromodeoxyuridine.

- One clinical study by the EORTC in head and neck cancer shows that fast-growing tumors $(T_{pot}$ less than 4 days) showed improved local control following accelerated fractionation compared with conventional therapy while slow-growing tumors did not.

- Predictive assays are in a developmental stage but show great promise in *selecting* groups of patients that may benefit from altered treatment protocols: accelerated treatment, hyperfractionation, bioreductive drugs, neutrons, and so on.

# BIBLIOGRAPHY

Brock W, Campbell H, Goepfert H, Peters LJ: Radiosensitivity testing of human tumor cell cultures: A potential method of predicting the response to radiotherapy. Cancer Bull 39:98–102, 1987

Cater DB, Silver IA: Quantitative measurements of oxygen tension in normal tissues and in the tumors of patients before and after radiotherapy. Acta Radiol 53:233–256, 1960

Chapman JD, Peters LJ, Withers HR (eds): Prediction of Tumor Treatment Response. New York, Pergamon Press, 1989

Deacon J, Peckham MJ, Steel GG: The radioresponse of human tumors and the initial slope of the cell survival curve. Radiother Oncol 2:317–323, 1984

Fertil B, Malaise EP: Intrinsic radiosensitivity of human cell lines is correlated with radiosensitivity of human tumors: Analysis of 101 published survival curves. Int J Radiat Oncol Biol Phys 11:1699–1707, 1985

Geara FB, Peters LJ, Ang KK, Wike JL, Sivon SS, Guttenberger R, Callender DL, Malaise EP, Brock WA: Cancer Res 52:6348–6352, 1992

Hockel M, Knoop C, Schlenger K, Vorndran B, Baumann E, Mitze M, Knapstein P, Vaupel P: Intratumoral $pO_2$ predicts survival in advanced cancer of the uterine cervix. Radiother Oncol, 26:45–50, 1993

Malaise EP, Fertil B, Chavaudra N, Guichard M: Distribution of radiation sensitivities for human tumor cells of specific histologic types: Comparison of in vitro to in vivo data. Int J Radiat Oncol 12:617–624, 1986

Mitchell JB: Potential applicability of nonoclonogenic measurements to clinical oncology. Radiat Res 114:401–414, 1988

Parliament MB, Chapman JD, Urtasun RC, McEwan AJ, Goldberg L, Mercer JR, Mannan RH, Wiebe LI: Noninvasive assessment of human tumour hypoxia with [123]I-iodoazomycin arabinoside: Preliminary report of a clinical study. Br J Cancer 65:90–95, 1992

Peters LJ, Brock WA, Johnson T, Meyn RE, Tofilon PJ, Milas L: Potential methods for predicting tumor radiocurability. Int J Radiat Oncol Biol Phys 12:459–467, 1968

Vaupel P, Schlenger K, Knoop C, Hockel M: Oxygenation of human tumors: Evaluation of tissue oxygen distribution in breast cancers by computerized $O_2$ tension measurements. Cancer Res 51:3316–3322, 1991

Weiss C, Fleckenstein W: Local tissue $pO_2$ measured with thick needle probes. Funktionsanal Biol Systeme 15:155–166, 1986

West CML, Davidson SE, Hendry JH, Hunter RD: Prediction of cervical carcinoma response to radiotherapy. Lancet 338:818, 1991

*Radiobiology for the Radiologist, Fourth Edition*, by Eric J. Hall
J. B. Lippincott Company, Philadelphia © 1994.

# 16

# *Hyperthermia*

Radiation Therapy

In Greek mythology the father of hyperthermia was Prometheus, a demigod who stole fire from Olympus and taught men to use it. For this act he was chained to a rock by Zeus, the chief of the gods, and a vulture fed daily on his liver (Fig. 16-1).

The use of hyperthermia for the treatment of cancer is certainly not new. The very first medical text known today contains a case study describing a patient with a breast tumor treated with hyperthermia. The case is found in the Edwin Smith Surgical Papyrus, an Egyptian papyrus roll, which dates from more than 5000 years ago. Later, heat was used in all cultures as one of the most prominent medical therapies for almost any disease, including cancer. Thus, Hippocrates (470–377 BC), in one of his aphorisms, states, *"Quae medicamenta non sanat, ferum sanat. Quae ferum non sanat, ignis sanat. Quae vergo ignis non sanat, insanobilia repotari oportet."* ("Those who cannot be cured by medicine can be cured by surgery. Those who cannot be cured by surgery can be cured by fire [hyperthermia]. Those who cannot be cured by hyperthermia, they are indeed incurable.")

The attempt in modern times to exploit elevated temperatures to treat cancer has a history longer than the use of ionizing radiations. In 1866, 30 years before Röntgen discovered "a new kind of ray," the German physician W. Busch described a patient with a sarcoma in the face that disappeared after a prolonged infection with erysipelas, an infectious disease normally characterized by high fever. This and similar cases led the New York surgeon William B. Coley to believe that the bacteria causing erysipelas may be effective against cancer. He extracted a toxin (Coley's toxin, or mixed bacterial toxin) with which he treated a number of patients.

Although it is difficult to evaluate the direct role of heat in this combined total-body hyperthermia and unspecific immunotherapy, the work by Coley initiated a number of other studies using local hyperthermia applied to patients and

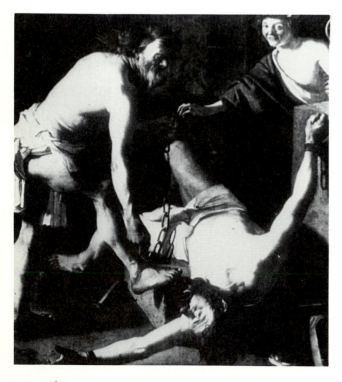

**Figure 16-1.** The chaining of Prometheus, from a painting by Dirck van Baburen in the Rijksmuseum, Amsterdam, The Netherlands.

tumors in experimental animals. In 1898, Westermark, a Swedish gynecologist, published a paper describing a marked regression of large carcinomas of the uterine cervix after local hyperthermia, although the treatments involved were poorly controlled and the cases largely anecdotal. The use of hyperthermia, either alone or in combination with radiation, has been attempted at irregular intervals over the years but has never in the past found a permanent place in the management of cancer. Historical reviews of the early clinical use of hyperthermia can be found in several excellent review articles (eg, by Dewey and colleagues, 1977, and by Overgaard, 1984).

The current revival of interest is likely to be more lasting because it is based on documented clinical evidence of tumor regression as well as a biological rationale and encouraging results from laboratory experiments.

## METHODS OF HEATING

In the clinic the applications of hyperthermia to the treatment of cancer can be divided into two broad categories: total-body systemic hyperthermia and localized hyperthermia. The patient receiving **total-body systemic hyperthermia** can be heated in an insulated suit resembling those used by astronauts in space or heated in an insulated chamber by infrared radiation; alternatively, the blood may be heated in an extracorporeal heat exchange. Earlier experience was obtained by immersing patients in a bath of hot wax. The control and measurement of temperature is relatively simple in this situation, although great care must be taken. The clinical use of total-body heating, sometimes in combination with chemotherapy, will be discussed later in this chapter.

**Localized heating** is much more difficult to achieve with any degree of control. Indeed a major obstacle to the development of clinical hyperthermia for cancer therapy has been the problem of designing and building equipment to heat designated tumor volumes accurately and precisely. Methods of local heating are (1) shortwave diathermy, (2) radiofrequency-induced currents, (3) microwaves, and (4) ultrasound.

Most of the work with cells cultured in vitro, as well as much of the early animal experimenta-

tion, involved heating by hot water baths. The simplest and most reliable way to heat a petri dish or a tumor transplanted into the leg of a mouse was to immerse it totally in a thermostatically controlled bath of water. Water temperature can be controlled within a fraction of a degree, and temperature measurement involves no problem, although even in this simplest of situations the tumor may not be at the same temperature as the skin.

When localized hyperthermia is achieved by microwaves, radiofrequency-induced currents, or ultrasound, there are serious technical problems and limitations. In the case of microwaves, good localization can be achieved at shallow depths, but at greater tumor depths, even when the frequency is lowered to allow deeper penetration, the localization is much poorer, and surface heating limits therapy. When ultrasound is used, the presence of bone or air cavities causes distortions of the heating pattern, but adequate penetration and good uniform temperature distributions can be achieved in soft tissues, particularly with ultrasound in focused arrays. In practice, then, tumors such as recurrent chest wall nodules can be treated adequately with microwaves, and it should theoretically be possible to heat deep-seated tumors below the diaphragm with focused ultrasound, regional microwave devices, or interstitial techniques.

In all cases, however, present methods of heating pose a problem, though progress has been made as a result of the clever application of focused arrays. The picture is complicated, and it is unlikely that one simple answer to all the complex problems will be found. This is the area, then, where engineering developments are needed and a breakthrough in basic science would be so welcome. Hyperthermia with today's equipment has been compared to "administering radiotherapy with a 40-kV x-ray machine, with the blood washing half of the rads away!" This is true, but it is only half of the story. Even in the 1930s, while struggling with radiotherapy equipment of 100 kV or so, the way to solve the limitations was already known: higher energies would improve penetration and remove the differential absorption in bone that used to be such a problem. The science was already known, and the improvement awaited only the engineering development that finally came as a spin-off from World

War II technology in the form of cobalt-60 units and linear accelerators. In hyperthermia, however, every current heating device suffers from serious limitations that are a direct result of basic physical characteristics that all the money in the world will not solve. The physics of hyperthermia is difficult and challenging and badly needs new ideas and new science.

One method of producing localized hyperthermia that suffers from fewer problems is the use of implanted microwave or radiofrequency sources. Good temperature distributions can be achieved and maintained when radiofrequency-induced currents or microwaves are applied to an array of wires actually implanted in the tumor and surrounding tissues. The "wires" used are frequently radioactive sources, so that heat and radiation can be combined. Alternatively, microwave coaxial antennae can be inserted into the catheters used to hold the radioactive iridium-192 wires and deep tumor volumes heated from

the inside out. Some of the most promising results have been obtained in this way, and for the small fraction of patients with cancer for whom an interstitial implant is practical, this may represent the treatment of choice. It does not, however, address the major problem of hyperthermia use in cancer therapy.

## CELLULAR RESPONSE TO HEAT

Heat kills cells in a predictable and repeatable way. Figure 16-2 shows a series of survival curves for cells exposed for various periods of time to a range of temperatures from 41.5°C to 46.5°C. The cell survival curves for heat are similar in shape to those obtained for x-rays (ie, an initial shoulder followed by an exponential region), except that the time of exposure to the elevated temperature replaces the absorbed dose of x-rays. For lower temperatures the picture is

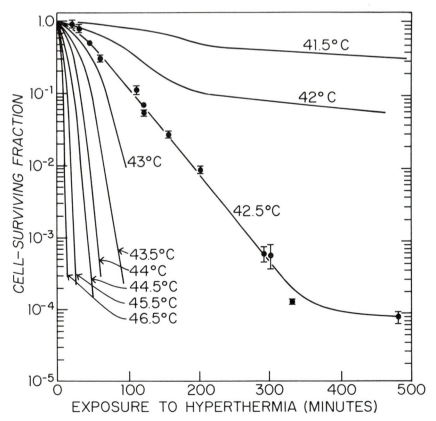

**Figure 16-2.** Survival curves for mammalian cells in culture (Chinese hamster CHO line) heated at different temperatures for varying lengths of time. (Redrawn from Dewey WC, Hopwood LE, Sapareto SA, Gerweck LE: Radiology 123:463–474, 1977)

complicated because the survival curves flatten out after a protracted exposure to hyperthermia, indicating the development of a resistance or tolerance to the elevated temperature. This will be discussed later. The similarity in the shape of the cell-survival curves for heat and x-rays is misleading. It is important, therefore, not to draw conclusions for heat based on the interpretation of radiation dose–response curves, because the amount of energy involved in cell inactivation is a thousand times greater for heat than for x-rays. This reflects the different mechanisms involved in cell killing by heat and x-rays.

Families of survival curves similar to those in Figure 16-2 have been obtained for many different cell types, and it is clear that cells differ widely in their sensitivity to hyperthermia. As with ionizing radiations, there is no consistent difference between normal and malignant cells, in spite of numerous individual reports claiming that tumor cells are inherently more sensitive to heat than their normal tissue counterparts.

Survival data for cells exposed to various levels of hyperthermia (taken from Figure 16-2) were replotted in Figure 16-3, with $1/D_0$ on the ordinate and $1/T$ on the abscissa. T is the absolute temperature, while $D_0$ is the reciprocal of the slope of the exponential region of the survival curve (ie, the time at a given temperature that is necessary to reduce the fraction of surviving cells to 37% of their former value). This type of presentation is known as an **Arrhenius plot;** its slope gives the activation energy of the chemical process involved in the cell killing. The dramatic *change* of slope that occurs at a temperature of about 43°C, which means that the activation energy is different above and below this temperature, may reflect different mechanisms of cell killing (ie, different targets for cytotoxicity above and below 43°C). On the other hand, it may

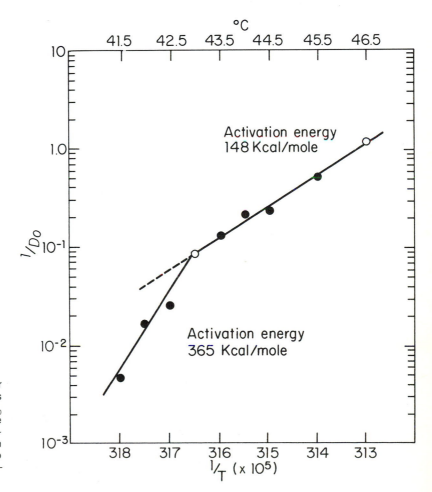

**Figure 16-3.** An Arrhenius plot for heat inactivation of mammalian cells in culture. The reciprocal of the $D_0$ values (obtained from Fig. 16-2) are plotted versus reciprocal of the absolute temperature. (Redrawn from Dewey WC, Hopwood LE, Sapareto SA, Gerweck LE: Radiology 123:463–474, 1977)

equally well be a manifestation of thermotolerance. Below 43°C, thermotolerance can develop gradually during the heating; above 43°C, it cannot. On this basis the intrinsic heat sensitivity is that observed above 43°C, while cell survival for continuous heating below this temperature is a combination of expression of heat sensitivity modified by the induction, development, and decay of thermotolerance. The similarity of the activation energy for protein denaturation to the activation energy for heat cytotoxicity, calculated from the Arrhenius analysis, led to the hypothesis that the target for heat cell killing may be a protein. The structural chromosomal proteins, nuclear matrix and cytoskeleton repair enzymes, and membrane components have all been identified as possible targets that are denatured by hyperthermia.

The Arrhenius plot for a given cell line can be modified by a number of things. For example, altering the pH of the cells **raises** the curves and the break point occurs at a **higher** temperature.

## SENSITIVITY TO HEAT AS A FUNCTION OF CELL AGE IN THE MITOTIC CYCLE

The age–response function for heat complements that for x-rays (Fig. 16-4). The phase of the cycle most *resistant* to x-rays, late in the DNA synthetic phase (late $S$), is most *sensitive* to hyperthermia treatment. On this basis, cycling tumor cells should be killed selectively by hyperthermia compared with the slowly turning over normal tissues responsible for late effects that are in a $G_1$ or $G_0$ state.

## EFFECT OF pH AND NUTRIENT DEFICIENCY ON SENSITIVITY TO HEAT

Cells at acid pH appear to be more sensitive to killing by heat. This is certainly true of cells heat treated soon after their pH is artificially altered by adjusting the buffer. Hahn, however, has shown that the pH dependence of cytotoxicity at elevated temperatures is affected by pH history. Cells can adapt to pH changes and avoid the

heat sensitivity shown for low pH. The time for adaptation is 80 to 100 hours.

Cells deficient in nutrients are certainly heat sensitive. This can be demonstrated with cells in culture in which sensitivity to heat increases progressively as cells have their energy supply compromised, either by depriving them of glucose or by the use of a drug that uncouples oxidative phosphorylation.

These conclusions about pH and nutrients, obtained under controlled conditions with cells in culture, led to the speculation that cells in tumors that are nutritionally deprived and at acid pH because of their location remote from a blood capillary may be particularly sensitive to heat. Because of their environment, it is likely that these cells will be out of cycle and possibly hypoxic, too. This conclusion certainly correlates with the observation that large necrotic tumors often shrink dramatically after a heat treatment. In this context, too, heat and x-rays appear to be complementary in their action, since the cells that are most resistant to x-rays (out of cycle and hypoxic because of their remoteness from a capillary) show enhanced sensitivity to heat. A further complicating factor here is that regions of a tumor in which the vasculature is poorly developed tend to be at an elevated temperature because the cooling effect of blood flow is reduced.

## HYPOXIA AND HYPERTHERMIA

The response of hypoxic cells constitutes a vital difference in response between x-rays and hyperthermia. Hypoxia protects cells from killing by x-rays. By contrast, hypoxic cells are *not* more resistant than aerobic cells to hyperthermia; indeed, the evidence suggests that under some conditions they may be slightly more sensitive.

Cells made *acutely* hypoxic and then treated with heat have a sensitivity similar to aerated cells. Cells subject to *chronic* hypoxia (ie, deprived of oxygen for prolonged periods) show a slightly enhanced sensitivity to heat. This increased sensitivity is probably not due to hypoxia per se but may be a consequence of the lowered pH and the nutritional deficiency that cells suffer as a result of prolonged hypoxia. Of utmost im-

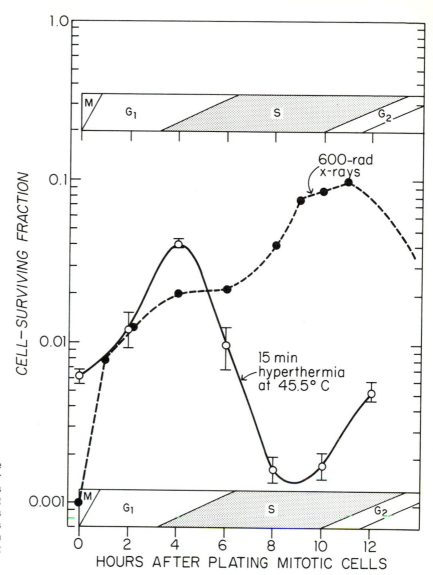

**Figure 16-4.** Comparison of the fraction of cells surviving heat or x-irradiation delivered at various phases of the cell cycle. The heat treatment consisted of 15 minutes at 45.5°C, and the x-ray dose was 600 rads (6 Gy). (Redrawn from Westra A, Dewey WC: Int J Radiat Biol 19:467–477, 1971)

portance in a practical situation is that hypoxic cells in tumors are often both acidic and nutrient deficient.

## RESPONSE OF ORGANIZED TISSUES TO HEAT

Normal tissues respond to heat in a way that is substantially different from their more familiar response to x-rays. The principal difference is that after irradiation, cells die only when attempting the next or a subsequent mitosis (except in very unusual circumstances), whereas heated cells die in interphase, so that heat damage is expressed *early*. In addition, heat affects differentiating as well as dividing cells. The familiar delay between exposure to x-rays and the subsequent response of a cell-renewal tissue is because moderate doses of x-rays kill the dividing stem cells and leave the differentiated cells functional; the response is delayed for a time that is related to the natural lifetime of the mature differentiated cells and the time it takes for stem cells to progress through the process of differentiation and become functional. This delay is absent in the case of heat because all cells are affected, differentiated, or dividing; the damage to the tissue is expressed immediately.

As a result of these considerations, experimental assay systems based on clonogenic survival may seriously underestimate the effect of hyperthermia.

## THERMOTOLERANCE

The development of a transient and nonheritable resistance to subsequent heating by an initial heat treatment has been variously described as **induced thermal resistance, thermal tolerance,** or, most commonly, **thermotolerance.** In 1976, Henle and Leeper and Gerner and Schneider independently showed that the resistance induced in cells by one heat exposure exceeded anything that could be expected from repair of sublethal damage or progression into a resistance phase of the cycle. Figure 16-5 illustrates the phenomenon of thermotolerance. If heating at 44°C is interrupted after 1 hour and resumed some 2 hours later, the dose–response curve is mucher shallower (ie, the cells have become resistant) than if heating had been continued. Operationally, there are two ways by which heating can induce thermotolerance. First, at lower temperatures of around 39°C to 42°C, thermotolerance is induced during the heating period after an exposure of 2 or 3 hours. This phenomenon is already apparent by the change of slope in the survival curves of Figure 16-2. Second, at higher temperatures of above 43°C, thermotolerance cannot be produced during the heating, and it takes some time to develop after the heating has been stopped. It then decays slowly.

Thermotolerance is a substantial effect; the slope of a survival curve may be altered by a factor of 4 to 10, which translates into a difference in cell killing of several orders of magnitude. It is a factor to be reckoned with in fractionated hyperthermia. For cells in culture the time taken for cells that have become thermotolerant to revert to their normal sensitivity (ie, the decay of thermotolerance) may be as long as 160 hours. The greater the degree of damage, the greater is the time to reach the level of thermotolerance, and the slower is the decay.

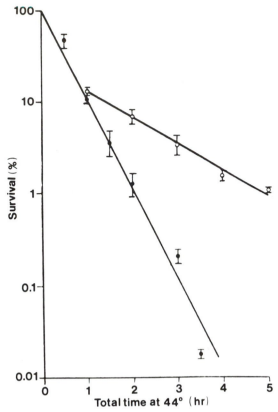

**Figure 16-5.** Development of thermotolerance in HeLa cells. Closed circles indicate cell survival to single heat exposures; open circles indicate response of cells treated at 44°C for 1 hour, returned to 37°C for 2 hours, and given second graded doses of 44°C for graded times. (From Gerner EW, Schneider MJ: Nature 256:500–502, 1975)

Groups led by Overgaard and by Urano have shown that thermotolerance can be induced in transplantable mouse tumors and that this thermotolerance also decays very slowly, requiring something of the order of 120 hours before the decay is complete.

There is evidence from the work of Field and Law and their colleagues at Hammersmith that in normal tissue systems, such as gut, skin, and cartilage, the appearance of thermotolerance may not reach a maximum until 1 or 2 days after heating, depending on the initiating treatment. It may take as long as 1 or 2 weeks to decay completely. Experimental studies suggest that a given heat treatment may produce more thermotolerance in the slowly cycling cells of the normal tissues responsible for late effects than in the tumor cells that may either be rapidly cycling or at low pH.

Thermotolerance is a serious problem in the clinical use of hyperthermia. Figure 16-6 illustrates why by contrasting heat and radiation. The top graph shows the familiar pattern for a multifraction regimen of x-rays given in daily doses, where the shoulder must be repeated each time and each dose produces about the same amount of cell killing. The bottom graph shows a strikingly different pattern for hyperthermia. The first heat dose kills a substantial fraction of cells, but subsequent daily treatments are comparatively ineffective because of the development of thermotolerance, which occurs a few hours after the first treatment and may take as much as a week to decay. Because of the problems and uncertainties involved, Field advises, "The best way to deal with thermotolerance is to avoid it." This advice has been generally followed in the clinical use of hyperthermia, which im-poses a limit of one or at most two heat treatments per week.

## HEAT-SHOCK PROTEINS

When cells are exposed to heat, proteins of a defined molecular weight are produced (mainly 70 and 90 kd). The appearance of these heat-shock proteins tends to coincide with the development of thermotolerance and their disappearance with the decay of thermotolerance. While the correlation is clear, it is not known if the heat-shock proteins are involved in the mechanism of the production of thermotolerance or an independent manifestation of the heat insult. In fact, although they have been given the name *heat-shock proteins*, they are produced after treatment with other agents including arsenite and

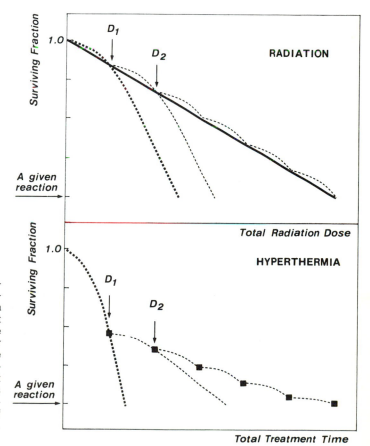

**Cell Survival after Multiple Doses**

Figure 16-6. Why the development of thermotolerance is such a problem in a daily fractionated regimen. (*Top*) X-rays. Each dose in a fractionated regimen has about the same effect (ie, kills the same proportion of cells). The shoulder of the curve must be reexpressed for each dose fraction. (*Bottom*) Hyperthermia. The first heat treatment results in a substantial biological effect but also triggers the development of thermotolerance, which may take as long as a week to decay. Subsequent daily heat treatments would be relatively ineffective because of the acquired thermoresistance of the cells. (From Urano M: Cancer Res 46:474–482, 1986)

ethanol. Proteins of roughly the same molecular weight are found in cells of many species and were, in fact, first discovered in the fruit fly *Drosophila*. They appear to be a ubiquitous cellular response to stress.

Heat-shock proteins are identified by gel electrophoresis, in which they show up as clearly defined bands of specific molecular weights. Methionine labeled with sulfur-75 is used to label the protein in the treated cells, which are then run on a polyacrylamide gel in an electric field. The proteins move a distance that depends on their molecular weight, with smaller proteins going farther. This separates out the various proteins in the cell (Fig. 16-7). After a treatment of 45°C for 20 minutes, proteins that are present only in small quantities before heat treatment are synthesized some hours later. Comparison with the control indicates a molecular weight of about 70 to 110 kd. The time of appearance of these proteins coincides with the development of thermotolerance.

The technique offers the possibility to monitor the development and decay of thermotolerance in individual patients, so that later fractions in a fractionated regimen can be given when the cells have regained their normal sensitivity.

## STEP-UP AND STEP-DOWN HEATING

When multiple hyperthermia treatments are given, cellular sensitivity to heat may be *increased* or *decreased*, compared with that seen for a single exposure, depending on the exposure conditions and the order of the different temperatures involved.

*Step-up heating* is a term used when a second heat exposure is at a higher temperature than the first. If the first treatment is at a temperature in the range of 39°C to 42°C, subsequent higher temperatures may be *less* cytotoxic than they would have been if no pretreatment had been given because of the development of thermotolerance. This strategy has no obvious clinical usefulness at present but could be used to exploit differences in thermotolerance between tumors and normal tissues, once they are known to exist!

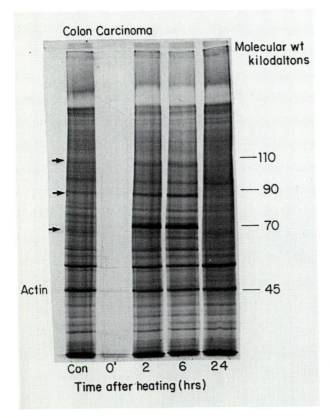

Figure 16-7. Autoradiograph of cells labeled with $^{35}$S methionine in a polyacrylamide gel to illustrate the synthesis of heat-shock proteins in cells derived from human colon carcinoma. The left column (Con) shows the normal pattern of protein synthesis in untreated cells. The other columns show patterns of protein synthesis at various times (0, 2, 6, and 24 hours) after a heat treatment of 20 minutes at 45°C. Immediately after treatment (0 hours), protein synthesis is completely shut down. At 2 and 6 hours after heat treatment, proteins of molecular weight 70, 90, and 110 kd are overexpressed, as evidenced by the dark bands. These are the heat-shock proteins whose appearance coincides with the development of thermotolerance. (Courtesy of Dr. Laurie Roizin-Towle)

*Step-down heating* is the term used to describe pretreatment by a short exposure at a high temperature (greater than 43°C), which sensitizes cells to a subsequent treatment at a lower temperature (less than 43°C). This was first shown by Henle and Leeper. The mechanism is not clear, but it is particularly interesting to note that marginally lethal or nonlethal temperatures become toxic when they are preceded by acute heat treatments at higher temperatures, such as 45°C; that is, an initial short heat exposure at a high temperature can act as a priming dose, so that further heating at temperatures below 42°C, which would be nontoxic if used alone, induce substantial cell killing. Step-down heating probably works because it inhibits the development of thermotolerance. This could, in principle, be exploited in a clinical situation, where it may be possible to maintain high temperatures for only a short period of time.

## HEAT AND TUMOR VASCULATURE

Tumors in general have a less organized and less efficient vasculature than most normal tissues. All functional capillaries in tumors are open and used to capacity, even under ordinary conditions, while in normal tissues many capillaries are closed under ambient conditions. Consequently, while blood flow may be greater in tumors (particularly those that are small) compared with normal tissues at physiological temperatures, the capacity of tumor blood flow to increase during heating appears to be rather limited in comparison with normal tissues. It is well documented that in normal tissues heat induces a prompt increase in blood flow accompanied by dilation of vessels and an increase in permeability of the vascular wall. As a result, heat dissipation by blood flow is slower in tumor than in normal tissues, and so it is often found that the temperature within a tumor is *higher* than in the surrounding normal tissues. In a practical situation, therefore, the difference in intrinsic sensitivity between normal and malignant tissues becomes a moot point, since the tumor is often hotter anyway. A postulated mechanism for the selective solid tumor heating is shown in Figure 16-8. Lest it should be thought that this is a function of the artificial "encapsulated" nature of most transplanted tumors in experimental animals, it should be noted here that differential heating of tumors relative to normal tissues has frequently been observed in humans in clinical trials of hyperthermia. It may well be one of the reasons why excessive normal tissue damage has

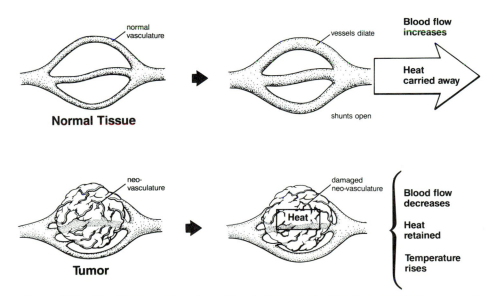

**Figure 16-8.** Possible mechanism to explain why tumors get hotter than surrounding normal tissues. Normal tissues have a relatively high ambient blood flow, which increases in response to thermal stress, thereby dissipating heat. Tumors, with relatively poor blood flow and unresponsive neovasculature, are incapable of augmenting flow (ie, shunting blood) and act as a heat reservoir. (Idea courtesy of Dr. F.K. Storm)

seldom been observed in clinical studies with heat.

There is, however, more to the story of heat and tumor vasculature. For reasons that are not fully understood, heat appears to preferentially damage the fragile vasculature of tumors; as a consequence, the heat-induced change in blood flow in at least transplantable tumors in animals is quite different from that in normal tissues. The relative change in blood flow in the skin and muscle of rats, as well as in various transplanted tumors, is graphically summarized in Figure 16-9. After hyperthermia, tumor blood flow in most cases goes *down*, while blood flow in representative normal tissues goes *up* by a factor of 8 to 10. This further exacerbates the difference in blood flow and further increases the temperature of the tumor compared with the surrounding normal tissues. Eddy has studied the microcirculation of tumors after hyperthermia at 41°C to 45°C. At the higher temperatures, particularly, compression, occlusion, hemorrhage, and stasis thrombosis were observed (Fig. 16-10). He concluded that pathophysiological changes in the tumor microvasculature during hyperthermia can play an important role in tumor response and may account for cure rates that are better than would be predicted from direct cell killing.

There is a complex interplay in tumors between hyperthermia, blood flow, and cell killing; this is illustrated in Figure 16-11. When a tumor is heated to an elevated temperature, there is direct cell killing, but there is also a *reduction* in blood flow. This causes the tumor to get even hotter because the reduced blood flow carries less heat away and at the same time the pH, $PO_2$ and nutrient status of the cells is affected, leading to enhanced cell killing.

Much has been written about the use of hydralazine to enhance the antitumor effect of both hyperthermia and bioreductive drugs. This drug is a vasodilator, the idea being that if blood flow to normal tissues is greatly increased, then blood flow to the tumor would be correspondingly reduced, leading to higher temperatures when external heating devices are used. This simple idea turns out to be difficult to exploit in practice. Song and colleagues studied the effects of hydralazine on blood flow in normal tissues and transplanted tumors in various sites in rats.

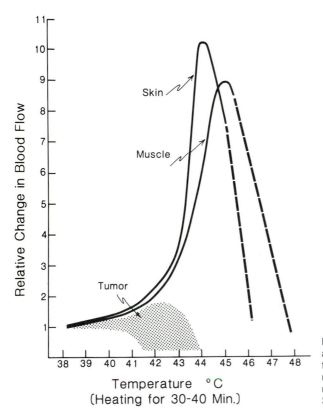

Figure 16-9. Relative changes in blood flow in the skin and muscle of SD rat and in various animal tumors at different temperatures. In general, blood flow *increases* in normal tissues during hyperthermia and *decreases* in tumors, often leading to differential tumor heating. (From Song CW: Cancer Res [Suppl] 44:4721S–4730S, 1984)

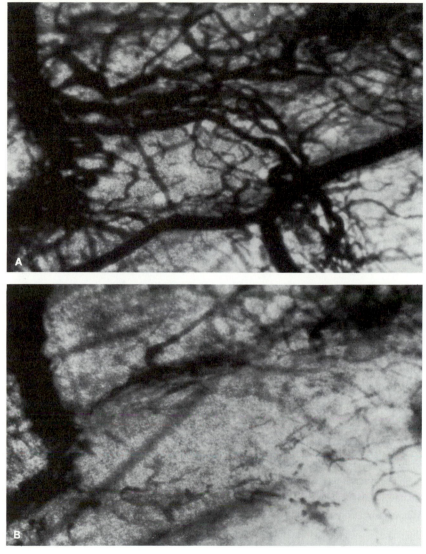

**Figure 16-10.** Hyperthermia-induced compression and occlusion of tumor vessels. (× 10). The photographs are of a squamous cell carcinoma grown in a transparent cheek pouch chamber of a Syrian hamster. **(A)** Vascular pattern at 34°C, before heating. Note the prominent feeding arteriole. **(B)** Occluded vascular network after 30 minutes of heating at 45°C. Blood flow to the area stopped because of marked constriction of the arteriole. Interstitial pressure then exceeded hydrostatic pressure to compress tumor vessels. (From Eddy HA: Radiology 137:515–521, 1980

Blood flow was *reduced* in most normal tissues and in tumors because of a diversion of blood to muscle with a marked increase in muscle blood flow. Its use to enhance hyperthermia or bioreductive drugs is therefore tricky.

Finally, a word of caution is in order here. The extensive experiments that have been performed with hyperthermia and blood flow have been with transplanted tumors in laboratory animals. It is by no means certain that the same results apply to spontaneous tumors in humans.

## TEMPERATURE MEASUREMENT

The control and measurement in tissues, when heating is achieved by an external source, is not a trivial problem. When microwaves, short-wave

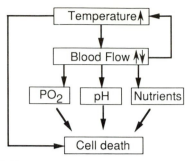

**Figure 16-11.** Diagram illustrating the complex interplay between hyperthermia and blood flow. An elevated temperature leads to direct cell killing, but it also causes a *reduction* in blood flow in tumors; this, in turn, causes changes in pH, PO₂, and nutrients, leading to enhanced cell killing. The reduction in blood flow also further elevates the temperature in the tumor because heat is not being carried away. (Based on the ideas of Dr. Chang Song)

diathermy, or radiofrequency-induced currents are used, accurate temperature measurements cannot be made with metal thermometers, such as thermocouples or thermistors, because of direct heating of the electrically conducting components and the perturbations of the electromagnetic field. These problems have been solved largely by the development of nonmetallic, temperature-sensitive crystal and fiberoptic probes. The remaining problem common to microwave and ultrasound heating is that current practical temperature measurement systems are invasive and involve measurements at a limited number of points within the heated volume, so that an accurate picture of the temperature distribution is difficult to achieve. Great strides have been made in noninvasive temperature distribution measurements by, for example, nuclear magnetic resonance (NMR), and this is likely to be the direction of future developments.

## HEAT DOSE OR THERMAL DOSE EQUIVALENT

The effects of heat are primarily dependent on *time of heating at a given temperature*. They are *not* primarily dependent on energy deposition. There appears to be no direct correlation between biological response and quantity of heat. Ironically, in contrast, there is a closer correlation for ionizing radiations, where the units of dose (gray or rads) are directly related to calories.

1 Gy = 100 rads = 1 joule/kg = 4.18 Cal/kg

In clinical hyperthermia one can use time as the unit of dose at a given temperature, but a problem arises when slightly different temperatures are achieved on different occasions or in different patients, or when the temperature varies during a protracted heat exposure. For example, if 43°C for 1 hour is prescribed as the standard protocol, what time should be used if the tumor temperature achieved is only 42°C?

The most widely used definition of heat dose at the present time is *the time in minutes for which the tissue would have to be held at 43°C to suffer the same biological damage as produced by the actual temperature, which may vary with time during a long exposure.*

The relationship between treatment time and temperature for a biological isoeffect (the Arrhenius plot, shown for cells in culture in Figure 16-3) has been confirmed in principal for a variety of normal tissues and tumors. A marked change of slope occurs somewhere between 42°C and 43°C. Above this transition temperature, the slope is consistent for a variety of cells and tissues. It is generally agreed that a 1°C rise of temperature is equivalent to a reduction of time by a factor of 2. Consequently, above this transition temperature

$$\frac{t_2}{t_1} = 2^{T_1 - T_2}$$

where $t_1$ and $t_2$ are the heating times at temperatures $T_1$ and $T_2$ to produce equal biological effect.

For temperature below the transition temperature an increase in temperature by 1°C requires that time be decreased by a factor of 4 to 6:

$$\frac{t_2}{t_1} = (4 \text{ to } 6)^{T_1 - T_2}$$

where $t_1$ and $t_2$ are the heating times at temperatures $T_1$ and $T_2$ to produce equal biological effect.

The equivalent heating time at 43°C—the **heat dose,** or **thermal dose equivalent**—may be calculated from one or the other of these expressions or a combination of both. In principle, at least, the heat dose associated with a changing temperature may be calculated as the sum of equivalent heating times at 43°C for each temperature.

It is generally recognized that, while equivalent time at 43°C is the best concept available, there are problems in its implementation:

- Nonuniformity of temperature occurs throughout the tumor.
- The concept relates only to cell killing by heat and does not include radiosensitization.
- It relates to one heat treatment, so it is not possible to add one treatment to the next given a few days later because of the problem of thermotolerance.

## CORRELATION OF TEMPERATURE AND BIOLOGICAL EFFECT

A second problem related to heat "dose" is the question of which temperature within the tumor determines the outcome. This problem is more acute for hyperthermia than for radiation, since the energy distributions are much more inhomogeneous to start with and suffer too from further temporal variations due to changes in blood flow. Based on first principles, tumor cure might be expected to correlate best with **minimum temperature** within the target volume, since clonogens surviving in any region of lower temperature may constitute a focus for the regrowth of the tumor. There is some experimental evidence to support this. On the other hand, the extent of tumor response and the time that this response lasts must be a function of the temperature distribution across the tumor volume and related in some way to the weighted mean or average temperature.

On the other hand, temperature *distribution* must be important, too, in determining treatment outcome. From an analysis of data from soft tissue sarcomas, superficial tumors, and deep tumors treated at Duke University, Oleson and his colleagues concluded that the $T_{90}$ and $T_{50}$ correlated with tumor response; the $T_{90}$ is the cumulative time for which 90% of the measured intratumoral temperatures exceeded 39.5°C, while $T_{50}$ is the cumulative time for which 50% of the measured intratumoral temperatures exceeded 41.5°C.

The concepts of $T_{90}$ and $T_{50}$ describe the temperature *distribution*, and can readily be integrated with the isoeffect formula described in the previous section.

## THE INTERACTION BETWEEN HEAT AND RADIATION

The biological effect of a combination of heat and radiation may be a consequence of

1. The independent but additive cytotoxic effects of the heat and radiation, with their complementary patterns of sensitivity through the cell cycle and the greater sensitivity to heat of nutritionally deprived cells at low pH or
2. The interaction between heat and radiation, in the form of sensitization of the radiation cytotoxicity by heat, resulting from the inhibition of repair of radiation-induced damage.

In a practical situation in the clinic, the interaction is most likely to be the independent and additive cytotoxic effects as described in No. 1 above, because of the modest heat levels that can be achieved, and the time interval usually used between hyperthermia and radiation treatment. Of course, both may occur simultaneously, in which case the combination of hyperthermia and x-rays results in a greater cytotoxicity than can be accounted for by the addition of the cytotoxic effects of the agents alone; that is, the interaction between the two modalities is **synergistic,** or supra-additive. This interaction has been studied with cells in culture and with experimental animal systems.

In the case of cells cultured in vitro, the **shape** of the x-ray survival curve is changed by the addition of heat.

For *acute* hyperthermia (ie, brief exposures to temperatures of about 45°C, which leads to a substantial amount of cell killing) the principal effect of hyperthermia is a steepening (ie, reduced $D_0$) of the x-ray survival curve. The change in the shoulder of the curve is minimal. On the other hand, when a more modest level of hyperthermia is used (40°C to 43°C), which involves little or no cell killing, the principal effect observed is a removal of the shoulder from the x-ray survival curve, and then heat treatment after irradiation is the more effective sequence. These differences between higher and lower temperatures, associated with the break in the Arrhenius plot at around 43°C, may reflect different critical targets or simply be a consequence of the fact that thermotolerance can develop *during* the treatment at lower temperatures.

Heat inhibits the repair of radiation-induced single-strand breaks and radiation-induced chromosome aberrations. This inability to repair molecular damage translates into the inability to repair both sublethal damage and potentially lethal damage produced by radiation. Repair of sublethal damage does not occur if hyperthermia is applied during the interval between the two doses of x-rays. Heat can also reduce the repair of x-ray–induced potentially lethal damage, but the sequence is of critical importance. Heat before irradiation does not inhibit potentially lethal damage, whereas heat afterward does. In other words, to inhibit potentially lethal damage, the heat must be applied when repair is taking place.

When heat and radiation are combined, an important consideration is the question of se-quencing. Sequencing in vitro is discussed first. Figure 16-12 shows the fraction of cells that survived a combination of 5 Gy (500 rads) of x-rays and 40 minutes of heating at 42.5°C when the sequence of the two treatments and the time interval between them were varied. The heat treatment did not itself kill any cells, but it potentiated the effect of the x-rays, even when given an hour or more before or after the radiation. The greatest reduction in cell survival was caused by irradiation *during* heating. Comparable data for mouse skin are shown in Figure 16-13. Heating at 43°C for 1 hour was given before or after a single 20 Gy (2000 rads) dose of x-rays. There was a marked variation in the normal tissue response after a given dose of x-rays, depending on the time interval between heat and irradiation and on the order in which the two treatments were given. Heating immediately before or immediately after irradiation produced a similar effect.

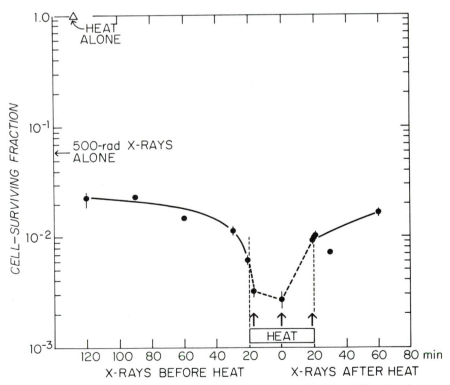

**Figure 16-12.** Survival of Chinese hamster cells irradiated with 5 Gy (500 rads) of x-rays before, during, or after a heat treatment of 40 minutes at 42.5°C. No killing was observed with this heat treatment alone (*open triangle*). The effect of 5 Gy (500 rads) of x-rays alone is shown by the arrow. There is a clear interaction between heat and x-rays, with the maximum effect being produced if the x-rays are delivered midway through the heat treatment. (Redrawn from Sapareto SA, Hopwood LE, Dewey WC: Radiat Res 43:221–233, 1978)

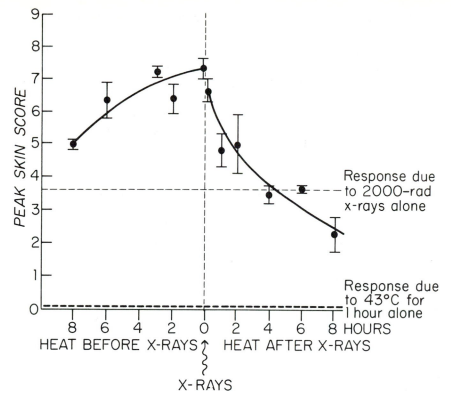

**Figure 16-13.** Response of mouse skin to the effect of combined heat and x-rays. The heat treatment was 43°C for 1 hour, and the x-ray dose was 20 Gy (2000 Rads). Heat was given before or after irradiation, and the time interval between the two was varied. (Redrawn from Field SB, Hume S, Law MP, Morris C, Myers R: International Symposium on Radiological Research Needed for the Improvement of Radiotherapy, Vienna, November 22–26, 1976)

Although many experiments have been performed with cultured cells and with laboratory animals to investigate the interaction of heat and radiation, when hyperthermia is used in the clinic as an adjunct to radiotherapy, their effects are probably not interactive at all. Because the daily doses used in conventional fractionated radiotherapy are small (2 Gy) and the levels of heating achieved are modest, the cytotoxicity of the heat and radiation are more probably independent but additive.

## THERMAL ENHANCEMENT RATIO

In the the case of either normal tissues or transplantable tumors in experimental animals, the extent of the interaction of heat and radiation is expressed in terms of the **thermal enhance-ment ratio** (TER), defined as the ratio of doses of x-rays required to produce a given level of biological damage with and without the application of heat.

The TER has been measured for a variety of normal tissues, including skin, cartilage, and intestinal epithelium. The data form a consistent pattern of increasing TER with increasing temperature, up to a value of about 2 for a 1-hour heat treatment at 43°C. The TER is more difficult to measure in transplanted tumors in laboratory animals because the direct cytotoxic effect of the heat tends to dominate. Heat can often control experimental tumors with acceptable damage to normal tissues, because cell killing by heat is strongly enhanced by nutritional deprivation and increased acidity, conditions that are typical of the poorly vascularized parts of solid tumors. Thus a moderate heat treatment, which can be tolerated by well-vascularized normal tissues, destroys a large proportion of the cells of many solid tumors in experimental animals. In those cases where thermal radiosensitization has been studied, typical TER values are 1.4 at 41°C, 2.7 at 42.5°C, and 4.3 at 43°C, where the heat was applied for 1 hour.

## HEAT AND THE THERAPEUTIC GAIN FACTOR

The **therapeutic gain factor** (TGF) can be defined as the ratio of the TER in the tumor to the TER in normal tissues. There is no advantage to using heat plus lower doses of x-rays if there is no therapeutic gain compared with the use of higher doses of x-rays alone. The answer to this question is equivocal at the present time.

The question of a therapeutic gain factor is complicated in the case of heat, because the tumor and normal tissues are not necessarily at the same temperature. When the statement is made that heat preferentially damages tumor cells compared with normal tissue, it is implied that they both are at the same temperature. In a practical situation, however, this is not always the case. For example, when a poorly vascularized tumor is treated with microwaves, it may reach a *higher* temperature than the surrounding normal tissue, because less heat is carried away by the flow of blood. In addition the overlying skin can be actively cooled by draft of air or even a cold water pack. In these circumstances the normal tissues may be at a significantly *lower* temperature than the tumor, which therefore exaggerates the differential response in a favorable direction.

With these reservations in mind, there are still good reasons for believing that the effects of heat, alone or in combination with x-rays, may be *greater* on tumors than on normal tissues for reasons discussed earlier.

## HEAT AND CHEMOTHERAPEUTIC AGENTS

The cell-killing potential of some but not all chemotherapeutic agents is enhanced substantially

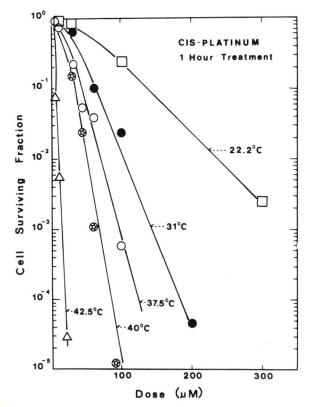

**Figure 16-14.** Effect of elevated temperatures on the cytotoxicity of cisplatin in V79 hamster cells in vitro. Cells were heated for 1 hour at the temperatures indicated. (From Roizin-Towle L, Hall EJ, Capuano L: NCI Monogr 61:149–151, 1982)

Table 16-1.
## Interaction of Heat and Chemotherapeutic Agents

| EFFECT | DRUG |
| --- | --- |
| Potentiated by heat | Melphalan |
| | Cyclophosphamide |
| | BCNU |
| | Cis DDP |
| | Mitomycin C |
| | Bleomycin |
| | Vincristine |
| Unaffected by heat | Hydroxyurea |
| | Methotrexate |
| | Vinblastine |
| Complex interaction | Doxorubicin |

*(From Kano E: Hyperthermia and drugs. In Overgaard J (ed): Hyperthermic Oncology, pp 277–282. London, Taylor & Francis, 1985)*

by a temperature elevation of even a few degrees. This is illustrated for cisplatin in Figure 16-14. There is also a striking synergism in cytotoxicity when hyperthermia (42°C to 43°C) is combined with either bleomycin or doxorubicin. It is probable that at least part of the cell's sensitization to bleomycin at 43°C is related to the inhibition of a repair mechanism. No such explanation can account for the sensitization to doxorubicin, but it has been shown clearly that the drug gets into the cells more easily at 43°C than at 37°C, possibly because of a change in the properties of the plasma membrane at the higher temperature. Once thermotolerance develops, *less* doxorubicin gets into the cell.

Whatever the mechanisms involved, the synergism between heat and drugs may prove very useful in the chemotherapy of solid tumors. There are two separate scenarios. In the case of total-body hyperthermia, an elevated temperature would increase drug cytotoxicity in both tumors and normal tissues; any possible advantage would of necessity accrue from an alteration in drug pharmakinetics resulting from the hyperthermia. The addition of local hyperthermia to a chemotherapy schedule would have the more obvious advantage of "targeting" and localizing the principal effect of the drug, allowing greater tumor cell killing for a given systemic toxicity. This would help to overcome one of the principal problems and limitations of chemotherapy. It is surprising that more has not been done in

this area in view of the substantial potential benefits. Table 16-1 is a listing of drugs that are potentiated by heat and those that are not. There are several different mechanisms that may be involved, some of which are listed in Table 16-2.

Urano investigated the activation energy of drug cytotoxicity in vitro of five chemotherapy agents, namely, carmustine (BCNU), cisplatin, bleomycin, mitomycin C, and 5-fluorouracil. The Arrhenius plots for these drugs are shown in Figure 16-15. They are well displaced one from another, and it appears that the break point is not at the same temperature for different agents. Urano also measured the TER for the same compounds using a transplantable mouse tumor. The interesting conclusion is that the activation energy (measured in vitro) appears to be a good indicator of TER. Drugs with a large activation energy show a large TER, and vice versa. This correlation is illustrated in Figure 16-16. These

Table 16-2.
## Mechanisms of Interaction of Hyperthermia and Drugs*

| MECHANISM | DRUG |
| --- | --- |
| Increased rate of alkylation | Thiotepa |
| | Nitrosoureas |
| | Mitomycin C |
| Single-strand DNA breaks | Bleomycin |
| Inhibition of repair | Methylmethane sulphonate |
| | Lonidamine |
| | Bleomycin |
| Altered drug uptake[†] | Doxorubicin +/− |
| | Bleomycin − |
| | Melphalan +/− |
| | Thiotepa − |
| | Cyclophosphamide − |
| | Methyl-CCNU − |
| | Fluorouracil + |
| | Methotrexate +/− |
| | Cisplatin +/− |
| | Dactinomycin +/− |
| Common membrane target | Polyene antibiotics |
| | Local anesthetics |
| | Alcohols |
| Energy metabolism | Several |
| Production of oxygen radicals | Several |

*Other mechanisms for the interaction of drugs and heat have been suggested, including increased ability of an agent to penetrate membranes and prolongation by drugs of the heat-sensitive cell-cycle phases.*
*[†] +, a reported increase from hyperthermia; −, a reported decrease.*
*(Based on Dahl O: Hyperthermia and drugs. In Watmougl DJ, Ross WM [eds]: Hyperthermia. Blackie, Glasson, 1986)*

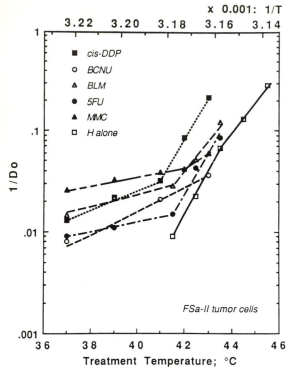

Figure 16-15. Arrhenius plots for five different chemotherapy agents (cisplatin [cis-DDP], carmustine [BCNU], bleomycin [BLM], 5-fluorouracil [5FU], and mitomycin C [MMC]), compared with heat (H) alone. The reciprocal of the $D_0$ of the survival curve is plotted against the reciprocal of the absolute temperature. The slope of the resulting line is a measure of the activation energy. Both the activation energy and the break point in the Arrhenius plot vary for different drugs. (Courtesy of Dr. Muneyasu Urano)

and other data indicate that alkylating agents in general may be the best drugs to use with moderate hyperthermia, antibiotics are controversial, while no antimetabolites appear to be enhanced by heat.

Stehlin and his colleagues used a combination of hyperthermia with regional perfusion of the anticancer agent melphalan for the treatment of melanoma of the extremities. In these studies the limb was isolated by means of a tourniquet, and the perfusion of the drug was combined with hyperthermia induced by heating the blood. Tumor response and survival of patients appear to be significantly improved by the heat. Side by side with the laboratory studies, this clinical investigation adds support to the notion that chemotherapy, as well as radiotherapy, may be significantly improved by the use of heat.

## HEAT AND CARCINOGENESIS

Hyperthermia has never been shown to be carcinogenic and is only weakly mutagenic. Several studies using in vitro oncogenic transformation assay systems have demonstrated no increase in the incidence of transformants over background levels for temperatures between 40°C and 45°C. The same is true of studies with experimental animals, in which no tumors have been produced

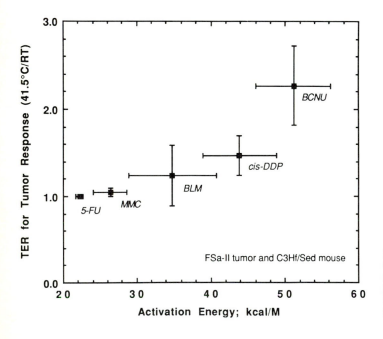

Figure 16-16. For a number of chemotherapy agents tested, the activation energy measured with cells cultured in vitro appears to predict the thermal enhancement ratio (TER) determined for tumors in laboratory animals. (Courtesy of Dr. Muneyasu Urano)

by heat alone. There is less agreement on the combination of heat and x-rays. In the case of oncogenic transformation, most studies indicate that heat *decreases* the number of transformants produced by x-rays depending on the time sequencing. Heat certainly increases the number of skin tumors produced in animals by a given dose of x-rays, but this is probably a consequence of cell division stimulated by tissue damage resulting from the hyperthermia.

There is also the case of erythema ab igne, a macular reticulated skin discoloration seen after chronic heat exposure, either conductive or radiative. It is a common finding on the anterior aspects of the legs of old persons who sit close to fires over a long period of time and is also seen after chronic direct conductive heating with hot water bottles or heating pads for pain relief in patients with cancer.

The documentation of premalignant and malignant changes in the skin where erythema ab igne has developed has come from many parts of the world: older persons in the United Kingdom; women exposed to peat fires in Ireland; the use of warming pans called kangri applied to the skin under clothes during the winter in Kashmir; and the use of hot brick beds (kang) in northwest China. This would appear to be an example of cancer induced by hyperthermia. It has been suggested, however, that the heat itself does not induce the malignant changes, but rather that the chronic stimulation of cells to divide caused by heat damage over a period of years allows the expression of accumulated genetic damage in elderly patients who are also subject to increased risk factors associated with aging, such as impaired immune surveillance.

These controversies notwithstanding, there is general agreement that heat itself is not carcinogenic in a few exposures and this is an attractive property of this new modality in an era of increasing concern for the induction of leukemia and solid tumors by chemotherapeutic agents and to a lesser extent by radiation.

## SPONTANEOUS TUMORS IN DOMESTIC ANIMALS

In general, the transplanted animal tumors that have been used so widely and successfully in ra-diation studies have proved to be unsuitable for comparable experiments with hyperthermia. This is unfortunate, since large experiments, which give repeatable and reproducible data and allow a number of variables to be investigated at reasonable cost and in a short time, are only possible with inbred strains of small rodents carrying transplantable tumors. Such systems were developed for radiation studies and have served well. Transplantable tumors are, however, often so readily curable by heat, especially when the elevated temperatures are produced by ultrasound, radiofrequency-induced currents, or microwaves, that they no longer represent a realistic model. This is probably a consequence of the encapsulated nature of transplanted tumors, which results in their reaching a higher temperature than the surrounding normal tissues. This has prompted a number of groups, notably at Stanford University in California, at the University of Arizona, and at Colorado State University, to study spontaneous tumors in domestic animals. Such studies are expensive and difficult to perform and interpret, since the number of animals that can be used is limited, and there is a tendency for every tumor to be unique. The results are by no means as spectacular as those obtained with transplanted tumors in mice, although it must be remembered that the animals, referred by veterinarians, tend to suffer from advanced malignancies.

These studies mirror the clinical experience that heat is a useful adjunct to radiotherapy. It turns out, however, that definitive trials with large domestic animals are as difficult to perform as those with patients!

## HUMAN APPLICATIONS

Hyperthermia has been widely used as a form of cancer therapy. Its use in the treatment of human tumors dates from early translations of Rama-jama (2000 BC). In 1891, Coley noted that the regression of an inoperable "round cell sarcoma of the neck" was associated with a febrile bout of erysipelas. At this stage it was not clear whether the shrinkage of the tumor was caused by fever or a direct effect of the bacterial toxins. In 1953, Nauts, Fowler, and Bogatko repeated Coley's work, and 25 of their 30 selected patients with soft tissue sarcoma, lymphosarcoma, and carcinoma of the cervix and breast were alive and disease free at 10 years. The earlier results of Coley with the highly pyrogenic agents was never equaled with lesser agents or systemic hyperthermia, however, perhaps because the fever rather than the toxin was the tumoricidal agent! Since the immune system was undoubtedly influenced by Coley's toxins, one can speculate that in those patients in whom permanent cures were obtained the cures could be the result of immune stimulation rather than direct thermal effect on the tumor alone.

In the past 2 decades many clinical studies of hyperthermia have been performed. At the Fourth International Conference of Hyperthermia at Aarhus in 1984, Overgaard estimated that more than 10,000 patients with cancer had been treated by hyperthermia from 1977 to 1984. These data are summarized in Table 16-3. The majority of the studies involve local hyperthermia.

## HYPERTHERMIA ALONE

It is generally agreed, based on a considerable body of data, that local hyperthermia has no role in the curative treatment of tumors. The available data have been summarized by Overgaard in Table 16-4. Regardless of treatment schedules, the complete response rate to heat alone does not exceed about 10% and seems to be of short duration. Local tumors can be sterilized only at high temperatures, which cause significant damage to surrounding normal tissues. This is in agreement with experimental studies in the laboratory, which suggest that tumor cells in a well-vascularized area under normal conditions have about the same sensitivity as normal tissues.

Nevertheless, local hyperthermia has been shown to be useful in palliation, for which it is effective in the relief of pain. Clinical studies with heat alone, therefore, play a limited role, and it is usually now recommended that they be performed only in patients who have a limited life expectancy or when conventional therapy is contraindicated.

## HEAT PLUS RADIATION

The use of hyperthermia as an adjuvant to radiation in the treatment of local and regional disease currently offers the most significant advantages. Numerous uncontrolled studies have been performed in which comparable lesions were treated with either radiation alone or combined with hyperthermia. The data have been summarized by Overgaard (Table 16-5). Although many of these studies are difficult to evaluate, they give strong evidence that adjuvant heat treatment increases the probability of complete response and, consequently, tumor control.

Table 16-3.
Clinical Studies with Hyperthermia, 1977 to 1984

| TREATMENT | NO. OF STUDIES | NO. OF PATIENTS |
|---|---|---|
| Local hyperthermia | | |
|   Heat alone | 38 | 1059 |
|   Heat and radiation | 65 | 2843 |
|   Heat and/or chemotherapy and/or radiation | 28 | 1853 |
|   Heat and radiation versus radiation alone | 20 | 1276 |
|   Heat + miscellaneous | 8 | 1093 |
| Regional hyperthermia | | |
|   Heat +/− chemotherapy (limb perfusion) | 17 | 1035 |
| Total-body hyperthermia | | |
|   Heat +/− chemotherapy | 37 | 1035 |
| All studies | 213 | 10,952 |

*(From Overgaard J [ed]: Hyperthermic Oncology 1984, vol 2, pp 325–338. London, Taylor & Francis, 1985)*

Table 16-4.
Effect of Local Hyperthermia Alone

| STUDY | NO. OF TUMORS | RESPONSE | | | RESPONSE RATE (CR + PR) |
|---|---|---|---|---|---|
| | | CR | PR | NR | |
| Luk et al. | 11 | 1 | 2 | 8 | 27% |
| U et al. | 6 | 0 | 3 | 3 | 50% |
| Overgaard | 13 | 0 | 5 | 8 | 38% |
| Fazekas et al. | 4 | 1 | 0 | 3 | 25% |
| Kim et al. | 19 | 4 | 6 | 9 | 53% |
| Perez et al. | 5 | 2 | 0 | 3 | 40% |
| Marmor et al. | 44 | 5 | 14 | 25 | 43% |
| Corry et al. | 28 | 5 | 11 | 12 | 57% |
| Israel et al. | 36 | 1 | 13 | 22 | 39% |
| Marchal et al. | 12 | 0 | 1 | 11 | 8% |
| Abe et al. | 6 | 0 | 1 | 5 | 17% |
| Okada et al. | 69 | 15 | 28 | 26 | 62% |
| Hall et al. | 35 | 4 | 19 | 12 | 66% |
| Hiraoka et al. | 9 | 0 | 2 | 7 | 22% |
| Lele | 36 | 6 | 20 | 10 | 72% |
| Dunlop et al. | 9 | 1 | 2 | 6 | 33% |
| Manning et al. | 11 | 2 | 3 | 6 | 45% |
| Dubois et al. | 27 | 1 | 8 | 18 | 33% |
| All studies | 380 | 48 (13%) | 138 (36%) | 194 (51%) | 49% |

CR, complete response; PR, partial response; NR, no response
(From Overgaard J: The design of clinical trials. In Field SB, Franconi C [eds]: Hyperthermic Oncology:
Physics and Technology of Hyperthermia. Amsterdam, Martinus Nijhuff Publishers, 1982)

The biological basis for combining hyperthermia and radiation consists of two different mechanisms, namely, hyperthermic radiosensitization and direct hyperthermic cytotoxicity.

Hyperthermic radiosensitization is expressed as increased damage from radiation when hyperthermia and radiation are applied concomitantly. This effect does not qualitatively alter the radiation response but only gives a quantitative enhancement. This hyperthermic radiosensitization occurs to an equal extent in normal tissues and in tumors.

Hyperthermic cytotoxicity is seen as direct heat killing of cells in a deprived microenvironment, characterized by insufficient blood supply with subsequent poor nutrition and increased acidity due to anaerobic metabolism and accumulation of lactic acid and other waste products. Cells situated in such an area are highly sensitive to hyperthermia and can be destroyed by a heat treatment that causes little damage to cells in a "normal" environment. Furthermore, the environmental parameters that enhance the hyperthermic damage are typically those that minimize the effects of radiation, such as hypoxia.

There are two possible strategies for applying hyperthermia as an adjuvant to radiotherapy. One is a radiosensitizing agent enhancing the effect of ionizing radiation in heated tissues. This strategy is only valid if hyperthermia and radiation are applied simultaneously. The other strategy utilizes the specific cytotoxic effect of heat against radioresistant cells, which results in damage to radioresistant areas of the tumors and is achieved by sequential treatment. Although hyperthermic radiosensitization with simultaneous treatment is able to yield the highest TER, the clinical applicability of this protocol is dubious owing to technical problems, and it is likely that the dominating effect is due to the hyperthermic cytotoxicity.

## CLINICAL PERSPECTIVES

The protocol that has emerged from the clinic is of the sequential application of radiation and

Table 16-5.
Effect of Adjuvant Hyperthermia on the Radiation Response

| SOURCE | NO. OF TUMORS | RADIATION ALONE (%) | RADIATION AND HEAT (%) | ISODOSE THERMAL ENHANCEMENT RATIO (TER) |
|---|---|---|---|---|
| Arcangeli et al. | 163 | 38 | 74 | 1.95 |
| Perez et al. | 154 | 41 | 69 | 1.68 |
| Overgaard et al. | 101 | 39 | 62 | 1.59 |
| U et al. | 14 | 14 | 86 | 6.14 |
| Gonzalez et al. | 46 | 33 | 50 | 1.52 |
| Kim et al. | 238 | 39 | 72 | 1.85 |
| Valdagni et al. | 78 | 36 | 73 | 2.03 |
| Bide et al. | 76 | 0 | 7 | >1 |
| van der Zee et al. | 71 | 5 | 27 | 5.40 |
| Corry et al. | 34 | 0 | 62 | >1 |
| Scott et al. | 62 | 39 | 87 | 2.23 |
| Lindholm et al. | 85 | 25 | 46 | 1.84 |
| Li et al | 124 | 29 | 54 | 1.86 |
| Steeves et al. | 90 | 31 | 65 | 2.10 |
| Dunlop et al. | 86 | 50 | 60 | 1.20 |
| Goldobenko et al. | 65 | 86 | 100 | 1.16 |
| Muratkhodzhaev | 313 | 25 | 63 | 2.52 |
| Hiraoka et al. | 33 | 25 | 71 | 2.84 |
| Bey et al. | 45 | 9 | 42 | 4.67 |
| Shidna et al. | 185 | 33 | 64 | 1.94 |
| Datta et al. | 65 | 46 | 66 | 1.43 |
| Uozumi et al. | 16 | 63 | 88 | 1.40 |
| Hornback et al. | 66 | 35 | 72 | 2.06 |
| Fuwa et al. | 24 | 63 | 83 | 1.32 |

Note: Complete response after treatment with the radiation given either alone or combined with hyperthermia.
(From Overgaard J: Int J Radiat Oncol Biol Phys 16:535–549, 1989)

heat, with one or two applications of heat interspersed with a normal multifraction course of radiotherapy.

The radiosensitizing effect of heat is most evident when the heat and radiation are applied simultaneously, but the effect is generally of the same magnitude in both tumors and normal tissues and will not improve the therapeutic ratio unless the tumor is heated to a higher temperature than the normal tissue. On the other hand, the hyperthermic cytotoxic mechanism predominates when heat follows radiation in a sequential procedure. The heat-sensitive cells are those found in a nutritionally deprived, chronically hypoxic and acidic environment, conditions that are found in tumors but not generally seen in normal tissues. In addition, as a result of heat killing the hypoxic radioresistant tumor cells, the actual radiation dose necessary to effectively control the tumor should be reduced. Thus, not only do we see a preferential enhancement occurring in tumors, but the overall radiation damage to normal tissues will also be decreased because the radiation dose is decreased. Consequently, an effective therapeutic gain should result.

A sequential administration of radiation and heat has several other advantages over a simultaneous treatment. The aim of giving heat is to improve the already existing radiotherapy treatment. When heat is combined in a simultaneous protocol, it has to be given with each radiation fraction. Thermotolerance then becomes a problem. This can be overcome by increasing the fraction interval, but that would be expected to reduce the effectiveness of the radiation alone. With a sequential heat and radiation treatment the heat can be administered once or twice, without interfering with the normal radiotherapy protocol. Last but not least, the sequential application of the two modalities is much more practical; to heat and irradiate simultaneously would be very difficult indeed.

The two situations where hyperthermia has been widely used with much success as an adjunct to palliative radiotherapy are (1) recurrent breast carcinoma in the chest wall after mastectomy and (2) malignant melanoma in which most of the lesions are superficial, either subcutaneous or lymph nodes.

Situations in which hyperthermia has been combined with radiation with curative intent include (1) advanced neck nodes associated with head and neck cancer, (2) advanced breast cancer in patients unable to undergo surgery, and (3) gastrointestinal tumors, particularly colorectal cancer. The results of these studies have been mixed, owing largely to the inadequate methods of heating available.

## HYPERTHERMIA AND LOW DOSE-RATE IRRADIATION

The dose-rate effect was described in detail in Chapter 7. In short, when x- or γ-rays are delivered at low dose rate, the biological effectiveness of a given dose is *reduced* because of the repair of sublethal damage that takes place during the protracted treatment time. Since heat inhibits the repair of sublethal damage, it is logical to predict that the effectiveness of low dose-rate irradiation would be enhanced by the simultaneous application of heat. This has been investigated in detail in vitro and confirmed in vivo, with TERs approaching 2. These reports inspired the use of hyperthermia and low dose-rate irradiation in implants in patients. Independent of the method used to produce the heating, some remarkable results have been obtained with interstitial heating combined with brachytherapy (Table 16-6). The reason for this superior response is likely to be the relatively homogeneous heating distribution, in general far better than can be achieved by external heating.

Figure 16-17 shows the technique of combining hyperthermia with a low dose-rate implant of iridium-192 wires. Brachytherapy catheters are implanted surgically and function as conduits for radioactive sources or microwave antennae. Results of these combined treatments are impressive, although no controlled study has been performed and it is not clear whether the results are better than could have been obtained with a conventional implant of radium needles or iridium-192 wires.

The earlier euphoria over heat and low dose-rate irradiation has been tempered somewhat. In 1983, Gerner and his colleagues concluded that the initial impression of a greater effect of hyperthermia combined with low dose-rate radiation, compared with the high dose-rate radiation obtained in our human clinical studies, was probably due to more effective tumor heating using invasive techniques, rather than to a greater degree of heat radiosensitization in interstitial thermoradiotherapy. A similar conclusion was reached by Dewey in his paper presented before

Table 16-6.
Interstitial Hyperthermia and Radiation

| SOURCE | EVALUABLE TUMORS (NO.) | COMPLETE RESPONSE (%) | PARTIAL RESPONSE (%) | NO RESPONSE (%) |
|---|---|---|---|---|
| Vora et al. | 15 | 73 | 7 | 20 |
| Oleson et al. | 52 | 39 | 42 | 19 |
| Cosset et al. | 23 | 83 | 17 | 0 |
| Puthawala et al. | 43 | 74 | 26 | 0 |
| Emani et al. | 44 | 59 | 27 | 14 |
| Lam et al. | 31 | 61 | 36 | 3 |
| French multicenter study (MINERVE) | 96 | 61 | 33 | 6 |

*(From Overgaard J: Int J Radiat Oncol Biol Phys 16:535–549, 1989)*

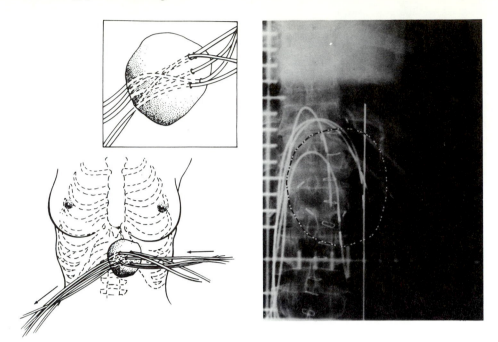

**Figure 16-17.** The use of a combination of hyperthermia and low dose-rate irradiation for the treatment of retrogastric squamous cell carcinoma. (*Left*) Standard 14-gauge brachytherapy catheters surgically implanted during an exploration laparotomy. Once exteriorized, they function as conduits through which radioactive iridium-192 wires or microwave antennae can be inserted. (*Right*) Anterior radiograph showing the microwave antennae in place. (From Coughlin CT, Wong TZ, Strohbehn JW, Culacchio TA, Sutton JE, Belch RZ, Douple EB: Int J Radiat Oncol Biol Phys 11:1673–1678, 1985)

the American Cancer Society: "Conceivably, the clinical results obtained with hyperthermia and brachytherapy appear to be best primarily because the best heat distribution can be obtained with interstitial hyperthermia implants."

The impressions of these two well-known researchers in the field of hyperthermia would certainly appear to be true. Implants with radioactive sources give good localized dose distributions. In addition, heating by means of implanted electrodes or antennae gives a better heat distribution than can usually be obtained by external microwave or ultrasonic devices. When the best heat distribution is combined with the best localized radiation dose distribution, it should come as no surprise that the clinical results are excellent. Therefore, although it cannot be denied that the combination of hyperthermia and interstitial implants represents a very promising development in the clinic and one that needs to be exploited further, it does not appear to be based on any unusual radiobiological properties of low dose-rate irradiation.

## MECHANISMS OF ACTION OF HYPERTHERMIA CYTOTOXICITY AND RADIOSENSITIZATION

Hyperthermia induces effects in both the nucleus and the cytoplasm. It is unclear whether heat effects in the nucleus, such as loss of polymerase activities, inhibition of DNA synthesis, and chromosomal aberrations, are a direct effect of heat within the nucleus or secondary to the effects on the membranes, intracellular structures, and cytoskeleton. Heat killing appears to be associated with degradation or denaturation of proteins (as judged by the activation energies from the Arrhenius plots), which is different from that for radiation killing, which clearly involves primarily damage to DNA.

Although the intermediate steps may be different, the ultimate effect of both heat and radiation is at the DNA level, especially for cells treated in the S phase of the cell cycle. Heat induces chromosomal aberrations in the S-phase, and, for a given level of cell killing induced by heat alone or heat plus radiation, the frequency and types of chromosomal aberrations correspond closely to those resulting from radiation alone. That is, one aberration corresponds to 37% survival.

The events associated with heat radiosensitiza-tion involve DNA damage and the inhibition of its repair. Hyperthermia has little effect on the *amount* of radiation-induced DNA damage in terms of single- or double-strand breaks. The role of heat appears to be to block the process of *repair* of these radiation-induced lesions.

► *Summary of Pertinent Conclusions*

- Total-body hyperthermia may be induced by a heated insulated suit. Earlier experience was gained by a hot wax bath.
- Localized hyperthermia using external devices can be induced by microwaves, ultrasound, or radiofrequency-induced currents.
- The best heat distributions can be obtained by implanting microwave or radiofrequency sources.
- Heat kills: survival curves for heat are similar in shape to those for radiation, except that time at the elevated temperature replaces absorbed dose.
- The inactivation energy is different above and below a break temperature of 42.5°C to 43°C; that is, change of sensitivity with temperature is more rapid below than above this temperature.
- Above the break point, the heating time required to produce a given level of cell killing is halved for every 1-degree temperature rise: below the break point, the time must be reduced by a factor of 4 to 6 for each 1-degree temperature rise.
- Different cells have very different sensitivities to heat. No *consistent* difference in inherent sensitivity exists between normal and malignant cells.
- The age–response function for heat complements that for x-rays. S-phase cells that are resistant to x-rays are sensitive to heat.
- Cells at low pH and nutritionally deprived (more likely to be in tumors) are more sensitive to heat, although cells can adapt to pH changes in 80 to 100 hours and lose their sensitivity to heat.
- Hypoxia does not protect cells from heat as it does from x-rays.
- Heat damage in normal tissues and tumors is expressed more rapidly than x-ray damage, because heat kills differentiated as well as dividing cells and, also, cells can die in interphase rather than at the next (or subsequent) mitosis, as in the case of x-rays.
- Thermotolerance is the induced resistance to a second heat exposure by prior heating.
- Thermotolerance can be induced during a heat exposure at temperatures below about 42.5°C but develops some hours after heating for temperatures above 42.5°C.
- The development of thermotolerance may be monitored by the appearance of heat-shock proteins.
- Thermotolerance is a complication in fractionated clinical hyperthermia. With our present state of knowledge the best way to deal with it may be to avoid it.
- Thermotolerance may be induced when a second exposure is at a higher temperature than the first (step-up heating). On the other hand, if the

*(continued)*

▶ *Summary of Pertinent Conclusions* (Continued)

temperature is reduced for the second exposure, heat treatments that would be nontoxic if used alone may now induce substantial cell killing (step-down heating), which may be due to the inhibition of thermotolerance.

- Heat preferentially damages tumor vasculature. After heating, blood flow goes down in tumors but increases in normal tissues. This may result in an enhanced temperature differential between tumors and normal tissues. There is good evidence for this in transplantable animal tumors, but it is less clear in spontaneous human tumors.

- Temperature measurement in vivo is difficult but improving with multiple nonmetallic thermometers. Great strides have been made in noninvasive temperature distribution measurements by, for example, nuclear magnetic resonance (NMR).

- Heat dose, or thermal dose equivalent, is often expressed in terms of equivalent minutes at 43°C. The concept is of limited usefulness, especially in the context of fractionated treatments, because of the development of thermotolerance. It is the best available concept.

- In experimental animals treated with heat alone, tumor cure correlates best with *minimum temperature*. When heat and radiation are combined, however, tumor response correlates best with some measure of temperature distribution.

- Hyperthermia interacts with radiation in a more than additive way and inhibits the repair of sublethal and potentially lethal damage.

- The thermal enhancement ratio (TER) is the ratio of radiation doses with and without heat to produce the same biological effects. TERs of 2 to 4 can be obtained in tumors and normal tissues in experimental animals.

- The therapeutic gain factor (TGF) is the ratio of the TER in the tumor to the TER in normal tissues.

- In a clinical situation, in which modest levels of hyperthermia are attained and small daily doses of radiation are delivered, the cytotoxic effects of the two modalities are probably independent and additive.

- Hyperthermia potentiates some chemotherapeutic agents. Local hyperthermia "targets" their action.

- Heat alone is not carcinogenic,and may even reduce the oncogenic potential of radiation combined with it.

- Many thousands of patients have been treated with hyperthermia.

- The general consensus is that hyperthermia alone is of limited use, except for palliation or re-treatment of recurrent tumors.

- Several clinical studies have shown that the combination of hyperthermia plus radiation produces more complete and partial tumor responses than radiation alone.

- Biological properties of heat appear favorable for its use in cancer therapy. Physical devices to produce uniform heating at a depth are not well developed, and adequate thermometry is also difficult.

- Microwaves provide good localization at shallow depths, but localization is poor at greater depths, where low frequencies are needed.

- With ultrasound, deep heating can be achieved with focused arrays but bones or air cavities cause distortions.

*(continued)*

▶ **Summary of Pertinent Conclusions** *(Continued)*

- In practice, breast tumors, including recurrences and melanomas, can be heated adequately with microwaves, and deep-seated tumors below the diaphragm can be heated adequately with ultrasound. In any other site present methods of heating pose a problem.
- The combination of interstitial implants of radioactive sources with hyperthermia generated by radiofrequency power applied to the implanted sources appears to be particularly promising, because a good radiation dose distribution is combined with a good heat distribution.
- Hyperthermia induced effects in both the nucleus and the cytoplasm. Probable mechanisms for heat killing include damage to the plasma membrane and inactivation of proteins, but these mechanisms may be different above and below the break temperature.
- Heat radiosensitization involves DNA damage and its repair.

# BIBLIOGRAPHY

Arcangeli G, Cividalli A, Nervi C, Creton G, Luvisulo G, Marm F: Tumor control and therapeutic gain with different schedules of combined radiotherapy and local external hyperthermia in human cancer. Int J Radiat Oncol Biol Phys 9:1125–1134, 1983

Arcangeli G, Nervi C, Cividalli A, Lovisolo GA: Problem of sequence and fractionation in the clinical application of combined heat and radiation. Cancer Res 44(suppl):4857–4863, 1984

Arrington JH, Lockman DS: Thermal keratoses and squamous cell carcinoma in situ associated with erythema ab igne. Arch Dermatol 115:1226–1228, 1979

Ashby MA: Erythema ab igne in cancer patients. J R Soc Med 78:925–926, 1985

Ashby MA, Carnochan P, Tait DM: Erythema ab igne: A model of hyperthermic skin damage and carcinogenesis in humans? Int J Hyperther 1:391–392, 1985

Bey P, Marchal C, Forchard JJ, Hoffstetter S: Potentialisation de la radiotherapie locale: A propos de 90 tumeurs superficielles comparables (abstr). Bull Cancer 71:263, 1984

Bide Z, Xiaoxiong W, Diven Z, Zhonghe G: Hyperthermia in combination with radiotherapy for middle- and late-stage bladder carcinoma. In Overgaard J (ed): Hyperthermic Oncology 1984, vol 1, pp 325–338. London, Taylor & Francis, 1984

Breasted JH: The Edwin Smith surgical papyrus. In Licht S (ed): Therapeutic Heat and Cold, 2nd ed, p 196. New Haven, Waverly Press, 1930

Bull JMC: An update on the anticancer effects of a combination of chemotherapy and hyperthermia. Cancer Res 44(suppl):4853S–4859S, 1984

Busch W: Uber den Einfluss, welchen heftigere Erysiipein zuweillen auf organisierte Neubildunge ausuben: Verhandlugen des naturhistorischen Vereines der preussischen Rheinlande und Westphalens 23:28, 1986

Butler ML, Erythema ab igne, a sign of pancreatic disease. Am J Gastroenterology 67:77–79, 1977

Coley WB: The treatment of malignant tumors by repeated inoculation of erysipelas: With a report of ten original cases. Am J Med Sci 105:487, 1893

Corry PM, Spanos WJ, Tilchen EJ, Barlogie B, Barkley HT, Armour EP: Combined ultrasound and radiation therapy treatment of human superficial tumors. Radiology 145:165–169, 1982

Cosset JM, Dutreix J, Haie C, Gerbaulet A, Janoray P, Dewars JA: Interstitial thermoradiotherapy: A technical and clinical study of 29 implantations performed at the Institut Gustave-Roussy. Int J Hypertherm 1:3–13, 1985

Coughlin CT, Wong TZ, Strohbehn JW, Culacchio TA, Sutton JE, Belch RZ, Douple EB: Intraoperative interstitial microwave-induced hyperthermia and brachytherapy. Int J Radiat Oncol Biol Phys 11:1673–1678, 1985

Crile G: The effects of heat and radiation on cancers implanted on the feet of mice. Cancer Res 23:372–380, 1963

Datta NR, Bose AK, Kapoor HK: Thermoradiotherapy in the management of carcinoma cervix (III B): A controlled clinical study. Indian Med Gazette 121:68–71, 1987

Dewey WC, Hopwood LE, Sapareto LA, Gerweck LE: Cellular responses to combinations of hyperthermia and radiation. Radiology 123:463–474, 1977

Dunlop PRC, Hand JW, Dickinson RJ, Field SB: An assessment of local hyperthermia in clinical practice. Int J Hypertherm 2:39–50, 1986

Eddy HA: Alterations in tumor microvasculature during hyperthermia. Radiology 137:515–521, 1980

Eddy, HA, Chmielewsky G: Effect of hyperthermia, radiation, and Adriamycin combination on tumor vascular function. Int J Radiat Oncol Biol Phys 8:1167–1175, 1982

Emami BH, Perez CA, Leybovich L, Straube W, Vongerichten D: Interstitial thermoradiotherapy in treatment of malignant tumours. Int J Hypertherm 3:107–118, 1987

Field SB, Morris CC: The relationship between heating time and temperature: Its relevance to clinical hyperthermia. Radiother Oncol 1:179–186, 1983

Fuwa N, Morita K, Kimura C, Aoyama K, Muroga M, Yamamoto A: A combined treatment of radiotherapy and local hyperthermia using 8 MHz RF-wave for advanced carcinoma of the breast. In Onoyama Y (ed): Hyperthermic Oncology '86. Proceedings of the third annual meeting of the Japanese Society of Hyperthermic Oncology, pp 337–338. Tokyo, Mag Bros Inc, 1986

Gautherie M, Cosset JM, Gerard JP, Horiot JC, Ardiet JM, El Akoum H, Alperovitch A: Interstitial hyperthermia using implanted electrodes: A multicentric program of technical evaluation and clinical trials over 96 patients. In Sugahara T (ed): Hyperthermic Oncology 1988, vol 2. London, Taylor & Francis, 1989

Gerner EW, Boon R, Conner WG, Hicks JA, Boon MLM: A transient thermotolerant survival response produced by single thermal does in HeLa cells. Cancer Res 36:1035–1040, 1976

Gerner EW, Schneider MJ: Induced thermal resistance in HeLa cells. Nature (London) 256:500–502, 1975

Gerweck LE, Nygaard TG, Burlett M: Response of cells to hyperthermia under acute and chronic hypoxic conditions. Cancer Res 39:966–972, 1979

Goldobenko GV, Durnov LA, Knnysh VI, Amiraslanov AT, Kondratieva AP, Matyakin GG, Tkachev SI, Tseitlin GY, Ivanov SM, Kozhushkov AI: Experience in the use of thermoradiotherapy of malignant tumors (in Russian). Med Radiol 32:36–37, 1987

Gonzalez Gonzalez D, van Dijk JDP, Blank LECM, Rumke Ph: Combined treatment with radiation and hyperthermia in metastatic malignant melanoma. Radiother Oncol 6:105–113, 1986

ter Haar GR, Stratford IJ, Hill CR: Ultrasonic irradiation of mammalian cells in vitro at hyperthermic temperatures. Br J Radiol 53:784, 1980

Hahn GM: Hyperthermia and Cancer. New York, Plenum Press, 1982

Hahn GM, Li GC: Thermotolerance and heat shock proteins in mammalian cells. Radiat Res 92:452–457, 1982

Hahn GM, Shiu C: Adaptation to low pH modifies thermal and thermo-chemical responses of mammalian cells. Int J Hyperther 2:379–387, 1986

Hall EJ: Cell proliferation, not cancer, produced ab igne? Int J Hyperther 1:392–393, 1985

Hall EJ, Roizin-Towle L: Biological effects of heat. Cancer Res (Suppl) 44:4708S–4713S, 1984

Hasegawa T, Song W: Effect of hydralazine on the blood flow in tumors and normal tissues in rats. Int J Radiat Oncol Biol Phys 20:1001–1007, 1991

Henle KJ: Sensitization to hyperthermia below 43°C induced in Chinese hamster ovary cells by step-down heating. JNCI 64:1479–1483, 1980

Henle KJ, Kramuz JE, Leeper DB: Induction of thermotolerance in Chinese hamster ovary cells by high (45°) or low (40°) hyperthermia. Cancer Res 38:570–574, 1978

Henle KJ, Leeper DB: Combination of hyperthermia (40°, 45°C) with radiation. Radiol 121:451–454, 1976

Hiraoka M, Jo S, Dodo Y, Ono K, Takahashi M, Nishida H, Abe M: Clinical results of radiofrequency hyperthermia combined with radiation in the treatment of radioresistant cancers. Cancer 54:2898–2904, 1984

Hornback NB: Clinical hyperthermia experience. In Hornback NB (ed): Hyperthermia and Cancer: Human Clinical Trial Experience, vol 2, pp 73–120. Boca Raton, FL, CRC Press, 1984

Hornback NB, Shupe RE, Shidnia H, Marshall CU, Lauer T: Advanced state IIIB cancer of the cervix treatment by hyperthermia and radiation. Gynecol Oncol 23:160–167, 1986

Kano E: Hyperthermia and drugs. In Overgaard J (ed): Hyperthermic Oncology, pp 277–282, London, Taylor & Francis, 1985

Kim J, Hahn EW: Clinical and biological studies of localized hyperthermia. Cancer Res 39:2258–2261, 1979

Kim J, Hahn E, Ahmed S: Combined hyperthermia and radiation therapy for malignant melanoma. Cancer (Philadelphia) 50:478–482, 1982

Lam K, Astraham M, Langholtz B, Jepson J, Cohen D, Luxton G, Petrovich Z: Interstitial thermoradiotherapy for recurrent or persistent tumors. Int J Hyperther 4:259–266, 1988

Law MP, Ahier RG, Field SB: The response of the mouse ear to heat applied alone or combined with x-rays. Br J Radiol 51:132–138, 1978

Leopold KA, Dewhirst M, Tucker JA, George L, Dodge K, Grant W, Clegg S, Prosnitz R, Oleson JR: Relationships among tumor temperature, treatment time, and histopathological outcome using preoperative hyperthermia with radiation in soft tissue sarcomas. Int J Radiat Oncol Biol Phys 22:989–998, 1992

Li GC, Hahn GM: A proposed operational model of thermotolerance based on effects of nutrients and the initial treatment temperature. Cancer Res 40:4501–4508, 1980

Li R-Y, Zhang T-Z, Lin S-Y, Wang HP: Effect of hyperthermia combined with radiation in the treatment of superficial malignant lesion in 90 patients. In Overgaard J (ed): Hyperthermic Oncology 1984, vol 1, pp 395–397. London, Taylor & Francis, 1984

Lindholm CE, Kjellen E, Nilsson P, Hertzman S: Microwave-induced hyperthermia and radiotherapy in human superficial tumours: Clinical results with a comparative study of combined treatment versus radiotherapy alone. Int J Hyperther 3:393–411, 1987

Mok DWH, Blumgart LH: Erythema ab igne in chronic pancreatic pain: A diagnostic sign. J R Soc Med 77:299–301, 1984

Muratkhodzhaev NK, Svetitsky PV, Kochegarov AA, Alimnazarov ShA, Kuznetsov VN, Shek BA: Hyperthermia in therapy of cancer patients (in Russian). Med Radiol 32:30–36, 1987

Nauts HC, Fowler GA, Bogatko FA: A review of the influence of bacterial infection and of bacterial products (Coley's toxins) on malignant tumors in man. Acta Med Scand 276:1–103, 1953

Oleson J, Heusinkveld A, Manning M: Hyperthermia by magnetic induction: II. Clinical experience with concentric electrodes. Int J Radiat Oncol Biol Phys 9:549–566, 1983

Oleson JR, Manning MR, Sim DA, Heusinkveld RS, Aristizabal RS, Aristizabal SA, Cetas TC, Hevezi JM, Connor WG: A review of the University of Arizona human clinical hyperthermia experience. In Vaeth JM (ed): Frontiers of Radiation and Oncology, vol 18, pp 136–143, Basel, Karger, 1984

Oleson JR, Dewhirst MW, Harrelson JM, Leopold KA, Samulski TV, Tso CY: Tumore temperature distributions predict hyperthermia effect. Int J Radiat Oncol Biol Phys 16:559–570, 1989

Oleson RR, Harrelson JM: Preoperative hyperthermia

(HT) and radiotherapy (RT) for extremity sarcoma: Initial results (abstract Bb7). Presented before the 34th annual meeting of the Radiation Research Society, Las Vegas, Nevada, 1986

Overgaard J: Fractionated radiation and hyperthermia: Experimental and clinical studies. Cancer 48:1116–1123, 1981

Overgaard J: The design of clinical trials. In Field SB, Franconi C (eds): Hyperthermic Oncology, Physics and Technology of Hyperthermia. Amsterdam, Martinus Nijhoff, 1982

Overgaard J: Experimental investigations on the possibility of using local hyperthermia alone or in combination with radiotherapy in the treatment of malignant tumors. In Field SB, Franconi C (eds): Hyperthermic Oncology, Physics and Technology of Hyperthermia. Amsterdam, Martinus Nijhoff, 1982

Overgaard J: Hyperthermia modification of the radiation response in solid tumors. In Fletcher G, Neroi C, Withers H (eds): Biological Basis and Clinical Implications of Tumor Resistance, pp 337–352. New York, Masson Publishing USA, 1983

Overgaard J: Historical perspectives of hyperthermia. In Overgaard J (ed): Introduction to Hyperthermic Oncology, vol 2, New York, Taylor & Francis, 1984

Overgaard J: Rationale and problems in the design of clinical studies. In Overgaard J (ed): Hyperthermic Oncology, vol 2, pp 325–338. London, Taylor & Francis, 1985

Overgaard J, Overgaard M: Hyperthermia as an adjuvant to radiotherapy in the treatment of malignant melanoma. Int J Hyperther 3:483–501, 1987

Perez CA, Kuske RR, Emani B, Fineberg B: Irradiation alone or combined with hyperthermia in the treatment of recurrent carcinoma of the breast in the chest wall: A nonradomized comparison. Int J Hypertherm 2:179–187, 1986

Peterkin GAG: Malignant change in erythema ab igne. Br Med J 2:1599–1602, 1955

Puthawala AA, Nisar Syed AM, Sheikh Khalid MA, Rafie S, McNamara CS: Interstitial hyperthermia for recurrent malignancies. Endocuriether Hyperther Oncol 1:125–131, 1985

Robinson JE, Wizenburg MJ: Thermal sensitivity and the effect of elevated temperatures on the radiation sensitivity of Chinese hamster cells. Acta Radiol 13:241–248, 1974

Roizin-Towle L, Hall EJ, Capuano L: Interaction of hyperthermia and cytotoxic agents. NCI Monogr 61:149–151, 1982

Sapareto SA, Dewey WC: Thermal dose determination

in cancer therapy. Int J Radiat Oncol Biol Phys 10:787–800, 1984

Sapareto SA, Hopwood LE, Dewey WC: Combined effects of x-irradiation and hyperthermia on CHO cells for various temperatures and orders of application. Radiat Res 43:221–233, 1978

Scott RS, Johnson RJR, Story KV, Clay L: Local hyperthermia in combination with definitive radiotherapy: Increased tumor clearance, reduced recurrence rate in extended follow-up. Int J Radiat Oncol Biol Phys 10:2119–2123, 1984

Shidnia H, Hornback NB, Shupe R, Shen R-N, Yune M: Correlation between hyperthermia and large dose per fraction in treatment of malignant melanoma (abstr). Presented before the annual meeting of the International Clinical Hyperthermia Society, Lund, Sweden, 1987

Song CW: Effect of local hyperthermia on blood flow and microenvironment: A review. Cancer Res (Suppl) 44:4721S–4730S, 1984

Steeves RA, Severson SB, Paliwal BR, Anderson S, Robins HI: Matched-pair analysis of response to local hyperthermia and megavoltage electron therapy for superficial human tumors. Endocuriether Hyperther Oncol 2:163–170, 1986

Stehlin JS: Hyperthermic perfusion for melanoma of the extremities: Experience with 165 patients, 1967 to 1979. Ann NY Acad Sci 335–352, 1980

Stewart JR: Past clinical studies and future directions. Cancer Res 44:4902–4904S, 1984

Storm FK (ed): Hyperthermia in Cancer Therapy. Boston, GK Hall Medical Publishers, 1983

Subjeck JR, Sciandra JJ, Chao CF, Johnson RJ: Heat shock proteins and biological response to hyperthermia. Br J Cancer 45(suppl V):127–131, 1982

U R, Noell T, Woodward KT, Worde BT, Fishburn RI,

Miller LS: Microwave-induced local hyperthermia in combination with radiotherapy of human malignant tumors. Cancer 45:638–646, 1980

Uozumi H, Baba Y, Yasunaga T, Ookura M, Takada C, Ueno S, Hoshiko N, Miyao M, Hatanaka Y, Takahashi M: Clinical evaluation of combined hyperthermia and radiation therapy of superficial malignant tumors. In Onoyama Y (ed): Hyperthermic oncology '86 in Japan. Proceedings of the 3rd annual meeting of the Japanese Society of Hyperthermic Oncology, pp 311–312, 1986

Urano M: Kinetics of thermotolerance in normal and tumor tissues: A review. Cancer Res 46:474–482, 1986

Urano M, Kenton A, Kahn J: The effect of hyperthermia on the early and late appearing mouse foot reactions and on the radiation carcinogenesis: Effect on early and late appearing reactions Int J Radiat Oncol Biol Phys 15:159–166, 1988

Valdagni R, Amichetti M, Pani G: Radical radiation alone versus radical radiation plus microwave hyperthermia for $N_3$ (TNM-UICC) neck nodes: A prospective randomized clinical trial. Int J Radiat Oncol Biol Phys 15:13–24, 1988

Valdagni R, Kapp DS, Valdagni C: $N_3$ (TNM-UICC) metastatic neck nodes managed by combined radiation therapy and hyperthermia: Clinical results and analysis of treatment parameters. Int J Hyperther 2:189–200, 1986

Vora N, Shaw S, Forell B, Desai K, Archambeau J, Penzer R, Lipsett J, Covell J: Primary radiation combined with hyperthermia for advanced (stage III–IV) and inflammatory carcinoma of breast. Endocuriether Hyperther Oncol 2:101–106, 1986

Westra A, Dewey WC: Variation in sensitivity to heat shock during the cell cycle of Chinese hamster cells in vitro. Int J Radiat Biol 19:467–477, 1971

*Radiobiology for the Radiologist, Fourth Edition*, by Eric J. Hall
J. B. Lippincott Company, Philadelphia © 1994.

*17*

# Chemotherapeutic Agents From the Perspective of the Radiation Biologist

BIOLOGICAL BASIS OF CHEMOTHERAPY
CLASSES OF AGENTS AND MODE OF ACTION
DOSE–RESPONSE RELATIONSHIPS
SUBLETHAL AND POTENTIALLY LETHAL DAMAGE
   REPAIR
THE OXYGEN EFFECT AND CHEMOTHERAPEUTIC
   AGENTS
PROLIFERATING AND NONPROLIFERATING CELLS
DRUG RESISTANCE
COMPARISON OF CHEMOTHERAPEUTIC AGENTS WITH
   RADIATION
ADJUNCT USE OF CHEMOTHERAPEUTIC AGENTS
ASSAYS FOR SENSITIVITY OF INDIVIDUAL TUMORS
SECOND MALIGNANCIES
SUMMARY OF PERTINENT CONCLUSIONS

Radiation Therapy

ALICE: There's no use trying—one can't believe impossible things.

THE QUEEN: I dare say you haven't had much practice. Why, sometimes I've believed as many as six impossible things before breakfast.

—*Alice in Wonderland*

This chapter was included after much thought and some equivocation. It was written in response to numerous requests that chemotherapeutic agents be compared and contrasted with radiation from the perspective of the experimental biologist. Many of the techniques and concepts used in chemotherapy were developed initially by radiation biologists, including quantitative tumor assay systems, the concept of cell cycle, sensitivity changes through the cell cycle, and, particularly, population kinetics. The term *growth fraction*, for example, was coined by a radiation biologist but never assumed the importance in radiotherapy that it has in chemotherapy.

The study of chemotherapeutic agents in the laboratory, as well as in the clinic, is vastly more complicated than the study of ionizing radiations. *Dose* is more difficult to define or to measure, and its meaning is less obvious. Variations in sensitivity through the cell cycle are more dramatic for chemicals than for radiation, assuming essentially an all-or-nothing effect for some agents, while there are many more factors involving the milieu that can influence cellular response.

The term *chemotherapy* was coined by Paul Erhlich around the turn of the century to describe the use of chemicals of known composition for the treatment of parasites. Erhlich synthesized an organic arsenic compound that was effective against trypanosome infections and rabbit syphilis. This was the first man-made chemical effective in the treatment of parasitic disease and was rather optimistically named *salvarsan*, which roughly translates to "the savior of mankind!" The next milestone was the discovery and clinical use of penicillin in the early years of World War II. Alkylating agents had been developed as a military weapon by both belligerents in World War I, but it was an explosion in Naples harbor and the exposure of seamen to these agents during World War II that led to the observation that they caused marrow and lymphoid hypoplasia. As a result, they were first tested in humans with Hodgkin's disease in 1943 at Yale University.

It has long since been shown beyond doubt that a single chemotherapeutic drug, used in the appropriate sequence, can cure patients with certain rapidly proliferating cancers. The initial demonstration of this was the use of methotrexate to cure patients with choriocarcinoma and, later, the use of cyclophosphamide for Burkitt's lymphoma.

The next major step forward was the use of combination chemotherapy in the treatment of acute lymphocytic leukemia in the early 1960s and, subsequently, in the treatment of Hodgkin's disease, diffuse histiocytic lymphoma, and testicular cancer in the mid 1970s. These trials verified that multiple non–cross-resistant drugs and different dose-limiting normal tissues could be used effectively in combination to cure tumors that were not curable with a single agent. The principle of combination therapy was then extended to combined modality treatment, in which chemotherapy was used in conjunction with surgery or radiotherapy, or both, to cure tumors such as pediatric sarcomas.

Today about 35 antineoplastic agents are routinely used in clinical oncology. Drug-induced cures are claimed for choriocarcinoma, acute lymphocytic leukemia of childhood, other childhood tumors, Hodgkin's disease, certain non-Hodgkin's lymphomas, and some germ cell tumors of the testes. Other evidence suggests that chemotherapeutic agents given in an "adjuvant" setting for clinically inapparent micrometastatic disease may prolong disease-free survival and possibly effect cure of breast cancer and osteogenic sarcoma.

The chemotherapy of cancer is the treatment of metastatic disease. With the exception of some leukemias and lymphomas, its function is one of retrieval—to treat and possibly to control a cancer that has become systemic and out of control. There are 13 types of cancer for which cures are claimed by chemotherapy; this accounts for about 10% of all cancers. The bad public image of chemotherapy is due in large part to the toxicities of normal tissue resulting from multidrug protocols used to induce remissions and achieve tumor cure. The lack of tumor-specific agents carries the burden of damage to self-renewing normal tissues, such as the gut, bone marrow, and scalp. Until drugs can be developed that discriminate between normal and neoplastic tissue, chemotherapy will continue to be a primitive form of cancer therapy—using the proverbial sledge hammer to crack a nut!

## BIOLOGICAL BASIS OF CHEMOTHERAPY

Almost all anticancer drugs work by affecting DNA synthesis or function, and they do not usually kill resting cells unless such cells divide soon after exposure to the drug. Consequently, the effectiveness of anticancer drugs is limited by the growth fraction of the tumor—by the fraction of cells in active cycle. Rapidly growing neoplasia with a short cell cycle, a large proportion of cells in S phase and therefore a large growth fraction, are more responsive to chemotherapy than large tumor masses in which the growth fraction is small. There is a strong tendency for growth fraction to decrease as tumor size increases, at least in experimental animal tumors.

Agents that are mainly effective during a particular phase of the cell cycle, such as S phase, are said to be **cell-cycle specific,** or **phase specific.** Those whose action is independent of the position of the cell in the cycle are said to be **cell-cycle nonspecific** or **phase nonspecific.** The distinction between cell-cycle specific and cell-cycle nonspecific is relative rather than absolute. Agents that are most effective against S phase cells will be relatively ineffective against slowly turning-over cell populations with a large proportion of dormant cells. On the other hand, alkylating agents and other drugs interacting primarily with macromolecular DNA are largely independent of the phase of the cell cycle and

may be effective against tumors with relatively low proliferative activity.

The other side of the coin is that the selective normal tissue toxicity of anticancer drugs is reflected in stem cells of the intestinal epithelium or hematopoietic stem cells, which have a high growth fraction.

Although many clinical oncologists claim that their thinking has been influenced by research on tumor growth kinetics, it is hard to point to clear advances in treatment that may be attributed to anything more than inspired clinical experimentation. This may be because the study of growth kinetics in human tumors is still in its infancy.

The effectiveness of at least some chemotherapeutic agents is dependent on the presence or absence of molecular oxygen in much the same way as x-rays. This is not surprising, at least for drugs whose action is mediated by free radicals.

## CLASSES OF AGENTS AND MODE OF ACTION

Most commonly used chemotherapeutic agents fall into one of three classes: alkylating agents, antibiotics, or antimetabolites. Some of the most important and most widely used agents, however, make up a fourth mixed class that can only be labeled "miscellaneous." This includes the platinum complexes, procarbazine, and the *Vinca* alkaloids.

An attempt to summarize the classification of drugs is presented in Table 17-1. A few of the most commonly used agents are briefly described, with emphasis on their characteristics and mechanism of action. A thorough discussion of their clinical usefulness is outside the scope of this book.

### Alkylating Agents

The alkylating agents are highly reactive compounds with the ability to substitute alkyl groups for hydrogen atoms of certain organic compounds, including DNA. There are five classes of alkylating agents:

Table 17-1.
Classes of Chemotherapeutic Agents

| CLASS OF COMPOUND | EXAMPLES | EXAMPLES OF DISEASES IN WHICH DRUGS ARE USEFUL |
|---|---|---|
| Alkylating agents | Nitrogen mustard, chlorambucil, cyclophosphamide, busulfan | Lymphomas, many solid tumors, chronic leukemia, multiple myeloma |
| Antimetabolites | Methotrexate | Acute leukemia |
| | 6-Mercaptopurine | Choriocarcinoma, head and neck cancer |
| | Cytarabine | |
| | 5-Fluorouracil | Carcinoma of breast, carcinoma of gastrointestinal tract |
| Antibiotics | Dactinomycin | Wilms' tumor, choriocarcinoma |
| | Doxorubicin | A wide spectrum of tumors |
| | Bleomycin | Lymphomas, testicular carcinoma |
| Plant alkaloids | Vincristine | Acute leukemia, lymphomas |
| | Vinblastine | Reticuloendothelial malignancy lymphomas, testicular carcinoma |
| Adrenocorticosteroids | Prednisone | Lymphocytic leukemias, lymphomas, carcinoma of breast |
| Other steroid hormones | Estrogens | Carcinoma of prostate |
| | Androgens | Carcinoma of breast |
| Antiestrogens | Progestins | Carcinoma of endometrium |
| | Tamoxifen | Carcinoma of breast |
| Enzymes | L-Asparaginase | Acute lymphatic leukemias, lymphomas |
| Miscellaneous agents | | |
| Methylhydrazine | Procarbazine | Lymphomas |
| Nitrosoureas | BCNU | Lymphomas |
| | CCNU | Brain tumors, many solid tumors |
| Hydroxyurea | Hydroxyurea | Chronic and acute leukemias |
| Cisplatin | Cisplatin | Testicular cancer |

*(Adapted from Cline MJ, Haskell CM: Cancer Chemotherapy. London, WB Saunders, 1980)*

1. Nitrogen mustard derivatives, such as cyclophosphamide, chlorambucil, and melphalan
2. Ethylenimine derivatives, such as thiotepa
3. Alkyl sulfonates, such as busulfan
4. Triazene derivatives, such as dacarbazine
5. Nitrosoureas, including BCNU, CCNU, and methyl CCNU

Most of these drugs contain more than one alkylating group and are therefore considered to be polyfunctional alkylating agents. The nitrosoureas and dacarbazine have mechanisms and cytotoxicity over and above their ability to alkylate nucleic acids. As a class, alkylating agents are considered to be cell-cycle nonspecific.

Nitrogen mustard is the prototype for three other useful alkylating agents: cyclophosphamide, chlorambucil, and melphalan. These drugs are given intravenously and interact rapidly with cells in vivo, producing their primary effect in seconds or minutes. By contrast, cyclophosphamide (Cytoxan) is inert until it undergoes biotransformation in the liver. Disappearance of injected cyclophosphamide from the plasma is biexponential, with an average half-life of 4 to 6½ hours. Like all useful alkylating agents, cyclophosphamide produces toxicity in rapidly proliferating normal tissues. Chlorambucil (Leukeran) is an aromatic derivative of nitrogen mustard and is the slowest acting alkylating agent in general use. Melphalan (Alkeran, L-PAM) is a phenylalanine derivative of nitrogen mustard.

The nitrosoureas are a group of lipophilic alkylating agents that undergo extensive biotransformation in vivo, leading to a variety of biological effects, including alkylation, carbamylation, and inhibition of DNA repair. The multiple mechanisms of action may explain why the nitrosoureas generally lack cross-resistance with other alkylating agents. These compounds are very lipid soluble and readily cross the blood–brain barrier. They disappear from plasma rapidly, but their metabolites may persist for days.

## Antibiotics

The clinically useful antibiotics are natural products of various strains of the soil fungus *Streptomyces*. They produce their tumoricidal effects by directly binding to DNA, and so their major inhibiting effects are on DNA and RNA synthesis. As a class, these drugs behave as cell-cycle nonspecific agents. Doxorubicin (Adriamycin) and daunomycin are closely related anthracycline antibiotics. After intravenous injection, both drugs undergo extensive bioreduction in the liver to active and inactive metabolites, are extensively bound in tissues, and persist in plasma for prolonged periods. Neither drug crosses the blood–brain barrier to any appreciable extent. Both doxorubicin and daunorubicin are highly toxic drugs, producing a variety of severe reactions; the major limiting toxicity, however, is cardiac damage.

Dactinomycin (Actinomycin D) inhibits DNA-primed RNA synthesis by intercalating with the guanine residues of DNA; at higher concentrations it also inhibits DNA synthesis. The net effect is cell-cycle nonspecific cytotoxicity. Dactinomycin must be administered intravenously. Its important longer plasma half-life is about 36 hours, and the drug is extensively bound to tissues.

Bleomycin sulfate (Blenoxane) affects cells by directly binding to DNA, resulting in reduced synthesis of DNA, RNA, and proteins. It can also lead to single-strand DNA breaks. Drugs acting by intercalation appear to augment the cytotoxic effects of bleomycin, as do x-rays and chemicals that generate superoxide radicals. Bleomycin is considered cell-cycle nonspecific. It is more damaging to nonproliferating than to most proliferating cells.

Mitomycin C (Mutamycin) is an extremely toxic antitumor antibiotic. Unlike most other antibiotics, it is activated in vivo to a bifunctional or trifunctional alkylating agent. It is cell-cycle nonspecific and is considerably more toxic to hypoxic than to aerated cells. Mitomycin C is almost always administered intravenously; it is rapidly cleared from the plasma with a half-life of 10 to 15 minutes, primarily by metabolism in the liver. It does not appear to cross the blood–brain barrier. The major toxicity of mitomycin C is myelosuppression.

## *Vinca* Alkaloids

Some of the most useful antineoplastic agents are produced from plants. Vincristine sulfate (Oncovin) and vinblastine sulfate (Velban) are alkaloids produced from the common periwinkle plant. The clinically useful alkaloids are large complex molecules that exert their major antitumor effect by binding to cellular microtubular proteins. Since these are essential compounds of the mitotic spindle of dividing cells, this binding leads to mitotic arrest.

## Antimetabolites

The antimetabolites are analogues of normal metabolites required for cell function and replication. They may interact with enzymes and damage cells by

1. *Substituting* for a metabolite normally incorporated into a key molecule
2. *Competing* successfully with a normal metabolite for occupation of the catalytic site of a key enzyme
3. *Competing* with a normal metabolite that acts at an enzyme regulatory site to alter the catalytic rate of the enzyme

Methotrexate is a folic acid antagonist. It works by competing for the folate binding site of the enzyme dihydrofolate reductase. This results in decreased synthesis of thymidine and purine nucleotides. The cytotoxicity of methotrexate can be reversed by leucovorin, which is readily converted to other forms of reduced folate within the cell and which can then act as methyl donors for a variety of biochemical reactions. The use of high-dose methotrexate with leucovorin rescue is based on the pharmacology of the two drugs, with the possibility of a differential effect between tumors and normal tissues in their ability to transport the two drugs across cell membranes. How true this turns out to be is another matter!

## 5-Fluorouracil

5-Fluorouracil is a structural analogue of the DNA precursor thymine. It works primarily as an irreversible inhibitor of the enzyme thymidylate synthetase but only after intracellular conversion to the active metabolite. It is also degraded by the liver and some other tissues. As a single agent, 5-fluorouracil is most useful in the treatment of carcinoma of the breast and gastrointestinal tract. The degradative enzymes are found in high concentrations in the gut but not in colonic carcinomas, and it has been suggested that this may explain in part the susceptibility of this tumor to 5-fluorouracil.

## Nucleoside Analogues

A variety of nucleoside analogues have been synthesized and tested for antineoplastic properties. They are readily transported into rapidly dividing cells and activated by the single metabolic step of phosphorylation. Two analogues of cytosine are useful in cancer chemotherapy.

Cytarabine (cytosine arabinoside) is an analogue of deoxycytidine in which the sugar moiety is altered. The active form of cytarabine is the triphosphate that functions as a competitive inhibitor of DNA polymerase. Cytarabine is cell-cycle specific and in clinical practice is almost always used in combination with other drugs in the treatment of acute myeloid leukemia.

5-Azacytidine contains a single nitrogen substitution in the pyrimidine ring of cytidine. It undergoes a sequence of biotransformation similar to cytarabine, with ultimate formation of an active triphosphate. The major biochemical effect of 5-azacytidine is believed to be the inhibition of the processing of large molecular weight species of RNA, with less important effects on DNA and protein synthesis. Like cytarabine, it is cell-cycle specific.

## Miscellaneous Agents

### Procarbazine

Procarbazine is a hydrazine derivative that must undergo biotransformation before it can exert its cytotoxic effects. The precise mechanism of action is not clear, since it interferes with a wide variety of biochemical processes. Procarbazine is well absorbed from the gastrointestinal tract and is cleared from the plasma with a half-life of about 10 minutes. The drug freely crosses the blood–brain barrier. It is used primarily in the treatment of advanced Hodgkin's disease.

### Hydroxyurea

Hydroxyurea was first synthesized as long ago as 1869 and was found to be bone marrow suppressive in 1928. It was not used in the treatment of cancer until the 1960s. It acts as an inhibitor of ribonucleotide reductase, an enzyme essential to DNA synthesis, and is consequently specifically cytotoxic to cells in the S phase of the cell cycle. In experimental biology hydroxyurea is used to synchronize cells, because in addition to killing S phase cells, it also causes survivors to pile up at a block at the $G_1$–S interface. Clinically, hydroxyurea is primarily used in the treatment of chronic myeloid leukemia.

### Cisplatin

Structurally, cisplatin (*cis*-dichlorodiammineplatinum, *cis*-DDP, *cis*-platinum) is an inorganic complex formed by an atom of platinum surrounded by chlorine and ammonium ions in the *cis* position of the horizontal plane. Cisplatin bears a resemblance to the bifunctional alkylating agents based on nitrogen mustard. It inhibits DNA synthesis to a greater extent than the synthesis of RNA or protein. It binds to DNA, causing both interstrand and intrastrand cross-linking.

Cisplatin is cell-cycle nonspecific. Its isomer, *trans*-platinum, is much less cytotoxic, presumably because of the different way that it cross-links to DNA. There is some evidence that cisplatin is more toxic to hypoxic than to aerated cells, that is, that it is a hypoxic cell radiosensitizer, though not as powerful in this regard as the nitroimidazoles.

# DOSE–RESPONSE RELATIONSHIPS

Dose–response relationships have been produced for a wide range of chemotherapeutic agents using techniques developed initially for radiation. Much less effort has been expended on fitting data to models than has been the case for ionizing radiations; from even a cursory examination of the data, however, it is evident that—with some clear exceptions—the shape of the survival curve is unremarkable and reminiscent of that of survival curves for ionizing radiations. When surviving fraction is plotted on a log scale against drug dose on a linear scale, the dose–response curve has an initial shoulder followed by a region that becomes steeper and straighter (Fig. 17-1). The antibiotics doxorubicin, bleomycin, and dac-

tinomycin are clear exceptions. For these agents the dose–response curve appears to have no shoulder, and the curve is concave **upward.** A dose–response curve with this shape is usually associated with a variation of sensitivity within the population (ie, nonuniform sensitivity of cells). This has never been demonstrated experimentally, however. For example, synchronously dividing cells likewise show the same upwardly concave dose–response curve. This shape must therefore remain unexplained at the present time.

Dose–response curves indicate that, at best, anticancer drugs kill by first-order kinetics; that is, a given dose of the drug will kill a constant *fraction* of a population of cells, regardless of its size. This assumes, of course, that the growth fraction and the proportion of sensitive to resis-

**Figure 17-1.** Dose–response relationships in vitro for six commonly used chemotherapeutic agents. Note the diverse shapes. Many have a shape similar to survival curves for x-rays, except that drug concentration replaces absorbed dose. The antibiotics bleomycin. (Adriamycin), and doxorubicin actinomycin D have dose-response relationships that are concave upward.

**(A)** Dose–response relationship for dividing CHO cells treated for 1 hour with graded doses of actinomycin D. (Redrawn from Barranco SC, Flournay DR: Cancer Res 36:1634–1640, 1976)

**(B)** Dose–response relationship for plateau-phase CHO cells treated for 1 hour with graded doses of bleomycin. (Redrawn from Barranco SC, Novak JK, Humphrey RM: Cancer Res 33:691–694, 1973)

**(C)** Dose–response relationship for CHO cells treated for 1 hour with graded doses of CCNU. (Redrawn from Barranco SC: Cancer Treat Rep 60:1799–1810, 1976)

**(D)** Dose–response relationship for human lung cancer cells exposed for 1 hour to graded doses of melphalan. (Unpublished data, courtesy of Dr. Laurie Roizin-Towle)

**(E)** Dose–response relationship for V79 Chinese hamster cells exposed for 1 hour to graded doses of doxorubicin. (Redrawn from Belli JA, Piro AJ: Cancer Res 37:1624–1630, 1977)

**(F)** Dose–response relationship for V79 Chinese hamster cells exposed for 1 hour to graded doses of cisplatin. (Unpublished data, courtesy of Dr. Laurie Roizin-Towle)

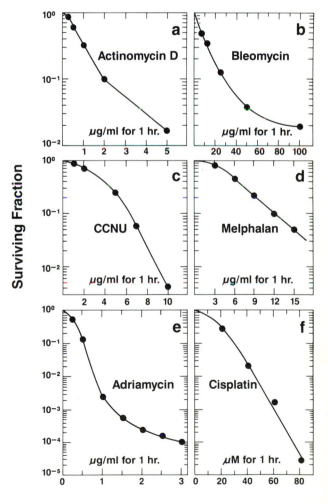

tant cells remains the same. This leads to the conclusion that the chance of eradicating a cancer is greatest when the population size is small, or that there is an inverse relationship between curability and the tumor-cell burden at the initiation of chemotherapy. This conclusion has been arrived at from long and bitter clinical experience, but in fact it is an inevitable consequence of the shape of the simplest dose–response relationship.

## SUBLETHAL AND POTENTIALLY LETHAL DAMAGE REPAIR

Studies with radiation led to the concepts of sublethal damage repair and potentially lethal damage repair, which are discussed in some detail in Chapter 7. These are still largely operational terms, although a notable exception is mitomycin C, in which the gene for repair of DNA damage has been identified and cloned (see Chapter 23). Sublethal damage repair is demonstrated by an increase in survival when a dose of radiation (or other cytotoxic agent) is divided into two or more fractions separated in time. There is a tendency for the extent of sublethal damage repair to correlate with the shoulder of the acute dose–response curve, but this is not necessarily always true. Potentially lethal damage repair is manifest as an increase in survival when cells are held in a nonproliferative state for some time after treatment.

Similar studies have been performed with a variety of chemotherapeutic agents. The results are confusing and not as clear cut as for radiation, partly because there are so many drugs and so many cell lines.

Potentially lethal damage repair is a significant factor in the antibiotics bleomycin and doxorubicin. Data for bleomycin are shown in Figure 17-2. Potentially lethal damage repair is also seen after treatment with dactinomycin. Sublethal damage repair is essentially absent with all of these drugs.

No potentially lethal or sublethal damage repair is seen with nitrosourea, even though the dose–response curves for single doses have a substantial shoulder. The breakdown products of

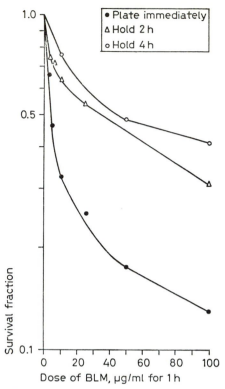

**Figure 17-2.** Potentially lethal damage repair (PLDR) in cultured Chinese hamster cells treated with bleomycin (BLM). An increase in survival is observed, interpreted as PLDR, when cells are held in depleted medium for 2 to 4 hours after the drug treatment. (From Barranco SC, Humphrey RM: Prog Biochem Pharmacol 11:78–22, 1976)

the nitrosoureas are known to inhibit DNA repair, and this may be a contributing factor.

Sublethal damage repair studies with drugs are complicated, because when a split-dose study is performed, decisions must be made about the equivalence of drug concentration and time. It is frequently assumed that biological response is determined by an integral dose (ie, the product of concentration and time), but this has not been checked and confirmed in all cases. There appears to be no correlation between the existence of a shoulder on the dose–response curve for single doses and the appearance of sublethal damage repair, as evidenced by an increase in survival in a split-dose experiment. It is possible that the presence of a shoulder in a survival curve does not have the same meaning for chemically induced damage as it does for radiation-induced damage. The presence of a shoulder on a

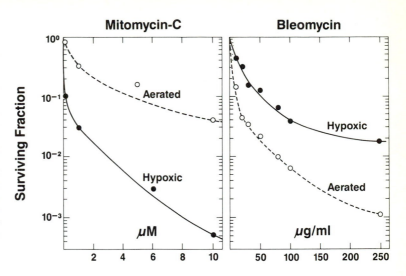

**Figure 17-3.** Molecular oxygen can be either a sensitizer or a protector, depending on the particular chemotherapeutic agent. **(A)** Survival curves for EMT6 cells treated for 1 hour with graded doses of mitomycin C under aerated or hypoxic conditions. In the absence of oxygen the cells are substantially more *sensitive*. (Data from Teicher BA, Laza TS, Santorelli AC: Cancer Res 41:73–81, 1981) **(B)** Survival curves for Chinese hamster cells in culture exposed for 4 hours to graded doses of bleomycin under aerated or hypoxic conditions. In the absence of molecular oxygen the cells are more *resistant*. (Redrawn from Roizin-Towle L, Hall EJ: Br J Cancer 37: 254, 1978)

survival curve for a chemotherapeutic agent may reflect more about drug concentrations and the time required for entry of the drug into the cells and interaction with a target molecule than it does about the accumulation and repair of sublethal damage.

## THE OXYGEN EFFECT AND CHEMOTHERAPEUTIC AGENTS

The importance of the oxygen effect for cell killing by radiation was discussed in an earlier chapter (see Chapter 8). It has been known for half a century that the presence or absence of molecular oxygen has a dramatic influence on the proportion of cells surviving a given dose of x-rays. Only in more recent years has the influence of oxygen on the cytotoxicity resulting from chemotherapeutic agents been studied. It is certainly more complicated than for ionizing radiations.

Some agents, such as bleomycin, are more toxic to oxygenated cells than to chronically hypoxic cells. Dose–response curves for cells exposed to graded concentrations of bleomycin in the presence or absence of oxygen are shown in Figure 17-3. At high concentrations of the drug there is an extra log of cell killing if oxygen is present, compared with hypoxic conditions. Other examples of agents that are more toxic to aerated than to hypoxic cells are procarbazine, streptonigrin, dactinomycin, and vincristine. It

should come as no surprise to those used to x-rays that oxygen is a factor in the response of cells to any chemotherapeutic agent in which the mechanism of cell killing is mediated by free radicals.

By contrast, agents such as mitomycin C are substantially more toxic to hypoxic than to aerated cells (see Fig. 17-3), because the drug undergoes bioreduction in the absence of oxygen. The same is true, of course, of misonidazole metronidazole, etanidazole, tirapazamine, and RB6145, which are discussed in Chapter 10, and of 5-thio-D-glucose.

A third group of drugs, including 5-fluorouracil, methotrexate, cisplatin, and the nitrosoureas, appear to be equally cytotoxic to aerated or hypoxic cells. This oversimplified classification only holds true if the level or duration of the hypoxia is not sufficient to disturb the movement of cells through the cell cycle. Table 17-2 is a summary of the classification of antineoplastic agents based on the effect of the presence or absence of molecular oxygen.

## PROLIFERATING AND NONPROLIFERATING CELLS

There are a number of reports in the literature that nonproliferating plateau-phase cells are more sensitive to a variety of antineoplastic agents than dividing cells in the exponential

Table 17-2.

## Classification of Antineoplastic Agents Based on Cellular Oxygenation

| PREFERENTIAL TOXICITY TO AEROBIC CELLS | PREFERENTIAL TOXICITY TO HYPOXIC CELLS | MINIMAL OR NO SELECTIVITY BASED ON CELLULAR OXYGENATION |
|---|---|---|
| Bleomycin | Mitomycin-C | 5-Fluorouracil[*] |
| Procarbazine | Doxorubicin | Methotrexate[*] |
| Streptonigrin | Misonidazole, metronidazole | Cisplatin |
| | Etanidazole | |
| | Tirapazamine | |
| | RB6145 | |
| Dactinomycin | 5-thio-D-glucose, 2-deoxy-D-glucose | BCNU, CCNU |

[*]*These conclusions are based on experiments in which hypoxic cells were still capable of DNA synthesis and cellular replication. These agents have cytotoxic effects primarily on cells in the S phase of the cell cycle. Thus, in hypoxic cells that are blocked in their progression through the cell cycle or cycling slowly, agents such as these that act on the S phase of the cell cycle would be expected to be relatively noncytotoxic.*
*(Based on Teicher BA, Laza JS, Sartorelli AC: Cancer Res 412:73–81, 1981)*

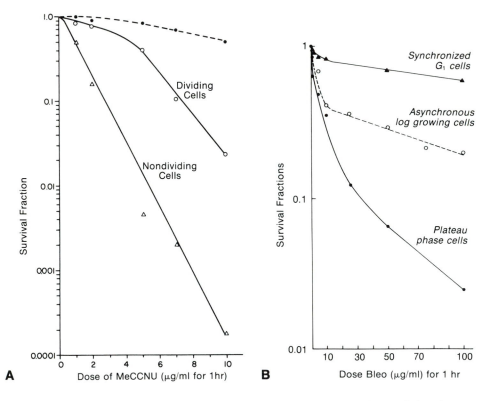

**Figure 17-4.** Dose–response curves for dividing and nondividing plateau-phase cells in culture exposed to two anticancer drugs: Me CCNU **(A)** and bleomycin **(B)**. In both cases the nondividing plateau-phase cells are more sensitive than the dividing cells in exponential growth. (From Barranco SC: In vitro responses of mammalian cells to drug-induced potentially lethal and sublethal damage. Cancer Treat Rep 60:1799–1810, 1976 and Barranco SC, Novak JK, Humphrey RM: Cancer Res 33:691–694, 1973)

phase of growth. Figure 17-4 shows data for bleomycin and methyl CCNU, for which this is clearly the case. At first sight this is a surprising result, and it is not possible to account for it in terms of the variation of sensitivity through the cycle. The most probable explanation is that cells in plateau phase have much lower levels of nonprotein thiols than actively dividing cells. Thiol content is known to have a marked influence of cellular sensitivity to a number of antineoplastic agents, particularly the alkylating agents.

# DRUG RESISTANCE

The biggest single problem in chemotherapy is drug resistance, which may either be evident from the outset or which may develop during prolonged exposure to a cytostatic drug. Cells resistant to the drug take over, and the tumor as a whole becomes unresponsive. The development of resistance can be demonstrated readily for cells in culture. Figure 17-5 shows a substantial resistance to doxorubicin developing as cells are grown continuously in a low concentration of the drug for a period of weeks.

Underlying this problem of drug resistance are genetic changes that can sometimes be seen in chromosome preparations. Figure 17-6 shows two illustrations involving gene amplification or the presence of multiple minute chromosome fragments.

Drug resistance is a big and important factor that occurs readily—a phenomenon quite alien to the radiobiologist. Radiation-resistant cells can be produced and isolated, but it is a difficult and time-consuming process. For instance, cells continuously irradiated at low dose rates do occasionally spawn a radioresistant clone. By contrast, resistance to chemotherapeutic agents is acquired quickly, uniformly, and inevitably.

If a resistant clone can arise by a chance mutation of a gene responsible for one of the important steps in drug action, then the probability of it occurring would be expected to increase rapidly as the tumor increases in size. The average mutation rate for mammalian genes is about $10^{-5}$ to $10^{-6}$ per division, so that in a tumor containing $10^{10}$ cells that go through many divisions the mutation is almost certain to occur,

especially in the presence of a powerful mutagen, which most chemotherapeutic agents are.

The usual strategy to overcome the problem of induced resistance is to use a battery of different drugs, applied sequentially and cyclically, that produce their cytotoxicity by diverse mechanisms. By this strategy, cells that develop resistance to drug A are killed by drug B, and so on.

The bigger problem is **pleiotropic resistance,** the phenomenon by which the development of resistance to one drug results in cross-resistance to other drugs, even those with different mechanisms of action. There are four interesting points to be made.

1. Multidrug resistance in tumor cells is due to extrusion of the drugs; that is, cells pump the drugs out as fast as they get in! This is mediated by increased expression of the product of the multiple drug resistance gene (*mdr*), a p-glycoprotein expressed in the cell membrane. This membrane protein is a polypeptide of 1280 amino acids composed of two similar domains, each containing six potential transmembrane segments and two putative adenosine triphosphate–binding regions. Its structure is similar to that of various transporters of ions, amino acids, peptides, or proteins in bacterial, yeast, and animal cells. Indeed, it has been reported that the multidrug resistance gene in human tumor cells shows considerable homology to the gene in yeast, which extrudes an attractant that is important in the reproductive cycle! The *mdr* gene has been mapped to human chromosome 7. Resistance by this means can be reversed by calcium channel blocking drugs, such as verapamil. This has been shown to be an important mechanism of resistance to doxorubicin in Chinese hamster ovary cells in culture, and there appears to be an expression of this same gene for resistance in cells from some human solid tumors that have acquired resistance.

2. Glutathione is a naturally occurring thiol in all cells. Elevated levels of glutathione have been observed in resistant cells, especially those made resistant by treatment with melphalan. Drugs are available that block the synthesis of glutathione and that can be used to lower the

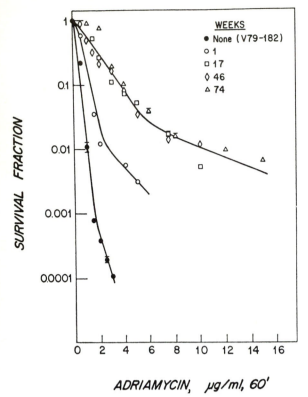

Figure 17-5. Change in survival response to doxorubicin (Adriamycin) of Chinese hamster cells grown in culture and exposed continuously to a low concentration of the drug (0.05 μg/mL) for prolonged periods of time, namely 1, 17, 46, or 74 weeks. The closed circles show the survival response for the parent cell line; a dramatic resistance to the drug develops by 17 to 74 weeks. (From Belli JA: Front Radiat Ther Oncol 13:9–20, 1979)

levels of this compound in tumors and normal tissues. The best known example is buthionine sulfoximine. Use of buthionine sulfoximine has been shown to reduce cross-resistance, particularly between melphalan and cisplatin in tumor-bearing mice. The use of buthionine sulfoximine would not be advisable in combination with doxorubicin or cisplatin because an increase in specific normal tissue toxicity (lung and kidney, respectively) would be expected.

3. A marked increase in DNA repair has been noted in some cells resistant to melphalan or cisplatin. If this proves to be a mechanism of induced resistance, drugs are available, such as aphidicolin, that block repair.
4. A debatable issue is whether cells that have acquired resistance to chemotherapeutic agents are also resistant to radiation. The con-

sensus is that they are not. There may be some data to suggest this from clinical experience, but the laboratory data show rather clearly that the acquiring of resistance to a drug does not necessarily result in radioresistance. This is illustrated in Figure 17-7, in which cells that have acquired extreme resistance to melphalan show a normal response to radiation. Radioresistance and chemoresistance may occur together, but radiation rarely induces chemoresistance and vice versa.

The evolving story of drug resistance has an impact on the development and screening of new drugs. In the past, the initial screening for new agents consisted of fast growing, highly drug-sensitive mouse tumors. Tests against specific patterns or types of drug resistance were not included. The screening systems, therefore, were weighted heavily in favor of producing more of the same types of drugs. This has now changed, and the screening of new drugs for activity is performed using a battery of cells of human origin cultured in vitro.

## COMPARISON OF CHEMOTHERAPEUTIC AGENTS WITH RADIATION

The title of this chapter includes the words, "from the perspective of the radiation biologist." This limited and specialized viewpoint must be borne in mind in what follows. A number of important differences are evident in the response of cells to chemotherapeutic agents versus ionizing radiation:

1. There is a much greater variation of sensitivity to chemotherapeutic agents than there is to radiation. In the case of x-rays the variation of $D_0$ from the most sensitive to the most resistant known mammalian cells may be a factor of about 4. By contrast, the response of a variety of cell lines to a given chemotherapeutic agent may differ by orders of magnitude. A particular cell line may be exquisitely sensitive to one drug and extremely resistant to another. A different cell line may have a different order of sensitivity to various drugs as well as a quite different absolute sensitivity. Different clones derived from a common stock may ex-

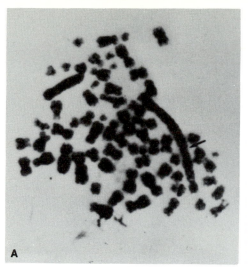

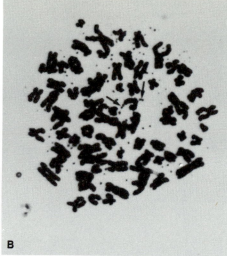

Figure 17-6.   Most forms of drug resistance probably have a genetic basis. A few extreme examples can be seen in chromosome changes. **(A)** The arrow indicates an elongated chromosome, which on banding shows the features of an extended homogeneously staining region. This karyotype was observed in the human breast cancer cell line (MCF-7), which is resistant to methotrexate. (From Cowan KH, Goldsmith ME, Levine R et al: Dihydrofolate reductase gene amplification and possible rearrangement in estrogen-responsive methotrexate-resistant human breast cancer cells. J Biol Chem 257:15079–15086, 1982) **(B)** Small cell lung carcinoma line derived from a patient treated with methotrexate. These cells are very resistant to the drug and contain numerous double-minute chromosomes. A pair is indicated by the arrows. (From Curt GA, Carney DN, Cowan KH et al: N Engl J Med 308:199–202, 1983)

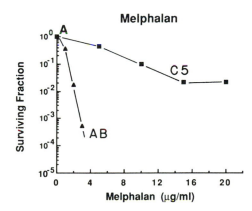

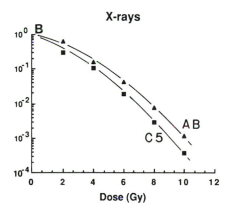

Figure 17-7.   Chinese hamster pleiotropic multidrug-resistant cells are not necessarily resistant to radiation. The parallel CHO cell line is designated AB. The drug-resistant cell line C5 was isolated by Dr. Victor Ling by exposing the parental line to the mutagen ethyl methane sulfonate, after which surviving cells were grown for an extended period of time in increasing concentrations of colchicine. A clone was isolated that is resistant to colchicine and to a variety of chemotherapeutic agents. (*Left*) C5 cells are resistant to melphalan, compared with the parental line (AB). They are also resistant to other agents, such as daunorubicin. (*Right*) The radiation responses of the parental and the chemotherapy-resistant cell lines are virtually indistinguishable. (From Mitchell JB, Gamson J, Russo A, Friedman N, Degraff W, Carmichael J, Glatstein E: NCI Monogr 6:187–191, 1988)

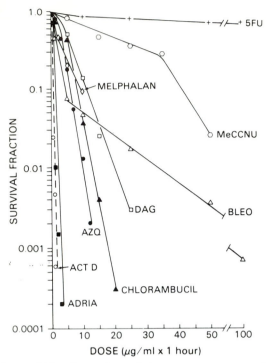

**Figure 17-8.** Comparison of dose–response curves of a stomach cancer cell line in culture exposed for 1 hour to graded doses of nine anticancer drugs. There is a wide variation in sensitivity and in the shape of the various curves. (From Barranco SC, Townsend CM, Quariashi MA, Nevill HC, Howell KH, Boerwinkle WR: Invest New Drugs 1:117–127, 1983)

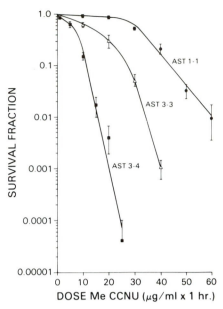

**Figure 17-9.** Dose–response data for three permanent clones derived from a single astrocytoma cell line exposed to the anticancer drug Me CCNU. Note the great variation in sensitivity. (From Rubin NH, Castartelli C, Macek BG, Boerwinkle WR, Barranco SC: Invest New Drugs 1:129–137, 1983)

hibit quite different sensitivity to a given agent. This variability is shown in Figure 17-8, which gives the response of one cell line to nine different cytotoxic agents, and in Figure 17-9, which shows the widely different response to CCNU of three clones derived from a common astrocytoma cell line.

2. The sensitivity of a given cell line to a given drug may be manipulated to a much greater extent than for radiation.

3. Repair of sublethal and potentially lethal damage is more variable and less predictable for drugs than for radiation.

4. The oxygen effect is more complex for drugs than for ionizing radiations. For radiation, the presence or absence of molecular oxygen has an important influence on the proportion of cells surviving a given dose of low linear energy transfer radiation, in which about two thirds of the damage is caused by indirect ac-

tion (ie, mediated by free radicals). As the linear energy transfer of the radiation increases and the balance shifts from indirect to direct action, the importance of oxygen decreases. For very high linear energy transfer radiations (above about 200 keV/μm) the biological effect for a given dose is independent of the presence or absence of molecular oxygen. Under no circumstances is oxygen protective in the case of ionizing radiations.

For drugs in which the biological effect involves free radicals, the presence or absence of oxygen is important in the same way as for low linear energy transfer ionizing radiations. The new factor in the case of drugs is that there is a whole class of antineoplastic agents that undergo bioreduction in the absence of oxygen, so that they are *more* effective in hypoxic cells. There is no parallel for ionizing radiations.

Other agents do not depend primarily on free radicals for their biological effects, nor do they undergo bioreduction under hypoxic conditions; consequently, the effect of a given treatment is independent of the presence or absence of molecular oxygen, a property these agents have in common with very densely ionizing radiations.

5. Resistance to drugs develops more quickly and more regularly than it does to radiation. Acquired resistance to drugs does not necessarily involve resistance to x-rays as well.

6. Drug resistance may be due to changes in thiol levels or to molecular changes observable at the chromosome level that result in the activation of a gene that functions to pump the drug out of the cells.

## ADJUNCT USE OF CHEMOTHERAPEUTIC AGENTS WITH RADIATION

The initial rationale for the combination of radiation and chemotherapeutic agents was what is usually known as "spatial cooperation." Radiation may be more effective for controlling the localized primary tumor, because it can be aimed and large doses given (Fig. 17-10), but it is ineffective against disseminated disease. Chemotherapy, on the other hand, may be able to cope with micrometastases, whereas it could not control the larger primary tumor. In other situations (see Fig. 17-10), chemotherapy is the primary treatment modality, and radiation is used only to treat "sanctuary" sites not reached by the drug.

Although spatial cooperation was the original rationale, it is no longer the only one. Radiation

and chemotherapeutic agents are combined in an attempt to achieve better local control.

A therapeutic gain requires differential effects between tumor and normal tissue. One or more of the following tumor characteristics may be exploited to achieve this difference:

1. Genetic instability of tumor cells
2. Rapid proliferation of some tumor cells
3. Cell age distribution of tumor cell populations
4. Hypoxia (characteristic of larger tumors)
5. pH (often low in tumors)

The strategy of combining the two modalities of radiation and cytotoxic drugs is to increase local tumor control, relapse-free survival, and overall survival and alter the pattern of relapse. Three obvious possibilities are to (1) start chemotherapy after the completion of the local treatment, (2) start chemotherapy before the local treatment, or (3) give chemotherapy during local treatment (simultaneous administration). Most cytotoxic agents do not provide enough differential sensitization of tumors compared with normal tissues; consequently, dose-limiting or life-threatening toxicity to critical tissues may be increased greatly.

Adjuvant chemotherapy has been found to materially increase the cure rate of a dozen or more experimental animal tumors. Emerging principles include the following:

1. The lower the body burden of the tumor, the better.
2. A maximally effective drug regimen should begin as soon as possible after surgery, with maximum practicable doses.

Improving local control improves overall survival and avoids uncontrolled local growth and the possible need for mutilating surgery. For this reason alone aggressive use of combined modalities to improve local control is warranted.

It has often been said that "you can only kill the sensitive cells once." There is no point in using a battery of different agents that all target the same subpopulation of sensitive cells. Rather, the *heterogeneity* of the tumor cell population should be acknowledged and exploited. One agent should be effective against cycling cells, another against resting cells, and a third perhaps against hypoxic cells; in other words, the strategy

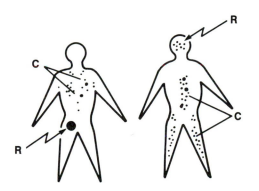

**Figure 17-10.** Spatial cooperation. In some instances radiation may be used to treat a large primary tumor with chemotherapy added to cope with systemic disease in the form of disseminated metastases. In other situations chemotherapy may be used as the primary treatment, with radiation added to treat "sanctuary" sites that the cytotoxic drug cannot reach.

should be to combine agents that will specifically attack the different subpopulations in the tumor.

A problem to be avoided is the triggering of "accelerated repopulation." This refers to triggering of surviving clonogens to divide and repopulate even more rapidly as a tumor shrinks after treatment with a cytotoxic agent. It is a phenomenon described in Chapter 13. It may be one of the reasons why radiotherapy after induction chemotherapy has shown disappointing results.

## With Hyperthermia

The combination of localized hyperthermia and chemotherapy is a possibility that has not been properly explored. Some drugs are potentiated dramatically by a temperature elevation of a few degrees; others are not. Local hyperthermia would serve to target drug action (ie, to increase tumor *cytotoxicity* without elevating systemic toxicity). This topic is discussed in more detail in Chapter 16.

## ASSAYS FOR SENSITIVITY OF INDIVIDUAL TUMORS

A great deal of effort has been expended to develop ways to assess which agents are likely to be effective for a particular tumor. The long-term goal would be to mimic the testing of a bacterial infection for sensitivity to a wide range of antibiotic drugs to select the one most suitable and effective.

One approach is to take biopsy specimens from a tumor in a patient, grow the cells in vitro, and subject the cells to a battery of chemotherapeutic agents in the petri dish. This approach has the advantages of not being too expensive to be practical and of providing answers quickly enough to influence the treatment and modify the protocol of the individual from whom the cells were taken. It does, of course, suffer from the obvious disadvantages of focusing attention solely on the question of inherent cellular sensitivity and not addressing the question of drug access, hypoxia, or any of the more complex factors involved as determinants of overall tumor response.

A different approach is to grow cells from human tumors as xenografts in immune-suppressed mice. This is a difficult and limited technique, which is beset with problems, some of which are discussed in Chapter 5. Human tumor cell xenografts do, however, maintain many characteristics of the clinical response of the donor tumors. Indeed, there is a good correlation between clinical remission in donor patients and growth delay in xenografts established from transplanted cells. Establishing xenografts and performing the necessary growth-delay experiments is sufficiently slow and time consuming that the technique cannot ever be expected to provide realistic input into deciding treatment strategy in individual patients, although it can provide guidance on the sensitivity of broad categories of human tumors to a battery of chemotherapeutic agents.

More recent assays to predict responsiveness of individual tumors to radiation, chemotherapy, or a combination of both include the scoring of chromosome aberrations (specifically, micronuclei) in cells from treated tumors. This avoids many of the artifacts of the systems just discussed. Cells are not required to grow well in culture, only to be able to move into metaphase to express chromosome defects.

An additional approach that may be employed in the future to identify tumors resistant to a particular chemotherapeutic agent might be to test for the presence of specific genes that confer resistance.

## SECOND MALIGNANCIES

Late effects are the key to the acceptance of combined treatments. The induction of second malignancies is one of the unfortunate late effects of treatment with radiation or cytotoxic drugs. In a large series of 3000 Hodgkin's disease patients treated with a combination of radiotherapy and chemotherapy, 114 developed second malignancies. The greatest risk was leukemia, but the greatest number were solid tumors.

Radiation is a relatively weak carcinogen; chemotherapeutic agents vary widely. There is a choice of many chemotherapeutic agents, and the variable potential for producing a second ma-

Table 17-3.
## Lesions Produced for a Given Level of Cell Killing by Various Cytotoxic Agents

| AGENT | $D_{37}$ | DNA LESION* | NUMBER OF LESIONS PER CELL PER $D_{37}$ |
|---|---|---|---|
| X-rays | 100 rads | SSB | 1000 |
| | | DSB | 40 |
| Bleomycin | 5.5 µg × 1 hour | SSB | 150 |
| | | DSB | 30 |
| Ultraviolet light | 10 joules/m² | TT dimer | 1,000,000 |
| | | SSB | 100 |
| Benzopyrene | | Adduct | 100,000 |

*SSB, single-strand DNA break; DSB, double-strand DNA break.*
*(Courtesy of Dr. John Ward, University of California at San Francisco)*

lignancy must be a factor influencing the choice of drug in patients who are likely to be long-term survivors.

Table 17-3 compares radiation, bleomycin, ultraviolet radiation, and benzopyrene in terms of the number of DNA lesions per cell necessary to kill 63% of the cell population, that is, to allow 37% to survive. Radiation is characterized by a relatively small number of double-strand breaks, only about 40 per cell on average, at a dose that allows 37% of the cells to survive. At the other extreme, ultraviolet light produces 1 million dimers, and benzopyrene produces 100,000 lesions for the same level of survival. These interesting figures show that radiation is a weak carcinogen because it is efficient at killing cells;

the same is true of bleomycin. By contrast, benzopyrene produces many more DNA lesions for a given level of cell killing and is therefore a powerful carcinogen; ultraviolet light is in the same category.

It is an interesting speculation, supported by these data, that the factor that determines whether an agent is a powerful or a weak carcinogen is the number of DNA lesions required to, on average, kill a cell. If the number is small, the agent is an efficient cytotoxic agent but is likely to be a weaker carcinogen. If the number is large, there will be many DNA lesions in cells that are not killed, and some of these lesions may involve the transformation to a neoplastic state.

► *Summary of Pertinent Conclusions*

- Single agents have been used successfully to cure a few rapidly proliferating tumors.
- Combinations of drugs are used routinely for the treatment of a variety of malignancies.
- Most anticancer drugs work by affecting DNA synthesis or function.
- Inevitably, anticancer drugs are toxic to stem cells of the intestinal epithelium and hematopoietic stem cells, since they have a high growth fraction.
- Agents that are mainly effective during a particular phase of the cell cycle, such as the S phase, are said to be cell-cycle specific, or phase specific.

*(continued)*

► *Summary of Pertinent Conclusions* (Continued)

- Agents whose action is independent of the position of the cell in the cycle are said to be cell-cycle nonspecific, or phase nonspecific.
- Most commonly used chemotherapeutic agents fall into one of three classes:
  1. *Alkylating agents,* which are highly active with the ability to substitute alkyl groups for hydrogen atoms in DNA. These include nitrogen mustard, cyclophosphamide, chlorambucil, melphalan, and the nitrosoureas (BCNU and CCNU).
  2. *Antibiotics,* which bind to DNA and inhibit DNA and RNA synthesis. These include dactinomycin, doxorubicin, daunorubicin, and bleomycin.
  3. *Antimetabolites,* which are analogues of the normal metabolites required for cell function and replication. These include methotrexate, 5-fluorouracil, cytarabine, and 5-azacytidine.
- Some important agents comprise a fourth "miscellaneous" group, including the platinum complexes, procarbazine, and the *Vinca* alkaloids.
- Dose-response relationships for most chemotherapeutic agents resemble those for radiation, with drug concentration replacing absorbed dose; that is, there is an initial shoulder followed by an exponential relationship between surviving fraction and dose. The exceptions are doxorubicin, bleomycin, and dactinomycin, which have dose–response curves that are concave upward.
- At best, anticancer drugs kill cells by first-order kinetics; that is, a given dose kills a constant fraction of cells. Consequently, the chance of eradicating a cancer is greatest when the population size is small (ie, there is an inverse relationship between curability and tumor cell burden).
- Studies of sublethal damage and potentially lethal damage are more confusing and less clear cut for drugs than for radiation.
- Potentially lethal damage repair is a significant factor for bleomycin and doxorubicin, but sublethal damage repair is essentially absent. Neither potentially lethal nor sublethal damage repair is reported for the nitrosoureas.
- The oxygen effect is more complex for drugs than for radiation.
- Some drugs (eg, bleomycin) are more toxic to aerated than to hypoxic cells. For these drugs, free radicals are involved in the mechanism of cell killing, as is the case for x-rays.
- Some drugs (such as mitomycin C) are more toxic to hypoxic than to aerated cells, because they undergo bioreduction. This also applies to etanidazole, tirapazamine, and RB6145 discussed in Chapter 10.
- Other drugs (including 5-fluorouracil, methotrexate, cisplatin, and the nitrosoureas) appear to be equally cytotoxic to aerated and hypoxic cells.
- In vitro studies indicate that nonproliferating cells are more sensitive than proliferating cells to some chemotherapeutic agents; this may be a result of lower thiol levels in nonproliferating cells.
- Drug resistance is the biggest single problem in chemotherapy. For example, cells exposed continuously to low levels of doxorubicin become very resistant to subsequent treatments with this drug.

*(continued)*

► **Summary of Pertinent Conclusions**   (Continued)

- The usual strategy to overcome resistance is to use a battery of drugs that produce cytotoxicity by diverse mechanisms.
- Pleiotropic resistance is when the development of resistance to one drug results in cross-resistance to other drugs with a different mechanism of action.
- Underlying acquired resistance are genetic changes.
- Resistance may be associated with the following:
  Decreased drug accumulation and the expression of P170 glycoproteins in the cell membrane from gene amplification
  Elevated levels of glutathione
  Marked increase in DNA repair

- Radioresistance and chemoresistance may occur together, but radiation rarely induces chemoresistance, and vice versa.
- The adjunct use of chemotherapy with radiation may involve sequential or simultaneous treatments.
- A therapeutic gain requires a differential between tumor and normal tissue. This may be achieved by exploiting one or more of the following tumor characteristics:

  Genetic instability
  Rapid proliferation
  Cell age distribution
  Hypoxia
  pH

- Sensitive cells can only be killed once. Tumor heterogeneity should be exploited by using a combination of drugs effective against different cell subpopulations.
- The adjunct use of chemotherapeutic agents with hyperthermia is a promising possibility.
- Some drugs are potentiated dramatically by a temperature elevation of a few degrees.
- Local hyperthermia targets drug action.
- Sensitivity of individual tumors to chemotherapeutic agents with or without radiation may be assessed by the following:

  In vitro clonogenic assays
  Xenografts in nude mice
  Micronuclei in treated cells

# BIBLIOGRAPHY

Barranco SC: In vitro responses of mammalian cells to drug-induced potentially lethal and sublethal damage. Cancer Treat Rep 60:1799–1810, 1976

Barranco SC, Fluorney DR: Modification of the response to actinomycin-D–induced sublethal damage by simultaneous recovery from potentially lethal damage in mammalian cells. Cancer Res 36:1634–1640, 1976

Barranco SC, Humphrey RM: Response of mammalian cells to bleomycin-induced potentially lethal and sublethal damage. Prog Biochem Pharmacol 11:78–92, 1976

Barranco SC, Novak JKJ, Humphrey RM: Response of mammalian cells following treatment with bleomycin and 1,3-BTS(2 chloroethyl)-1-nitrosourea during plateau phase. Cancer Res 33:691–694, 1973

Barranco SC, Townsend CM Jr, Quraishi MA, Burger NL, Nevill HC, Howell KH, Boerwinkle WR: Heterogeneous responses of an in vitro model of human stomach cancer to anticancer drugs. Invest New Drugs 1(2):117–127, 1983

Belli JA: Radiation response and Adriamycin resistance in mammalian cells in culture. Front Radiat Ther Oncol 13:9–20, 1979

Belli JA, Piro AJ: The interaction between radiation and Adriamycin damage in mammalian cells. Cancer Res 37:1624–1630, 1975

Boice JD, Greene MH, Killen JY et al: Leukemia and preleukemia after adjuvant treatment of gastrointestinal cancer with semustine (methyl CCNU). N Engl J Med 309:1079–1084, 1983

Bonadonna G, Valagussa P: Dose–response effect of CMF in breast cancer. Proc Am Soc Clin Oncol 21:413, 1980

Carney DN, Winkler CF: In vitro assays of chemotherapeutic sensitivity. In DeVita VT Jr, Hellman S, Rosenberg SA (eds): Important Advances in Oncology, vol 1. Philadelphia, JB Lippincott, 1984

Chabner BA: The oncologic end game. J Clin Oncol 4:625–638, 1986

Chabner BA, Sponzo R, Hubbard S, Canellos GP, Young RC, Schein P, DeVita VT: High-dose intermittent intravenous infusion of procarbazine. Cancer Chemother Rep 57:361–363, 1973

Chan HSL, Haddad G, Thorner PS, DeBoer G, Lin YP, Ondrusak N, Yeger H, Ling V: P-glycoprotein expression as a predictor of the outcome of therapy for neuroblastoma. N Engl J Med 325:1608–1614, 1991

Cowan KH, Goldsmith ME, Levine R et al: Dihydrofolate reductase gene amplification and possible rearrangement in estrogen-responsive methotrexate-resistant human breast cancer cells. J Biol Chem 257:15079–15086, 1982

Curt GA, Carney DN, Cowan KH, Jolivet J, Bailey BD, Drake JC, Kao-Shan CS, Minna JD, Chabner BA: Unstable methotrexate resistance in human small-cell carcinoma associated with double minute chromosomes. N Engl J Med 308:199–202, 1983

Debenham PG, Kartner H, Simonovitch L et al: DNA-mediated transfer of multiple drug resistance and plasma membrane glycoprotein expression. Mol Cell Biol 2:881–889, 1982

DeVita VT: Cell kinetics and the chemotherapy of cancer: III. Cancer Chemother Rep 2:23–33, 1971

DeVita VT Jr: The James Ewing lecture: The relationship between tumor mass and resistance to chemotherapy—implications for surgical adjuvant treatment of cancer. Cancer 51:1207–1220, 1983

DeVita VT, Henney JE, Hubbard SM: Estimation of the numerical and economic impact of chemotherapy in the treatment of cancer. In Burchenal JH, Oettgen HS (eds): Cancer Achievements, Challenges, and Prospects for the 1980s, pp 857–880. New York, Grune & Stratton, 1981

DeVita VT, Henney JE, Stonehill E: Cancer mortality: The good news. In Jones SE, Salmon SE (eds): Adjuvant Therapy of Cancer II, pp xv–xx. New York, Grune & Stratton, 1979

DeVita VT, Oliverio VT, Muggia FM et al: The Drug Development Program and Clinical Trials Programs of the Division of Cancer Treatment, National Cancer Institute. Cancer Clin Trials 2:195–216, 1979

DeVita VT, Serpick AA, Carbone PP: Combination chemotherapy in the treatment of advanced Hodgkin's disease. Ann Intern Med 73:881–895, 1970

Elkiind MM, Kano E, Sutton-Gilbert H: Cell killing by actinomycin D in relation to the growth cycle of Chinese hamster cells. J Cell Biol 42:366–377, 1969

Endicott JA, Ling V: The brochemistry of p-glycoprotein-mediated drug resistance. Annu Rev Biochem 58:137–171, 1989

Fine RL, Patel J, Allegra CJ et al: Increased phosphorylation of a 20,000 M.W. protein in pleiotropic drug-resistant MCH-7 human breast cancer lines. Proc Am Assoc Cancer Res 26:345, 1985

Frei E: The clinical use of actinomycin. Cancer Chemother Rep 58:49–54, 1974

Frei E III, Canellos GP: Dose: A critical factor in cancer chemotherapy. Am J Med 69(4):585–594, 1980

Frei E III, Freireich EJ, Gehan E et al: Studies of sequential and combination antimetabolite therapy in acute leukemia: 6-Mercaptopurine and methotrexate—from the acute leukemia group. Blood 18:431–454, 1961

Gottesman MM, Pastan I: The multidrug transporter, a double-edged sword. J Biol Chem 263:12163–12166, 1988

Gottesman MM, Schoenlien PV, Currier SJ, Bruggemann EP, Pastan I: In Pretlow TG, Pretlow TP (eds): Biochemical and Molecular Aspects of Selected Cancers, pp 339–371. San Diego, CA, Academic Press, 1991

Hamburger AW, Salmon SE: Primary bioassay of human tumor stem cells. Science 197:461–463, 1977

Hutchinson DJ: Cross-resistance and collateral sensitivity studies in cancer chemotherapy. In Haddow A, Weinhouse S (eds): Advances in Cancer Research, vol 7, pp 235–350. New York, Academic Press, 1983

Hyde SC, Emsley P, Hartshorn MJ, Mimmack MM, Gileadi U, Pearce SR, Gallagher MP, Gill DR, Hubbard RE, Higgins CF: Structural model of ATP-binding proteins associated with cystic fibrosis, multidrug resistance and bacterial transport. Nature 346:362–365, 1990

Juranka PF, Zastawny RL, Ling V: P-glycoprotein: Multidrug-resistance and a superfamily of membrane-associated transport proteins. FASEB J 3:2583–2592, 1989

Lee IP, Dixon RL: Mutagenicity, carcinogenicity, and teratogenicity of procarbazine. Mutat Res 55:1–14, 1978

Ling V, Kartner N, Sudo T, Siminovitch L, Riodan JR: Multidrug-resistance phenotype in Chinese hamster ovary cells. Cancer Treat Rep 67:869–874, 1983

Ling V, Thompson LH: Reduced permeability in CHO cells as a mechanism of resistance to colchicine. J Cell Physiol 83(1):103–116, 1976

Madoc-Jones H, Mauro F: Interphase action of vinblastine and vincristine: Differences in their lethal action through the mitotic cycle of cultured mammalian cells. J Cell Physiol 72:185–196, 1968

Mitchell JB, Gamson J, Russo A, Friedman N, DeGraff W, Charmichael J, Glatstein E: Chinese hamster pleiotropic multidrug resistant cells are not radioresistant. NCI Monogr 6:187–191, 1988

Roizin-Towle L, Hall EJ: Studies with bleomycin and misonidazole on aerated and hypoxic cells. Br J Cancer 37:254–260, 1978

Rubin NH, Casantelli C, Maerk BG, Boerwinkle WR, Barranco SC: In vitro cellular characteristics and survival responses of human astrocytoma clones to chloroethyl-nitrosoureas and idanhydrogalactical. Invest New Drugs 1:129–137, 1983

Salmon SE: Application of the human tumor stem cell assay in the development of anticancer therapy. In Burchenal JF, Oettgen HS (eds): Cancer Achievements, Challenges, and Prospects for the 1980s. New York, Grune & Stratton, 1981

Salmon SE, Hamburger AW, Soehnlen BJ et al: Quantitation of differential sensitivity of human tumor stem cells to anticancer drugs. N Engl J Med 298:1321–1327, 1978

Sartorelli AC: Approaches to the combination chemotherapy of transplantable neoplasms. Prog Exp Tumor Res 6:228, 1965

Skipper HE: Reasons for success and failure in treatment of murine leukemias with the drugs now employed in treating human leukemias. In Cancer Chemotherapy, vol 1, pp 1–166. Ann Arbor, MI, University Microfilms International, 1978

Skipper HE, Hutchison DJ, Schabel FM Jr et al: A quick reference chart on cross-resistance between anticancer agents. Cancer Treat Rep 56:493–498, 1972

Skipper HE, Schabel FM Jr, Wilcox WS: Experimental evaluation of potential anticancer agents: XII. On the criteria and kinetics associated with "curability" of experimental leukemia. Cancer Chemother Rep 35:1–111, 1964

Tannock I: Cell kinetics and chemotherapy: A critical review. Cancer Treat Rep 62:1117–1133, 1978

Teicher BA, Lazo JS, Sartorelli AC: Classification of antineoplastic agents by their selective toxicities toward oxygenated and hypoxic tumor cells. Cancer Res 41:73–81, 1981

Trent JM, Buick RN, Olson S et al: Cytologic evidence for gene amplification in methotrexate-resistant cells obtained from a patient with ovarian adenocarcinoma. J Clin Oncol 2:8–15, 1984

Weinstein JM, Magin RL, Cysyk RL et al: Treatment of solid L1210 murine tumors with local hyperthermia and temperature-sensitive liposomes containing methotrexate. Cancer Res 40:1388–1396, 1980

*Radiobiology for the Radiologist, Fourth Edition,* by Eric J. Hall
J. B. Lippincott Company, Philadelphia © 1994.

# 18

# *Acute Effects of Total-Body Irradiation*

Diagnostic Radiology
Nuclear Medicine
Radiation Therapy

The effect of ionizing radiation on whole organisms is discussed in this chapter. Data on the acute radiation syndrome have been drawn from many sources. Animal experiments provide the bulk of the data and result in a significant understanding of the mechanisms of death after exposure to total-body irradiation. At the human level, data have been drawn from experiences in radiation therapy and studies of the Japanese survivors of Hiroshima and Nagasaki, the Marshallese accidentally exposed to fallout in 1954, and the victims of the limited number of accidents at nuclear installations, including Chernobyl. From these various sources the pattern of events that follow a total-body exposure to a dose of ionizing radiation has been well documented.

## EARLY LETHAL EFFECTS

**Early radiation lethality** is generally considered to be death occurring within a few weeks that can be attributed to a specific high-intensity exposure to radiation. Soon after irradiation, early symptoms appear, which last for a limited period of time; this is referred to as the **prodromal radiation syndrome.** The eventual survival time and mode of death depend on the magnitude of the dose. In most mammals three distinct modes of death can be identified, although in actual accidental exposures some overlap is frequently seen. At very high doses, in excess of about 100 Gy (10,000 rads), death occurs 24 to 48 hours after exposure and appears to result from neurologic and cardiovascular breakdown; this mode of death is known as the **cerebrovascular syndrome.** At intermediate dose levels, on the order of 5 to 12 Gy (500 to 1200 rads), death occurs in a matter of days and is associated with extensive bloody diarrhea and destruction of the gastrointestinal mucosa; this mode of death is known as the **gastrointestinal syndrome.** At low dose levels, on the order of 2.5 to 5 Gy (250 to 500 rads), death occurs several weeks after exposure and is due to effects on the blood-forming organs; this mode of death

has come to be known as **bone marrow death,** or the **hematopoietic syndrome.**

The exact cause of death in the cerebrovascular syndrome is by no means clear. In the case of both of the other modes of death—the gastrointestinal and the hematopoietic syndromes—the principal mechanisms that lead to the death of the organism are understood. Death is due to the depletion of the stem cells of a critical self-renewal tissue: that of the epithelium of the gut or that of the circulating blood cells, respectively. The difference in the dose level at which these two forms of death occur and the difference in the time scales involved reflect variations in the population kinetics of the two cell-renewal systems involved and differences in the amount of the damage that can be tolerated in these different systems before death ensues.

## THE PRODROMAL RADIATION SYNDROME

The various symptoms making up the human prodromal syndrome vary with respect to time of onset, maximum severity, and duration, depending on the size of the dose. With doses of a few tens of gray, all persons can be expected to show all phases of the syndrome within 5 to 15 minutes of exposure. Reaction might reach a maximum by about 30 minutes and persist for a few days, gradually diminishing in intensity until the prodromal symptoms merge with the universally fatal vascular syndrome or, after a lower dose, with the fatal gastrointestinal syndrome. Dose-response predictors are difficult to make because of the interplay of many different factors. Although it is not always so, a severe prodromal response indicates a poor clinical prognosis and portends at the least a prolonged period of acute hematologic aplasia accompanied by potentially fatal infection, anemia, and hemorrhage.

The signs and symptoms of the human postirradiation syndrome can be divided into two main groups: gastrointestinal and neuromuscular. The gastrointestinal symptoms are anorexia, nausea, vomiting, diarrhea, intestinal cramps, salivation, fluid loss, dehydration, and weight loss. The neuromuscular symptoms include easy fatigability, apathy or listlessness, sweating, fever, headache, and hypotension. All of these signs and symptoms are not seen unless the exposure is in the supralethal range. At doses that would be fatal to 50% of the population, the principal symptoms of the prodromal reaction are anorexia, nausea, vomiting, and easy fatigability. Immediate diarrhea, fever, and hypotension are frequently associated with supralethal exposure (Table 18-1). One of the Soviet firefighters at the Chernobyl reactor accident vividly described the onset of these symptoms as he accumulated a dose of several gray working in a high dose-rate area.

# THE CEREBROVASCULAR SYNDROME

A total-body dose on the order of 100 Gy (10,000 rads) of $\gamma$-rays and correspondingly less of neutrons results in death in a matter of hours. At these doses all organ systems will also be seriously damaged; the gastrointestinal and the hematopoietic systems will both of course be severely damaged and would fail if the person lived long enough, but cerebrovascular damage brings death very quickly, so that the consequences of the failure of the other systems do not have time to be expressed. The symptoms that are observed vary with the species of animal involved and also with level of radiation dose; they are summarized briefly as follows. There is

the development of severe nausea and vomiting, usually within a matter of minutes. This is followed by manifestations of disorientation, loss of coordination of muscular movement, respiratory distress, diarrhea, convulsive seizures, coma, and finally death. Only few instances of accidental human exposure have involved doses high enough to produce a cerebrovascular syndrome; two such cases will be briefly described.

In 1964 a 38-year-old man, working in a uranium-235 recovery plant, was involved in an accidental nuclear excursion. He received a total-body dose estimated to be about 88 Gy (8800 rads) made up of 22 Gy (2200 rads) of neutrons and 66 Gy (6600 rads) of $\gamma$-rays. He recalled seeing a flash and was hurled backward and stunned; he did not, however, lose consciousness and was able to run from the scene of the accident to another building 200 yards away. Almost at once he complained of abdominal cramps and headache, vomited, and was incontinent of bloody diarrheal stools. The next day the patient was comfortable but restless. On the second day his condition deteriorated; he was restless, fatigued, apprehensive, and short of breath and had greatly impaired vision; his blood pressure could only be maintained with great difficulty. Six hours before his death he became disoriented, and his blood pressure could not be maintained; he died 49 hours after the accident.

In a nuclear criticality accident at Los Alamos in 1958, one worker received a total-body dose of mixed neutron and $\gamma$ radiation estimated to be between 39 and 49 Gy (3900 to 4900 rads). Parts of his body may have received as much as 120 Gy (12,000 rads). This person went into a state of shock immediately and was unconscious within a few minutes. After 8 hours, no lymphocytes were found in the circulating blood and there was virtually a complete urinary shutdown despite the administration of large amounts of fluids. The patient died 35 hours after the accident.

The exact and immediate cause of death in what is known as the cerebrovascular syndrome is not at all fully understood. Although death is usually attributed to events taking place within the central nervous system, much higher doses are required to produce death if the head alone is irradiated, rather than the entire body; this would suggest that effects on the rest of the body

Table 18-1.
Symptoms of the Prodromal Syndrome

| NEUROMUSCULAR | GASTROINTESTINAL |
|---|---|
| **Signs and Symptoms to be Expected at About LD$_{50}$** | |
| Easy fatigability | Anorexia |
| | Vomiting |
| **Additional Signs to be Expected After Supralethal Doses** | |
| Fever | Immediate diarrhea |
| Hypotension | |

are by no means negligible. It has been suggested that the immediate cause of death is an increase in the fluid content of the brain owing to leakage from small vessels, resulting in a buildup of pressure within the bony confines of the skull.

## THE GASTROINTESTINAL SYNDROME

A total-body exposure of more than 10 Gy (1000 rads) of γ-rays or its equivalent of neutrons commonly leads in most mammals to symptoms characteristic of the gastrointestinal syndrome, culminating in death some days later (usually between 3 and 10 days). The characteristic symptoms are nausea, vomiting, and prolonged diarrhea. Persons lose their appetites and appear sluggish and lethargic. Prolonged diarrhea, extending for several days, is usually regarded as a bad sign because it indicates that the dose received has been more than 10 Gy (1000 rads), and it will inevitably prove fatal. After a few days, the person shows signs of dehydration, loss of weight, emaciation, and complete exhaustion; death usually occurs in a few days. There is no instance on record of a human having survived a dose in excess of 10 Gy (1000 rads).

The symptoms that appear and the death that follows are attributable principally to the depopulation of the epithelial lining of the gastrointestinal tract by the radiation. The normal lining of the intestine is a classic example of a self-renewing tissue; Figure 18-1 shows the general characteristics of such a tissue that are common in all forms of life, from plants to mammals. They are composed of a stem-cell compartment, a differentiating compartment, and mature functioning cells. The structure of the intestinal epithelium was described in some detail in Chapter 4 and illustrated in Figures 4-4, 4-5, and 4-6. Dividing cells are confined to the crypts, which provides a continuous supply of new cells; these cells move up the villi, differentiate, and become the functioning cells. The cells at the top of the folds of villi are slowly but continuously sloughed off in the normal course of events, and the villi are continuously replaced by cells that originate from mitoses in the crypts.

A dose of radiation on the order of 10 Gy (1000 rads) will sterilize a large proportion of the dividing cells in the crypts; a dose of this order of magnitude will not seriously affect the differentiated and functioning cells. As the surface of the villi is sloughed off and rubbed away by normal use, there will be no replacement cells produced in the crypt. Consequently, after a few days, the villi will begin to shorten and shrink, and eventually the surface lining of the intestine will be completely denuded of villi. The rate of cell loss and shrinkage depends on dose. It occurs faster at higher doses than at lower doses.

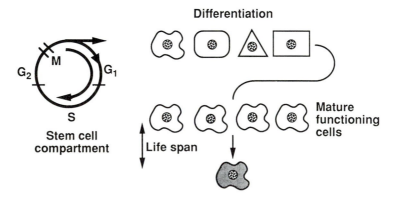

**Figure 18-1.** The classic self-renewal tissue. The stem cell compartment contains the dividing cells. Of the new cells produced, some maintain the pool and some go on to differentiate and produce mature functioning cells. When exposed to radiation, the "Achilles heel" is the stem cell compartment. Huge doses of radiation are needed to destroy differentiated cells and prevent them from functioning, but modest doses kill some or all of the stem cells, in the sense that they lose their reproductive integrity. Irradiation does not produce an immediate effect on the tissue because it does not affect the functioning cells. The delay between the time of irradiation and the onset of the subsequent radiation syndrome is dictated by the normal life span of the mature functioning cells.

At death the villi are very clearly flat and almost completely free of cells.

The precise time schedule of these events and the time required before the intestine is entirely denuded of cells varies with the species. In small rodents this condition is reached between 3 and 4 days after the dose of radiation is delivered. In large animals, such as the monkey, and probably in humans, too, it does not occur until 5 to 10 days after irradiation. All of the persons who have received a dose large enough for the gastrointestinal syndrome to result in death have already received far more than enough radiation to result in hematopoietic death. Death from a denuding of the gut occurs, however, before the full effect of the radiation on the blood-forming organs has been expressed because of difference in the population kinetics of the stem cell systems involved.

Before Chernobyl there was probably only one example in the literature of a human suffering a gastrointestinal death. In 1946, a 32-year-old white man was admitted to the hospital within 1 hour of a radiation accident in which he received a total-body dose of neutrons and γ-rays. The dosimetry is very uncertain in this early accident, and various estimates of total-body exposure range from 11 to 20 Gy (1100 to 2000 rads). In addition, the man's hands received an enormous dose, possibly as much as 300 Gy (30,000 rads). The patient vomited several times within the first few hours of the exposure. On admission, his temperature and pulse rate were slightly elevated; the remainder of the results of his physical examinations were within normal limits. His general condition remained relatively good until the sixth day, when signs of severe paralytic ileus developed, which could only be relieved by continuous gastric suction. On the seventh day, liquid stools that were guaiac positive for occult blood were noted. The patient developed signs of circulatory collapse and died on the ninth day after irradiation. At the time of death, jaundice and spontaneous hemorrhages were observed for the first time.

At autopsy, the small intestine showed the most striking change. The mucosal surface was edematous and erythematous, and the jejunum was covered by a membranous exudate. Microscopically, there was complete erosion of the epithelium of the jejunum and ileum as well as loss of the superficial layers of the submucosa. The duodenal epithelium was lost, except in the crypts, while the colon epithelium was somewhat better preserved. The denuded surfaces were covered everywhere by a layer of exudate in which masses of bacteria were seen, and in the jejunum the bacteria had invaded the intestinal wall. Blood cultures postmortem yielded *Escherichia coli*.

Several of the firefighters at Chernobyl, including those who had received bone marrow transplants, died between a week and 10 days after exposure, suffering from symptoms characteristic of the gastrointestinal syndrome.

## THE HEMATOPOIETIC SYNDROME

At doses of 3 to 8 Gy (300 to 800 rads), death, if it occurs, is a result of radiation damage to the hematopoietic system. Mitotically active precursor cells are sterilized by the radiation, and the subsequent supply of mature red blood cells, white blood cells, and platelets is thereby diminished. The time of potential crisis, when the number of circulating cells in the blood reaches a minimum value, is delayed for some weeks. It is only when the mature circulating cells begin to die off and the supply of new cells from the depleted precursor population is inadequate to replace them that the full effect of the radiation becomes apparent.

The concept of the 50% lethal dose as an end point for scoring radiation death from this cause has been borrowed from the field of pharmacology. The 50% lethal dose ($LD_{50}$) is defined as the dose of any agent or material that causes a mortality of 50% in the experimental group within a specified period of time.

Within a given population of humans or animals, there are many factors that influence the response of the individual to total-body irradiation. For example, the very young and the old appear to be more radiosensitive than the middle-aged individual or young adult. The female, in general, appears to have a greater degree of tolerance to radiation than does the male. Figure 18-2 shows a typical relationship between the dose of radiation and the percentage of monkeys killed by total-body irradiation. Up to a dose exceeding 2 Gy (200 rads), no animals die, whereas a dose of about 8 Gy (800 rads) kills all

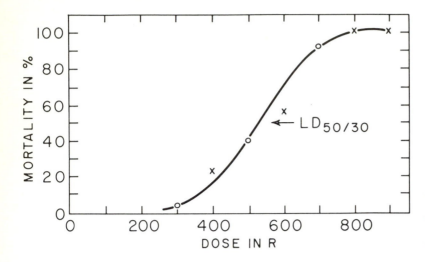

Figure 18-2. Mortality of rhesus monkeys at 30 days after a single total-body exposure to x-rays. (From Henschke UK, Morton JL: AJR 77: 899–909, 1957)

the animals exposed. Between these two doses, there is a very rapid increase in the percentage of animals killed as the dose increases, and it is a simple matter by visual inspection of the graph or by a more sophisticated statistical analysis to arrive at a precise estimate of the $LD_{50}$ dose, which in this case is 5.3 Gy (530 rads).

Humans develop signs of hematologic damage and recover from it much more slowly than all other mammals. The peak incidence of human deaths from hematologic damage occurs at about 30 days after exposure, but deaths continue for up to 60 days. The $LD_{50}$ estimates for hematopoietic death for humans are therefore expressed as the $LD_{50/60}$, in contrast to the $LD_{50/30}$ for animals, in which peak incidence of death occurs 10 to 15 days after exposure, and is complete by 30 days.

A dose of radiation close to the $LD_{50}$ results in the prodromal syndrome already described, the chief symptoms of which are nausea and vomiting. A symptom-free interval of time, known as the *latent period*, follows. This is, in fact, a very inappropriate name, since during this period the most important consequences of the radiation exposure, leading to its lethal effects, are in progress. About 3 weeks after the radiation exposure there is an onset of chills, fatigue, petechial hemorrhages in the skin, and ulceration of the mouth; epilation also occurs at this time. These symptoms are a manifestation of the depression of blood elements: infections and fever from granulocyte depression and impairment of immune mechanisms, bleeding, and possibly anemia caused by hemorrhage resulting from platelet depression. Anemia from red blood cell depression does not usually occur. Death occurs at this stage unless the bone marrow has begun to regenerate in time. Infection is an important cause of death, but it may be controlled to a large extent by antibiotic therapy.

As a consequence of the reactor accident at Chernobyl, 203 operating personnel, firemen, and emergency workers were hospitalized suffering from the early radiation syndrome, having received doses in excess of 1 Gy (100 rads). Of these, 35 had severe bone marrow failure and 13 of them died. The remainder recovered with conservative medical care.

## MEAN LETHAL DOSE ($LD_{50}$) AND BONE MARROW TRANSPLANTS

Studies of total-body irradiation have been performed on many species; a few $LD_{50}$ values are listed in Table 18-2, ranging from mouse to human. Such studies were popular and important in the 1950s and 1960s, supported largely by the military. In more recent years, total-body irradiation has been of interest from the point of view of bone marrow transplantation. This interest may stem from the treatment of radiation accidents, such as the Chernobyl disaster, or from the rescue of patients receiving cancer therapy

Table 18-2.
The LD$_{50}$ for Various Species From Mouse to Human and the Relation Between Body Weight and the Number of Cells That Need to be Transplanted for a Bone Marrow "Rescue"

| SPECIES | AVERAGE BODY WEIGHT (kg) | LD$_{50}$ TOTAL-BODY IRRADIATION (Gy) | RESCUE DOSE PER kg $\times$ 10$^{-8}$ | RELATIVE HEMATOPOIETIC STEM CELL CONCENTRATION |
|---|---|---|---|---|
| Mouse | 0.025 | 7 | 2 | 10 |
| Rat | 0.2 | 6.75 | 3 | 6.7 |
| Rhesus monkey | 2.8 | 5.25 | 7.5 | 7.3 |
| Dog | 12 | 3.7 | 17.5 | 1.1 |
| Humans | 70 | 4 | 20 | 1 |

*(Data from Vriesendorp HM, van Bekkum DW: In Broerse JJ, MacVittie T (eds): Response to Total Body Irradiation in Different Species. Amsterdam, Martinus Nijhoff, 1984)*

with total-body irradiation, radiolabeled antibodies, or cytotoxic drugs.

Many attempts have been made to estimate the LD$_{50/60}$ for humans based on the experiences at Hiroshima and Nagasaki, the total-body irradiation of patients with malignant disease, and the accidents that have occurred at nuclear installations. In a careful summary of all of the available data, Lushbaugh claims that the best estimate is around 3.25 Gy (325 rads) for young healthy adults without medical intervention. There does exist in the literature a surprising number of instances in which young men and women have received total-body irradiation up to a dose of around 4 Gy (400 rads) and recovered under conservative care in a modern well-equipped hospital. The LD$_{50}$ for humans quoted in Table 18-2 is the estimate of Vriesendorp and van Bekkum in the Netherlands. In addition to LD$_{50}$ data for a number of species, this table also shows estimates of the bone marrow rescue "dose" required in a bone marrow transplant, that is, the number of transplanted bone marrow cells that are required for a person to recover from a supralethal dose. Larger species are clearly more susceptible to hematopoietic damage than smaller species, as reflected by a lower LD$_{50}$. The bone marrow transplant experience indicates that this is due to a negative correlation between body weight and hematopoietic stem cell concentration, that is, the number of hematopoietic stem cells per body unit. The correlation between body weight and the number of

bone marrow cells needed for a rescue is illustrated in Figure 18-3 for a range of species, from mouse to human. Humans require 10 times as many bone marrow cells per kilogram of body weight as the mouse for a successful bone marrow rescue after supralethal total-body irradiation because of the lower concentration of hematopoietic stem cells.

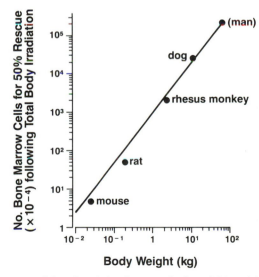

**Figure 18-3.** Correlation between body weight and bone marrow dose for 50% rescue (ie, number of hematopoietic stem cells required to be transplanted) following supralethal total-body irradiation. (From Vriesendorp HM, van Bekkum DW: In Thierfelder S, Rodt H, Kolb HJ [eds]: Immunobiology of Bone Marrow Transplantation, pp 349–364, Berlin, Springer Verlag, 1980)

# TREATMENT OF RADIATION ACCIDENT VICTIMS EXPOSED TO DOSES CLOSE TO THE LD$_{50/60}$

If the radiation exposure is known to be less than 4 to 5 Gy (400 to 500 rads), most experts recommend that the patient be watched carefully but only treated in response to specific symptoms, such as antibiotics for an infection, fresh platelets for local hemorrhage, and so on. Petechial hemorrhages in skin were commonly observed in the Japanese irradiated in 1945 but are not so commonly reported among young white persons exposed accidentally in nuclear power installations. Blood transfusions should not be given prophylactically because it would delay the regeneration of the blood-forming organs.

If the dose is known to have exceeded about 5 Gy (500 rads), then death from the hematopoietic syndrome 3 to 4 weeks later is a real possibility. In some countries, notably Germany, isolation and barrier nursing is recommended. The victim of a radiation accident is "sterilized" externally by repeated bathing in antiseptic solutions and then given a large dose of antibiotics. He is then isolated in an airtight plastic unit and fed sterilized food so that he does not come into contact with pathogens in the environment during the period in which his blood elements are depressed. It has been shown in animals that the LD$_{50}$ can be raised by a factor of about 2 by the use of antibiotics, and there is no reason to suppose that the same is not true in humans. The important thing is to avoid infection, bleeding, or physical trauma during the period when the circulating blood elements reach a nadir and give opportunity for the bone marrow to regenerate.

The area of most discussion and disagreement is the use of bone marrow transplantation. This technique was used on four Yugoslav scientists who were accidentally exposed in the 1950s to doses initially estimated to be about 7 Gy (700 rads). All of the grafts were rejected, but the exposed persons survived anyway, probably because later estimates indicated that the dose received was much lower, in the region 4 Gy (400 rads). In fact, many observers claim that the scientists survived in spite of the transplantations, rather than because of them! Figure 18-4 shows the depression and recovery of blood elements in the Yugoslav scientists and also in victims of the famous Y12 accident at Oak Ridge, Tennessee, who received about 4 Gy (400 rads).

In more recent years, bone marrow transplantation techniques have been greatly improved and are used routinely to "rescue" patients given supralethal doses of radiation for the treatment of leukemia or in preparation for organ transplants. In such cases, of course, the dosimetry is accurate and the doses are just enough to suppress the immunologic response.

Of the Chernobyl accident victims, 13 received bone marrow transplants (some matched for immune compatibility and some not). In addition, 6 received fetal liver transplants, but these patients all died early, some of gastrointestinal symptoms. Of the 13 who received bone marrow transplants, only 2 survived and 1 showed autologous bone marrow repopulation. There was, therefore, only one successful transplant that saved a life.

The situation was made difficult because the doses to which persons had been exposed were not known with any precision. After doses close to the LD$_{50}$, and certainly for higher doses, peripheral lymphocytes disappear before 24 hours and so it is not then possible to estimate total-body doses by counting chromosome aberrations in stimulated lymphocytes taken from peripheral blood. Since the US transplant team did not arrive in Chernobyl for some time, biological dosimetry was never possible for those exposed to higher doses. Consequently, some victims who received bone marrow transplants were already doomed to die of the gastrointestinal syndrome, having received doses in excess of 10 Gy (1000 rads).

In fact, the window of dose within which a bone marrow transplant is useful is very small. Below about 8 Gy (800 rads) an exposed person is likely to survive with careful nursing and an antibiotic screen since the LD$_{50}$ can be approximately doubled by such conservative measures. In such cases, therefore, a transplant is not necessary. Above about 10 Gy (1000 rads), death from the gastrointestinal syndrome is inevitable and so a bone marrow transplant is of no use. This highlights the narrow "window" of dose within which a transplant can be effective (about 8 to 10 Gy or 800 to 1000 rads). This is illustrated in Figure 18-5. The urgent need is to de-

## COMPARISON OF PLATELET COUNTS IN THE Y-12 PATIENTS AND IN 4 VICTIMS OF THE VINČA ACCIDENT

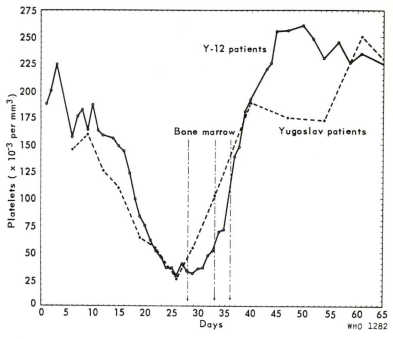

## COMPARISON OF GRANULOCYTE COUNTS IN THE Y-12 PATIENTS AND IN 4 VICTIMS OF THE VINČA ACCIDENT

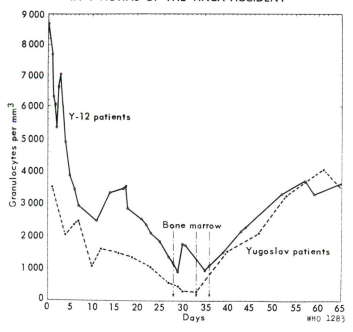

**Figure 18-4.** Depression and recovery of circulating blood elements in victims of the Y12 reactor accident at Oak Ridge, Tennessee, and four accidentally exposed Yugoslav scientists. (From Andrews GA, Sitterson BW, Kretchmar AL, Brucer M: Diagnosis and treatment of acute radiation injury, pp 27–48. Geneva, World Health Organization, 1961)

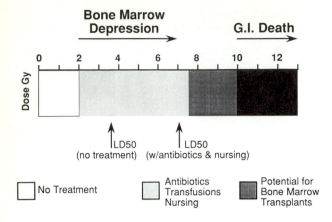

**Figure 18-5.** Illustrating the narrow window of dose over which bone marrow transplants might be useful following total-body irradiation. Up to about 8 Gy (800 rads) most persons would survive with antibiotics and careful nursing. Above about 10 Gy (1000 rads) most persons would die as a consequence of the gastrointestinal syndrome.

velop better methods of in vivo biological dosimetry, since chromosome aberrations in lymphocytes is not always useful in this dose range.

## SURVIVORS OF SERIOUS RADIATION ACCIDENTS IN THE UNITED STATES

Over the past 50 years there have been a number of accidents in which small numbers of persons employed in the nuclear program were exposed to total-body, or partial-body, irradiation. Most occurred in the early days of the nuclear program and involved criticality accidents. The number involved in the United States is about 70 workers in 13 separate accidents.

The long-term survivors have been exhaustively studied over the years, and the most recent report appeared in 1990. The medical history of these heavily irradiated persons mirrors that of any aging population. The expected high incidence of shortened life span, of early malignancies after a short latent period, and of rapidly progressing lenticular opacities has *not* been observed. The numbers in any group are small, but the several malignancies, cataracts and degenerative diseases that have been seen are no more than might be expected in a similar group of unirradiated persons of the same age.

The survivors of the 1958 criticality accident at the Oak Ridge Y12 plant are a case in point. Their blood cell counts are shown in Figure 18-4. A group of 8 workers, ranging in age from 25 to 56 years, received total-body doses of 0.23 to 3.65 Gy; 5 of them received doses above 2 Gy. Nevertheless, as of 1990, over 30 years after the acci-

dent, only 3 had died of cancer, and 2 of those involved lung cancer in very heavy smokers. Three of the workers who received the biggest doses of 2 or 3 Gy are retired and in good health.

This highlights the problem of detecting an excess cancer incidence in any small irradiated population. For example, if a group of workers receive a total-body exposure of 3 Gy, the biggest dose possible with suffering early death from the hematopoietic syndrome, the excess cancer incidence would be expected to be about 20%. (The cancer risk estimates of the Committee on Biological Effects of Ionizing Radiation [BEIR V] and the United Nations Scientific Committee on the Effects of Atomic Radiation [UNSCEAR] based on the Japanese A-bomb survivors amount to about 7% per sievert.) Thus, the biggest dose to which humans can be exposed and survive will just double the spontaneous cancer incidence. This is difficult to detect in a small group of persons and is likely to be masked by other biological factors. That is not to say that heavily irradiated persons are not at increased risk, but an excess cancer incidence can only be observed by a careful study of a large population.

## RADIATION EMERGENCY ASSISTANCE CENTER

In the context of radiation accidents, it should be noted that the Medical Sciences Division of the Oak Ridge Institute for Science and Education operates a Radiation Emergency Assistance Center/Training Site (REAC/TS). This is operated on behalf of the US Department of Energy.

REAC/TS provides 24-hour direct or consultative assistance with medical and health physics problems associated with radiation accidents in local, national, and international incidents. The resources of REAC/TS consist of expertise in cytogenetics for dose assessment, calculation of doses from internally deposited radionuclides, and laboratory facilities that include total-body counting capabilities. The regular telephone number is (615) 576-3131, and the 24-hour emergency number is (615) 481-1000.

## ► Summary of Pertinent Conclusions

- The prodromal syndrome varies in time of onset, severity, and duration.
- At doses close to the $LD_{50}$ the principal symptoms of the prodromal syndrome are anorexia, nausea, vomiting, and easy fatigability.
- Immediate diarrhea, fever, or hypertension indicate a supralethal exposure.
- The cerebrovascular syndrome results from a total-body exposure to about 100 Gy (10,000 rads) of $\gamma$-rays and results in death in 30 to 50 hours. The cause of death may be changes in permeability of small blood vessels in the brain.
- The gastrointestinal syndrome results from a total-body exposure to about 10 Gy (1000 rads). Death occurs in about 9 days in humans because of depopulation of the epithelial lining of the gastrointestinal tract.
- The hematopoietic syndrome results from total-body exposure to 3 to 8 Gy (300 to 800 rads). The radiation sterilizes some or all of the mitotically active precursor cells. Symptoms result from lack of circulating blood elements 3 weeks or more later.
- The $LD_{50}$ for humans (ie, the dose that would be lethal to 50% of the population) is 3 to 4 Gy (300 to 400 rads) for young adults without medical intervention. It may be less for the young or the old.
- Some persons who would otherwise die may be saved by antibiotics, platelet infusions, or bone marrow transplants.
- In animals, the $LD_{50}$ can be raised by a factor of 2 by appropriate treatment, including careful nursing and antibiotics.
- The dose window over which bone marrow transplants may be useful is narrow, namely, 8 to 10 Gy (800 to 1000 rads).
- Heavily irradiated survivors of accidents in the nuclear industry have been followed for many years; their medical history mirrors that of any aging population. A high incidence of shortened life span, early malignancies after a short latency, and rapidly progressing cataracts have *not* been observed.

## BIBLIOGRAPHY

Bacq ZM, Alexander P: Fundamentals of Radiobiology, 2nd ed. New York, Pergamon Press, 1961

Bond VP, Fliedner TM, Archambeau JO: Mammalian Radiation Lethality: A Disturbance in Cellular Kinetics. New York, Academic Press, 1965

Fry SA, Littlefield G, Lushbaugh CC, Sipe AH, Ricks RC, Berger ME: Follow-up of survivors of serious radiation accidents in the United States. In Ricks R, Fry SA (eds): The Medical Basis for Radiation Accident Preparedness. New York, Elsevier Science Publishing Co, 1990

Hemplemann LH, Lisco H, Hoffman JG: The acute radiation syndrome: A study of nine cases and a review of the problem. Ann Intern Med 36:279–510, 1952

Henschke UK, Morton JL: The mortality of rhesus monkeys after single total-body radiation. AJR 77:899–909, 1957

Karas JS, Stanbury JB: Fatal radiation syndrome from an accidental nuclear excursion. N Engl J Med 272:755, 1965

Langham WH (ed): Radiobiological Factors in Manned Space Flight: Report of the Space Radiation Study Panel of the Life Sciences Committee, publication No. 1487. Washington, DC, National Academy of Sciences—National Research Council, 1967

Lushbaugh CC: Reflections on some recent progress in human radiobiology. In Augenstein LG, Mason R, Zelle M (eds): Advances in Radiation Biology, pp 277–314, New York, Academic Press, 1969

Shipman TL, Lushbaugh CC, Peterson D, Langham WH, Harris PS, Lawrence JNP: Acute radiation death resulting from an accidental nuclear critical excursion. J Occup Med 3(suppl):145–192, 1961

Vriesendorp HM, van Bekkum DW: Bone marrow transplantation in the canine. In Shifrine M, Wilson FD (eds): The Canine as a Biomedical Research Model: Immunological, Hematological and Oncological Aspects. Washington, DC, Department of Energy, Office of Health and Environmental Research, 1980

Vriesendorp HM, van Bekkum DW: Role of total-body irradiation in conditioning for bone marrow transplantation. In Thierfelder S, Rodt H, Kolb HJ (eds): Immunobiology of Bone Marrow Transplantation, pp 349–364. Berlin, Springer Verlag, 1980

Vriesendorp HM, van Bekkum DW: Susceptibility to total-body irradiation. In Broerse JJ, MacVittie T (eds): Response to Total-Body Irradiation in Different Species. Amsterdam, Martinus Nijhoff, 1984

Vriesendorp HM, Zurcher C: Late effects of total-body irradiation in dogs treated with bone marrow transplantation. In Fliedner TM, Grossner W, Patrick G (eds): Proceedings of the Meeting of the European Late Effects Project Group of EURATOM, Report EUR 8078. Luxembourg, Commission of the European Communities, 1982

*Radiobiology for the Radiologist, Fourth Edition*, by Eric J. Hall
J. B. Lippincott Company, Philadelphia © 1994.

# 19

# *Radiation Carcinogenesis*

Diagnostic Radiology
Nuclear Medicine
Radiation Therapy

## DETERMINISTIC
## AND STOCHASTIC EFFECTS

If cellular damage occurs as a result of radiation that is not adequately repaired, it may (1) prevent the cell from surviving or reproducing or (2) result in a viable cell that has been modified, that is, suffered a change or mutation that it retains as a legacy of the radiation exposure.

The two outcomes have profoundly different implications for the person of whom the cell is a part.

Most organs or tissues of the body are unaffected by the loss of a few cells; but if the number lost is sufficiently large, there will be observable harm, reflecting the loss of tissue function. The probability of causing such harm will be zero at small radiation doses; but above some level of dose, called the threshold dose, the probability will increase rapidly with dose to 100%. Above the threshold the severity of harm will also increase with dose. Effects such as this, previously called nonstochastic, are now called *deterministic*. A deterministic effect has a threshold of dose, and the severity of the effect is dose related. Radiation-induced cataracts are an example.

The outcome is very different if the irradiated cell is viable but modified. Carcinogenesis and hereditary effects fall into this category. If somatic cells are exposed to radiation, the probability of cancer increases with dose, probably with no threshold. But the severity of the cancer is not dose related. A cancer induced by 1 Gy (100 rads) is no worse than one induced by 0.1 Gy (10 rads), but of course the probability of its induction is increased. This category of effect is called *stochastic*, a word that has been given a special meaning in radiation protection but, in general, just means "random." If the radiation damage occurs in germ cells, mutations may occur that could cause deleterious effects in future generations. Again, there is probably no threshold and the severity of hereditary effects is not dose related, although the probability of it occurring is.

The belief that stochastic effects have no dose threshold is based on the molecular mechanisms involved. There is no reason to believe that even a single x-ray photon could not result in a base change leading to a mutation that could cause cancer or a hereditary defect. For this reason it is considered prudent to assume that no dose is too small to be effective.

## CARCINOGENESIS: THE
## NATURE OF THE PROBLEM

Cancer induction is the most important somatic effect of low dose ionizing radiation. In sharp contrast to the case for the hereditary effects of radiation (see Chapter 20), information on risk estimates for leukemogenesis and carcinogenesis does not rely on animal data but can be based on experience in humans. There is a long history of a link between radiation exposure and an elevated incidence of cancer. Figure 19-1 is a beautiful picture of Marie Curie and her daughter Irene, who both are thought to have died of leukemia as a result of the radiation they received in their experiments with radioactivity. Figure 19-2 is a photograph of the hand of a dentist in New York who held films in patients' mouths for many years and who suffered malignant changes as a result. Quantitative data on cancer induction by radiation come from populations irradiated for medical purposes and exposed deliberately or inadvertently to nuclear weapons. Persons exposed therapeutically received comparatively high doses, and their susceptibility to the effects of radiation might have been influenced by the medical condition for which treatment was being given. Those exposed to $\gamma$-rays and neutrons from nuclear weapons represent a wider cross section in terms of health and also received a wider range of doses, including low doses. In both cases dose-rates were high and exposure times brief. There are a few groups of exposed persons to whom these generalizations do not apply. Examples include pitchblende and uranium miners who inhaled the radioactive gas

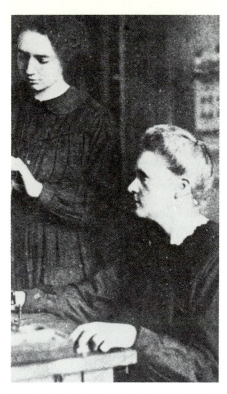

**Figure 19-1.** Marie Curie (seated) at work with her daughter Irene. Both are thought to have died of leukemia as a consequence of the radiation exposure they receive during their experiments with radioactivity. (Courtesy of the Austrian Radium Institute and the International Atomic Energy Bulletin)

noted in the uranium miners in the central Colorado plateau. In both cases the mines were poorly ventilated and there was a buildup of radon gas in the atmosphere of the mine; radon and its daughter products were breathed in by the miners, depositing atoms of radioactive material in their lungs. The intense local α-radiation was responsible for inducing lung tumors.

3. Bone tumors were observed in the radium dial painters. The painters were mostly young women who worked in factories where the luminous dials on clocks and watches were painted with a special paint preparation containing a radioactive material. The workers dipped their brush into the radium paint and used their tongue to shape the brush into a sharp point to paint the small dials on watches. As a result, some radium was ingested, which, because it is in the same group of the periodic table as calcium, was deposited in the tips of the growing bones. The intense α-irradiation produced bone tumors. There is also history of bone tumors in persons who, in the 1920s and 1930s, received injections of radium salts for the treatment of tuberculosis or ankylosing spondylitis.

radon and its daughter products over a prolonged period of time, patients injected with radium chloride for medical purposes, and persons who ingested radionuclides while painting luminous dials on clocks and watches with a paint containing radium. A large number of workers have been exposed occupationally, but they have so far yielded little useful quantitative data on cancer risk estimates.

The human experience of radiation-induced cancer may be summarized as follows:

1. Skin cancer was common in early x-ray workers, principally physicists and engineers who worked around accelerators before radiation safety standards were introduced.
2. Lung cancer was found to be a frequent problem in pitchblende miners in Saxony, who dug out the ore from which radium was extracted. In later years, lung cancer was also

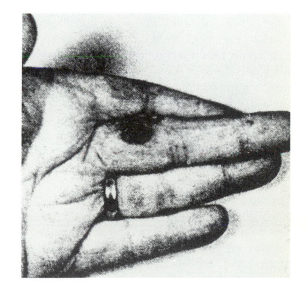

**Figure 19-2.** Hand of a dentist who for 35 years held x-ray films in place in patients' mouths. The thumb has been partially amputated. Damaged skin on the fingers has been replaced by grafts. The lesion on the finger is a skin cancer subsequently removed. (Courtesy of Dr. Victor Bond, Brookhaven National Laboratory)

4. An excess incidence of liver tumors was reported in patients in whom the contrast material Thorotrast was used. This contains radioactive thorium, which, when deposited in the liver, produced a small incidence of liver tumors by α-irradiation.

These early examples are interesting and historical but largely anecdotal. None of these examples involved situations that now constitute a public health hazard; these problems will never happen again, and the dosimetry in each instance is so uncertain that it is rarely possible to deduce any quantitative relationship between the dose of radiation involved and the tumor incidence.

More recent examples of the human experience of radiation-induced cancer and leukemia include the following:

1. The Japanese survivors of the A-bomb attacks on Hiroshima and Nagasaki are the most important single group studied because of their large number, the care with which they have been followed, and the fact that persons of all ages and both sexes received a wide range of doses. About 120,000 persons have been followed carefully, of whom 90,000 were exposed to significant doses of radiation. By 1990, there had been 6000 deaths due to cancer, of which about 400 were considered to be an excess incidence due to radiation. The weapons used on the two cities were very different. The one used on Nagasaki was of a type that would be expected to emit γ-rays with few neutrons and had been previously tested, so that dosimetry is based partly on measurements. The weapon used at Hiroshima was of a type never tested before or since, so that all dose estimates are based on computer simulations. The radiation from this weapon was a mixture of neutrons and γ-rays. In 1986, the dosimetry relating to the A-bombs was revised. Computer simulations indicated that the proportion of neutrons, especially at Hiroshima, was lower than previously thought, while the γ-rays doses at large distances were higher. The net effect was to substantially *increase* cancer risk estimates. The United Nations Scientific Committee on Effects of Atomic Radiation (UNSCEAR) report in 1988 and the report of the Committee on Biological Effects of Ionizing Radiation (BEIR V) in 1990 summarized the new estimates. The numerical values are discussed later in this chapter.

2. In Britain, from 1935 to 1944, some 14,000 patients suffering from ankylosing spondylitis were given radiotherapy to various regions of their spine to relieve pain. A small incidence of leukemia has been reported in these persons. Although the spondylitic series provides one of the largest bodies of data on leukemia in humans after exposure to x- or γ-radiation, and the dosimetry is quite good, it is far from ideal, because it lacks a proper control, consisting of patients with the same disease who did not receive x-ray therapy but whose treatment was otherwise the same. A possible contribution of carcinogenic drugs to the tumor incidence has also been suggested.

3. There is also allegedly an elevated incidence of leukemia in radiologists who joined learned societies before about 1922, before the introduction of safety standards.

4. Thyroid cancer has been observed in children who received radiotherapy for what was thought to be an enlarged thymus. The thyroid was included in the treatment field, and both malignant and benign thyroid tumors have been observed.

5. As recently as the 1950s, it was common practice to use x-rays to epilate children suffering from tinea capitis (ringworm of the scalp). Thyroid cancer from this practice was first reported by Modan and his colleagues in Israel, who treated a large number of immigrant children from North Africa in whom ringworm of the scalp reached epidemic proportions.

A comparable group of children in New York for whom x-rays were used for epilation before the treatment of tinea capitis show quite different results. There are *no* malignant thyroid tumors, although there are some benign tumors. There is, however, an incidence of skin cancer around the face and scalp in those areas also subject to sunlight. The skin tumors arose only in white children, and there were no tumors in black children in the New York series. In the Israeli series, no skin tumors were reported, but this may be because the children were all of North African descent and dark skinned.

6. Patients with tuberculosis, who were fluoroscoped many hundreds of times during artificial pneumothorax, have an elevated incidence of breast cancer. This was first reported in Nova Scotia, but the report has been confirmed by a similar study in New England. The doses are uncertain but must have been quite high, since some of the women involved had skin changes in the chest wall on the side frequently fluoroscoped. Patients who received radiotherapy for postpartum mastitis also show an excess incidence of breast cancer.

## CARCINOGENESIS IN LABORATORY ANIMALS

Radiation carcinogenesis in small experimental animals is well documented. A bewildering array of different dose–response relationships has been obtained. Figure 19-3 shows the results of a typical experiment in which the incidence of leukemia production is plotted against the dose of radiation absorbed. Many such curves have a characteristic shape: the incidence of malignancy increases with dose up to a maximum, which usually occurs between 3 and 10 Gy (300 and 1000 rads), to be followed by a subsequent decrease with further increases in dose.

The usual interpretation of such a shape postulates the concurrent presence of two different phenomena: (1) a dose-related increase of the proportion of normal cells that are transformed into malignant ones and (2) a dose-related decrease of the probability that such cells may survive the radiation exposure. Both of these phenomena are normally operating in the region of doses where data are available but to a different degree for various doses and different types of cancer. With this interpretation some of the cells that would otherwise show transformation are killed, so that the fraction actually seen as transformed is reduced at high doses.

It is important to note that tumor incidence does not necessarily continue to increase indefinitely with increasing total-body dose. A *qualitatively* similar pattern has been observed for a number of tumors in different animals, and there is every reason to suppose that the same would be true in humans if sufficiently detailed data were available for a given type of tumor. This

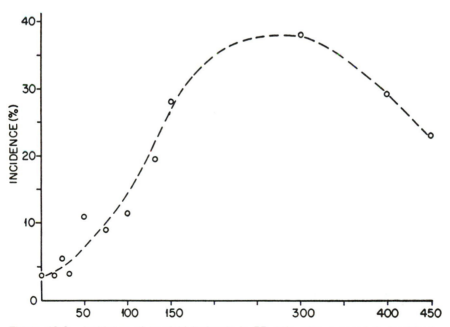

**Figure 19-3.** Incidence of myeloid leukemia in RF male mice exposed to total body x-irradiation. (From Upton AC: Cancer Res 21:717–729, 1961)

should be kept in mind when considering the human data.

## THE LATENT PERIOD

The time interval between irradiation and the appearance of a malignancy is known as the **latent period.**

Leukemia has the shortest latent period. Excess cases began to appear in the survivors of Hiroshima and Nagasaki a few years after irradiation, reached a peak by 7 to 12 years, and essentially disappeared by 20 years. Solid tumors show a longer latency than the leukemias of anything from 20 to 50 years. For example, an excess incidence of solid tumors is still evident in Japanese survivors exposed to radiation from the A-bombs in 1945.

As the Japanese data have matured, ideas concerning latency have changed. The concept of a fixed time interval between irradiation and the appearance of the malignancy has been replaced by the concept of "age at expression." Regardless of the age at the time of exposure, radiation-induced tumors tend to be expressed later in life at the same time as spontaneous tumors of the same type. Breast cancer in women is a good example. This suggests that while radiation may initiate the carcinogenic process at a young age, additional steps are required later in life, some of which may well be hormone dependent.

## ASSESSING THE RISK

Most data on carcinogenesis in humans involve relatively small numbers of persons who received relatively large doses of radiation. To use the available data to estimate risks as a function of dose, it is necessary to fit the data to a model. There are several reasons for this.

1. Data obtained at relatively high doses must be extrapolated to the low doses of public health concern.
2. No large human population exposed to radiation has yet been studied for its full life span, and so estimates must be projected into the future.
3. The best data pertain to the Japanese irradi-

ated by the A-bombs, and risk estimates based on this must be transferred to other populations that have quite different characteristics, including their natural cancer incidence.

There are two types of models that are conceptually quite different. First, the **absolute risk model** assumes that radiation induces a "crop" of cancers over and above the natural incidence and unrelated to it. This model was used widely in the past. Second, the **relative risk** model assumes that the effect of radiation is to increase the natural incidence **at all ages** subsequent to exposure by a given factor. Since the natural or spontaneous cancer incidence rises significantly in old age, the relative risk model predicts a large number of radiation-induced cancers in old age, too.

The model favored for the most recent assessment of the cancer risks from the Japanese A-bomb survivors is a **time-dependent relative risk model.** The excess incidence of cancer was assumed to be a function of dose, $(dose)^2$, age at exposure, and time since exposure. For some tumors, sex must be added as a variable, for example, in the case of breast cancer.

## COMMITTEES CONCERNED WITH RISK ESTIMATES AND RADIATION PROTECTION

There are two series of reports that analyze available data and come up with risk estimates for radiation-induced cancer. The first is the United Nations Scientific Committee on the Effects of Atomic Radiation (UNSCEAR). This committee reports to the General Assembly at regular intervals; the most recent report appeared in 1988. The second is the committee of the US National Academy of Sciences known as the Committee on the Biological Effects of Ionizing Radiations (BEIR). Reports appeared periodically the most recent (BEIR V) appearing in 1990. To a large extent these are "scholarly" committees, in as much as they are under no compulsion to draw conclusions when data are not available.

On the other hand, there are committees involved with radiation protection that cannot afford to be scholarly in as much as they must make recommendations whether or not adequate data are available. First, there is the International

Commission on Radiological Protection (ICRP). This commission was originally set up and funded by the first International Congress of Radiology. Over the years, the funding base of this commission has broadened and it has assumed the role of an independent self-propagating committee. At a national level in the United States, there is the National Council on Radiological Protection and Measurements (NCRP). This is an independent body chartered by Congress and funded from industry, government grants, and professional societies. The NCRP formulates policies for radiation protection in the United States, often but not always following the lead of the ICRP. The recommendations of the NCRP carry no weight in law but are almost always adopted and enforced by the regulatory agencies.

## LEUKEMIA

The incidence of chronic lymphocytic leukemia does not appear to be affected by radiation. Acute and chronic myeloid leukemia are the types chiefly responsible for the excess incidence observed in irradiated adults, while susceptibility to acute lymphatic, or stem cell, leukemia seems to be highest in childhood and to decrease sharply during maturation.

Two principal population groups are available for study:

1. Survivors of the A-bomb attacks on Hiroshima and Nagasaki
2. Patients treated for ankylosing spondylitis

## THYROID CANCER

The thyroid gland is an organ of high sensitivity for radiation carcinogenesis. Indeed, in view of the small mass of the gland, the sensitivity per cell must be higher than for any other tissue. The malignant tumors that have been produced have, however, consistently been of a histologically well-differentiated type, which develop slowly and can often be completely removed by surgery or treated successfully with radioactive iodine if metastasized; consequently, they show low mortality. It is estimated that about 5% of those with radiation-induced thyroid cancer will die as a result.

The principal population groups available for the derivation of risk estimates for thyroid cancer are listed below:

1. Survivors of the A-bomb attacks on Hiroshima and Nagasaki
2. Residents of the Marshall Islands exposed to external radiation and ingested iodine-131 from fallout after the 1954 testing of a thermonuclear device, in whom there was a high incidence of nodule formation and some thyroid cancer (ie, benign as well as malignant tumors)
3. Children treated with x-rays for an enlarged thymus
4. Children treated for diseases of the tonsils and nasopharynx
5. Children epilated with x-rays for the treatment of *tinea capitis*

Figure 19-4 shows the incidence of thyroid cancer per person-year as a function of thyroid dose.

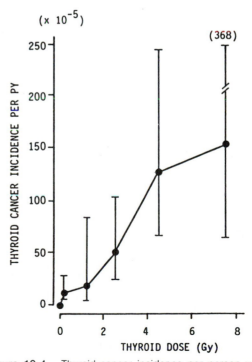

**Figure 19-4.** Thyroid cancer incidence per person year (PY) as a function of the radiation dose in the thyroid. Rates adjusted for sex, ethnicity, and interval after irradiation. Error bars represent 90% confidence limits. (From Shore RE, Woodard E, Hildreth N et al: JNCI 74:1177–1184, 1985)

# BREAST CANCER

Breast cancer may be induced with relatively high frequency by radiation. The cancer is of the type arising initially from duct cells but is commonly found to infiltrate breast tissue.

There are three principal exposed populations from which the risk of breast cancer incidence may be derived:

1. Japanese female survivors of the A-bomb attacks on Hiroshima and Nagasaki.
2. Female patients in a Nova Scotia sanatorium subjected to multiple fluoroscopies during artificial pneumothorax for pulmonary tuberculosis. There is doubt about the dosimetry, but the dose to breast tissue per fluoroscopy is estimated to be 0.04 to 0.2 Gy (4 to 20 rads). The number of examinations commonly exceeded 100, and in some instances women received more than 500 fluoroscopies; three patients, in fact, developed radiation dermatitis! This group of exposed women probably constitutes the most convincing evidence of the production of cancer by fractionated x-rays used for diagnosis. This Canadian study was later confirmed by the follow-up of patients discharged from two tuberculosis sanatoria in Massachusetts. These patients were examined fluoroscopically an average of 102 times over a period of years and subsequently were found to be 80% more likely to develop breast cancer than a comparable unexposed population.
3. Females treated for postpartum mastitis and other benign conditions. Patients typically received 1 to 6 Gy (100 to 600 rads) and showed an excess incidence of breast cancer compared with the general female population of New York state. A legitimate objection to the use of these data for risk estimates is the uncertainty as to whether postpartum mastitis predisposes to breast cancer.

The data for excess incidence of breast cancer in these populations is shown in Figure 19-5. A number of interesting points are immediately apparent. First, the data from the New York series of postpartum mastitis patients are so poor that they do not give any clue as to the shape of the dose–response relationship. Second, there is marked difference in the natural incidence of breast cancer in Japanese women, in whom it is low, compared with American and Canadian women, in whom it is high; nevertheless, in all cases incidence rises with radiation dose. Third, the data for breast cancer are reasonably well fitted by a straight line, giving more credence to the linear extrapolation than any of the other types of cancer.

# LUNG CANCER

Radiation is but one of a long list of carcinogens for lung cancer; cigarette smoking, asbestos, chromium salts, mustard gas, hematite, and asphalt derivatives have all been implicated, too. Risk estimates come from two principal sources:

1. Persons exposed to external sources of radiation, including the Japanese survivors and those with the ankylosing spondylysis.
2. Underground miners exposed to radon in the mine atmosphere. The naturally occurring deposits of radioactive materials in the rocks of the earth decay through a long series of steps until they reach a stable isotope of lead. One of these steps involves radon, which, unlike the other elements in the decay series, is a gas. In the closed environment of a mine, workers breathe in radon gas, and some radon atoms decay to the next member of the radioactive series, a solid, which is consequently deposited on the bronchial epithelium. Subsequent steps in the radioactive decay series take place in the lungs, causing intense α-irradiation of the localized surrounding tissue.

There is a clear excess of lung cancer among workers in the uranium mines of the Colorado plateau in the United States, the uranium mines in Czechoslovakia, nonuranium mines in Sweden, and fluorspar mines in Newfoundland. It remains difficult to separate adequately the contributory effects of radon and cigarette smoking in causing the cancers, since there are too few nonsmoking miners to form an adequate control group. Determination of the radiation dose is complicated by uncertainties inherent in the circumstances of irradiation. The average duration of exposure has usually spanned 15 to 20 years, during which standards of safety and ventilation have changed

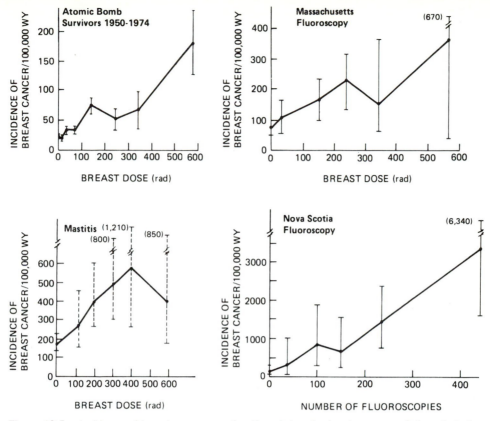

**Figure 19-5.** Incidence of breast cancer as a function of dose for four human populations that allow risk estimates to be made. Note that the natural incidence of breast cancer is low in Japanese women and high in American and Canadian women. (From Boice JD, Land CE, Shore RE, Norman JE, Tokunaga M: Radiology 131:589–597, 1979)

substantially. In any case it is no easy matter to estimate the dose to the critical cells in the basal layer of the epithelium of the lung from a knowledge of the radon concentration in the air that is breathed.

## BONE CANCER

There is some evidence of bone cancer induced by external x-irradiation in children epilated for the treatment of *tinea capitis* and in patients treated for ankylosing spondylitis. The numbers are small and the risk estimates poor. The largest body of data comes from two populations, both of whom ingested isotopes of radium that emit high linear energy transfer α-particles and that follow the metabolic pathways of calcium in the body to become deposited in the bone. The populations include

1. Young persons, mostly women, employed as dial painters, who ingested radium as a result of licking their brushes into a sharp point while applying luminous paint to watches and clocks. In this group there have been bone sarcomas and carcinomas of epithelial cells lining the paranasal sinuses and nasopharynx. None of these tumors occurred at doses below 5 Gy (500 rads); above this level, the incidence rose sharply, particularly the sarcomas. The radium in these paints consisted of the isotopes radium-226 and radium-228, with half-lives of 1600 years and 6 to 7 years, respectively.
2. Patients given injections of radium-224 for the treatment of tuberculosis or ankylosing spondylitis.

Three points need to be emphasized. First, the dose is made up of α-particles, which have a short range and deposit their energy close to the site where the isotope is deposited; α-particles are also more effective than x-rays by a factor of about 20. Second, osteosarcomas arise predominantly from endosteal cells, and the relevant dose for estimating the risk of sarcoma is the dose to these cells, which lie at a distance of up to 10 μm from the bone surface, rather than the mean dose throughout the bone. Radium-224 has a short half-life (3.6 days), and its radiation is therefore largely delivered while it is still present on the bone surface. This contrasts sharply to radium-226 and radium-228, which have long half-lives and consequently become distributed throughout bone during the period of its radioactive decay. The dose to endosteal cells from radium-224 is about nine times larger than the dose averaged throughout bone, whereas it is about two thirds of the mean bone value from radium-226. Consequently, it is difficult to compare data from the two groups of persons who ingested these very different isotopes of radium. Third, age at the time of exposure is an important factor in the development of bone cancer. For young persons and possibly also for those exposed in utero, the rapid deposition of bone-seeking radioisotopes during active bone growth might confer a higher risk of cancer than in adults. There is, in general, poor agreement among the risk estimates derived from the various groups of persons showing an excess of bone cancer, so that risk estimates must be very crude. Figure 19-6 shows the incidence of bone sarcoma in female dial painters as a function of activity of radium ingested. These data imply that a linear extrapolation from high to low doses would overestimate risks at low doses.

## SKIN CANCER

The first neoplasm attributed to x-rays was an epidermoid carcinoma on the hand of a radiologist, which was reported in 1902. In the years that followed several hundred such cases arose among physicians, dentists, physicists, and x-ray technicians, in an era when safety standards were virtually nonexistent. In most cases the onset of neoplasms followed chronic radiodermatitis and a long latent period. Squamous cell and basal cell carcinomas have been most frequently observed and occasionally a sarcoma of the subcutaneous tissues. Since the evolution of modern safety standards, epidermoid carcinoma has ceased to be an occupational disease of radiation workers.

Radiation-induced skin cancers are readily diagnosed and treated at an early stage of development, and there is a large difference between incidence and mortality. There have been no reports of an increased incidence of skin cancer among the Japanese survivors of the atomic attacks. It may be that the Japanese are less susceptible to radiation-induced skin cancer or that tumors are infrequent at moderate doses.

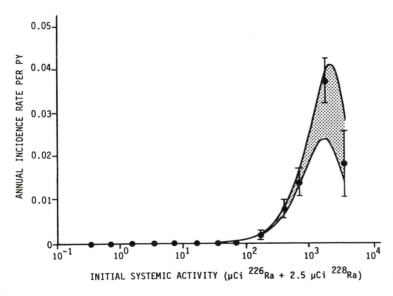

Figure 19-6. A semi-logarithmic plot of bone sarcoma incidence rate as a function of systemic intake for female dial painters employed before 1950, showing a dose-squared exponential fit. The shaded band indicates the range covered by the fitted function when the coefficients are allowed to vary by ± 1 standard deviation. (From Rowland R, Stehney AF, Lucas HF: Health Phys 44:15–31, 1983)

## OTHER TUMORS

The diversity of neoplasms reported in irradiated populations is such that radiation must be considered to be potentially carcinogenic for essentially all tissues of the body under the appropriate conditions of dose and host responsiveness. It does not follow, of course, that all types of tumors will be included in any given population in a practical situation. There are the special circumstances (eg, in the uranium miners or the radium dial painters) in which a specific type of tumor appears because the tissue of origin is irradiated from local deposition of an ingested radionuclide. This does not mean that a particular tissue was particularly sensitive but rather that it was preferentially irradiated. On the other hand, in the case of more generalized irradiation, some tissues appear to be more susceptible than others, the thyroid, breast, and lung being perhaps the clearest examples. A word of caution is in order at this point, however. The total carcinogenic potential of radiation delivered to a population will not be fully evident until all members of that population are followed up until their death. This has not yet been done, so that the picture that has emerged may be subject to change as time goes on. For example, in the 1950s it was thought that leukemia was the dominant malignancy to follow irradiation of humans. Because of leukemia's short latent period, it was the first to appear in the A-bomb survivors. As the period of follow-up has been extended, however, a whole spectrum of solid tumors has appeared, which were delayed because of their longer latencies but which are now far more numerous than the leukemias. By the time an irradiated population has lived out its life span, it is estimated that the ratio of solid tumors to leukemias will be in the range 4 to 6.

## THE DOSE–RESPONSE RELATIONSHIP FOR RADIATION-INDUCED CANCER

For acute doses of low linear energy transfer radiation, the most likely form of the relationship between dose to an organ and the probability of an induced cancer (Fig. 19-7) is an initial proportional response at low doses, followed by a steeper rate of increase that can be represented by a quadratic dependence on dose, followed finally by a flattening of the curve and a subsequent decrease with dose as cell killing of some target cells becomes important. A dose–response relationship having this general shape has already been shown to apply for leukemia in mice (see Fig. 19-3). There are no adequate grounds for assuming a threshold in dose; rather, the molecular mechanisms for cancer induction argue against a threshold.

In practice, the data available from the Japanese survivors cover a limited range of intermediate to high doses (illustrated schematically in Figure 19-7). Both the UNSCEAR 88 and BEIR V committees found that for solid tumors, the excess incidence appeared to be a linear function of dose. This is probably a consequence of the limited dose range over which data are available and the bending over of the curve at higher doses, also illustrated in Figure 19-7. At low dose rate, the dose–response relationship is essentially an extension of the initial portion of the complex

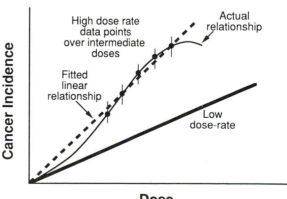

**Figure 19-7.** Graph illustrating the shapes of dose–response curves for radiation-induced carcinogenesis. For high dose and high dose-rate exposures, the actual relationship is likely to have a complex shape; excess cancer incidence is a linear-quadratic function of dose and bends over at high doses as cell killing of target cells becomes important. Since human data points are available over a limited dose range (and are of poor quality), they may be adequately fitted by a straight line, that is a linear function of dose. For exposures at low dose rate, the dose–response curve for excess cancer incidence is shallower and is an extrapolation of the initial region of the high dose-rate curve. (Drawn from the ideas of Dr. Warren Sinclair)

overall dose response relationship and is shallower than that characteristic of acute exposures.

## QUANTITATIVE RISK ESTIMATES FOR RADIATION-INDUCED CANCER

Despite a diverse collection of data for cancer in humans from medical sources, both the BEIR V and the latest UNSCEAR report elected to base their risk estimates almost entirely on the data from the survivors of the A-bomb attacks on Hiroshima and Nagasaki.

Table 19-1 summarizes the cancer risk estimates from the BEIR V and UNSCEAR reports. The two committees considered slightly different groupings of cancer sites, but in general the agreement between the two is more remarkable than the differences. The risk estimates for these principle tumor types that have been shown to be radiogenic differ only by a factor of 2 or 3. It should be noted that cancer risks in other organs or tissues are much lower or too low to be detectable.

As the data from Japan have matured, and more detailed information has become available, it is evident that the risk of radiation induced cancer varies considerably with age at the time of exposure. Table 19-2 summarizes excess cancer mortality in males and females, as a function of age at time of exposure. In most cases those exposed at an early age are much more susceptible than at later times. The difference is most dramatic for breast cancer in females; females exposed before 15 years of age are most susceptible, while women of 50 or more show little or no excess. There are exceptions to this general rule. Susceptibility to radiation-induced leukemia is relatively constant throughout life, while susceptibility to respiratory cancers increases in middle age.

## DOSE AND DOSE-RATE EFFECTIVENESS FACTOR (DDREF)

The Japanese data relate only to high doses and high dose rates because they are based on the A-bomb survivors. Both the UNSCEAR 88 and BEIR V committees considered that there is a dose-rate effect for low linear energy transfer radiations; that is, that fewer malignancies are induced when a given dose is spread out over a period of time at low dose rate than when it is delivered in an acute exposure. There are insufficient data, however, in the human to be certain of a quantitative value for the magnitude of the dose-rate effect; consequently, a range of 2 to 10 was proposed, based on animal data. For purposes of radiation protection, the ICRP recommend a dose and dose-rate effectiveness factor (DDREF) of 2 for doses below 0.2 Gy at any dose rate and higher doses when the dose rate is less than 0.1 Gy/h. This corresponds to the shallower straight line in Figure 19-7. It is, in effect, an

Table 19-1.
**Excess Cancer Mortality: Lifetime Risk/100,000, 0.1 Sv**

| | BEIR V (US Population) | | UNSCEAR 88 (Japanese Population) | |
|---|---|---|---|---|
| | Males | Females | | |
| Breast | | 70 | Breast | 60 |
| Respiratory | 190 | 150 | Lung | 151 |
| Digestive | | | Stomach | 126 |
|   system | 170 | 290 | Colon | 79 |
| Other solid | 300 | 220 | Other solid | 194 |
| Leukemia | 110 | 80 | Leukemia | 100 |
| Total | 770 | 810 | Total | 710 |

Table 19-2.
Cancer Excess Mortality by Age at Exposure and Site for 100,000 Persons of Each Age Exposed to 0.1 Sv (10 rem)

| AGE AT EXPOSURE | TOTAL | LEUKEMIA | NONLEUKEMIA | | RESPIRATORY | DIGESTIVE | OTHER |
|---|---|---|---|---|---|---|---|
| **Males** | | | | | | | |
| 5 | 1276 | 111 | 1165 | | 17 | 361 | 787 |
| 15 | 1144 | 109 | 1035 | | 54 | 369 | 612 |
| 25 | 921 | 36 | 885 | | 124 | 389 | 372 |
| 35 | 566 | 62 | 504 | | 243 | 28 | 233 |
| 45 | 600 | 108 | 492 | | 353 | 22 | 117 |
| 55 | 616 | 166 | 450 | | 393 | 15 | 42 |
| 65 | 481 | 191 | 290 | | 272 | 11 | 7 |
| 75 | 258 | 165 | 93 | | 90 | 5 | |
| 85 | 110 | 96 | 14 | | 17 | | |
| Average | 770 | 110 | 660 | | 190 | 170 | 300 |
| **Females** | | | | | | | |
| 5 | 1532 | 75 | 1457 | 129 | 48 | 655 | 625 |
| 15 | 1566 | 72 | 1494 | 295 | 70 | 653 | 476 |
| 25 | 1178 | 29 | 1149 | 52 | 125 | 679 | 293 |
| 35 | 557 | 46 | 511 | 43 | 208 | 73 | 187 |
| 45 | 541 | 73 | 468 | 20 | 277 | 71 | 100 |
| 55 | 505 | 117 | 388 | 6 | 273 | 64 | 45 |
| 65 | 386 | 146 | 240 | | 172 | 52 | 16 |
| 75 | 227 | 127 | 100 | | 72 | 26 | 3 |
| 85 | 90 | 73 | 17 | | 15 | 4 | |
| Average | 810 | 80 | 730 | 70 | 150 | 290 | 220 |

*(Adapted from Committee on the Biological Effects of Ionizing Radiation: Health Effects of Exposure to Low Levels of Ionizing Radiation. Washington, DC, National Academy Press, 1990)*

extrapolation of the initial linear portion of the actual dose response relationship.

## SUMMARY OF RISK ESTIMATES

In summarizing all of these risk estimates for practical purposes of radiation protection, the ICRP recommends the following figures, listed in Table 19-3. For a working population composed of both sexes, the lifetime risk of fatality from cancer is $8 \times 10^{-2}$ per sievert for high doses and dose rates, and $4 \times 10^{-2}$ per sievert for low doses and low dose rates. The comparable values for the whole population are a little higher because of the sensitivity of the young at $10 \times 10^{-2}$ per sievert for high doses and dose rates, and $5 \times 10^{-2}$ per sievert for low doses and dose

rates. Based on all of the assumptions inherent in the relative risk projection model, the ICRP has estimated that **on average** 13 to 15 years of life are lost for each radiation-induced cancer, but that again on average, death will occur at 68 to 70 years of age!

## SECOND MALIGNANCIES IN RADIOTHERAPY PATIENTS

The risk of second malignancies after radiotherapy is a subject not without controversy. Some investigators report that doses between 40 and 60 Gy (4000 to 6000 rads) to limited areas do not significantly increase the incidence of second cancers. In contrast, others report excess carcinogenesis when substantial doses are given

Table 19-3.
## ICRP Summary of Risks of Cancer Lethality by Radiation

|  | HIGH DOSE<br>HIGH DOSE RATE | LOW DOSE<br>LOW DOSE RATE |
|---|---|---|
| Working population | $8 \times 10^{-4}$ per Sv | $4 \times 10^{-4}$ per Sv |
| Whole population | $10 \times 10^{-4}$ per Sv | $5 \times 10^{-4}$ per Sv |

*(International Commission on Radiological Protection: Recommendations. Annals of the ICRP Publication 60. Oxford, Pergamon Press, 1990)*

to healthy organs. One of the reasons for the uncertainty is that radiotherapy patients are often at high risk of a second cancer because of their lifestyle, and this factor is more dominant than the radiation risk. Now that the combination of chemotherapy and radiotherapy is so commonly used, it is even more difficult to dissect out the risk of radiation alone. For this reason, two large studies reported recently are of particular importance, both of which involve large numbers of patients with carcinoma of the uterine cervix. These form an ideal study group since survival is good, accurate dosimetry is possible, chemotherapy is rarely given, and surgically treated patients are available for comparison. Boice and his colleagues reported on a study of 150,000 patients worldwide treated for carcinoma of the uterine cervix. Doses of the order of several hundred gray were found to increase the risk of cancer of the bladder, rectum, and vagina and possibly of bone, uterine corpus, and cecum, as well as the risk of non-Hodgkin's lymphoma. For all female genital cancer taken together, a sharp dose–response gradient was observed reaching a fivefold increase for doses more than 150 Gy (15,000 rads). Irradiation with several gray increased the risk of stomach cancer and leukemia. Cancer of the kidney was significantly increased among 15-year survivors. The situation concerning breast cancer was complex. For most cancers commonly associated with radiation, risks were highest among long-term survivors and appeared to be concentrated among women irradiated at relatively younger ages. Arai and his colleagues surveyed over 11,000 patients in Japan treated

for cancer of the uterine cervix with radiotherapy alone, surgery alone, or postoperative radiotherapy. They concluded that organs in the irradiated field, such as the rectum and bladder, showed an evident increase in the incidence of second cancers. The incidence of leukemia was also increased after radiotherapy.

It would appear, therefore, that when a sufficiently large number of patients are studied, with adequate controls, radiotherapy does induce a small but significant incidence of second malignancies, both in heavily irradiated tissues and in organs more remote from the target area that receive few gray. Radiation is a known carcinogen, and it should come as no surprise that elevated risks are seen after radiotherapy. It is noteworthy that despite the large number of patients studied, at most about 5% of all second cancers could be convincingly linked to the radiation treatment.

## INDUCED CANCER IN HUMANS AFTER "LOW" DOSES

The data used to derive risk estimates for radiation-induced cancer (principally the Japanese survivors of the A-bomb attacks and secondarily those exposed to medical x-rays) all relate to high doses and high dose rates.

There are numerous studies in the literature of human populations exposed to low doses and at low dose rates. These include the following:

- Studies of high natural background radiation in areas such as India, Brazil, or even Denver, Colorado.
- Occupational exposure such as the study of the Hanford workers in the United States or the employees of the Atomic Energy Agency in the United Kingdom.
- Studies of persons exposed to fallout from nuclear weapons testing or exposed as a result of living near nuclear reactors or full reprocessing plants.

Studies of this kind would be especially useful if they yielded unequivocal results, but all have one or more serious problems, such as

- Small sample size
- Inadequate dosimetry
- Lack of suitable controls

- Extraneous confounding factors
- "Positive" reporting

Some studies yield risk estimates for radiation-induced cancer that are higher and some that are lower than the estimates derived from the Japanese survivors for high doses and high dose rates. Some even yield negative values, implying a beneficial effect of low doses of radiation! The BEIR V committee considered all the studies carefully and judged that none were useful to supplement, much less replace, the current estimates.

## CHILDHOOD CANCER AFTER RADIATION EXPOSURE IN UTERO

In a widely publicized British study, Stewart and her colleagues reported an excess of leukemia and childhood cancer in children irradiated in utero as a consequence of diagnostic x-ray examinations involving the pelvis of the mother. An association between childhood malignancies and x-rays in utero was confirmed in the United States by MacMahon.

This has been a highly controversial topic. It is discussed in more detail in Chapter 21. Taken at face value, the data imply a high susceptibility to radiation-induced cancer during development in utero. A few diagnostic films may increase the natural or spontaneous cancer incidence by a factor of 1.5 to 2.0.

## MECHANISMS OF CARCINOGENESIS

During the past 2 decades, substantial progress has been made toward an understanding of the molecular genetics of cancer. The control of cell proliferation is the consequence of signals affecting cell division and differentiation. These signals may be positive or negative, and the acquisition of tumorigenicity results from changes that affect these control points. The conversion of a cell to a malignant state may result from the turning on (activation) of an oncogene or by the loss of a suppressor gene. There may be examples in which a combination of both is involved in the expression of the malignant phenotype.

## ONCOGENES

Oncogenes were first discovered from a study of retroviruses (ie, viruses whose genome is composed of RNA) that cause cancers in animals. The retroviruses contain modified cellular genes captured from the genomes of their vertebrate hosts. Cancer caused by a retrovirus, then, is mediated through cellular genes that have been mutated or changed. Normal versions of these genes (proto-oncogenes) are present in every mammalian cell and many have been shown to function in regulating cell growth. Infection of cells by these viruses leads to integration of the viral oncogene into the host genome, where it is expressed at high levels leading to overproliferation, the signature of cancer. Although a virus causes cancer by *inserting* an oncogene from its own genome into that of the cell, the mechanism of transformation by radiation and/or chemicals is to cause *changes* in a normal proto-oncogene indigenous to that cell, causing it to be activated. The notion of oncogenes helps explain why agents as diverse as radiations, chemicals, and viruses can all produce tumors that are indistinguishable one from another. This is illustrated in Figure 19-8.

The critical feature of oncogenes is that they act in a dominant fashion, which means that the presence of a single copy of the gene in the cell is sufficient to produce the transformed phenotype, even in the presence of normal copies of the same oncogene. Activated cellular oncogenes can often be detected by transfecting high molecular weight DNA from a tumor into a recipient cell line in culture, such as NIH 3T3 or $C_3H$ 10T½. A cell that picks up a DNA fragment containing an activated oncogene becomes transformed, detected by a loss of contact inhibition leading to piling up of cells to form a "focus," which is readily visible in the petri dish; cells from a focus form a tumor when injected into immune-suppressed animals.

About 50 oncogenes have been identified. Members of the *ras* family are found most frequently: H-*ras*, K-*ras*, and N-*ras*. Activated *ras* oncogenes have been identified in most forms of human cancer; the overall incidence is only 10% to 15% but tends to be higher in leukemias and lymphomas while lower in solid tumors.

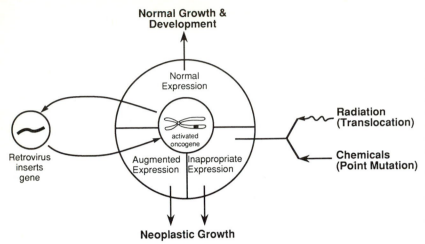

**Figure 19-8.** Diagram illustrating the way in which the concept of oncogenes provides a ready answer for how agents as diverse as viruses, radiations, or chemicals can all induce tumors that are essentially indistinguishable one from another. The retrovirus inserts a gene; a chemical may activate an endogenous oncogene by a point mutation; radiation may do the same by, for example, a translocation. (Adapted and redrawn from Bishop JM: Annu Rev Biochem 52: 301–354, 1983)

There are three principal mechanisms by which proto-oncogenes can be activated to produce a malignant cell:

1. A point mutation can occur, changing a single base pair, which subsequently produces a protein with a single amino acid change. For example, a point mutation in N-*ras* is found in the cancer cells of most patients suffering from acute leukemia.
2. A chromosomal rearrangement or translocation can occur, often placing a proto-oncogene next to a strong promotor sequence, leading to its overexpression, or producing a new fusion gene whose product acquires a new transforming activity. Ionizing radiations are effective at producing DNA breaks. These breaks may rejoin in such a way as to form a dicentric, which is almost always lethal to the cell. An approximately equal number of symmetrical translocations may occur, which are not lethal and are much more difficult to see except with the new techniques of chromosome painting. (Dicentrics and Translocations are explained in Chapter 2.) Translocations have been shown to be associated with several human cancers involving *myc* genes. For example, a translocation between chromosomes 2 and 8 is responsible for *myc* activation in Burkitt's lymphoma. Alternatively, the chromosome rearrangement may involve a partial deletion as in the activation of c-*fos*.
3. Gene amplification, in which many extra copies of a proto-oncogene exist in a cell, is associated with the activation of oncogene in several cancers. The presence of multiple copies of a proto-oncogene leads to its overexpression. Gene amplification of N-*myc* is characteristic of many neuroblastomas.

Table 19-4 is a summary of some known oncogenes and the human cancers associated with them, as well as the characteristic chromosomal changes seen.

Radiation readily causes oncogenic transformation in assays based on short-term explants of embryo cells derived from rodents or established cell lines such as NIH 3T3 or $C_3H$ 10T½ cells. In these assay systems, transformation can be shown to occur by direct damage to DNA. For example, DNA isolated from radiation-transformed $C_3H$ 10T½ cells was shown to transmit the malignant phenotype by transfection into recipient cells.

## SUPPRESSOR GENES

It was discovered in the 1970s that the tumorigenicity of tumor cells could be suppressed by hybridization with normal cells (Harris, 1971; Stanbridge, 1976). Specifically, the fusion of a normal human fibroblast with a HeLa cell suppressed the expression of the malignant phenotype of the HeLa cell (Fig. 19-9). These experiments, which preceded the notion of oncogenes by several years, led to the hypothesis that normal cells contain a gene or genes that can

Table 19-4.
Chromosomal Changes Leading to Oncogene Activation and the Human Malignancies Associated With Them

| ONCOGENE | CHROMOSOMAL CHANGES | HUMAN CANCERS |
|---|---|---|
| N-*ras* | Deletion (1) | Neuroblastoma |
| Blym | Deletion (1) | Neuroblastoma |
| *fms* | Deletion (5) | Acute nonlymphocytic leukemia |
| H-*ras* | Deletion (11) | Sarcoma |
| c-*abl* | Translocation (9-12) | Chronic myelogenous leukemia |
| c-*myc* | Translocation (8-14) | B-cell lymphoma |
|  | Translocation (2-8) | Burkitt's lymphoma |
| N-*myc* | Translocation (2-8) | Burkitt's lymphoma |
| raf | Translocation (3-8) | Parotid gland tumor |
| myb | Translocation (6-14) | Carcinoma |
| mas | Translocation (3-8) | Acute myelocytic leukemia |
| abl | Translocation (9-22) | Chronic myelogenous leukemia |
| sis | Translocation (9-22) | Chronic myelogenous leukemia |
|  | Translocation (8-22) | Burkitt's lymphoma |
| N-*myc* | Gene amplification | Neuroblastoma |
| neu | Gene amplification | Breast carcinoma |

**suppress** the neoplastic potential of tumor cells. The putative suppressor genes have been mapped to specific chromosomes, notably chromosome 11 in the example quoted, by analyzing which chromosomes were lost from those hybrids that reexpress tumorigenicity.

Later experiments, illustrated in Figure 19-10, involved the use of microcells, each containing a single human chromosome. By introducing these microcells into tumor cells by microinjection, investigators were able to demonstrate that the suppressor gene was carried on chromosome 11.

The human fibroblast–HeLa hybrid cells referred to above can be used as a basis of an assay for radiation induced transformation. When irradiated, a proportion of these hybrids express a tumor-associated antigen in a time-dependent manner, corresponding to the loss of the long arm of chromosome 11, which includes the suppressor gene.

# THE PARADIGM OF RETINOBLASTOMA

Retinoblastoma is present in the human population as sporadic or familial forms. The sporadic form is relatively rare at one in 20,000 children. Malignancy results from the absence of a functional copy of the retinoblastoma (Rb) gene. Unlike oncogenes, which act in a dominant fashion, the Rb gene is recessive-acting since its pres-

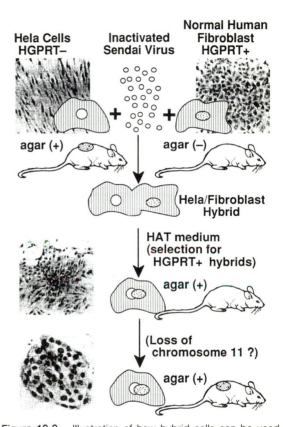

Figure 19-9. Illustration of how hybrid cells can be used to demonstrate the way in which tumorigenicity may result from the loss of a suppressor gene. HeLa cells are tumorigenic, while normal human fibroblasts are not. HeLa cells are transformed, as indicated by their ability to grow in soft agar, and tumorigenic, as evidenced by their ability to form tumors in immune-suppressed animals. Normal human fibroblasts do not show either property of malignancy. A hybrid formed by the fusion of a HeLa cell and a normal human fibroblast will grow in soft agar but does not form tumors; the malignant phenotype of the HeLa cell is suppressed by the normal fibroblast. If, however, chromosome 11 from the normal fibroblast is lost, tumorigenicity is restored, indicating that the suppressor gene or antioncogene is located on that chromosome. (Illustrating the experiments of Stanbridge EJ: Nature 260:17–20, 1976)

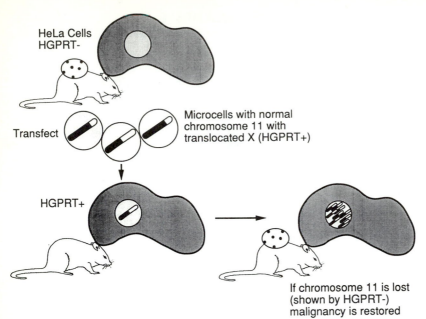

Figure 19-10. Illustrating of the effect of the suppressor gene on human chromosome II. HeLa cells are tumorigenic in nude mice. If a microcell is introduced containing chromosome II from a normal human fibroblast, the malignant phenotype of the HeLa cell is suppressed. If during culture chromosome II is lost, tumorigenicity is restored. The chromosome in the microcell is number II translocated with part of the X chromosome containing the HGPRT gene as a marker of the presence or absence of the chromosome in the HeLa cell. (Illustrating the experiments of Saxon PJ et al: Mol Cell Biol 5:140–146, 1985 and of Saxon PJ et al: EMBO J 5:3461–3466, 1986)

ence, even in a single copy, inhibits formation of the associated cancer. As early as 1971, Knudson had postulated that all types of retinoblastoma involve two separate mutations that are carried by all retinoblastoma tumor cells. In the case of sporadic retinoblastoma, he argued that both mutations occur somatically, in the same retinal precursor cell, that is, after conception during in utero life or early childhood, which then leads to a tumor in the absence of a functioning Rb gene. In the heritable form, in contrast, Knudson proposed that one of the two mutations is inherited from a parent and is therefore present at concep-

tion in all cells of the developing retina, whereas the second mutation occurs spontaneously. The mechanisms of familial and sporadic retinoblastoma are illustrated in Figure 19-11. By the early 1980s the location of the suppressor gene involved in retinoblastoma was shown to be on the short arm of chromosome 13, and by the late 1980s the gene had been cloned and sequenced.

The Rb gene itself has now been implicated in several other human cancers, which indicates that it may play a generalized role in growth suppression in a variety of tissues. For example, patients who are cured of familial retinoblastoma

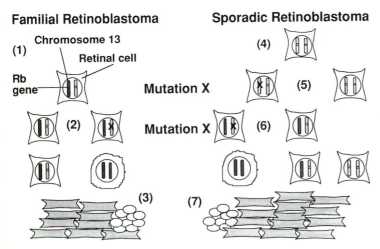

Figure 19-11. Rb mutations in familial and sporadic retinoblastoma. In familial retinoblastoma, one normal and one mutated Rb are inherited (1). Subsequent mutation in any retinal cell inactivates the remaining RB (2), leading to loss of growth control in a clone of tumor cells (3). In sporadic retinoblastoma, two normal Rb are inherited (4). First, a mutation inactivates one copy of Rb (5). A subsequent mutation within the same retinal cell inactivates the remaining copy of Rb (6), leading to loss of growth control in a clone of tumor cells. (Illustrating the concepts proposed by Knudsen AG: Proc Natl Acad Sci USA 68:820–823, 1971)

are at increased risk of osteosarcoma, small cell lung cancer, and breast cancer; while the loss of the Rb gene alone is sufficient for retinoblastoma, further changes in addition are required for the development of these other tumors.

Wilms' tumor turned out to be more complex than retinoblastoma. Wilms' tumor is a kidney cancer in children that can occur in unilateral and early-onset bilateral forms (ie, sporadic or familial in the same way as retinoblastoma). Initially, one suppressor gene was mapped to chromosome 11p13, but a second genetic locus mapping to 11p15 has been implicated. More recently, in three larger studies of familial Wilms' tumor, genetic linkage analysis excluded both 11p13 and 11p14, leading investigators to search for yet a third gene.

Table 19-5 summarizes the six suppressor genes considered to be most common and important at the present time and the wide range of human solid tumors associated with their loss or inactivation. There are likely to be many families of suppressor genes not yet discovered.

The most common cancer-related genetic change known at the gene level is the p53 mutation. The normal allele of this autosomal gene encodes a 53-kd nuclear phosphoprotein involved in the control of cell proliferation. Various mutant alleles with only single base substitutions in p53 code for proteins with altered growth-regulating properties. In addition, other alterations in p53 in human tumors have been detected, including deletions and rearrangements.

The spectrum of mutations observed in p53 differs among cancers of the lung, esophagus, breast, liver, and brain. These differences may reflect the variety of both exogenous and endogenous factors that cause human cancers.

One report has described a study of lung cancer in uranium miners exposed to high levels of radon and tobacco smoke. Of 19 patients studied, no mutations were found in K-*ras*, but nine p53 mutations, including two deletions, were found in 7 patients by direct DNA sequencing. None of the mutations were of the type most frequently associated with tobacco smoking, and none were found at the hot-spot codons described in lung cancer. The mutations appear to be characteristic of radiation.

## SOMATIC HOMOZYGOSITY

Both copies of a suppressor gene in the sporadic form of retinoblastoma and other solid tumors may result from two independent mutations in the two alleles, but in practice it occurs more often by the process of somatic homozygosity. This is illustrated in Figure 19-12. This process occurs for chromosome 13 in the case of retinoblastoma, chromosome 11 in Wilms' tumor, chromosome 3 for small cell lung cancer, and chromosome 5 for colon cancer. Most interesting of all, perhaps, is the case of astrocytomas in which somatic homozygosity is observed for chromosome 10 in grade II and III astrocytoma

Table 19-5.
## Currently Identified Suppressor Genes

| SUPPRESSOR GENE | SITE | CHROMOSOME | ASSOCIATED TUMOR |
|---|---|---|---|
| p-105 Rb | Nucleus | 13q | Retinoblastoma |
| WT | Nucleus | Three different loci, llp | Wilms' tumor |
| NFI | Cytoplasm | 17q | Neurofibroma, sarcoma |
| FAP | ? | 5q | Familial adenomatosis polyposis |
| p-53 | Nucleus | 17p | Breast cancer, small cell lung cancer, cervical cancer, bladder cancer |
| DCC | Cell surface | 18q | Colon cancer |

## Somatic Homozygosity

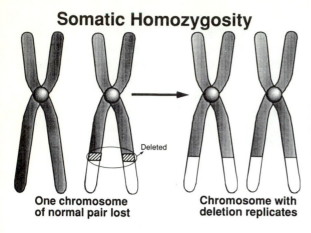

**One chromosome of normal pair lost**

**Chromosome with deletion replicates**

Deleted

**Figure 19-12.** The process of somatic homozygosity. In a normal cell, there are two copies of each chromosome, one inherited from each parent. For a given suppressor gene to be inactivated, the copy must be lost from *both* chromosomes. This could, of course, occur by independent deletions from the two chromosomes, but in practice it is more common for a single deletion to occur in one chromosome while the second chromosome is lost completely. The remaining chromosome, with the deletion, then replicates. The cell is thus homozygous, rather than heterozygous, for that chromosome.

and for *both* chromosomes 10 and 17 for grade IV glioblastoma.

The steps appear to be as follows: one chromosome of a pair is lost, a deletion then occurs in the remaining chromosome, and the deleted chromosome replicates. Instead of having one allele from each parent, the cell has both alleles from *one* parent, with a vital piece containing the suppressor gene missing.

## COOPERATING GENES

There is much evidence in vivo that carcinogenesis is a multistep process. At least two steps are involved, often described operationally as *initia-*

*tion* and *promotion*. These defined steps may be followed by a less well-defined period, which itself may be made up of several different components. At the cellular level, transformation experiments support the notion of multiple steps.

In general *two* cooperating oncogenes are required to result in the expression of the malignant phenotype. For example, as illustrated in Figure 19-13 the *ras* oncogene alone will not elicit transformation when transfected into a primary rat fibroblast but will produce transformation in an established cell line (such as NIH 3T3) that is already immortalized. Although neither transfection of *myc* or *ras* alone will lead to transformation of a primary embryonic cell line, the combination of *myc* and *ras* will produce on-

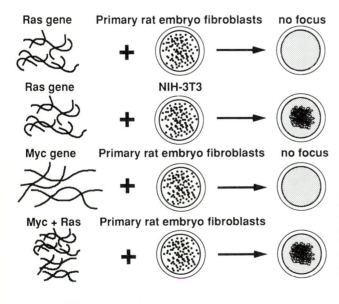

Ras gene + Primary rat embryo fibroblasts → no focus

Ras gene + NIH-3T3 →

Myc gene + Primary rat embryo fibroblasts → no focus

Myc + Ras + Primary rat embryo fibroblasts →

**Figure 19-13.** Schematic illustration of the cotransfection studies that showed that cooperation between the *ras* and *myc* genes is required to transform primary nonimmortalized rat embryo fibroblasts, whereas the *ras* gene is responsible for the morphologic changes associated with oncogenic transformation. (Illustrating the experiments of Land H, Pavada LF, Weinberg RA: Nature 304:596–602, 1983)

cogenic transformation in a primary embryonic fibroblast cell line. The interpretation of this experiment is that in the in vitro transformation assays, the *myc* oncogene confers immortality, while the *ras* oncogene confers the loss of contact inhibition and the morphologic changes associated with the neoplastic state.

Cooperating oncogenes activate distinct signal pathways, and it is generally found that oncogene products that act in the nucleus (typically immortalizing) cooperate best with those that act in the cytoplasm (typically cause loss of contact inhibition). It should also be mentioned here that activated *ras* may also cooperate with an inactivated p53 suppressor gene to transform primary rat fibroblasts.

Cancer has long been thought of as a multistep process, described operationally in terms of *initiation, promotion,* and *progression.* In at least one human malignancy, namely, colon cancer, Vogelstein and his colleagues have documented multiple steps at the chromosomal and molecular level between the normal epithelium and a carcinoma with metastatic potential. These steps, illustrated in Figure 19-14, involve the activation of oncogenes, the loss of suppressor genes, as well as less specific chromosomal changes. It is not clear which of these events are causative and necessary and which are part of a cascade of events resulting from genomic instability.

## ATAXIA-TELANGIECTASIA AND CANCER

There are a number of genetically transmitted repair deficiencies in humans. One of the most well-known and most extensively studied is **ataxia-telangiectasia** (AT).

Homozygotes have distinctive neurologic disorders and oculocutaneous telangiectasia. It has long been known that the AT gene predisposes those carrying it to cancer with a risk 61 to 184 times higher than the general population. The AT gene is also associated with an unusual sensitivity to ionizing radiation. Homozygotes suffer devastating tissue necrosis when exposed to conventional radiotherapy, and cultured cells from homozygotes are more sensitive than control cells to x-rays by a factor of about 3. What has long been debated is whether heterozygotes, persons carrying one copy of the gene, are likewise radiosensitive and susceptible to cancer. Although on average cells cultured from AT heterozygotes are more sensitive to x- or γ-rays, there is so much overlap with the wide range of sensitivities of normal cells that radiosensitivity itself cannot be used as a means of identifying a heterozygote in any individual case.

Striking evidence of the increased sensitivity to cancer of AT heterozygotes comes from a review by Swift of 161 families affected by AT. In this prospective study, new cases of cancers were

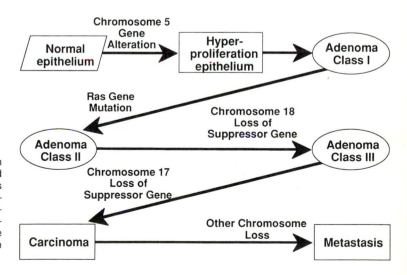

**Figure 19-14.** Cancer has long been thought to be a multistep process and has been described in operational terms such as *initiation, promotion,* and *progression.* In at least one human malignancy, namely, colon cancer, the molecular events during the progress of the disease have been identified. (Based on the work of Vogelstein)

**Table 19-6.**
**New Cases of Cancer Occurring at Age 20 or Older During Follow-up of 161 Families Affected by Ataxia-Telangiectasia**

| PRIMARY SITE | BLOOD RELATIVES | | SPOUSES |
| | Obligate Heterozygotes | All Others | |
| --- | --- | --- | --- |
| Breast | 5 | 18 | 3 |
| All other | 13 | 55 | 16 |
| Total | 18 | 73 | 19 |

$$91/1599 = 5.7\% \qquad 19/821 = 2.3\%$$

*(From Swift M, Morrell D, Massey RB, Chase CL: N Engl J Med 325:1831–1836, 1991)*

**Table 19-8.**
**Breast Cancer and Radiation in 161 Families With Ataxia-Telangiectasia**

| | BLOOD RELATIVES WITH CANCER | BLOOD RELATIVES WITHOUT CANCER |
| --- | --- | --- |
| **Number** | 19 | 57 |
| **Percent With Radiation History** [*] | 10/19 = 53% | 11/57 = 19% |

[*]*Radiation history includes fluoroscopy of chest, back, or abdomen; therapeutic radiation; and occupational exposure.*
*(From Swift M, Morrell D, Massey RB, Chase CL: N Engl J Med 325:1831–1836, 1991)*

observed in blood relatives of AT sufferers (of whom about half may be AT heterozygotes), in those who are definite heterozygotes (obligates), and in spouses who were assumed to be normal but who lived in the same environment. The crude results are shown in Table 19-6 and converted to rate ratios in Table 19-7. It is quite clear that heterozygotes are at an increased risk for all types of cancer, with breast cancer in women being prominent. Although AT heterozygotes may comprise only 1% to 3% of a white population, these persons may account for a substantial proportion (9% to 18%) of *all* breast cancer in younger women.

This extensive study also divided blood relatives of AT homozygotes into those with, and those without, a "radiation history." A radiation history was loosely interpreted as fluoroscopy of the chest, back, or abdomen, therapeutic irradiation, or occupational exposure. Table 19-8 shows the results of the survey. Fifty-three percent of blood relatives with cancer had a radiation history compared with 19% of those without cancer.

From these data the study purported to show that AT heterozygotes are very sensitive to radiation-induced cancer. A case-control study of this kind does not provide proof of this, but nevertheless the possibility exists. It is a challenging and sobering thought to the diagnostic radiologists that a proportion of the women routinely screened by mammography may be exquisitely sensitive to radiation-induced carcinogenesis because of repair deficiencies associated with

**Table 19-7.**
**Rate Ratios and Estimates of the Risk of Cancer Among Persons 20 to 79 Years Old in Families Affected by Ataxia-Telangiectasia**

| SEX AND TYPE OF CANCER | RATE RATIOS | | ESTIMATED RISK IN HETEROZYGOTES |
| | All Blood Relatives | Obligate Heterozygotes[*] | |
| --- | --- | --- | --- |
| Men, all types | 2.5 | 3.9 | 3.8 |
| Women | | | |
| All types | 2.1[*] | 2.7[*] | 3.5[*] |
| Breast | 3.3[*] | 3.8[*] | 5.1 |

[*]*Estimated risk refers to cases of cancer per 1000 person-years (From Swift M, Morrell D, Massey RB, Chase CL: N Engl J Med 325:1831–1836, 1991)*

being AT heterozygotes. This study has triggered a renewed debate concerning the use of mammography to screen for breast cancer because of the risk of inducing cancer by the x-rays in this sensitive group of women and highlights the urgent need to identify and sequence the defective gene involved in AT so that heterozygotes in the population can be identified.

## ► *Summary of Pertinent Conclusions*

- Radiation carcinogenesis is a **stochastic** effect; that is, the probability of an effect increases with dose, with no dose threshold, but the severity of the effect is not dose related. Hereditary effects are also stochastic.
- A **deterministic** effect has a threshold of dose, and the severity of the effect is dose related. Cataracts are an example of a deterministic effect.
- The human experience of radiation-induced carcinogenesis includes the survivors of the A-bomb attacks on Hiroshima and Nagasaki, patients exposed to medical irradiation, and early workers exposed occupationally. Some examples are listed below:

  Leukemia and solid tumors in Japanese survivors of the A-bomb
  Leukemia in patients irradiated for ankylosing spondylitis
  Thyroid cancer in children irradiated for enlarged thymus and children epilated for tinea capitis
  Breast cancer in patients treated with x-rays for postpartum mastitis and patients fluoroscoped repeatedly during management of tuberculosis
  Lung cancer in uranium miners
  Bone cancer in dial painters who ingested radium and patients who had injections of radium for tuberculosis or ankylosing spondylitis

- Latency refers to the time interval between irradiation and the appearance of the malignancy.
- The shortest latency is for leukemia (5 to 7 years). For solid tumors, the latency may extend for 45 years or more.
- Regardless of the age at exposure, radiation-induced malignancies tend to appear at the same age as spontaneous malignancies of the same type.
- To determine risk estimates for radiation-induced cancer from observed data (the Japanese A-bomb survivors), a model must be assumed because

  1. Data must be projected out to a full life-span, since no exposed population has yet lived out its life-span
  2. Data must be extrapolated from high to low doses
  3. Risks must be "transferred" from (for example) a Japanese to Western population with different natural cancer rates.

- There are two principal models. The **absolute risk model** assumes that radiation produced a discrete "crop" of cancers, over and above the spontaneous level and unrelated to the spontaneous level. The **relative risk model** assumes that radiation increases the spontaneous incidence by a factor. Since the natural cancer incidence increases with age, this model predicts a large number of excess cancers appearing late in life after irradiation.
- The most recent reassessment of radiation-induced cancer risks by the BEIR V committee was based on a time-related relative risk model. Ex-

*(continued)*

► **Summary of Pertinent Conclusions** *(Continued)*

cess cancer mortality was assumed to depend on dose, (dose)$^2$, age at exposure, time since exposure, and, for some cancers, sex.

- For solid tumors, excess mortality was found to be a linear function of dose. Leukemia best fitted a linear-quadratic function of dose.
- Based on reports of the UNSCEAR 88 and BEIR V committees, the ICRP suggests a risk estimate of excess cancer mortality in a working population of $8 \times 10^{-4}$ per sievert for high doses and high dose rates, and $4 \times 10^{-4}$ per sievert for low doses and low dose rates.
- For the general population, slightly higher risks apply because of the increased susceptibility of the young. The estimates are $10 \times 10^{-4}$ per sievert for high doses and dose rates and $5 \times 10^{-4}$ per sievert for low doses and dose rates.
- The ICRP estimates that, *on average*, 13 to 15 years of life are lost for each radiation-induced cancer and that death will occur at age 68 to 70 years.
- Studies of hundreds of thousands of radiotherapy patients show an incidence of second malignancies of at most 5%. Such tumors may occur in heavily irradiated tissues or in organs more remote from the target area.
- Irradiation in utero by diagnostic x-rays appears to increase the spontaneous incidence of leukemia and childhood cancers in children up to 15 years of age by a factor of 1.5 to 2.

### Mechanisms of Carcinogenesis

- Cell proliferation and differentiation is under positive and negative controls.
- Tumorigenesis may result from the activation of an oncogene, the loss of a suppressor gene, or a combination of both.
- Proto-oncogenes are present in every cell, and many have been shown to function in regulating cell growth or differentiation.
- Radiation or chemicals may activate a normal proto-oncogene indigenous to the cell. Alternatively a retrovirus may insert an activated oncogene from its own genome into that of the mammalian cell.
- Oncogenes act in a dominant fashion; that is, the presence of a single copy is sufficient to produce the malignant phenotype.
- About 50 oncogenes have been identified so far. Activated *ras* oncogenes have been identified in 10% to 15% of human cancers but tend to be higher in leukemias and lymphomas and lower in solid tumors.
- Proto-oncogenes can be activated by three mechanisms: (1) a point mutation, (2) a chromosomal rearrangement such as a translocation, and (3) gene amplification.
- Suppressor genes are recessive; that is, both copies must be lost or inactivated for the malignant phenotype to be expressed.
- Retinoblastoma was the first human tumor to be shown to be associated with the loss of a suppressor gene.
- At present there are six principal suppressor genes involved in a wide spectrum of human cancers.
- Mutations in the p53 gene is the most common expression of a suppressor gene.

*(continued)*

► **Summary of Pertinent Conclusions** *(Continued)*

- In general, two cooperating oncogenes are required to result in the expression of the malignant phenotype. Oncogene products that act in the nucleus (causing immortality) cooperate best with those that act in the cytoplasm (causing loss of contact inhibition). For example, *ras* plus *myc* causes transformation of primary rat fibroblasts, as does *ras* plus an inactivated p53 suppressor gene.

- A number of repair-deficient syndromes have been identified in the human; ataxia-telangiectasia (AT) is the most well known.

- AT homozygotes are sensitive to cell killing by radiation. They also show a very high spontaneous incidence of cancer.

- AT heterozygotes may be, on average, more sensitive to cell killing than normal, but there is too much overlap for persons to be diagnosed on this basis.

- AT heterozygotes show an elevated incidence of spontaneous cancer, particularly breast cancer.

- AT heterozygotes comprise only 1% of the population; they may account for 20% of breast cancer especially in younger women. It has been *suggested,* but not proven, that AT heterozygotes may be sensitive to radiation-induced cancer. This raises concerns about x-ray screening programs such as mammography.

# BIBLIOGRAPHY

Alberts B, Broy D, Lewis J, Raff M, Roberts K, Watson JD (eds): The Molecular Biology of the Cell, 2nd ed, pp 1187–1218, New York, Garland, 1989

Arlett CF, Harcourt SA, Lehman AR, Stevens S, Bridges BA: Ataxia-telangiectasia: A human mutation with abnormal radiation sensitivity. Nature 258:427–429, 1975

Bishop JM: Cellular oncogene retroviruses. Annu Rev Biochem 52:301–354, 1983

Bishop JM, Varmus HE: Functions and origins of retroviral transforming genes. In Weiss R, Teich N, Varmus H, Coffin J (eds): RNA Tumor Viruses: Molecular Biology of Tumor Viruses, pp 990–1108. New York, Cold Spring Harbor Laboratory, 1984

Blomberg R, Larsson LE, Lindell B, Lindren E: Late effects of Thorotrast in cerebral angiography. Acta Radiol [Diagn] 1:995–1006, 1963

Boice JD, Hutchison GB: Leukemia in women following radiotherapy for cervical cancer: Ten-year follow-up of an international study. JNCI 65:115–129, 1980

Boice JD Jr, Engholm G, Kleinman RA, Blettner M, Stovall M, Lisco H, Moloney WC, Austin DF, Bosch A, Cookfair DL, Krementz ET, Latourette HB, Merrill JA, Peters LJ, Schulz MD, Storm HH, Bjorkholm E,

Pettersson CM, Bell J, Coleman MP, Fraser P, Neal FE, Prior P, Won Choi N, Hislop TG, Koch M, Kreiger N, Robb D, Robson D, Thomson DH, Lochmuller H, von Fournier D, Frischkorn R, Kjorstat E, Rimpela A, Pejovic M-h, Kirn VP, Stankusova H, Berrino F, Sigurdsson K, Hutchison GB, McMahon B: Radiation dose and second cancer risk in patients treated for cancer of the cervix. Radiat Res 116:3–55, 1988

Boice JD Jr, Land CE, Shore RE, Norman JE, Tokunaga M: Risk of breast cancer following low-dose exposure. Radiology 131:589–597, 1979

Boice JD, Monson RR: X-ray exposure and breast cancer. Am J Epidemiol 104:349–350, 1976

Bond VP, Thiessen JW (eds): Re-evaluation of Dosimetric Factors: Hiroshima and Nagasaki. Springfield, VA, US Department of Energy/US Department of Commerce, 1982

Bos JL: The *ras* gene family and human carcinogenesis. Mutat Res 195:255–271, 1988

Brodeur GM, Seeger RC, Schwab M, Varmus HE, Bishop JM: Amplication of N-*myc* in untreated human neuroblastomas correlates with advanced disease stage. Science 224:1121–1124, 1984

Cavanee WK: Tumor progression stage: Specific losses of heterozygosity. Int Symp Princess Takamatsu Cancer Res Fund 20:33–42, 1989

Cavanee WK, Hansen MF, Nordenskjold M, Kock E, Maumenee I, Squire JA, Phillips RA, Gallie BL: Genetic origin of mutations predisposing to retinoblastoma. Science 228:501–503, 1985

Cole J, Arlett CF, Green MH et al: Comparative human cellular radiosensitivity: II. The survival following gamma-irradiation of unstimulated ($G_0$) T-lymphocytes, T-lymphocyte lines, lymphoblastoid cell lines and fibroblasts from normal donors, from ataxia-telangiectasia patients and from ataxia-telangiectasia heterozygotes. Int J Radiat Biol 54:929–943, 1988

Coleman CN: Second malignancy after treatment of Hodgkin's disease: An evolving picture. J Clin Oncol 4:821–824, 1986

Committee on the Biological Effects of Ionizing Radiation: The Effects on Populations of Exposure to Low Levels of Ionizing Radiations. Washington, DC, National Academy of Sciences/National Research Council, 1972

Committee on the Biological Effects of Ionizing Radiation: The Effects on Populations of Exposure to Low Levels of Ionizing Radiations. Washington, DC, National Academy of Sciences/National Research Council, 1980

Committee on the Biological Effects of Ionizing Radiation: Health Effects of Exposure of Low Levels of Ionizing Radiations. Washington, DC, National Academy of Sciences/National Research Council, 1990

Cooper GM: Cellular transforming genes. Science 217:801–806, 1982

Court-Brown WM, Doll R: Mortality from cancer and other causes after radiotherapy for ankylosing spondylitis. Br Med J 2:1327–1332, 1965

Court-Brown WM, Doll R, Hill AB: The incidence of leukemia following exposure to diagnostic radiation in utero. Br Med J 2:1539, 1960

Czesnin K, Wronkowski Z: Second malignancies of the irradiated area in patients treated for uterine cervix cancer. Gynecol Oncol 6:309–315, 1978

Dalla-Favera RS, Martinotti S, Gallo R, Erikson J, Croce D: Translocation and rearrangement of the c-*myc* oncogene locus in human undifferentiated B-cell lymphomas. Science 219:963–997, 1983

Doll R, Smith PG: The long-term effects of x irradiation in patients treated for metropathia haemorrhagica. Br J Radiol 41:362–368, 1968

Dryja TP, Mukai S, Peterson R, Rapport JM, Walton D, Yandell DW: Parental origin of mutations of the retinoblastoma gene. Nature 339:556–558, 1989

Fearon ER, Choi R, Nigro JM et al: Identification of a chromosome 18 gene that is altered in colorectal cancers. Science 247:49–56, 1990

Finkel AI, Miller CE, Hasterlik RJ: Radium-induced tumors in man. In Mays C, Jee W, Lloyd R, Stover B, Dougherty J, Taylor G (eds): Delayed Effects of Bone-Seeking Radionuclides, pp 195–224. Salt Lake City, University of Utah Press, 1969

Fournier REK, Ruddle FH: Microcell-mediated transfer of murine chromosomes into mouse, Chinese hamster, and human somatic cells. Proc Natl Acad Sci USA 74:319–323, 1977

Fujita S. Awa AA, Pierce DA, Kato H, Shimiza Y: Re-evaluation of the biological effects of atomic bomb radiation by the changes of estimation (sic) dose. In Proceedings of the International Symposium on the Biological Effects of Low-Level Radiation With Special Regard to Stochastic and Nonstochastic Effects. Vienna, IAEA, 1983

Green M, Wilson GM: Thyrotoxicosis treated by surgery of iodine-131: With special reference to development of hypothyroidism. Br Med J 1:1005–1010, 1964

Hall EJ, Freyer GA: The molecular biology of radiation carcinogenesis. In Glass WA, Varma MN (eds): Physics and Chemical Mechanisms in Molecular Biology, pp 3–25, New York, Plenum Press, 1991

Harris H: Cell fusion and the analysis of malignancy. Proc R Soc Lond Biol 179:1–20, 1971

Hempelmann LH, Pifer JW, Burke GJ, Terry R, Ames WR: Neoplasms in persons treated with x-rays in infancy for thymic enlargement: A report of third follow-up survey. JNCI 38:317–341, 1967

Hollstein M, Sidvansky, D, Vogelstein B, Harris CC: Mutations in human cancers. Science 253:49–53, 1991

International Commission on Radiological Protection: Recommendations. Annals of the ICRP Publication 60. Oxford, England, Pergamon Press, 1990

International Commission on Radiation Units and Measurements: Radiation Quantities and Units, report 33. Washington, DC, ICRU, 1967

Jablon S, Belsky JL, Tachikawa K, Steer A: Cancer in Japanese exposed as children to atomic bombs. Lancet 1:927–932, 1971

Jablon S, Kato H: Childhood cancer in relation to prenatal exposure to atomic bomb radiation. Lancet 2:1000–1003, 1970

Kapp DS, Fisher D, Grady KJ, Schwartz PE: Subsequent malignancies associated with carcinoma of uterine cervix, including an analysis of the effects of patient and treatment parameters on incidence and site metachronous malignancies. Int J Radiat Oncol Biol Phys 8:192–205, 1982

Knudson AG: Mutation and cancer: Statistical study of retinoblastoma. Proc Natl Acad Sci USA 68:820–823, 1971

Land H, Parada LF, Weinberg RA: Tumorigenic conversion of primary embryo fiobroblasts requires at least two cooperating oncogenes. Nature 304:596–602, 1983

Lee JY, Perez CA, Ettinger N et al: The risk of second primaries subsequent to irradiation for cervix cancer. Int J Radiat Oncol Biol Phys 8:207–211, 1982

Lee WH, Bookstein R, Hong F, Young LH, Shew JY, Lee EY-HP: Human retinoblastoma susceptibility gene: Cloning identification and sequence. Science 235:1394–1399, 1987

MacKenzie I: Breast cancer following multiple fluoroscopies. Br J Cancere 19:1–8, 1965

MacMahon B: Prenatal x-ray exposure and childhood cancer. JNCI 28:1173–1191, 1962

Messerchmidt GL, Hoover R, Young RC: Gynecologic cancer treatment: Risk factors for therapeutically induced neoplasia. Cancer 48:442–450, 1981

Mettler FA, Hempelmann LH, Dutton AM, Pifer JW, Toyooka ET, Ames WR: Breast neoplasms in women treated with x-rays for acute postpartum mastitis: A pilot study. JNCI 43:803–811, 1969

Modan B, Baidatz D, Mart H, Steinitz R, Levin SG: Radiation-induced head and neck tumors. Lancet 1:277, 1974

Mole RH: Endosteal sensitivity to tumor induction by radiation in different species: A partial answer to an unsolved question? In Mays C, Jee W, Lloyd R, Stover B, Dougherty J, Taylor G (eds): Delayed Effects of Bone-Seeking Radionuclides, pp 249–258. Salt Lake City, University of Utah Press, 1969

Morrell D, Cromartie E, Swift M: Mortality and cancer incidence in 263 patients with ataxia-telangiectasia. JNCI 77:89–92, 1986

Myrden JA, Hiltz JE: Breast cancer following multiple fluoroscopies during artificial pneumothorax treatment of pulmonary tuberculosis. Can Med Assoc J 100:1032–1034, 1969

Pederson BJ, Larson SD: Incidence of acute nonlymphocytic leukemia, preleukemia and acute myeloproliferative syndrome up to 10 years after treatment of Hodgkin's disease. N Engl J Med 307:965–975, 1982

Rotblat J, Lindop P: Long-term effects of a single whole-body exposure of mice to ionizing radiations: II. Causes of death. Proc R Soc Lond [Biol] 154:350–368, 1961

Rowland RE, Stehney AF, Lucas HF: Dose–response relationships for female radium dial workers. Radiat Res 76:368–383, 1978

Saenger EL, Thoma BE, Tompkins EA: Leukemia after treatment of hyperthyroidism. JAMA 205:855–862, 1968

Saxon PJ, Srivatsan ES, Leipzig GV, Sameshima JH, Stanbridge EJ: Selective transfer of individual human chromosomes to recipient cells. Mol Cell Biol 5:140–146, 1985

Saxon PJ, Srivatsan ES, Stanbridge EJ: Introduction of normal human chromosome 11 via microcell transfer controls tumorigenic expression of HeLa cells. EMBO J 5:3461–3466, 1986

Stanbridge EJ: Suppression of malignancy in human cells. Nature 260:17–20, 1976

Stewart A, Kneale GW: Changes in the cancer risk associated with obstetric radiography. Lancet 1:104–107, 1968

Stewart A, Webb J, Giles D, Hewitt D: Malignant disease in childhood and diagnostic irradiation in utero. Lancet 2:447, 1956

Stewart A, Webb J, Hewitt D: A survey of childhood malignancies. Br Med J 1:1495–1508, 1958

Swift M, Morrell D, Massey RB, Chase CL: Incidence of cancer in 161 families affected by ataxia-telangiectasia. N Engl J Med 325:1831–1836, 1991

Tatsuo A, Takashi N, Fukushia K, Kasamatsu T, Tsunematsu R, Masubuchi K, Yamauchi K, Hamada T, Fukuda T, Nofuchi H, Murata M: Second cancer after radiation therapy for cancer of the uterine cervix. Cancer 67:398–405, 1991

Taylor AMR, Harnden DG, Arlett CF et al: Ataxia-telangiectasia: A human mutation with abnormal radiation sensitivity. Nature 258:427–429, 1975

United Nations Scientific Committee on the Effects of Atomic Radiation: Sources and Effects of Ionizing Radiation. New York, UNSCEAR, 1988

Upton AC: The dose–response relation in radiation-induced cancer. Cancer Res 21:717–729, 1961

Vahakangas KH, Samet JM, Metcalf RA, Welsh JA, Bennett WP, Lane DP, Harris CC: Mutation of *p53* and *ras* genes in radon-associated lung cancer from uranium miners. Lancet 339:576–580, 1992

Varmus HE: The molecular genetics of cellular oncogenes. Annu Rev Genet 18:553–612, 1984

Vogelstein B: A deadly inheritance. Nature 348:681, 1990

Wall PL, Clausen KP: Carcinoma of urinary bladder in patients receiving cyclophosphamide. N Engl J Med 293:271–273, 1975

Wanebo CK, Johnson KG, Sato K, Thorsland TW: Lung cancer following atomic radiation. Am Rev Respir Dis 988:778–787, 1968

Wanebo CK, Johnson KG, Sato K, Thorsland TW: Breast cancer after exposure to the atomic bombings of Hiroshima and Nagasaki. N Engl J Med 279:667–671, 1968

Watson JD, Hopkins NH, Roberts JW, Steitz JA, Weiner AM (eds): Molecular Biology of the Gene, 4th ed, Scientific American Books, New York, 1987

Wood JW, Tamagaki H, Neriishi S, Sato T, Sheldon WF, Archer PG, Hamilton HB, Johnson KG: Thyroid carcinoma in atomic bomb survivors, Hiroshima and Nagasaki. Am J Epidemiol 89:4–14, 1969

*Radiobiology for the Radiologist, Fourth Edition*, by Eric J. Hall
J. B. Lippincott Company, Philadelphia © 1994.

# 20

# *Hereditary Effects of Radiation*

Diagnostic Radiology
Nuclear Medicine
Radiation Therapy

## GERM CELL PRODUCTION IN THE MALE AND FEMALE

In the male mammal, spermatozoa arise from the germinal epithelium in the seminiferous tubules of the testes, and their production is continuous from puberty to death. The spermatogonial (stem) cells consist of several different populations that vary in their sensitivity to radiation. The postspermatogonial cells pass through several stages of development: primary spermatocytes, secondary spermatocytes, spermatids, and finally spermatozoa. The division of a spermatogonium to the development of mature sperm involves a period of 6 weeks in the mouse and 10 weeks in the human. The effect of radiation on fertility is not apparent immediately because the postspermatogonial cells are relatively resistant compared with the sensitive stem cells. After exposure to a moderate dose of radiation, the individual remains fertile as long as mature sperm cells are available, but decreased fertility or even temporary sterility follows when these are used up. The period of sterility lasts until the spermatogonia are able to repopulate by division.

The threshold for temporary sterility in men exposed to a single absorbed dose in the testes is about 0.15 Gy (15 rads). Under prolonged exposure conditions, the threshold dose rate is about 0.4 Gy/y (40 rads/y). The corresponding values for permanent sterility are about 3.5 to 6 Gy (350 to 600 rads) and 2 Gy/y (200 rads/y). The induction of sterility by radiation in human males does not produce significant changes in hormone balance, libido, or physical capability.

The production of mature germ cells in the female mammal follows a different time course than in the male. All cells in the oogonial stages progress to the oocyte stage in the embryo. By 3 days after birth, in the mouse or human, all of the oocytes are in a resting phase and there is no cell division. Consequently, in the adult there are no stem (oogonial) cells, but there are three types of follicles: immature, nearly mature, and mature.

The threshold for permanent sterility in women is an acute absorbed dose in the range 2.5 to 6 Gy (250 to 600 rads) or a protracted dose rate over many years of more than 0.2 Gy/y (20 rads/y). Pronounced hormonal changes, comparable to those associated with the natural menopause, accompany radiation-induced sterilization in females.

## REVIEW OF BASIC GENETICS

**Genetics** is the study of the inheritance of observable characteristics, which include molecular as well as morphologic and behavioral traits. The chromosomes carry in code form all of the information that specifies a particular human with all of his or her individual characteristics. The **chromosomes** are long threadlike structures, the essential ingredient of which is DNA, itself a long complex molecule with a sugar phosphate backbone. Attached to each sugar molecule is an organic base; these come in four varieties: thymine, adenine, guanine, and cytosine. This whole configuration is tightly coiled in a double helix, rather like a miniature spiral staircase, with chains of sugar molecules linked by phosphates forming the rail on either side, bridged at regular intervals by pairs of bases, which form the steps. The order, or sequence, of the bases contains the genetic information in code form.

A **gene** is a finite segment of DNA specified by an exact sequence of bases. Genes occur along chromosomes in linear order like beads on a string, and the position of a gene is referred to as its **locus.**

The human genome is composed of the DNA of chromosomes and, to a minute extent, mitochondria. The 46 chromosomes contain about 6 $\times$ $10^9$ base pairs of DNA, with each chromosomal arm including a single supercoiled molecule of DNA associated with chromosomal proteins. With contemporary cytogenetic techniques, fixed chromosomal metaphase spreads reveal 500 or so bands, although refined technique can reveal about 2000 bands, per haploid set of chromosomes. The total number of genes is unknown but may be in the range of 0.5 to 1 $\times$ $10^5$ per haploid set of chromosomes. This genetic material recombines in each generation, at a frequency that is measured at 30 to 40 morgans (recombination units). Thus a visible chromosomal band (assuming a haploid number of 500) may include 6 to 8 centimorgans (cM) of recombining genome, 100 to 200 genes, and about $6 \times 10^3$ kilobase pairs (kb) of DNA. The average gene would thereby contain 30 to 60 kb of DNA if no DNA is unrelated to genes. The study of individual genes has hardly begun, but it is apparent that some genes are smaller than this while at least one, that whose mutation can cause Duchenne type muscular dystrophy, has been reported to contain more than $10^3$ kb of DNA. Since most protein products of genes are less than 300,000 daltons, the translated portions of genes are seldom larger than 10 kb, so a major part of the genome appears to be untranslated. Some of this DNA appears to be transcribed but not translated. Much of the untranslated DNA consists of introns that reside between translated exons. In addition, much of the DNA outside the exons is involved in gene function, through regulation and RNA polymerase attachment.

Not only does this genome recombine in each generation, but it also undergoes *mutation,* a term applied here to denote all changes in chromosomes, their genes, and their DNA. Thus, alterations in chromosome number and structure would be included along with changes not visible microscopically. These latter changes include an array of changes in DNA, such as deletion, rearrangement, breakage in the sugar-phosphate backbone, and base alterations. Gene function can be disturbed not only by loss or modification of translated exons but also through alteration of nonexonic sites that regulate transcription and translation. Mutation occurs in both germ cells and somatic cells, although it is much less apparent in the latter, unless it occurs under conditions of clonal proliferation, as happens with cancer. On the other hand, many mutations in the germline will be lethal during embryonic development.

In humans, every normal cell has 46 chromosomes, 23 derived from the mother and 23 from the father. Each of a pair of chromosomes normally has the same genes for given characteristics lined up in the same sequence. In this case the two chromosomes are said to be **homologous.** The pair of chromosomes that determine sex are XX in the female and XY in the male; in the case of the male, therefore, the two chromosomes of this pair are **heterologous**—they do not contain parallel genes. When the two members of a pair of genes are alike, the person is said to be **homozygous** for that pair of genes; when they are different, the person is said to be heterozygous.

The fact that pairs of chromosomes contain corresponding sets of genes introduces the idea of **dominant** and **recessive genes.** A dominant gene, by definition, expresses itself when its corresponding gene is recessive, the recessive gene in this case being either ineffective or suppressed. A completely recessive gene will only be expressed in a person when both the corresponding genes of a pair of chromosomes are recessive (ie, the person must be homozygous for the recessive gene) or when the recessive gene is on the X chromosome in a male. Eye color is the simplest example. The gene for blue eyes is recessive, while that for brown eyes is dominant. A child will have blue eyes only if he receives the gene for blue eyes from both parents. If both or only one of the genes that determine eye color is for brown eyes, then the child will have brown eyes, because this gene is dominant. It should be pointed out that not all genes are completely dominant; some permit expression of the recessive counterpart to a varying extent, depending on the particular characteristics involved.

The Y sex chromosome in humans has genes that determine maleness but appears to have few other genes. The X chromosome, on the other hand, has many genes. If a mother carries a recessive mutant gene on the single X chromosome that she donates to her son, there will be no matching gene from the father, and consequently the recessive gene will be expressed. If the offspring is a daughter, there may well be a dominant gene on the X chromosome supplied by the father, which would suppress the expression of the recessive mutant. The daughter could, however, transmit the mutant gene to *her* sons, in whom it would be expressed. Characteristics that are due to recessive genes on the X chromosome, so that they are expressed almost exclusively in male children, are said to be **sex-linked.** The most common examples are color blindness and hemophilia.

An elementary discussion of genetics, such as that presented here, may give the impression that each characteristic of a person is determined by a single pair of genes. On the contrary, this is the exception rather than the rule, since most characteristics are the result of an interplay in the expression of many genes.

## MUTATIONS

It is a commonly held view that radiation produces bizarre mutants and monsters, as illustrated in Figure 20-1. This view is absolutely false. Radiation does not result in genetic effects that are new or unique but rather increases the frequencies of the same mutations that already occur spontaneously or naturally in that species.

Radiation-induced genetic changes, like mutations from any other agent, may be a consequence of a gene mutation or chromosomal changes. The causes are summarized in Table 20-1.

## GENE MUTATIONS

A gene mutation is a change in the *structure* of DNA, which may involve either the base composition, the sequence, or both. An alteration so small that it involves the substitution, gain, or loss

of a single base can be the cause of significant inheritable changes. A striking example is sickle cell anemia, which results from the substitution of only one base. A *dominant* gene mutation is expressed in the first generation after its occurrence. More than 700 such conditions have been identified with certainty, and an additional 700 or more are less well established. Some examples are polydactyly, achondroplasia, Huntington's chorea, and retinoblastoma.

*Recessive* mutations, unless sex-linked, require that the gene be present in duplicate to produce the trait, which means that the mutant gene must be inherited from each parent; consequently, many generations may pass before it is expressed. More than 500 recessive diseases are known, and another 600 are suspected. Some examples are sickle cell anemia, cystic fibrosis, and Tay-Sachs disease.

The best known examples of sex-linked disorders are hemophilia, color blindness, and a severe form of muscular dystrophy, but altogether there are more than 80 well-established and another 60 probable conditions of this sort. Because males have only one X chromosome, a sex-linked recessive mutation can be expressed if only a single gene complement is present; therefore, like dominant mutations, they are expressed soon after mutation occurs.

Some dominant and some recessive mutant genes cause traits that are regarded by society as normal or acceptable, such as different eye colors or blood groups. The majority, however, cause diseases ranging from mild to severe in their impact on the person.

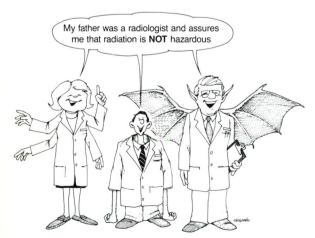

Figure 20-1. It is a commonly held view that radiation produces bizarre mutations or monsters that may be readily recognized. This is not true. Radiation increases the incidence of the same mutations that occur spontaneously in a given population. The study of radiation genetics is difficult, because the mutations produced by the radiation must be identified on a statistical basis in the presence of a high natural incidence of the same mutations.

Table 20-1.
Heritable Effects of Radiation

| HERITABLE EFFECT | | | EXAMPLE |
|---|---|---|---|
| **Gene Mutations·** | | | |
| Single dominant | 736 | (753) | Polydactyly, Huntington's chorea, retinoblastoma |
| Recessive | 521 | (596) | Sickle cell anemia, Tay-Sachs disease, cystic fibrosis |
| Sex-linked | 80 | (60) | Color blindness, hemophilia |
| **Chromosome Changes** | | | |
| Too many or too few | | | Down's syndrome (extra chromosome 21), mostly embryonic death |
| Chromosome aberrations, physical abnormalities Robertsonian translocation | | | Embryonic death or mental retardation |
| **Frequent but Mild Mutations** | | | |
| Most frequent class of mutation in Drosophila; can only be detected statistically | | | Lower probability of survival from egg to adult |

·*The number following gene mutations refers to the number of human diseases known to be caused by such a mutation. The number in parentheses refers to additional possible diseases.*

There is an additional class of mutations, the importance of which is difficult to assess, because they cause effects that are so mild that they cannot be detected individually, and their existence can only be demonstrated statistically in experiments involving a huge number of animals. It is tempting to ignore them, but in *Drosophila* they are by far the most frequent class of mutations. An example of such a mutation is a change in the probability of surviving from the egg to the adult stage; it is clearly impossible to detect such differences in humans, and even in the laboratory they can be revealed only in *Drosophila*, with which experiments of mammoth proportions are feasible.

## CHROMOSOMAL ABERRATIONS

Errors in chromosome distribution can result in cells containing too many or too few chromosomes. Down's syndrome is the best-known example; it results from an extra chromosome 23. Most of the time, however, an incorrect chromosome number, whether a deficiency or an excess, leads to embryonic death. It is estimated that at least 40% of the spontaneous abortions that occur from the 5th to the 28th week of gestation and about 6% of stillbirths are associated with chromosomal anomalies. This kind of chromosome error is not believed to be strongly influenced by radiation, particularly at low doses. Chromosome breakage is less frequent than aberrations among spontaneous instances of severe human anomalies, but radiation is much more effective at breaking chromosomes than in causing errors in chromosome distribution. Chromosomes that are broken may rejoin in various ways (see Chapter 2). A translocation, for example, involves the reciprocal exchange of parts between two or more chromosomes and is not necessarily harmful as long as both rearranged chromosomes are present and contain the full gene complement. Children of a person with a translocation often receive only one of the rearranged chromosomes, and their cells are therefore genetically unbalanced. The nature and extent of the abnormality varies enormously, and the harm to the person ranges from rather mild to very severe. Chromosome imbalance, if it does not cause the death of the embryo, typically leads to physical abnormalities, usually accompanied by mental deficiency.

Robertsonian translocations are the most common type found in *normal* humans. These are fusions of two chromosomes, each having a spindle attachment at the end of the chromosome, to produce a single chromosome with the spindle attachment in the center. The children of a person with this type of translocation are usually normal, since they inherit either the translocated pair or a pair of normal chromosomes. Radiation does not appear to be a major cause of Robertsonian translocations but rather tends to induce those of the reciprocal exchange type.

## RADIATION-PRODUCED GENETIC EFFECTS

The fact that mutants produced by man-made radiations cannot be recognized or identified as different, compared with the natural spontaneous types, makes their study particularly difficult. Sample sizes must be large to detect a small increase caused by radiation.

Few human data are available on the genetic effects of radiation, except the observations of genetic consequences in the children of Japanese survivors of the A-bomb attacks on Hiroshima and Nagasaki. Consequently, the estimation of genetic risks in the human must be based almost entirely on animal data.

## RELATIVE VERSUS DIRECT (OR ABSOLUTE) MUTATION RISK

There are essentially two ways to estimate the genetic risks of radiation. The first is to compare radiation-induced mutations with those that occur spontaneously and to express the results in terms of the doubling dose—the dose required to double the spontaneous mutation rate. This is the *relative mutation risk*. The alternative approach is to ignore the natural or spontaneous rate and simply to quote the incidence of disorders resulting from mutations in the first generation. This is the *direct* or *absolute* mutation risk. They correspond to relative and absolute risks of radiation carcinogenesis. Both of these approaches have been used in experiments with mice and will be discussed in turn.

## RELATIVE MUTATION RISK ASSESSED IN THE MEGAMOUSE PROJECT

The husband and wife team of Russell and Russell, working at Oak Ridge National Laboratory, mounted an experiment of heroic proportions to determine specific locus mutation rates in the mouse under a variety of irradiation conditions. These experiments are often referred to as the "megamouse project" because of the enormous number of animals involved. Before the study ended, 7 million mice had been used.

An inbred mouse strain was chosen in which seven specific-locus mutations occur, six of which involve a change of coat color, one expressed as a stunted ear. Figure 20-2, kindly supplied by Dr. W. L. Russell, shows three coat color variations: a piebald, a light honey, and a darker brown. These mutations occur spontaneously, and their incidence is increased by radiation.

These extensive studies included the irradiation of both male and female mice with a range of doses, dose rates, and fractionation patterns. Of particular interest was a comparison of mutation rates induced by radiation in different stages of spermatogenesis. The results obtained are exceedingly complex; only the briefest summary is presented in this chapter. Five major conclusions are pertinent to the radiologist:

1. The radiosensitivity of different mutations varies by a significant factor of about 35, so that it is only possible to speak in terms of average mutation rates.
2. In the mouse there is a substantial dose-rate effect, so that spreading the radiation dose over a period of time results in fewer mutations for a given dose than in an acute exposure. This is in complete contrast to the data on *Drosophila*. In the male there is a big dose-rate effect, between 90 and 0.8 R/min (about 90 and 0.8 cGy/min), which Dr. Russell Russells attribute to a repair process. The data are shown in Figure 20-3. In oocytes, the incidence of mutations produced by radiation delivered at a low dose rate is not distinguishable from the incidence in control animals.
3. The male is much more radiosensitive than the female. This is particularly true at a low dose rate, where it is doubtful if there is any

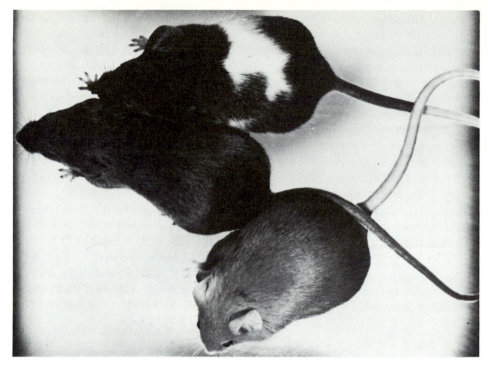

**Figure 20-2.** In the megamouse project seven specific-locus mutations were used to study radiation-produced genetic effects. This picture shows three of the mutations, which involve changes of coat color. (Courtesy of Dr. William L. Russell, Oak Ridge National Laboratory)

increase in mutations in the female, even after a dose of several gray (several hundred rads). The difference between the sexes is so pro-

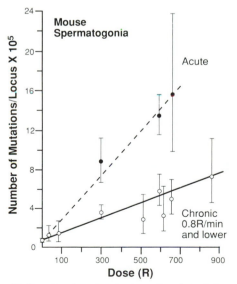

**Figure 20-3.** Mutations in mice as a function of dose, delivered at high and low dose rates. (Courtesy of Dr. William L. Russell, Oak Ridge National Laboratory)

nounced that, for practical purposes, at a low dose rate almost all of the radiation-induced genetic burden in a population is carried by the males.

4. The genetic consequences of a given dose can be greatly reduced if a time interval is allowed between irradiation and conception. This was first noticed in the male and a correlation found to exist with the stage of spermatogenesis at which the radiation was delivered. If animals were irradiated and used immediately for mating in genetic experiments, so that the sperm used for fertilization had been irradiated in a mature state, then a relatively large number of mutations were produced. In contrast, if animals were irradiated and mating delayed for a number of weeks, so that the sperm used for fertilization had been irradiated in a primitive state, then fewer mutations were produced. Consequently, it is inferred that this decrease in mutation rate with time after irradiation is the consequence of some repair process. Whatever the explanation, it is an important empirical observation

that the genetic consequences of a given dose of radiation can be reduced if a time interval is allowed between irradiation and conception. This information is already used in genetic counseling. In the mouse, a time interval between irradiation and conception of 2 months in the male and rather longer in the female is sufficient to produce a maximum reduction in the effect of radiation. Although data are not available for humans, by analogy a period of 6 months is usually recommended. Consequently, if persons are exposed to a significant dose of radiation, either accidentally or as a result of their occupation, it is recommended that 6 months be allowed to elapse between the exposure to the radiation and a planned conception to minimize the genetic consequence.

This would be good advice to a person accidentally exposed to, say 0.1 Gy (10 rads), to young patients with Hodgkin's disease receiving radiotherapy, or even to patients subjected to diagnostic x-ray procedures involving the lumbar spine or the lower gastrointestinal tract, in which a large exposure is used and the gonads must be included within the radiation field.

5. The estimate of the doubling dose favored by the latest reports of the Committee on the Biological Effects of Ionizing Radiation (BEIR V) and the United Nations Scientific Committee on the Effects of Atomic Radiation (UNSCEAR 88) is 1 Gy (100 rads) based on low dose-rate exposure. This is a *calculated* rather than a *measured* quantity, based on the *measured* mutation rate per locus in the mouse, *adjusted* for the estimated comparable number of loci in the human. It involves a number of uncertainties. Earlier reports quoted a range of doses, rather than a single dose, including 0.2 to 2 Gy (20 to 200 rads) and 0.5 to 2.5 Gy (50 to 250 rads).

## DIRECT OR ABSOLUTE MUTATION RISK: ESTIMATE OF THE FIRST-GENERATION INCIDENCE OF MUTATIONS FROM MOUSE SKELETAL DEFORMITIES

A second set of experiments performed with mice, also at Oak Ridge National Laboratory, focused attention on a species of mice in which 37 skeletal abnormalities resulting from mutations can be observed. Most are subtle changes that can only be readily detected by an experienced "mouse radiologist," but one of the more obvious, involving an extra rib, is shown in Figure

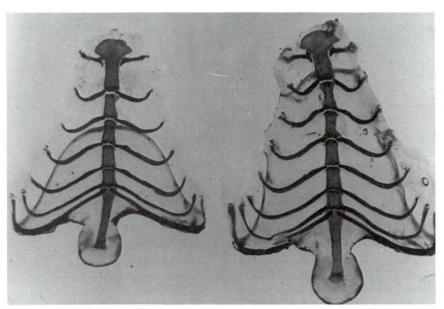

**Figure 20-4.** One of the skeletal anomalies in mice, the extra rib, used for the direct estimate of first generation genetic risks of radiation. (Courtesy of Dr. P.B. Selby, Oak Ridge National Laboratory)

20-4. The animals were irradiated and mated, and skeletal anomalies were observed in the first-generation offspring by means of radiographs. Since the offspring were not sacrificed, subsequent breeding experiments could be performed to check that the observed skeletal abnormalities "breed true," that is, that they were, in fact, mutations. The mutation rate produced by acute exposures was then reduced by a factor of 3 to allow for the lower efficiency of irradiation delivered at low dose rate and increased by a factor of 10 to allow for the fact that in humans only 10% of known genetic disorders involve the skeleton. This, of course, involves the implicit assumption that the average radiation sensitivity of all mutations is not different from those involving mutations that produce skeletal deformities.

Other estimates of direct risks involve the induction of dominant mutations producing cataracts in the mouse and the induction of congenital malformed births due to chromosome aberrations. These calculations do not rely on a knowledge of the natural prevalence of such genetic disorders in the population, but other assumptions are needed to bridge the gap between the species.

# HEREDITARY EFFECTS OF RADIATION IN HUMANS

The little human data available suggest that the doubling dose, deduced largely from the megamouse experiments, is about right for humans also. The lowest possible doubling dose is 0.03 Sv (3 rems), for this is the average amount of radiation received from natural sources during the typical reproductive lifetime of 30 years. Such a value for the doubling dose would imply that *all* spontaneous mutations are caused by background radiation, which is most unlikely. The survivors of the A-bomb attacks on Hiroshima and Nagasaki constitute the largest irradiated human population studied carefully for genetic effects. Four genetic indicators have been studied for more than 40 years in children born to survivors of the A-bomb attacks:

1. Untoward pregnancy outcomes, including stillbirths, major congenital defects, or death during the first postnatal week
2. Occurrence of death in live-born children through an average life expectancy of 17 years

3. Frequency of children with sex chromosome abnormalities
4. Frequency of children with a mutation resulting in an electrophoretic variant in blood proteins. (Each child born to irradiated parents was studied for rare electrophoretic variants of 28 proteins of the blood plasma and red blood cell and for activity variants of a subset of eight erythrocyte enzymes.)

Parents of children studied came from both cities and from low-dose (0.01 to 0.09 Gy, or 1 to 9 rads) and high-dose (1 Gy, or more than 100 rads) groups. Persons from outside the cities were studied as controls.

For these four measures of genetic effects, the differences between the children of proximally and distally exposed survivors is in the direction expected if a genetic effect did result from the radiation, but in fact none of the findings is statistically significant. Nevertheless, the differences between these groups of children were used to calculate doubling doses. It is argued that it is permissible to use those data to estimate doubling doses, even in the absence of a statistically significant effect, since the link between radiation exposure and genetic anomalies is not in doubt, having been established unequivocally by animal data. In addition, of course, the chromosomal damage seen in the survivors suggests that this is the case.

Only three of the four indicators lend themselves to estimate of doubling dose, and the results are shown in Table 20-2. The simple average of the three estimates is 1.56 Sv (156 rems). The fourth set of data on electrophoretic variants is

Table 20-2.
**Doubling Dose (Gametic) in the Offspring of Survivors of the A-bomb Attacks on Hiroshima and Nagasaki**

| GENETIC INDICATOR | DOUBLING DOSE (REMS)* |
|---|---|
| Untoward pregnancy outcome | 69 |
| Childhood mortality | 147 |
| Sex chromosome aneuploidy | 252 |
| Simple average | 156 |

*Divide by 100 to obtain doubling dose in sievert.
(From Schull WJ, Otake M, Neal JV: Science 213:1220–1227, 1981)

consistent with a wide range of possibilities and is omitted at present.

This estimate for humans should be compared with the comparable figure of about 0.39 Gy (30 rads) for the doubling dose in the mouse for an acute exposure to low-LET radiation. (The figure of 1 Gy for the doubling dose quoted earlier refers to low dose rate.) The sparse human data do not provide estimates that are statistically significant but do allow upper bounds to be set on the estimate of risk. They also indicate that the estimates based on the mouse may not be too far wrong.

The guiding principles for assessing genetic risk in humans may be summed up as follows:

1. Most mutations, whether spontaneous or induced by radiation, are harmful.
2. Any dose of radiation, however small, entails some genetic risk.
3. The number of mutations produced is proportional to the dose, so that a linear extrapolation from high-dose data provides a valid estimate of low-dose effects.
4. Risk estimates based on experiments with the mouse are not too far off for humans.

The conditions under which humans are exposed to radiation, whether as members of the general public or in the course of their occupations, are such that mutation rates are low. Either the dose rate is very low in conditions of continuous exposure or, when high dose rates are involved, the dose per exposure is small. In either case, the mouse data indicate a low yield of mutations. On the rare occasions when a large dose is absorbed in an acute exposure, as, for example, in a radiation accident, a significant proportion of the deleterious genetic consequences can be avoided if conception is deferred. For a male 2 months is sufficient; the comparable period for females is not known with any certainty, but it is probably longer than for males. As suggested earlier, a prudent and conservative approach might be to recommend to both males and females that planned conception should be delayed for a least 6 months after a significant irradiation exposure to minimize the hazard of genetic anomalies.

## NUMERICAL VALUES OF GENETIC RISK

The results of both major mouse experiments, involving the specific locus mutations and the skeletal deformity mutations, are summarized in Table 20-3, reproduced in modified form from the BEIR III report. In this table the number of mutations occurring spontaneously, together with those produced by radiation, are expressed per million live-born children. The spontaneous or natural incidence is listed in the second column. Of every 1 million live-born humans, 107,000 (about 10%) carry a spontaneous mutation of

Table 20-3.
Genetic Effects of an Average Population Exposure of 1 Rem (10 mSv) per 30-Year Generation Compared With the Spontaneous Levels

| TYPE OF GENETIC DISORDER | SPONTANEOUS INCIDENCE PER MILLION LIVEBORN OFFSPRING | EFFECT OF 1 REM (10 mSv) PER GENERATION PER MILLION LIVE OFFSPRING | |
| | | First Generation | Equilibrium |
| --- | --- | --- | --- |
| Autosomal dominant and X-linked | 10,000 | 5–65 | 40–200 |
| Irregularly inherited | 90,000 | 5–65 | 20–900 |
| Recessive | 1100 | Very few; effects in heterozygotes accounted for in top row | Very slow increase |
| Chromosomal | 6000 | Fewer than 10 | Increases only slightly |

*(From Committee on the Biological Effects of Ionizing Radiation (BEIR III): The Effects on Populations of Exposure to Low Levels of Ionizing Radiation. Washington, DC, National Academy of Sciences, 1980)*

some sort, ranging from very mild to very serious. One third to one half of all the known naturally occurring hereditary disorders may be deemed severe and equivalent in severity to fatal cancer, either because they occur early in life or because they are as detrimental as lethal diseases in adult life. The table attributes some of these to gene mutations, either recessive or dominant, and some to chromosome aberrations, but the vast majority are "irregularly inherited," meaning that the mechanism by which they occur is not understood. The figures for radiation in the last two columns are quoted in terms of a dose of 10 mSv (1 rem) per 30-year generation. The number of mutations that can be scored in the first generation is very small, only about 50, because, of course, only dominant mutations are apparent at this stage. At equilibrium (ie, when the radiation dose is delivered to each generation and allowed to come into equilibrium genetically, so that all

forms of mutations are scored) the numbers are higher: 60 to 1100 mutations per million live-born offspring by a dose of 10 mSv (1 rem) per generation. This compares with 107,000 spontaneous mutations per million offspring.

Table 20-3 lists the conclusions of the BEIR III report. The latest BEIR (BEIRV) and UNSCEAR (88) reports do not include any allowance for a genetic component to multifactorial disorders; both committees feel that this may be an important effect of radiation but were unable to make a realistic estimate.

For a working population, the International Commission on Radiological Protection (ICRP) estimates the probability per caput for radiation-induced hereditary disorders to be $0.6 \times 10^{-2}$ per sievert. This is based on the doubling dose of 1 Gy (100 rads), plus an approximate allowance for multifactorial diseases. This risk, of course, is additional to that for cancer.

► ***Summary of Pertinent Conclusions***

- Radiation does not produce new, unique mutations but increases the incidence of the same mutations that occur spontaneously.
- Information on the genetic effects of radiation comes almost entirely from animal experiments.
- First-generation mutations in mice have been measured by observing skeletal anomalies in the offspring of irradiated mice. This is the direct or absolute method.
- Relative mutation rates have been measured in the megamouse project by observing specific locus mutation. This leads to an estimate of the doubling dose.
- The doubling dose is the dose required to double the spontaneous mutation incidence; put another way, it is the dose required to produce an incidence of mutations equal to the spontaneous rate. Based on the mouse data, the doubling dose for low dose-rate exposure in humans is estimated to be 1 Gy (100 rads).
- Not more than 1% to 6% of spontaneous mutations in humans may be ascribed to background radiation.
- Children of the survivors of the A-bomb attacks on Hiroshima and Nagasaki have been studied for (1) untoward pregnancy outcomes, (2) death of live-born children, (3) sex chromosome abnormalities, and (4) electrophoretic variants of blood proteins. Although no genetic indicator is statistically significant, the average doubling dose is 1.58 Sv (158 rem).
- Humans are not more sensitive and are probably less sensitive than mice to radiation-induced genetic effects.
- Based on the limited human data, it is concluded that the mouse data for radiation-induced genetic effects can be applied to humans with some measure of confidence.

*(continued)*

▶ *Summary of Pertinent Conclusions* *(Continued)*

- In terms of detriment, expressed in years of life lost or impaired, congenital anomalies (ie, resulting from effects on the developing embryo and fetus) are much more important than genetically transmitted disorders.
- For a working population, the ICRP estimates the probability per caput for radiation-induced hereditary disorders to be $0.6 \times 10^{-2}$ per Sv. This is based on a doubling dose of 1 Gy, plus an approximate allowance for multifactorial diseases.

# Bibliography

Bacq ZM, Alexander P: Fundamentals of Radiobiology, 2nd ed, pp 436–450. New York, Pergamon Press, 1961

Committee on the Biological Effects of Ionizing Radiation: The Effects on Populations of Exposure to Low Levels of Ionizing Radiation. Washington, DC, National Academy of Sciences/National Research Council, 1972

Committee on the Biological Effects of Ionizing Radiation: The Effects on Populations of Exposure to Low Levels of Ionizing Radiation. Washington, DC, National Academy of Sciences/National Research Council, 1980

Committee on the Biological Effects of Ionizing Radiation: Health Effects of Exposure to Low Levels of Ionizing Radiation. Washington, DC, National Academy of Sciences/National Research Council, 1990

International Commission on Radiological Protection and International Commission on Radiation Units and Measurements: Exposure of man to ionizing radiation arising from medical procedures. Phys Med Biol 2:107–151, 1957

McKusick VAP: Human Genetics. Englewood Cliffs, NJ, Prentice-Hall, 1969

Pochin EE: Sizewell 13 inquiry: The biological basis of the assumption made by NRPB in the calculation of health effects and proof of evidence. NRPB/P/2 (Rev). Chilton, Oxon, UK, National Radiological Protection Board, 1983

Russell LB, Russell WL: The sensitivity of different stages in oogenesis to the radiation induction of dominant lethals and other changes in the mouse. In Mitchell JS, Holmes BE, Smith CL (eds): Progress in Radiobiology, pp 187–192. Edinburgh, Oliver & Boyd, 1956

Russell WL: Genetic hazards of radiation. Proc Am Phil Soc 107:11–17, 1963

Russell WL: The effects of radiation dose rate and fractionation on mutation in mice. In Sobels FH (ed): Repair of Genetic Radiation Damage, pp 205–217, New York, Pergamon Press, 1963

Russell WL: Studies in mammalian radiation genetics. Nucleonics 23:53–56, 1965

Russell WL: Effect of the interval between irradiation and conception on mutation frequency in female mice. Proc Natl Acad Sci USA 54:1555–1556, 1965

Schull WL, Otake M, Neal JV: Genetic effects of the atomic bomb: A reappraisal. Science 213:1220–127, 1981

Searle GH, Phillips RJS: Genetic effect of high LET radiation in mice. Space Radiol Biol Radiat Res 7(suppl):294–303, 1967

Selby PB: Induced skeletal mutations. Genetics 92(suppl):127–133, 1979

Selby PB: Radiation-induced dominant skeletal mutations in mice: Mutation rate, characteristics, and usefulness in estimating genetic hazard to human from radiation. In Okada S, Imamura M, Terasima T, Yamaguchi M (eds): Radiation Research: Proceedings of the Sixth International Congress of Radiation Research, pp 537–544. Tokyo, Toppan Printing Co, 1979

Selby PB, Selby PR: Gamma-ray–induced dominant mutations that cause skeletal abnormalities in mice: I. Plan, summary of results, and discussion. Mutat Res 43:357–375, 1977

Spencer WP, Stern C: Experiments to test the validity of the linear R-dose mutation frequency relation in *Drosophila* at low dosage. Genetics 33:43–74, 1948

United Nations Scientific Committee on the Effects of Atomic Radiation: Genetic Effect of Radiation. New York, United Nations, 1977

United Nations Scientific Committee on the Effects of Atomic Radiation: Ionizing Radiation Sources and Biological Effects. New York, United Nations, 1982

United Nations Scientific Committee on the Effects of Atomic Radiation: Ionizing Radiation Sources and Biological Effects. New York, United Nations, 1988

*Radiobiology for the Radiologist, Fourth Edition*, by Eric J. Hall
J. B. Lippincott Company, Philadelphia © 1994.

# 21

# *Effects of Radiation on the Embryo and Fetus*

Diagnostic Radiology
Nuclear Medicine
Radiation Therapy

## OVERVIEW OF RADIATION EFFECTS ON THE EMBRYO AND FETUS

Among the somatic effects of radiation other than cancer, developmental effects on the unborn child are of greatest concern. The classic effects are listed below:

1. Lethal effects, induced by radiation before or immediately after implantation of the embryo into the uterine wall or induced after increasingly higher doses during all stages of intrauterine development, to be expressed either before birth (prenatal death) or at about the time of birth (neonatal death)
2. Malformations, characteristic of the period of major organogenesis, when the main body structures are formed, and especially of the most active phase of cell multiplication in the relevant structures
3. Growth disturbances without malformations, induced at all stages of development but particularly in the latter part of pregnancy

The principal factors of importance are the dose and the stage of gestation at which it is delivered. Dose rate is also of significance, since many pathologic effects on the embryo are reduced significantly by reducing the dose rate.

It should be recognized that congenital anomalies arise in all animal species, even in the absence of any radiation beyond that received from natural sources. The incidence depends to a large extent on the time at which the anomalies are scored. The incidence of malformed infants at birth is about 6%, averaged for the human species. Some malformations disappear after birth, but more become evident later that are not scored at birth. The global incidence roughly doubles to 12% if grown children rather than infants are examined. Any assessment of the effectiveness of radiation in inducing damage in utero must be viewed against this natural level of inborn defects and its variable expression.

## DATA FROM RATS AND MICE

Most experimental data on the effect of radiation in the developing embryo or fetus have been obtained with the mouse or rat, animals that reproduce in quantity with relatively short gestation periods. Russell and Russell divided the total developmental period in utero into three stages: (1) preimplantation, which extends from fertilization to the time when the embryo attaches to the wall of the uterus; (2) organogenesis, the period during which the major organs are developed; and (3) the fetal stage, during which growth of the structures already formed takes place. There is a very large variability in the relative duration of these periods among animal species, as well as in the total duration of intrauterine life. Also, at any given stage of development, the state of differentiation or maturation of any one structure, with respect to all the others, varies considerably in different species.

In the mouse, preimplantation corresponds to days 0 to 5; organogenesis to days 5 to 13; and the fetal period from day 13 to full term, which is about 20 days. The effect of 2 Gy (200 rads) delivered at various times after conception is illustrated in Figure 21-1. The lower scale contains Rugh's estimates of the equivalent ages for human embryos, based solely on comparable stages of organ development. It is a nonlinear match, since preimplantation, organogenesis, and the fetal period in the mouse are about equal in length, whereas the fetal period in the human is proportionately much longer.

Figure 21-2 is taken from the work of Brent and Ghorson, who have performed an extensive series of experiments with rats. It shows the various periods during gestation when the principal effects of radiation are most evident. The horizontal scale refers to the times of the major events during gestation for the rat and gives an estimate of the comparable stages for the human. The following discussion of the principal effects of radiation delivered during preimplantation, organogenesis, and the fetal stages represents a

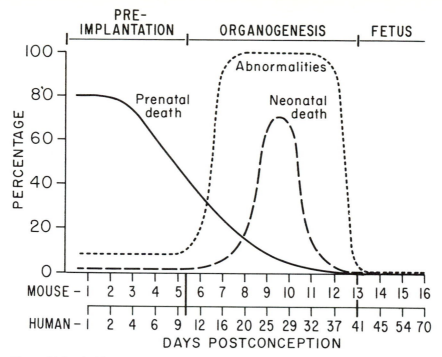

**Figure 21-1.** Incidence of abnormalities and of prenatal and neonatal death in mice given a dose of 200 R at various times after fertilization. The lower scale consists of Rugh's estimates of the equivalent stages for the human embryo. (Curves redrawn from Russell LB, Russell WL: J Cell Physiol [Suppl 1] 43:103, 1954)

consensus view, combining conclusions from various experiments with either rats or mice.

## Preimplantation

Preimplantation is the most sensitive stage to the *lethal* effects of radiation. This high incidence of prenatal death may be expressed in a decrease in litter size. Growth retardation is not observed after irradiation at this stage; if the embryo survives, it grows normally in utero and afterward. Few if any abnormalities are produced by irradiation at this stage. Rugh has shown in mice that a dose of 0.05 to 0.15 Gy (5 to 15 rads) can kill the fertilized egg. Brent and Ghorson have shown in the rat that about 0.1 Gy (10 rads), delivered on the first day of gestation, increases the rate of embryonic resorption to 11.9% compared with 4.7% in unirradiated controls.

Thus the irradiated preimplanted embryo that survives until term grows normally in the prepartum and postpartum periods, that is, there is

an "all-or-nothing" effect of radiation because when the number of cells in the conceptus is small and their nature is not yet specialized, the effect of damage to these cells is most likely to take the form of a failure to implant or an undetected death of the conceptus. This is illustrated in the remarkable pictures produced by Pedersen and reproduced in Figure 21-3. If too many cells are killed by irradiation, the embryo dies and is resorbed. If only a few cells are killed, one or two cell divisions can make good the damage.

## Organogenesis

During organogenesis, the principal effect of radiation in small rodents is the production of a variety of congenital anomalies of a structural nature. As seen from Figure 21-1, a dose of about 2 Gy (200 rads) to the mouse embryo during the period of maximum sensitivity can result in a 100% incidence of malformations at birth. A similar result is seen for rats exposed to about 1

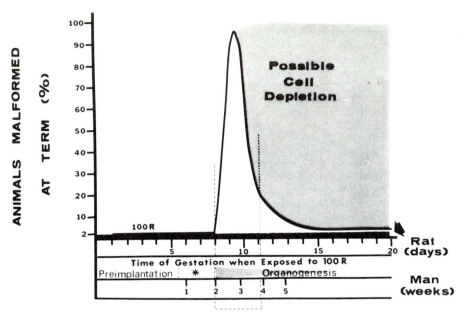

**Figure 21-2.** Relative incidence of congenital malformations in the rat after an x-ray exposure of 100 R, delivered at various stages during gestation. The control incidence in this species is about 2%, indicated by the arrow on the right. The incidence of malformation after irradiation before the ninth day is not detectably different from controls. A large incidence, approaching 100%, occurs if the radiation is delivered during early organogenesis, corresponding to the third and fourth week of a human pregnancy. The number of malformations produced falls off rapidly as organogenesis diminishes, though some organogenesis of the central nervous system continues to term. During the fetal stage, a dose of 100 R causes an irreversible loss of cells that is expressed as growth retardation persisting to adulthood. The asterisk shows the stage in implantation when radiation causes growth retardation that is expressed as a decrease in weight at term. (From Brent RL, Ghorson RO: Curr Probl Radiol 2:1–48, 1972)

Gy (100 rads) in Figure 21-2. During organogenesis, most of the embryonic cells are in their blastula, or differentiating, stage and are particularly sensitive. This is the period in the human when the tranquilizer thalidomide produced such disastrous effects (at about 35 days after conception) and is also the time of maximum risk of deleterious effects from the rubella virus.

Examples of gross anomalies resulting from irradiation during the period of organogenesis are shown in Figures 21-4 and 21-5. It is characteristic of mice and rats that a wide variety of structural malformations are seen. The production of a specific defect is associated with a definite time during this period of organogenesis, usually the time of the first morphologic evidence of differentiation in the organ or portion of the organ involved.

Embryos exposed during early organogenesis also exhibit the greatest intrauterine growth retardation. This is expressed as a weight reduction at term and is a phenomenon resulting from cell depletion. Animals show a remarkable ability to recover from the growth retardation produced by irradiation during organogenesis, and while they may be smaller than usual at birth they may achieve a normal weight as adults. There is an association between growth retardation and teratogenesis: irradiated embryos that show major congenital anomalies also suffer an overall reduction of growth. In animals a dose about 1 Gy (100 rads) will produce growth retardation when delivered at any stage of gestation (except during preimplantation), while 0.25 Gy (25 rads) does not produce an observable effect even at the most sensitive stage.

If death occurs as a result of irradiation in organogenesis, it is likely to be neonatal death—occurring at or about the time of birth. The transition from prenatal death from irradiation during preimplantation to neonatal death resulting from irradiation in organogenesis is very clear from Figure 21-1. In this case, neonatal deaths peak at 70% for mice receiving about 2 Gy (200 rads) on the tenth day. The deaths probably occur because some grossly abnormal fetuses are unable to develop to term.

## The Fetal Period

The remainder of pregnancy, the fetal period, extends from about day 14 onward in the mouse; this corresponds to 6 weeks onward in the human. A variety of effects have been documented in the experimental animal after irradiation during the fetal stages, including effects on the hematopoietic system, liver, and kidney, all occurring, however, after fairly high radiation doses. The effects on the developing gonads have been particularly well documented, both morphologically and functionally. There appears to be at present little correspondence between the cellular and functional damage as a function of dose, but doses of a few tenths of a gray as a minimum are necessary to produce fertility changes in various animal species.

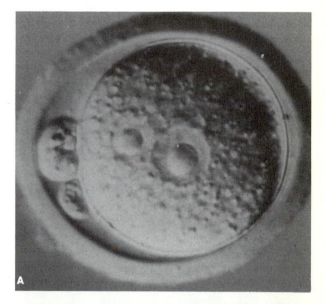

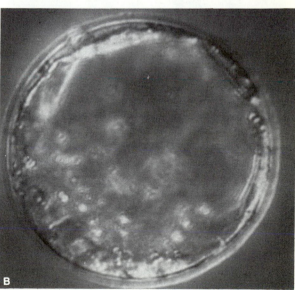

**Figure 21-3.** During preimplantation, the embryo consists of a limited number of cells. **(A)** Newly fertilized mouse egg. **(B)** By the third day, the mouse embryo consists of only 16 cells. About 5 days after conception in the mouse, which corresponds to 9 or 10 days in the human, the embryo becomes embedded in the wall of the uterus, and at about this time cells begin to differentiate to form specific tissues and organs. (Courtesy of Dr. Pedersen, University of California at San Francisco)

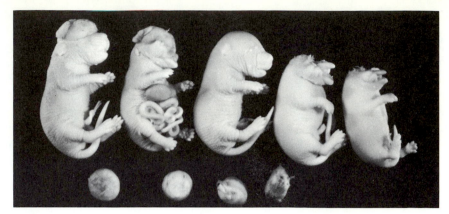

**Figure 21-4.** Litter from a female mouse irradiated with x-rays and sacrificed at 19 days. At least four different anomalies are demonstrated in this litter. There are four resorbed fetuses (*below*) and five fetuses alive. From left to right, the first shows exencephaly; the second, exencephaly and evisceration; the third is apparently normal, and the remaining two are anencephalics with stunting. (Photograph by Dr. Roberts Rugh)

Much higher doses of radiation are required to cause lethality during this period than at earlier stages of development, although the irradiated early fetus exhibits the largest degree of *permanent* growth retardation, in contrast to the embryo in early organogenesis, which exhibits the most *temporary* growth retardation, which is evident at term but from which the animal is able to recover later.

## EXPERIENCE IN HUMANS

Information on the irradiation of human concepti come from two major sources: (1) medical exposures (particularly therapeutic irradiations), especially during the early part of the century, when hazards were not yet fully appreciated, and (2) studies of A-bomb survivors in Japan.

The list of human abnormalities reported after

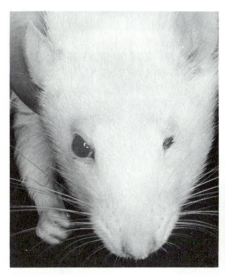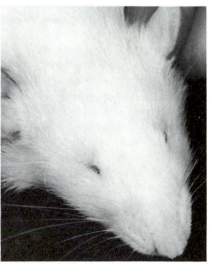

**Figure 21-5.** Two rats from the same litter exposed to a dose of 100 R of x-rays $9\frac{1}{2}$ days after conception. The rat on the left has a normal right eye and microphthalmus of the left. The rat on the right shows anophthalmia of both eyes. (From Rugh R, Caveness WF, Duhamel L, Schwarz GS: Milit Med 128:392, 1963)

in utero irradiation is long. Most commonly reported are microcephaly (sometimes combined with mental retardation), some other central nervous system defects, and growth retardation.

## SURVIVORS OF THE A-BOMB ATTACKS ON HIROSHIMA AND NAGASAKI IRRADIATED IN UTERO

The growth to maturity of children exposed in utero at Hiroshima and Nagasaki has been carefully studied. There are difficulties associated with the dosimetry, but the conclusions have far-reaching implications.

Data on those children exposed in utero in Hiroshima and Nagasaki show too few persons who were younger than 4 weeks of gestational age at the time the bomb was dropped. This deficiency is presumably due to increased fetal loss or infant mortality. This stage of development is so early that damage to a single cell, or a group of cells, is likely to impair the function of all the progeny and lead to death of the embryo. In accord with this reasoning is the observation that no birth defects were found as a result of irradiation before 15 days of gestational age. This is in accord with the experimental data for rats and mice in which exposure during preimplantation had an all-or-none effect: death of the embryo or normal development.

Exposure to radiation resulted in growth retardation (Table 21-1). Children exposed as embryos closer than 1500 meters from the hypo-

Table 21-1.
Growth Retardation at Hiroshima From in Utero Irradiation*: Comparison of Those Exposed Within 1500 m† of the Hypocenter With Those More Than 3000 m From the Hypocenter

| Height | 2.25 cm shorter |
|---|---|
| Weight | 3 kg lighter |
| Head diameter | 1.1 cm smaller |

*80% of 1613 children exposed in utero followed to age 17 years.
†Average kerma, 25 rads (0.25 Gy), but doses are subject to modification. (Data from Committee on the Biological Effects of Ionizing Radiations BEIR III: The Effects on Populations of Exposure to Low Levels of Ionizing Radiation. Washington, DC, National Academy of Sciences, 1980)

center of the atomic explosion were shorter, weighed less, and had head diameters significantly smaller than children who were more than 3000 meters from the hypocenter and received negligibly small doses. It is of interest to note that there was no catch-up growth, since the smallness in head size was maintained into adulthood.

The principal effects of irradiation in utero of the Japanese at Hiroshima and Nagasaki are small head size (microcephaly) and mental retardation. Figure 21-6 is one of the few photographs available of a young Japanese adult, exposed in utero to radiation from the A-bomb, whose head circumference is evidently smaller than normal. A three-dimensional graphic portrayal of the Hiroshima data (Fig. 21-7) shows the frequency of small head circumference with respect to dose and gestational age. It should be noted that

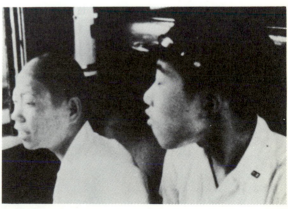

Figure 21-6. One of the few photographs available of a Japanese youth with reduced head circumference as a result of radiation exposure in utero from the A-bomb. (From Committee for the Compilation of Materials on Damage Caused by the Atomic Bomb in Hiroshima and Nagasaki: Hiroshima and Nagaski, The Physical, Medical and Social Effects of the Atomic Bombings. New York, Basic Books, 1981)

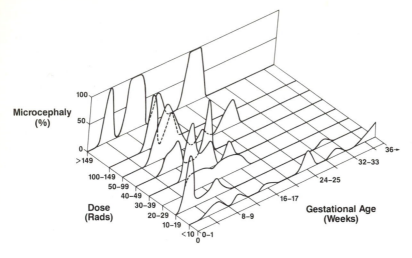

**Figure 21-7.** Incidence of micro-cephaly as a function of dose and gestational age among children in Hiroshima exposed in utero to the A-bomb. (Redrawn from Miller RW, Mulvihill JJ: In Sever JL, Brent RL [eds]: Teratogen Update: Environmentally Induced Birth Defect Risks, pp 141–143. New York, Alan R. Liss, 1986)

each point is based on only a few observations. The frequency of small head circumference is most pronounced in the most heavily exposed group (1.5 Gy, ie, 150 rads or more), but that the effect is seen in those whose maternal exposure was 0.1 to 0.19 Gy (10 to 19 rads).

The prevalence of mental retardation in children exposed in utero to the A-bombs in Hiroshima and Nagasaki has also been reevaluated in reference to gestational age and tissue dose in the fetus. The study involved about 1600 children and confirmed that about 30 of them showed clinically severe mental retardation. A child was deemed to be mentally retarded if he or she was "unable to perform simple calculations, to make simple conversation, to care for himself or herself, or if he or she was completely unmanageable or has been institutionalized." Most of these children were never enrolled in public schools,

but among the few who were, the highest IQ was 68.

Of the 30 children judged to be severely mentally retarded, 5 were considered to be the consequences of causes other than radiation, including Down's syndrome, neonatal jaundice, encephalitis, or birth trauma; nevertheless, the remaining number represents an incidence far higher than normal. Severe mental retardation was *not* observed to be induced by radiation before 8 weeks after conception or after 25 weeks. The most sensitive period is 8 to 15 weeks after conception; for exposure during weeks 16 to 25, the risk is four times smaller. Figure 21-8 shows the relation between the incidence of mental retardation and absorbed dose for this most sensitive period. The relationship appears to be linear, and the data are consistent with a probability of occurrence of mental retardation of 40% at a

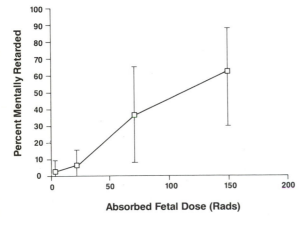

**Figure 21-8.** The frequency of mental retardation as a function of dose among those exposed in utero to A-bomb radiation. The data are pooled from Hiroshima and Nagasaki for those exposed at 8 to 15 weeks' gestational age. The vertical bars represent the 90% confidence intervals. There was no risk at 0 to 8 weeks after conception, and for exposure at later periods during gestation the excess is barely significant, even at the higher doses. (Redrawn from Otake M, Schull WJ: Br J Radiol 57:409–414, 1984)

dose of 1 Gy (100 rads). The possibility of a dose threshold cannot be excluded. By using the most recent dosimetry and discarding two cases of mental retardation for which in utero irradiation was unlikely to be the cause, the dose–response relationship is consistent with a threshold of 0.12 to 0.2 Gy (12 to 20 rads). A linear, nonthreshold response is unlikely in view of the presumed deterministic nature of mental retardation that would require the killing of a minimum number of cells to be manifest. The highest risk of mental retardation occurs at a gestational age when the relevant tissue, that is, the brain cortex, is being formed. It is thought to be associated with impaired proliferation, differentiation, and, most of all, migration of cells from their place of birth to their site of function. Cells killed before 8 weeks of gestation can cause small head size without mental retardation because the neurons that lead to the formation of the cerebrum are at a stage not yet sensitive to impairment by radiation. Glial cells that provide structural support for the brain are, however, susceptible to depletion. Magnetic resonance images of individuals irradiated in utero at 8 to 15 weeks' gestational age show evidence of massive impairment of cells to migrate from proliferative zones. Atypical distribution of gray matter is often seen in patients with mental retardation, but it is usually *unilateral*; that due to radiation exposure is *bilateral*.

Although severe mental retardation requiring the children to be institutionalized has been known for some time in those exposed in utero at Hiroshima, more recent studies have shown mental impairment of less severity, indicated by IQ test scores. During the sensitive period of 8 to 15 weeks after conception the observed shift in intelligence test scores corresponds to about 30 IQ points per gray (100 rads). Extrapolating these data to the situation in which a fetus is knowingly or unwillingly exposed to diagnostic radiology, resulting in a dose of perhaps 0.05 Gy (5 rads), the loss of IQ, using a linear model, would be too small to be detected.

## EXPOSURE TO MEDICAL RADIATION

A relationship between microcephaly and x-irradiation during intrauterine life has been recognized since Murphy and Goldstein first focused attention on the subject in 1930. The numbers are small and the doses are not known with any certainty, though most were in the therapeutic range. Microcephaly was reported as well as mental retardation and a variety of defects including spina bifida, bilateral clubfoot, ossification defects of the cranial bones, deformities of the upper extremities, hydrocephaly, alopecia of the scalp, divergent squint, and blindness at birth.

Dekaban has surveyed the literature for instances of pelvic x-irradiation in pregnant women. On the basis of the available data, the following generalizations were proposed:

1. Large doses of radiation (2.5 Gy [250 rads]) delivered to the human embryo before 2 to 3 weeks of gestation are not likely to produce severe abnormalities in most children born, although a considerable number of the embryos may be resorbed or aborted.
2. Irradiation between 4 and 11 weeks of gestation would lead to severe abnormalities of many organs in most children.
3. Irradiation between 11 and 16 weeks of gestation may produce a few eye, skeletal, and genital organ abnormalities; stunted growth, microcephaly, and mental retardation are frequently present.
4. Irradiation of the fetus between 16 and 20 weeks of gestation may lead to a mild degree of microcephaly, mental retardation, and stunting of growth.
5. Irradiation after 30 weeks of gestation is not likely to produce gross structural abnormalities leading to a serious handicap in early life but could cause functional disabilities.

## COMPARISON OF HUMAN AND ANIMAL DATA

Figure 21-9 is an attempt to summarize the data for the effects of radiation on the developing embryo and fetus, comparing and contrasting the information from animals and humans.

Exposure to radiation during preimplantation leads to a high incidence of embryonic death, but embryos that survive develop normally. This has been shown clearly in experiments with both

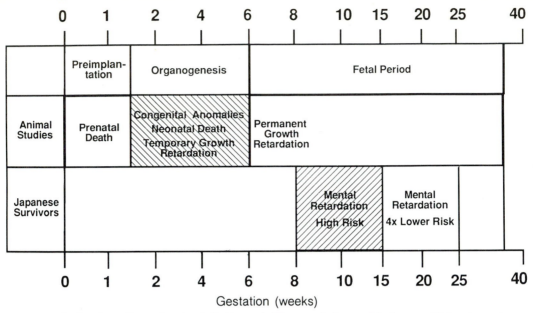

Gestation (weeks)

Figure 21-9. Chart illustrating the similarities and differences between data from small laboratory animals, and data from the Japanese survivors of the A-bomb attacks. Both agree that irradiation early in gestation may result in the death of the embryo but that malformations do not occur. The animal data show a high incidence of a wide spectrum of malformations during organogenesis. The principal finding in the Japanese is microcephaly and mental retardation, which occurred most frequently following irradiation at 8 to 15 weeks of gestation and, to a lesser extent, at 15 to 25 weeks.

rats and mice and is consistent with the data from Japan. In animals, irradiation during organogenesis leads to neonatal death, temporary growth retardation, and, above all, a wide range of malformations affecting many different limbs and organs. By contrast, the principal effect in the Japanese survivors of the A-bomb attacks is microcephaly with or without mental retardation, and this begins in the eighth week, that is, after the period classically described as organogenesis. The wide array of congenital malformations found in rats and mice irradiated in organogenesis was *not* reported in the Japanese survivors. Much has been made of this difference. On the one hand, it has been suggested that the gross structural deformities in Japan were simply not recorded in the chaos that followed the dropping of the A-bombs. On the other hand, it is argued that humans differ from rats and mice in that the period of susceptibility to a wide array of congenital malformations (10 to 32 days of gestation) is short compared with the 8 weeks during which mental retardation can be induced and the 16 weeks during which irradiation can result in a reduced head diameter. Since the number of

children involved is quite small, it might be expected that effects on the central nervous system, which is developing over a larger period of time, would dominate. The situation is different in laboratory animals; their susceptibility to radiation-induced small head size is of similar duration to that for the induction of other deformities. The data from patients exposed to therapeutic doses of medical radiation show a range of congenital malformations that more closely mirror the animal results, although the numbers are small and the doses high. To be on the safe side, it must be assumed that the entire period of gestation from about 10 days to 25 weeks is sensitive to the induction of malformations by radiation.

Table 21-2 summarizes the lowest doses at which effects on the embryo and fetus have been observed. This table summarizes the conclusions of third report of the Committee on the Biological Effects of Ionizing Radiation (BEIR III). Readily measurable damage can be observed at doses below 0.1 Gy (10 rads) delivered at sensitive stages of gestation. The principal abnormalities produced by radiation are almost certainly the consequence of

Table 21-2.
**Minimum Doses at Which Effects on the Embryo and Fetus Have Been Observed**

**Animal Data**

| | |
|---|---|
| Oocyte killing (primates) | $LD_{50}$ at 5 rads (0.5 Gy) |
| Central nervous system damage (mouse) | Threshold at 10 rads (0.1 Gy) |
| Brain damage and behavioral damage (rat) | Threshold at 6 rads (0.06 Gy) |

**Human Data**

| | |
|---|---|
| Small head circumference | Air kerma 10 to 19 rads (0.1 to 0.19 Gy) Fetal dose 6 rads (0.06 Gy) |

**Summary**
Readily measurable damage caused by doses below 10 rads (0.1 Gy) (acute exposure) delivered at sensitive stages

*(Summarized from Committee on the Biological Effects of Ionizing Radiation: The Effects on Populations of Exposure to Low Levels of Ionizing Radiation. Washington, DC, National Academy of Sciences, 1980)*

Table 21-3.
**Childhood Cancer and Irradiation In Utero**

| | |
|---|---|
| Number of children with leukemia or cancer before age 10 years | 7649 |
| Number x-rayed in utero | 1141 |
| Number of matched controls | 7649 |
| Number of controls irradiated in utero | 774 |
| Number of films | 1 to 5 |
| Fetal dose per film | 0.46 to 0.2 rad (4.6 to 2 mGy) |
| Relative cancer risk estimate, assuming radiation to be the causative agent | 1.52 |

*(Based on Stewart A, Kneale GW: Lancet 1:1185–1188, 1970)*

damage to many cells (ie, a *deterministic* effect) and would therefore be consistent with a threshold in dose. There is some indication of this in the data for mental retardation.

## CANCER IN CHILDHOOD AFTER IRRADIATION IN UTERO

The Oxford Survey of Childhood Cancers, published by Stewart and Kneale in the 1950s, suggested an association between the risk of cancer, principally leukemia, up to 15 years of age and exposure in utero to diagnostic x-rays. This was a retrospective case-controlled study and is summarized in Table 21-3. Of 7649 children who died of leukemia or childhood cancers, 1141 had been x-rayed in utero. Of an equal number of controls who did not develop childhood cancer, only 774 had been irradiated prenatally. The irradiated children received one to five films. A subsequent study in New England by MacMahon also reported an association between prenatal x-rays and childhood cancer. It has been argued for years whether radiation is causative or whether the excess risk could be attributed to other factors or was limited to a particular

subpopulation. The initial follow-up of prenatally exposed A-bomb survivors did not support the Oxford study, but a more recent follow-up involving 1630 in utero exposed survivors show two cases of childhood cancer, both in persons heavily exposed. The dose estimates to the A-bomb survivors have been revised *downward* in recent years, while the estimated in utero doses in the Oxford study have been revised *upward* recently, and so the two studies no longer conflict.

The most compelling evidence supporting the idea that radiation may be the causative agent in childhood cancer after prenatal exposure comes from the study of twins. In years gone by the radiographic examination of women with twins was usually performed because of the twin pregnancy rather than for other diagnostic concerns. Studies in both Great Britain and the United States show as many cases of leukemia and childhood cancer in irradiated dizygotic and monozygotic twins as in irradiated singleton births, with a clear excess over those not exposed.

Because of the comparatively small radiation doses to the fetus from diagnostic radiology, these data prompt the tentative conclusion that susceptibility to the carcinogenic effects of radiation is high during in utero life. The data suggest that a few diagnostic exposures increase the natural cancer incidence by a factor of 1.5 to 2.0. This corresponds to a risk estimate of 200 to 250 excess cancer deaths per 10,000 person-Gy in the first 10 years of life, with half being leukemia. There is also now some suggestion of an increased cancer mortality in the Japanese survivors more than 40 years after they were exposed in utero. This group of survivors is only now reaching the age when the natural cancer incidence begins to rise, and it will be of great interest to see whether in utero irradiation so many years ago will carry a legacy of increased cancer incidence in old age as the preliminary data suggest.

## OCCUPATIONAL EXPOSURE OF WOMEN

The maximum permissible dose to the fetus during the entire gestation period from occupational exposure of the mother should not exceed 5mSv (0.5 rem) with a monthly exposure not to exceed 0.5mSv (0.05 rem). This is the recommendation of the National Council on Radiological Protection and Measurements (NCRP). Once a pregnancy is declared, the radiation worker should be interviewed by the radiation safety officer or the chairman of the radiation safety committee to decide whether duties need to be changed or curtailed. There are only a few occupations in which the possibility of an unplanned radiation exposure, which while not being more than that allowed a radiation worker, would exceed the more stringent limits suggested for the unborn child. The 5mSv (0.5 rem) limit is based on the premise that the unborn child is sensitive to the production of defects and/or to an increased risk of leukemia, which is not warranted in the performance of the mother's occupation, although it may be acceptable in the course of delivering her health care.

## THE PREGNANT OR POTENTIALLY PREGNANT PATIENT

Most practicing radiologists at some time in their career will be faced with a patient who has discovered in retrospect that she was pregnant at a time when extensive x-ray procedures were performed that involved the pelvis or lower abdomen.

The only completely satisfactory solution to this problem is to ensure that the situation never occurs in the first place. Patients should always be asked if they are, or may be, pregnant, and in the case of procedures involving larger doses of radiation to the pelvis, a pregnancy test may be in order.

Despite the best-laid plans and the most careful precautions, there will still be occasional instances when, because of clinical urgency or unusual accident, an early developing embryo will have been exposed to a substantial dose of radiation amounting to several centigray (rads) or more. The first step is to estimate the dose involved. It is sometimes useful to solicit the help of an experienced medical physicist to make measurements in a phantom after carefully reconstructing the setup that was used. No dose level can be regarded as completely safe. Congenital abnormalities occur in 5% to 10% of the human population anyway, and so it is impossible in retrospect to attribute a given anomaly to a small dose of radiation received by an embryo or fetus. All that can be said is that radiation increases the probability of an anomaly and that this increase is a function of dose.

The figure of 0.1 Gy (10 rads) is often mentioned as the cutoff point above which a therapeutic abortion should be considered if the developing embryo or fetus received this dose at a gestational age sensitive to the induction of congenital malformations, including reduced head diameter and mental retardation. This period extends from about 10 days to 26 weeks of gestation. The basis of this recommendation is as follows. The data from Japan for severe mental retardation could be interpreted as having a threshold, and the mechanism of the radiation effect is consistent with this conclusion. At the same time, the loss of IQ measured at 1 Gy (100 rads) would be undetectable if extrapolated linearly to 0.1 Gy (10 rads).

Not everyone would agree with this view, and the cutoff point is clearly not sharp. When a dose approaching this value has been given during the sensitive period, however, it is prudent to consider the relative merits of terminating the pregnancy in consultation with the referring physician as well as with the patient and her family. There are a number of factors to consider in conjunction with the dose. These include the hazard of the pregnancy to the expectant mother, the probability of future pregnancies, the extent to which the prospective parents want the unborn infant, their mental outlook on the possibility of a deformed child, and the ethnic and religious background of the family. The exact dose level at which it is justifiable to terminate the pregnancy may be flexible within broad limits around the guideline figure depending on a combination of these other circumstances.

There are special problems involved in the use of nuclear medicine procedures in pregnant or potentially pregnant females. This is particularly true in the case of radionuclides that are able to cross the placenta. This topic is discussed in Chapter 24.

► *Summary of Pertinent Conclusions*

- Moderate doses of radiation can produce catastrophic effects on the developing embryo and fetus.
- The effects depends on the stage of gestation, the dose, and also the dose rate.
- Gestation is divided into preimplantation, organogenesis, and the fetal period. In humans, these periods correspond to about 0 to 9 days, 10 days to 6 weeks, and 6 weeks to term, respectively.
- The principal effects of radiation on the developing embryo and fetus are (1) growth retardation; (2) embryonic, neonatal, or fetal death; and (3) congenital malformations, and functional impairment such as mental retardation.
- Irradiation during preimplantation leads to death of the embryo. Growth retardation or malformations are not seen in animals at this time. The human data are consistent with this conclusion.
- In animals, embryos exposed to radiation in early organogenesis exhibit the most severe intrauterine growth retardation, from which they can recover later (ie, temporary growth retardation). Irradiation in the fetal period leads to the greatest degree of permanent growth retardation.
- In animals, lethality from irradiation varies with stage of development. The embryonic $LD_{50}$ dose is lowest during early preimplantation; at this stage, embryos killed by radiation suffer a prenatal death and are resorbed. In organogenesis, prenatal death is replaced by neonatal death—death at or about the time of birth. During the fetal stage the $LD_{50}$ approaches that of the adult.
- In animals, the peak incidence of teratogenesis, or gross malformations, occurs when the fetus is irradiated in organogenesis.
- Contrary to what is observed in experimental animals, radiation-induced malformations of body structures other than the central nervous system are uncommon in the Japanese survivors irradiated in utero, although they have been reported in patients exposed to therapeutic doses of medical radiation.
- In the Japanese survivors, irradiation in utero resulted in small head size (microcephaly) and mental retardation.
- Mental retardation occurred primarily at 8 to 15 weeks of gestational age, with a smaller excess at 16 to 25 weeks. It is thought to be due to radiation effects on cell migration within the brain.
- Cells killed before 8 weeks of gestational age cause small head size without mental retardation.

*(continued)*

► *Summary of Pertinent Conclusions* *(Continued)*

- Small head circumference was three times more common than mental retardation.
- Data on A-bomb survivors indicate that microcephaly can result from an air dose (kerma) of 0.1 to 0.19 Gy (10 to 19 rads)
- The incidence of severe mental retardation as a function of dose is reported to be apparently linear without threshold at 8 to 15 weeks, with a risk coefficient of 0.4 per Gy (0.4 per 100 rads). The incidence is about four times lower at 16 to 25 weeks. The data are consistent with a dose threshold of 0.12 to 0.2 Gy (12 to 20 rads).
- A variety of effects have been documented in experimental animals after irradiation during fetal stages, including effects on the hematopoietic system, liver, and kidney, all occurring, however, after quite high radiation doses.
- The effects on the developing gonads have been well documented both morphologically and functionally. Doses close to 1 Gy (100 rads) are needed to produce fertility changes in various species.
- There is an association between exposure to diagnostic x-rays in utero and the subsequent development of childhood malignancies.
- The original study of diagnostic x-ray exposure in utero and subsequent malignancies was done by Stewart and Kneale at Oxford University, but the same association was observed in the United States by MacMahon. If x-rays are the causative agent, these studies imply that radiation at low doses in utero increase the spontaneous cancer incidence in the first 10 to 15 years of life by a factor of 1.5 to 2.
- Initially the Japanese data on A-bomb survivors did not support this conclusion, but a more recent study has reported two childhood leukemias and the data no longer conflict.
- It has been argued for years whether radiation is the causative agent or whether there are other factors involved.
- The strongest evidence for radiation as a causative agent is that twins show an excess of cancer, too, and in times past the radiographic examination of women with twins was performed because of the twin pregnancy rather than for other diagnostic concerns.
- The data prompt the tentative conclusion that susceptibility to the carcinogenic effects of radiation is high during in utero life.
- Preliminary evidence suggests that the Japanese survivors irradiated in utero show an excess of adult cancers more than 4 decades later.
- The maximum permissible dose to the fetus during gestation is 5mSv (0.5 rem), with a monthly limit of 0.5mSv (0.05 rem).
- Once a pregnancy is declared, the duties of a radiation worker should be reviewed to ensure that this limit is not exceeded.
- A dose of 0.1 Gy (10 rads) to the embryo during the sensitive period of gestation (10 days to 26 weeks) is often regarded as the cutoff point, above which a therapeutic abortion should be considered to avoid the possibility of an anomalous child. The decision to terminate a pregnancy should be flexible and must depend on many factors in addition to dose.

# BIBLIOGRAPHY

Balakier H, Pedersen RA: Allocation of cells to inner cell mass and trophectoderm lineages in preimplantation mouse embryos. Dev Biol 90:352–362, 1982

Bithel JF, Stiller CA: A new calculation of the carcinogenic risk of obstetric x-raying. Stat Med 7:857–864, 1988

Brent RL: Irradiation in pregnancy. In Sciarra JJ (ed): Davis' Gynecology and Obstetrics, vol 2, pp 1–32. New York, Harper & Row, 1972

Brent RL, Ghorson RO: Radiation exposure in pregnancy. Curr Probl Radiol 2:1–48, 1972

Committee on the Biological Effects of Ionizing Radiation: The Effects on Populations of Exposure to Low Levels of Ionizing Radiation. Washington, DC, National Academy of Sciences, 1980

Committee on the Biological Effects of Ionizing Radiation: Health Effects of Exposure to Low Levels of Ionizing Radiations. Washington, DC, National Academy of Sciences/National Research Council, 1990

Dekaban AS: Abnormalities in children exposed to x-radiation during various stages of gestation: Tentative timetable of radiation to the human fetus: I. J Nucl Med 9:471–477, 1968

Goldstein L, Murphy DP: Microcephalic idiocy following radium therapy for uterine cancer during pregnancy. Am J Obstet Gynecol 18:189–195, 281–282, 1929

Hammer-Jacobsen E: Therapeutic abortion on account of x-ray examination during pregnancy. Dan Med Bull 6:113–121, 1959

Harvey EB, Boice JD, Honeyman M, Fannery JT: Prenatal x-ray exposure and childhood cancer in twins. N Engl J Med 312:541–545, 1985

Jablon S, Kato H: Childhood cancer in relation to prenatal exposure to atomic-bomb radiation. Lancet 2:1000–1003, 1970

MacMahon B: Prenatal x-ray exposure and childhood cancer. JNCI 28:1173–1191, 1962

MacMahon B, Hutchinson GB: Prenatal x-ray and childhood cancer: A review. Acta Univ Int Contra Cancrum 20:1172–1174, 1964

Miller RW: Effects of prenatal exposure to ionizing radiation. Health Phys 59:57–61, 1990

Miller RW, Blot WJ: Small head size after in utero exposure to atomic radiation. Lancet 2:784, 1972

Miller RW, Mulvihill JJ: Small head size after atomic irradiation. In Sever JL, Brent RL (eds): Teratogen Update: Environmentally Induced Birth Defect Risks, pp 141–143. New York, Alan R Liss, 1986

Mole RH: Antenatal irradiation and childhood cancer: Causation or coincidence? Br J Cancer 30:199–208, 1974

Murphy DP: Congenital Malformations. Philadelphia, JB Lippincott, 1947

Murphy DP, Goldstein L: Micromelia in a child irradiated in utero. Surg Gynecol Obstet 50:79–80, 1930

Otake M, Schull WJ: In utero exposure to A-bomb radiation and mental retardation: A reassessment. Br J Radiol 57;409–414, 1984

Plummer G: Anomalies occurring in children exposed in utero to the atomic bomb in Hiroshima. Pediatrics 10:687–693, 1952

Rugh R: Ionizing radiations: Their possible relation to the etiology of some congenital anomalies and human disorders. Milit Med 124:401–415, 1959

Rugh R: Low levels of x-irradiation and the early mammalian embryo. AJR 87:559–566, 1962

Rugh R: The impact of ionizing radiation on the embryo and fetus. AJR 89:182–190, 1963

Rugh R, Caveness WF, Duhamel L, Schwarz GS: Structural and functional (electroencephalographic) changes in the post-natal mammalian brain resulting from x-irradiation of the embryo. Milit Med 128:392, 1959

Rugh R, Grupp E: Ionizing radiations and congenital anomalies in vertebrate embryos. Acta Embryol Exp (Palermo) 2:257–268, 1959

Russell LB, Montgomery CS: Radiation sensitivity differences within cell-division cycles during mouse cleavage. Int J Radiat Biol 10:151–164, 1966

Russell LB, Russell WL: Radiation hazards to the embryo and fetus. Radiology 58:369–376, 1952

Russell LB, Russell WL: An analysis of the changing radiation response of the developing mouse embryo. J Cell Physiol 43(suppl 1):1030–149, 1954

Russell WL: Effect of the interval between irradiation and conception on mutational frequency in female mice. Proc Natl Acad Sci USA 54:1552–1557, 1965

Seigel DG: Frequency of live births among survivors of Hiroshima and Nagasaki atomic bombs. Radiat Res 28:278–288, 1966

Stewart A: The carcinogenic effects of low level radiation: A reappraisal of epidemiologists' methods and observations. Health Phys 24:223–240, 1973

Stewart A, Kneale GW: Radiation dose effects in relation to obstetric x-rays and childhood cancers. Lancet 1:1185–1188, 1970

Stewart A, Webb J, Hewitt D: A survey of childhood malignancies. Br Med J 1:1495–1500, 1958

United Nations Scientific Committee on the Effects of Atomic Radiation Report A/3838, General Assembly Official Records, Thirteenth Session, Suppl No. 17. New York, United Nations, 1958

United Nations Scientific Committee on the Effects of Atomic Radiation Report A/5216, General Assembly Official Records, Seventeenth Session, Suppl No. 16. New York, United Nations, 1962

United Nations Scientific Committee on the Effects of Atomic Radiation Report A/8314, General Assembly Official Records, Twenty-first Session, Suppl No. 144. New York, United Nations, 1966

United Nations Scientific Committee on the Effects of Atomic Radiation Report A/6314, General Assembly Official Records, Twenty-fourth Session, Suppl No. 13. New York, United Nations, 1969

United Nations Scientific Committee on the Effects of Atomic Radiation Report A/8725, General Assembly Official Records, Twenty-seventh Session, Suppl No. 25. New York, United Nations, 1972

United Nations Scientific Committee on the Effects of Atomic Radiation Report A/3240, General Assembly Official Records, Thirty-second Session, Suppl No. 40. New York, United Nations, 1977

United Nations Scientific Committee on the Effects of Atomic Radiation: Sources and Effects of Ionizing Radiation. New York, UNSCEAR, 1986

Wood JW, Johnson KG, Omori Y: In utero exposure to the Hiroshima atomic bomb: Follow-up at 20 years. Pediatrics 39:385–392, 1967

Wood JW, Johnson KG, Omori Y, Kawamoto S, Keehn RJ: Mental retardation in children exposed in utero to the atomic bomb in Hiroshima and Nagasaki. Am J Public Health 57:1381–1390, 1967

Yamazaki JW, Wright SW, Wright PM: Outcome of pregnancy in women exposed to the atomic bomb in Nagasaki. Am J Dis Child 87:448–463, 1954

Yoshimoto Y, Kato H, Schull WJ: Risk of cancer among children exposed in utero to A-bomb radiation, 1950–1984. Lancet 2:665–669, 1988

*Radiobiology for the Radiologist, Fourth Edition*, by Eric J. Hall
J. B. Lippincott Company, Philadelphia © 1994.

# 22

# *Radiation Cataractogenesis*

Diagnostic Radiology
Nuclear Medicine
Radiation Therapy

## CATARACTS OF THE OCULAR LENS

The word **cataract** is used to describe any detectable change of the normally transparent lens of the eye. The effect may vary from tiny flecks in the lens to almost complete opacification, resulting in total blindness. Cataracts are most usually associated with old age or less commonly with some abnormal metabolic disorder, chronic ocular infection, or trauma. It is also well known that sufficient exposure to ionizing radiations (such as x- or γ-rays, charged particles, or neutrons) may cause a cataract.

The ocular lens is enclosed in a capsule (Fig. 22-1); the lens itself consists largely of fiber cells and is covered with an epithelium anteriorly. The lens has no blood supply. Dividing cells are limited to the pre-equatorial region of the epithelium. The progeny of these mitotic cells differentiate into lens fibers and accrete at the equator.

Cell division continues throughout life, and so the lens may be regarded as a self-renewal tissue. It is, however, a most curious cellular system in that there appears to be no mechanism for cell removal. If dividing cells are injured by radiation, the resulting abnormal fibers are not removed from the lens but migrate toward the posterior pole; because they are not translucent, they constitute the beginning of a cataract.

## LENS OPACIFICATION IN EXPERIMENTAL ANIMALS

Some species of animals, especially the mouse, are very sensitive to radiation as far as lens opacification is concerned. A dose of a few centigray of x-rays or a fraction of a centigray of fast neutrons will produce readily discernible changes in the lens. A large proportion of a mouse population naturally develops opacifications as they become older. As the dose is increased, the **latent period**—the time that elapses before an opacity of given severity is evident—becomes shorter. Put another way, radiation advances in time, a process that occurs normally.

Neutrons and other densely ionizing radiations are *very* effective at inducing cataracts, as evidenced by the number of physicists and engineers who developed cataracts as a result of working around high energy accelerators in the early days. The relative biological effectiveness (RBE) of the fast neutrons is a strong function of dose, with a value of about 10 pertaining to high dose levels on the order of several gray (several hundreds of rads), relative to x-rays, but rising to 50 or more for small doses of a fraction of a centigray (rad). Worgul and his associates have reported similar RBEs for lens damage in rat eyes exposed to accelerated heavy ions. The increase in RBE at low doses is due largely to a sharply

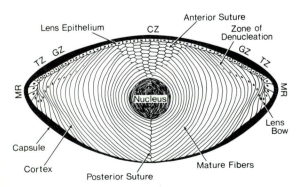

**Figure 22-1.** Diagram of a sagittal section of a human lens illustrating the various cellular relationships. Cells are produced by mitosis in the germination zone of the epithelium (GZ). They begin to differentiate into lens fibers at the meridional rows (MR) and accumulate at the equator. Cells in the central zone (CZ) do not normally divide. (From Merriam GR, Worgul BV: Bull NY Acad Med 59:372–392, 1983)

declining effectiveness of x-rays with decreasing dose, rather than an increase in effect per unit dose of neutrons or charged particles.

## CATARACTS IN HUMANS

Radiologists have known for many years that the lens of the eye may be damaged by radiation. A study of patients treated with x- or γ-rays, in which a proportion of the dose reached the eye, has provided some insight into radiation cataractogenesis in humans. Figure 22-2 shows a typical cataract in a patient on radiotherapy. An early radiation cataract viewed through an ophthalmoscope may appear as a dot, usually situated at the posterior pole. As it enlarges, small granules and vacuoles appear around it. With further enlargement to the point at which the opacity is several millimeters in diameter, it may develop with a relatively clear center, so that it is shaped like a doughnut. At the same time, granular opacities and vacuoles may appear in the anterior subcapsular region, usually in the pupillary area. Depending on dose, the cataract frequently remains stationary at this stage, confined to the posterior subcapsular region. If it continues to progress, it becomes nonspecific and cannot be distinguished from other types of cataracts.

## THE DEGREE OF OPACITY

At low doses, the opacity may become stationary at a level that involves little or no impairment of vision. At higher doses, the opacity may progress until it results in a significant loss of vision. Of those patients on radiotherapy who received low dose levels to the eye (2.2 to 6.5 Gy [220 to 650 rads]), only about 12% developed *progressive* opacities. Conversely, in the higher dose groups (6.5 to 11.5 Gy [650 to 1150 rads]), only 12% had *stationary* opacities.

## THE LATENT PERIOD

The time period between irradiation and the appearance of lens opacities in humans has been variously reported in the literature to be from 6

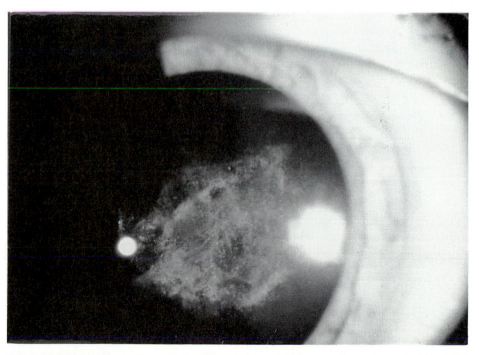

**Figure 22-2.** Cataract in the posterior subcapsular region 4 years after a dose of 24 Gy (2400 rads) of x-rays to a patient on radiotherapy. (From Merriam CR, Worgul BV: Bull NY Acad Med 59:372–392, 1983)

months to 35 years. In patients who had received 2.5 to 6.5 Gy (250 to 650 rads) the average latent period was about 8 years. At higher doses of between 6.51 to 11.5 Gy (651 to 1150 rads), the average latent period was reduced to about 4 years. This and other evidence indicate that the latent period becomes shorter as dose is increased.

## DOSE–RESPONSE RELATIONSHIP FOR CATARACTS IN HUMANS

Merriam, Szechter, and Focht carefully reviewed the case histories of 233 patients on radiotherapy who received radiation to the lens of the eye and for whom dose estimates were available. Of these, 128 developed cataracts, while 105 did not.

No opacities were observed with doses of less than 2.5 Gy (250 rads) of x-rays; there were two cases of minimum static opacities in patients who had received this minimum dose in a single exposure. The lowest single dose at which a progressive cataract was observed was 5 Gy (500 rads).

The lens seemed able to tolerate a higher dose with increased fractionation and overall treatment time. For a multifraction treatment spread over 3 weeks to 3 months or over periods in excess of 3 months the minimum cataractogenic doses rose to 4 to 5.5 Gy (400 to 550 rads), respectively.

Figure 22-3 is deduced from accumulated clinical experience. It represents a dose–time relationship for the production of cataracts. A combination of a dose and a treatment time that falls *below* the shaded band will *not* produce injury to the lens. A dose and overall time that falls *above* the shaded area *would* be expected to produce a progressive opacity with impairment of vision. Within the shaded zone a cataract may or may not be produced. The probability of a progressive cataract increases with increasing dose.

Britten and his colleagues reported 14 cases of radiation-induced cataracts in 38 patients treated with radon gold seed implants for tumors of the eyelid; in 6 visual acuity was seriously affected. These cataracts were thought to be progressive between 6 and 11 years after treatment. Doses were calculated to the center of the lens, and it appeared that 4 Gy (400 rads) produced a cataract in all cases, whereas 20 Gy (2000 rads) resulted in no cataracts at all. In a parallel series treated by superficial x-rays, only one case of radiation cataract was observed in 57 patients treated; this was in the contralateral eye, which received a dose of 9.5 Gy (950 rads) in a single

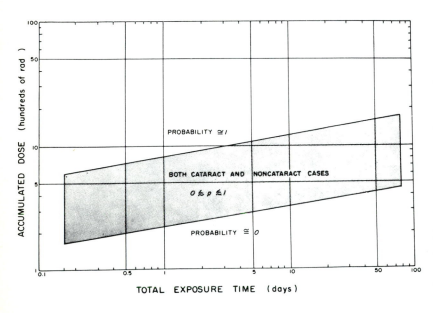

Figure 22-3. Time–dose relationship indicating radiation dosage for cataract production in humans with a probability between zero and one. A combination of a total dose and overall treatment time that falls above the shaded area would produce a progressive vision-impairing opacity. A dose and treatment time falling below the shaded area would not be expected to produce injury to the lens. Within the shaded area a cataract may or may not be produced; the probability increases with increasing dose. (From Merriam GR, Szechter A, Focht EF: Front Radiat Ther Oncol 6:346–385, 1972)

exposure, which was presumably transmitted through the nose to the opposite eye. The lens dose on the treated side that was shielded with lead was only 0.16 Gy (16 rads).

Observations of the survivors of Hiroshima and Nagasaki have been consistent with the data from patients on radiotherapy. Large doses of radiation are required to produce vision-impairing cataracts. Physicists exposed to neutrons during the operation of cyclotron accelerators and survivors of reactor accidents have also developed cataracts, but the numbers are too small and the doses are not known with sufficient certainty to allow a meaningful construction of a dose–response relationship.

The available information appears to indicate the existence of a threshold for the induction of detectable lens opacification in humans. This does not exclude the possibility that the smallest doses do produce some damage, but in practical terms a dose of several gray (several hundred rads) is required to result in a demonstrable effect and even larger doses to produce a cataract that impairs vision. Great care should be exercised in the use of neutrons and indeed all forms of high linear energy transfer radiations, since animal experiments indicate that they have a high RBE for lens opacification.

Radiation-induced cataracts are a deterministic (nonstochastic) late effect, since there is a practical threshold dose below which they do not occur and above the threshold the severity of the biological response is dose related.

► *Summary of Pertinent Conclusions*

- A cataract is an opacification of the normally transparent lens of the eye.
- Dividing cells are limited to the pre-equatorial region of the epithelium. Progeny of these mitotic cells differentiate into lens fibers and accrete at the equator. It is the failure of these cells to differentiate correctly that leads to a radiation cataract.
- The minimum dose required to produce a progressive cataract is about 2 Gy (200 rads) in a single exposure, with larger doses necessary in a fractionated regimen.
- The latent period between irradiation and the appearance of a lens opacity is dose related. The latency is about 8 years after exposure to a dose in the range of 2.5 to 6.5 Gy (250 to 650 rads).
- The RBE of neutrons or heavy ions is about 10 at high doses but rises to 50 or more for small doses.
- A radiation-induced cataract is a deterministic (nonstochastic) late effect. There is a practical threshold dose below which cataracts are not produced, and above this threshold the severity of the biological response is dose related.

# BIBLIOGRAPHY

Bateman JL, Bond VP: Lens opacification in mice exposed to fast neutrons. Radiat Res 7(suppl) 239–249, 1967

Britten MJA, Halnan KE, Meredith WJ: Radiation cataract: New evidence on radiation dosage to the lens. Br J Radiol 39:612–617, 1966

Langham WH (ed): Radiobiological Factors in Manned Space Flight, publication No. 1487. Washington, DC, National Academy of Sciences/National Research Council, 1967

Merriam GR, Focht EF: Clinical study of radiation cataracts and the relationship to dose. AJR 77:759–785, 1957

Merriam GR, Focht EF: Radiation dose to the lens in treatment of tumors of the eye and adjacent structures: Possibilities of cataract formation. Radiology 71:357–369, 1958

Merriam GR, Szechter A, Focht EF: The effects of ionizing radiations on the eye. Front Radiat Ther Oncol 6:346–385, 1972

Merriam GR, Worgul BV: Experimental radiation cata-ract: Its clinical relevance. Bull NY Acad Med 59:372–292, 1983

Worgul BV, Merriam GR, Medvedovsky C: Accelerated heavy particles and the lens: II. Cytopathological changes. Invest Ophthalmol Vis Sci 27:108–114, 1985

*Radiobiology for the Radiologist, Fourth Edition*, by Eric J. Hall
J. B. Lippincott Company, Philadelphia © 1994.

# 23

# *Molecular Techniques in Radiobiology*

Optional

# HISTORICAL PERSPECTIVES

Recombinant DNA technology has revolutionized research in biology. It allows questions to be asked that, a few years ago, were unthinkable. It is also a technology that is moving fast; we are in the midst of a whirlwind revolution, so that anything written in a book is likely to be out of date before it appears in print. This technology is invading every field of biological research, and radiobiology is no exception. To keep abreast with developments in the field it is essential to know what recombinant DNA technology is and how it works. A detailed description is beyond the scope of this book; for a more exhaustive account, the interested reader is referred to several excellent volumes that have appeared in recent years and are listed in the bibliography. The goal here is to provide an overview and to illustrate the way in which recombinant techniques have been used to solve specific problems in radiobiological research.

The birth of molecular biology could be ascribed to the one-page publication in *Nature* in 1953 by Watson and Crick, describing the structure of DNA. In short order, this work led the way toward breaking the genetic code and toward understanding the process of transcription of DNA to mRNA and the translation of mRNA into proteins.

These remarkable discoveries were followed by a period of limited progress focusing mainly on simple systems such as viruses, bacteriophage, and bacteria until new tools and techniques to work with DNA were perfected.

The start of recombinant DNA technology was the first successful cloning experiment of Stanley Cohen, in which he joined two DNA fragments together (a plasmid containing a tetracycline resistance gene with a karamycin resistance gene), introduced this recombinant molecule into *Escherichia coli,* and demonstrated that the bacteria now had dual antibiotic resistance.

This simple experiment was only possible because of the simultaneous development of several techniques for (1) cutting DNA with restriction enzymes and joining the fragments with ligases and (2) using *E. coli* as a host with the ability to take up foreign DNA through the use of plasmid vectors.

What follows is a brief and simplified description of these techniques and those that followed, together with some examples of their application to problems in radiobiology.

# RESTRICTION ENDONUCLEASES

Restriction enzymes are endonucleases found in bacteria that have the property of recognizing a specific DNA sequence and cleaving at or near that site. These enzymes can be grouped into three categories, types I, II and III. The restriction enzymes commonly used are of type II, meaning that they have endonuclease activity only (ie, they cut the DNA, without modification) at a predictable site within or adjacent to the recognition sequence. Types I and III have properties that make them impractical for use in molecular biology.

More than a thousand type II enzymes have been isolated, and more than 70 are commercially available. Some examples are shown in Table 23-1. They are named according to the following system.

1. The first letter comes from the genus of the organism from which the enzyme was isolated.
2. The second and third letters follow the organism's species name.
3. If there is a fourth letter, it refers to a particular strain of the organism
4. The Roman numerals, as often as not, refer to the order in which enzymes were discovered, although the original intent was that it would indicate the order in which enzymes of the same organism and strain are eluted from a chromatography column.

Restriction endonucleases scan the DNA molecule, stopping when they recognize a particular nucleotide sequence. Some endonucleases, such

Table 23-1.
## Examples of Type II Restriction Enzymes

| ***Hind*III** | H | = | genus *Haemophilus* |
| | in | = | species *influenzae* |
| | d | = | strain Rd |
| | III | = | third endonuclease isolated |
| ***Eco*RI** | E | = | genus *Escherichia* |
| | co | = | species *coli* |
| | R | = | strain RY13 |
| | I | = | first endonuclease isolated |
| ***Bam*HI** | B | = | genus *Bacillus* |
| | am | = | species *amyloliquefaciens* |
| | H | = | strain H |
| | I | = | first endonuclease isolated |

Table 23-2.
## Specificities of a Few Typical Restriction Endonucleases

| RESTRICTION ENZYME | RECOGNITION SEQUENCE |
| --- | --- |
| *Eco*RI | G⌊AATTC |
| *Bam*HI | G⌊GATCC |
| *Hind*III | A⌊AGCTT |
| *Sma*I | CCC⌊GGG |
| *Not*I | GC⌊GGCCGC |

*The arrows indicate cleavage sites. Recognition sequences are written 5′ to 3′. Only one strand is represented.*

as *Hind*II for example, produce blunt-ended fragments because they cut cleanly through the DNA, cleaving both complementary strands at the same nucleotide position, most often near the middle of the recognition sequence. Other endonucleases cleave the two strands of DNA at positions two to four nucleotides apart, creating exposed ends of single-stranded sequences. The commonly used enzymes *Eco*RI, *Bam*HI, and *Hind*III, for example, leave 5′ overhangs of four nucleotides, which represent "sticky" ends, very useful for making recombinant molecules. Table 23-2 shows the recognition sequence and point of cutting of five commonly used restriction enzymes. This specificity is the same, regardless of whether the DNA is from a bacterium, a plant, or a human cell.

Most restriction recognition sites have symmetry in that the sequence on one strand is the same as on the other. For example, *Eco*RI recognizes the sequence 5′ GAATTC 3′; the complementary strand is also 5′ GAATTC 3′. *Eco*RI cuts the DNA between the G and A on each strand leaving a 5′ single-strand sequence of AATT on each strand. The strands are complementary. Therefore, all DNA fragments generated with *Eco*RI are complementary and can "base pair" with each other. This is illustrated in Figure 23-1.

## VECTORS

A vector is a self-replicating DNA molecule that has the ability to carry another foreign DNA molecule into a host cell. In the context of this chapter, the object of the exercise is usually to insert a fragment of human DNA (perhaps containing a

## DNA Cutting by *Eco* RI

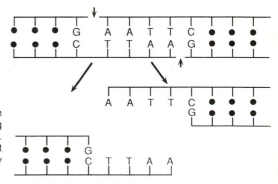

**Figure 23-1.** Illustration of how some endonucleases cleave each strand of the DNA off center in the recognition site, creating fragments with exposed ends of short, single-stranded sequences. These "sticky" ends are extremely useful in making recombinant molecules because they will rejoin only with complementary sequences.

gene of interest) into a bacterium so that it can be replicated and grown into quantities suitable for study.

There are many types of vectors:

1. Plasmids
2. Bacteriophage λ
3. Cosmids
4. Yeast artificial chromosomes (YACs)
5. Viruses

## Plasmids

The simplest bacterial vectors are **plasmids,** which are circular DNA molecules that can exist and replicate inside a bacterium, independent of the host chromosome. A piece of foreign DNA can be inserted into a plasmid, which in turn is introduced into a bacterium. As the bacteria grow and replicate, so, too, will the foreign DNA. The plasmid also contains a gene for resistance to an antibiotic (eg, ampicillin), so that when the bacteria are subsequently grown in a culture medium containing antibiotic, only those bacteria that have taken up a plasmid will survive and replicate. This is illustrated in Figure 23-2.

It is a relatively simple matter, subsequently, to harvest the recombinant plasmids. There are two limitations to this technique. First, plasmids are useful only for relatively small DNA inserts up to about 10,000 bp. Second, the plasmids do not transfect into bacteria with high efficiency.

## Bacteriophage λ

Bacteriophage are bacterial viruses. The bacteriophage most commonly used as a cloning vector is bacteriophage λ. It has two advantages compared with other vectors. As a bacteriophage particle, bacteriophage λ can infect its host at a much higher efficiency than a plasmid and it can accommodate a large range of DNA fragments from a few to up to 24,000 bp, depending on the specific vector used. Many vectors derived from bacteriophage λ exist. Some have been modified to be used to clone small DNAs, usually cDNAs, and some have been modified to clone large DNA molecules. When bacteriophage λ is used to clone large DNA molecules, the central portion of the bacteriophage DNA is deleted. This is to allow the foreign DNA to be accommodated within the bacteriophage particle, which has an upper limit of 55,000 bp. Once the bacteriophage DNA is ligated with the DNA to be cloned, the total DNA is mixed with extracts containing empty bacteriophage particles. The ligated DNA is taken up into the bacteriophage, which is then used to infect *E. coli.*

To insert itself into the *E. coli* chromosome, it circularizes by the base pairing of the complementary single-strand tails that exist at its two ends—the **cos** sites. The resulting circular λ DNA then recombines into the *E. coli* chromosome.

If part of the wild type DNA of the bacteriophage is removed, room can be made for a piece of human DNA to be inserted, again together with a gene that confers resistance to an antibi-

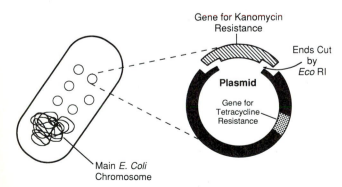

**Figure 23-2.** A plasmid is the simplest bacterial vector, that is, a means of carrying foreign DNA sequences into *Escherichia coli*. A plasmid is a circular DNA molecule, capable of autonomous replication, that typically carries one or more genes encoding an antibiotic resistance. Foreign DNA (eg, from a human cell) can also be incorporated into the plasmid. When inserted into a bacterium, the plasmid replicates along with the main chromosome.

otic to allow selection. The bacteriophage can then be used to infect bacteria that multiply their own DNA as well as the integrated piece of human DNA. The bacteriophage λ will accommodate DNA inserts up to about 24,000 bp.

## Cosmids

A cosmid is a plasmid that contains a cos site. This is the sequence within bacteriophage that leads to its encapsulation within a bacteriophage particle. Cosmid vectors can accommodate up to 45 kb of DNA, which is packaged within a bacteriophage particle for efficient transfer into a bacterial cell. Once in the cell, cosmids grow like a plasmid. Cosmids contain an antibiotic resistance gene to allow selection of infected cells. The use of cosmids is illustrated in Figure 23-3.

## Yeast Artificial Chromosomes

Yeast artificial chromosomes (YACs) represent a recent development. Basically a YAC is a vector containing a centromere and telomeres, which are incorporated into large DNA fragments (up to $10^6$ bp). These DNAs are introduced into the yeast *Saccharomyces cerevisiae*, where they replicate as a chromosome.

## Viruses

Viruses are highly efficient vectors for introducing foreign genes into mammalian cells. SV40 was the first one employed, but it is limited in its usefulness. Retroviruses are ideal vectors for introducing a gene into a mammalian cell in a stable fashion. In using retroviruses as a vector,

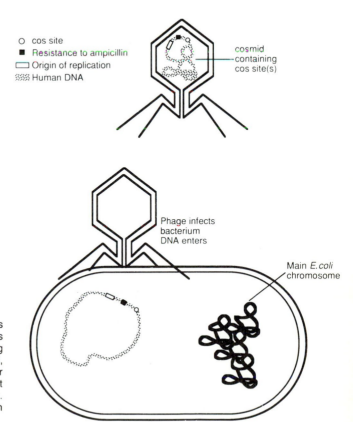

**Figure 23-3.** A bacteriophage is a virus that infects bacteria. It represents a much more efficient means of inserting foreign DNA into a bacterium than using a plasmid. If part of the wild type DNA is removed, room can be made for a piece of "foreign" DNA, for example, from a human cell as well as a gene that confers resistance to an antibiotic to allow selection. The DNA of the bacteriophage replicates along with that of the bacterium.

the gene of interest is cloned into a virus that lacks most viral genes and is expressed under the control of strong viral promoter sequences. The genetic material of retroviruses is RNA, so that when they infect cells, their RNA genomes are converted to a DNA form (by the viral enzyme reverse transcriptase). The viral DNA is efficiently integrated into the host genome where it permanently resides, replicating with the host DNA every cell cycle. Retroviruses can infect virtually every type of mammalian cell, making them very versatile.

## LIBRARIES

### Genomic Library

A genomic library is a compilation of DNA fragments that make up the entire genome. Making a genomic library is frequently the starting point of a gene isolation experiment. DNA is extracted from a tissue sample, or from cultured cells, and a partial digest is made using *Eco*RI, for example. This enzyme has a six nucleotide recognition sequence, so if the digest is complete, it would cut the DNA into pieces about 4000 bp long. By reducing the enzyme concentration and incubation time, a partial digest is obtained so that the *Eco*RI enzyme cuts at only about one in five restriction sites, resulting in fragments of about 40,000 bp.

The genomic DNA fragments are then ligated into a cosmid (or other suitable vector), and "packaged" inside infective bacteriophage particles. The assembled bacteriophage particles are used to infect *E. coli* cells, which are spread on plates and incubated in growth medium containing the appropriate antibiotic (eg, ampicillin), so that only bacteria that have taken up the cosmid survive and grow into colonies. Each colony will contain millions of copies of a single ge-

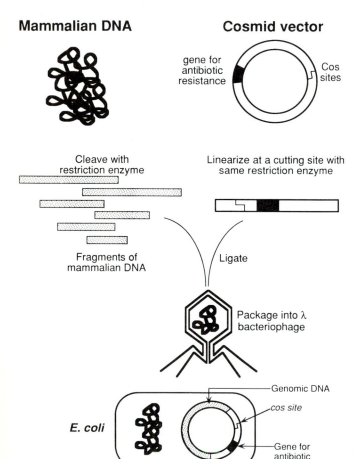

Figure 23-4. Illustration of the construction of a genomic DNA library. The genomic DNA is partially digested with a restriction enzyme, to produce DNA fragments with an average size of about 40,000 base pairs. These fragments are inserted into cosmids that have a cos site and markers for drug resistance to allow subsequent selection. The cosmids are packaged into bacteriophage, which in turn are used to infect *E. coli*. In this way the DNA fragments are amplified.

nomic DNA insert. About 75,000 colonies will encompass the entire genome. If the equivalent of several genomes worth of colonies are screened, then one or more should contain the gene of interest. The trick is to identify that particular colony out of hundreds of thousands! The process is illustrated in Figure 23-4.

## cDNA Library

As an alternative to making a genomic DNA library, it is sometimes more useful to make a cDNA library. cDNA is DNA that is complementary to the messenger RNA (mRNA) and therefore includes only the expressed genes of a particular cell. For eukaryotic cells, the mRNA is usually much shorter than the total size of the gene because the coding sequences in the genome are split into **exons** separated by noncoding regions of DNA called **introns.**

cDNA libraries are made in either plasmids or bacteriophage λ. Often these vectors have been modified such that the cDNA can be transcribed into mRNA and then translated into protein. When this type of vector is used, the library can be screened using an antibody that recognizes the protein of the gene of interest, since the cells are expressing the gene. This type of cDNA library is called an **expression library.**

## HOSTS

Recombinant DNA molecules can be constructed and manipulated to some extent in the test tube, but amplification and expression ideally require a host.

### *Escherichia coli*

*E. coli* is the most widely used organism in molecular biology because it is relatively simple and well understood. It contains a single chromosome consisting of about 5 million bp.

In addition to their main chromosome(s), many bacteria, including *E. coli*, possess large numbers of tiny circular DNA molecules that may contain only a few thousand base pairs. They are called episomes, a subset of which are known as plasmids. Plasmids are autonomously replicating "minichromosomes." They were first identified as genetic elements separate from the main chromosome and carrying genes that conveyed resistance to antibiotics. Foreign DNA can readily be introduced into *E. coli* in the form of plasmids.

Since the DNA of all organisms is made of identical subunits, *E. coli* will accept foreign DNA from any organism. The DNA of bacteria, *Drosophila,* plants, and humans consist of the same four nucleotides, adenine, cytosine, guanine, and thymine. A foreign gene inside *E. coli* is replicated in essentially the same way as its own DNA.

### Yeast

Yeasts are simple eukaryotes that have many characteristics in common with mammalian cells but can be grown almost as quickly and inexpensively as bacteria.

The study of yeasts has frequently and consistently provided insights into similar phenomena and functions in mammalian cells that are much more difficult to address. Yeasts have been of particular value in radiobiology because the availability of a wide array of mutants that are sensitive to ultraviolet or ionizing radiations has made the study of the genes responsible for radiosensitivity/radioresistance much simpler than if studies were conducted just in mammalian cells. Complementation of many yeast mutants with mammalian genes has proven to be a powerful screening method.

Yeasts have also proven to be good systems for studying cell cycle control. Since it appears that the cell cycle machinery of all eukaryotes is very similar, it makes sense to concentrate on the simplest and most easily manipulated system. The availability of temperature sensitive mutants is of particular value with yeasts. This led to the discovery of checkpoint genes, as will be described later. The yeasts *Saccharomyces cerevisiae* (budding yeast, baker's yeast or brewer's yeast) and *Schizosaccharomyces pombe* (fission yeast) have been widely used. They grow rapidly and have been well characterized genetically.

## Mammalian Cells

The limited number of cell systems used in radiation and chemical transformation studies can be separated broadly into two categories. The first category includes short-term explants of cells derived from rodent or human embryos with a limited life-span. These include:

Hamster embryo cells
Rat embryo cells
Human skin fibroblasts
Human foreskin cells
Human embryo cells

These cell assay systems can be used to assess the expression or activity of foreign genes transfected into them, or they may be used in studies of oncogenic transformation induced by radiation or chemicals.

In practice, the bulk of the experimental work has been performed with hamster or rat embryo cells. One advantage of such systems is that they consist of diploid cells, so that parallel cytogenetic experiments can be performed. Cell survival and cell transformation can be scored simultaneously in the same dishes.

The experimental methodology is illustrated in Figure 23-5. Cells are seeded at low density into dishes or flasks and treated with radiation or chemicals. They are allowed to grow for 8 to 10 days, and the resultant colonies are fixed and stained. Transformed colonies are identifiable by dense multilayered cells, random cellular arrangement, and haphazard cell-to-cell orientation accentuated at the colony edge. Normal counterparts are flat, with an organized cell-to-cell orien-

tation and no piling up of cells. An example of the contrast between a normal and a transformed colony is shown in Figure 23-6.

The second category of experimental systems includes established cell lines that have an unlimited life span. The karyotype of these cells shows various chromosomal rearrangements and heteroploidy. The two most widely used established cell lines for transformation studies are the BALB/C-3T3 cell line and the $C_3H$ 10T½ cell line. Both originated from mouse embryos, are transformable by a variety of oncogenic agents, and have been used extensively in transformation studies. The advantage of these established cell lines lies in the fact that they are "immortal," so that a particular passage can be used over a long period of time and maintained in banks of frozen cells. The transformation assay is a focal assay. Cells are treated with radiation or chemicals and then allowed to grow for 6 weeks. The "normal" cells stop growing after confluence is reached, and transformed foci can be identified against a background of the contact-inhibited normal cells because they are densely stained, tend to pile up, and show a crisscross random pattern at the edge of the focus. Transformed cells, identified by their characteristic morphology, will grow in soft agar, which indicates that they have lost anchorage dependence, and produce fibrosarcomas when injected into suitably prepared animals. This is illustrated in Figure 23-7.

The in vitro assay systems based on mammalian cells have two quite different uses in radiobiology. First, they may be used to accumulate data and information that are essentially pragmatic in nature; for example, they may be used to compare and contrast the oncogenic potential of a

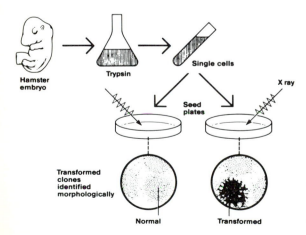

**Figure 23-5.** Protocol for the assay of oncogenic transformation in hamster embryo cells by radiation. Midterm hamster embryos are removed, minced, enzymatically dissociated, and seeded as single cells on feeder layers. They are then treated with either radiation or chemicals, and the resultant colonies (normal and transformed) are scored after 8 to 10 days of incubation.

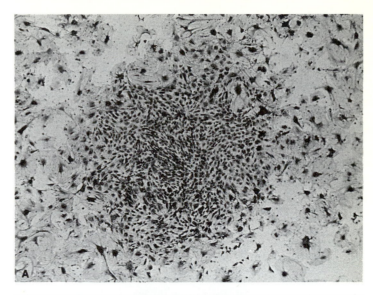

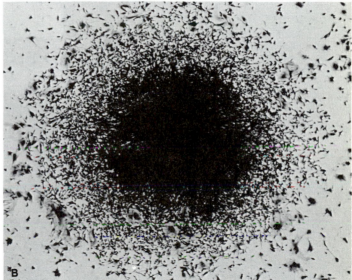

Figure 23-6. **(A)** A normal untransformed colony of hamster embryo cells. The cells are orderly and show contact inhibition. **(B)** A colony of radiation-transformed hamster embryo cells. Note the densely stained, piled up cells and the crisscross pattern at the periphery of the colony.

variety of chemical and physical agents. As such, they occupy a useful intermediate position between the bacterial mutagenesis assays, which are quick and inexpensive but score mutagenesis rather than carcinogenesis, and animal studies, which may be more relevant to humans but are quite cumbersome and inordinately expensive. Second, they can be used to study the mechanisms of carcinogenesis. In this context, transformation assays have played a vital role in unfolding the oncogene story, since transfecting DNA from human tumors into one or the other of the established cell lines used for transformation, most often 3T3 or rat-2 cells, and observing the

induction of transformed foci is one way to detect the expression of an oncogene, as illustrated in Figure 23-8.

## DNA-Mediated Gene Transfer

Gene transfer is now a routine tool for studying gene structure and function. Gene transfer into mammalian cells is an inefficient process, so that an abundant source of starting cells is necessary to generate a workable number of **transfected** cells, that is, cells containing a transferred gene.

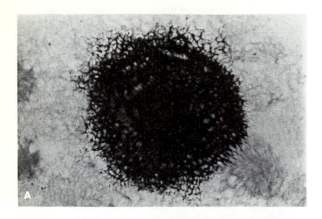

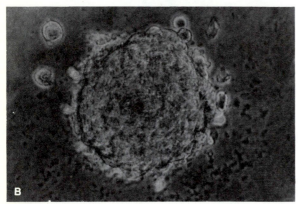

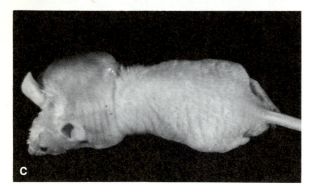

**Figure 23-7.** **(A)** A type III transformed focus of $C_3H$ 10T1/2 cells induced by the hypoxic cell sensitizer etanidazole (SR 2508). Note the multilayered growth and the crisscrossing of cells at the periphery of the clone over a contact-inhibited background of nontransformed cells. **(B)** When cells from the above focus were plucked, expanded in culture, and plated into semisolid medium, they formed colonies indicating that they had lost anchorage dependence. This is an indication of malignancy. **(C)** The ultimate test of malignancy is when cells from a type III transformed clone injected into a suitably prepared animal produce a tumor (a fibrosarcoma) that eventually kills the animal.

Mammalian cells do not naturally take up foreign DNA; indeed, they try to protect themselves from invading DNA. Consequently, one of several tricks must be used to bypass natural barriers.

1. *Microinjection.* This is the most direct, but most difficult procedure to accomplish. DNA can be injected, cell by cell, directly into the nucleus through a fine glass needle.
2. *Calcium phosphate precipitation.* Cells take up DNA relatively efficiently in the form of a pre- cipitate with calcium phosphate. The efficiency varies markedly from one cell line to another. For example, NIH 3T3 cells are particularly receptive to foreign DNA introduced by this technique. This is the most widely used method of gene transfer and is illustrated in Figure 23-9. High-molecular-weight DNA is mixed with insoluble calcium phosphate as a carrier and layered onto cells in petri dishes. Typically, a plasmid containing a selectable marker, such as G418 resistance, is co-pipetted and co-trans-

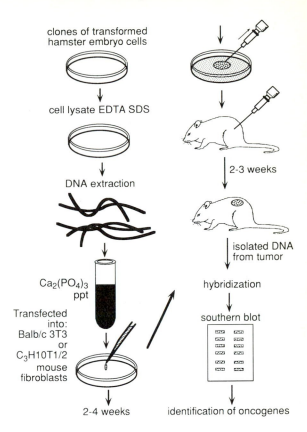

clones of transformed
hamster embryo cells

cell lysate EDTA SDS

DNA extraction

2-3 weeks

isolated DNA
from tumor

$Ca_2(PO_4)_3$
ppt

hybridization

Transfected
into:
Balb/c 3T3
or
$C_3H10T1/2$
mouse
fibroblasts

southern blot

2-4 weeks

identification of oncogenes

**Figure 23-8.** Schematic diagram of a typical DNA transfection protocol in which oncogenes can be isolated from cells transformed in vitro by either radiation or chemical carcinogens. DNA sequences are then characterized by using a Southern blot hybridization.

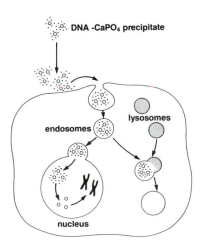

DNA -$CaPO_4$ precipitate

lysosomes

endosomes

nucleus

**Figure 23-9.** The technique of transfection DNA from a mammalian cell, cut into fragments, can be introduced into another cell as part of calcium phosphate precipitate. The donor DNA is integrated at low frequency into the genome of the recipient cell.

fected into cells. In this way cells that take up DNA can be selected. Of the cells that take up DNA, only a small percentage ultimately integrate the DNA into their genomes **(stably transfected).** When a fragment of DNA containing an activated oncogene is transfected into NIH 3T3 cells, morphologic transformation of the cell occurs, leading to loss of contact inhibition, and the cells produce tumors when injected into immune-suppressed animals.

3. *Electroporation.* This technique is useful for cells that are resistant to transfection by calcium phosphate precipitation. Cells in solution are subjected to a brief electrical pulse that causes holes to open transiently in the membrane, allowing foreign DNA to enter.

4. *Viral vectors.* The ultimate means of transfection involves the use of a retrovirus—this is essentially the analogue of using bacteriophage to get DNA into bacteria. The genetic material of a retrovirus is RNA, so that when it infects a mammalian cell their RNA genomes are

converted to DNA by the viral enzyme **reverse transcriptase.** The viral DNA is efficiently incorporated into the host genome, replicating along with the host DNA at each cell cycle. If a foreign gene is incorporated into the retrovirus, it will be permanently maintained in the infected mammalian cell. Oncogenes, genes that can cause cancer, and their counterpart, tumor suppressor genes, can be studied by incorporating them into retroviral vectors.

## AGAROSE GEL ELECTROPHORESIS

The purpose of agarose gel electrophoresis is to separate pieces of DNA of different size. This technique is based on the fact that DNA is negatively charged. Under the influence of an electric field, DNA molecules move from negative to positive poles and are sorted by size in the gel. In a given time, small fragments migrate through the gel farther than large fragments.

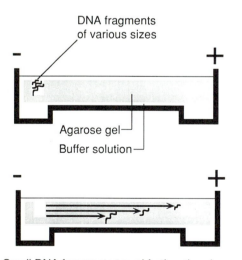

Small DNA fragments travel further than large

**Figure 23-10.** Illustrating agarose gel electrophoresis, DNA is negatively charged so that under the influence of an electric field it migrates toward the anode. During electrophoresis, DNA fragments sort by size, small molecules moving farther than larger molecules. Since smaller molecules move farther than larger molecules in a given time, polyacrylamide gel electrophoresis is often employed to separate smaller DNA fragments.

The technique, illustrated in Figure 23-10, is as follows: Molten agarose is poured into a tray in which a plastic comb is suspended near one end to form wells in the gel after it has solidified like jello. The concentration of the agarose is varied according to the size of the DNA fragment to be separated and visualized: high concentration for small fragments, lower concentration for larger fragments. The solidified gel is immersed in a tray containing an electrolyte to conduct electricity. The DNA samples, mixed with sucrose and a visible dye, are pipetted into the wells and the electric field is connected. Electrophoresis is monitored by observing the movement of the dye in the electric field. After separation is complete, the gel is soaked in ethidium bromide, which intercalates into DNA and fluoresces under ultraviolet light to make the position of the DNA visible. Several examples are shown later in the chapter.

## POLYMERASE CHAIN REACTION

The polymerase chain reaction (PCR) uses enzymatic amplification to increase the number of copies of a DNA fragment of up to about 6000 bp. The principle is based on primer extension by DNA polymerases, which was discovered in the 1960s. First, primers, which are complementary to the 5' end of the double-stranded DNA sequence to be amplified are synthesized. The two primers are mixed in excess with a sample of DNA that includes the fragments to be amplified, together with a heat-stable Taq DNA polymerase from *Thermus aquaticus*, a bacterium that inhabits hot springs. The four deoxyribonucleotide triphosphates are also provided in excess, one or more of which may be radioactively labeled. The power of the technique is that it can be used to amplify a DNA fragment from total genomic DNA. The PCR technique is illustrated in Figure 23-11.

The amount of the sequence is doubled in each cycle, which takes about 7 minutes. During each cycle the sample is heated to about 94°C to denature the DNA strands, then cooled to about 50°C to allow the primers to anneal to the template DNA, and then heated to 72°C, the optimal

## Illustrating the polmerase chain reaction for the amplification of a DNA fragment

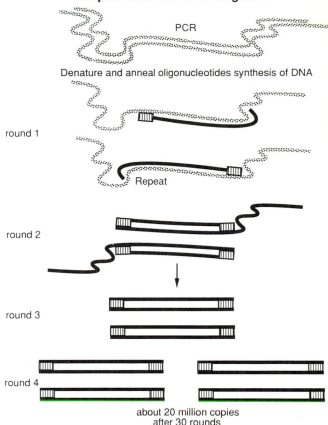

PCR

Denature and anneal oligonucleotides synthesis of DNA

round 1

Repeat

round 2

round 3

round 4

about 20 million copies
after 30 rounds

**Figure 23-11.** The polymerase chain reaction (PCR) for the amplification of DNA fragments. The number of DNA molecules is doubled in each cycle, which takes about 7 minutes, so that in a matter of several hours, millions of copies of a DNA fragment can be made. (Courtesy of Dr. Greg Freyer)

temperature for Taq polymerase activity. In a matter of a few hours, a million copies of the DNA fragment can be obtained in an essentially automated device. PCR has found many applications in both basic research and clinical settings. For example, it has been used to detect malignant cells in patients with leukemias that are characterized by consistent translocation breakpoints. Primers that span the breakpoint are added to a bone marrow sample and subjected to multiple cycles of PCR. Even one cell in a million with the translocation can be detected.

## GENE CLONING STRATEGIES

In the most general terms, there are *three* steps involved in cloning a gene:

1. Choose a source of DNA, which may be genomic DNA or cDNA.
2. Construct a library, which is a collection of DNA fragments inserted into an appropriate vector.
3. Screen the library to locate the gene of interest.

The first two steps have already been described. There are four principle methods to screen for a gene.

### Functional Complementation

This technique depends on the DNA segment producing its corresponding protein within the cell, thereby giving the host a specific and detectable phenotype. For example, in screening for a repair gene that confers resistance to radiation or to a particular chemical agent (eg, mitomycin C), a sensitive line of cells that lacks the functional gene is transfected with a library of genomic DNA from cells that contain the active gene.

Only one in many thousands of cells will have taken up the gene of interest, but these cells will acquire resistance and can be selected by long-term treatment with the cytotoxic agent (eg, x-rays, mitomycin C).

During DNA transfection many genes enter the cell, so it is necessary to first determine which of the introduced sequences contain the repair gene. The DNA fragment from the library can be identified by its association with the vector sequence. If this is a cosmid, the incoming DNA can be rescued from total genomic DNA. Once all of the library sequences are isolated they must be screened individually to determine which contains the repair gene or genes. This can be done by reintroducing the purified vector genomic DNA clones into the sensitive cell line to determine which clone confers resistance.

## Hybridization

Double-stranded DNA can be denatured; that is, the hydrogen bonds between the base pairs can be disrupted, causing the complementary strands to disassemble. DNA denatures under a variety of conditions, such as in the presence of high pH or high temperature. Under the right conditions, the two single-stranded molecules can re-form the original duplex DNA molecule. This process of complementary single-stranded molecules lining up to form a double-stranded molecule is known as **hybridization**. Under "low stringency" conditions, partial hybridization takes place if the strands have a lesser degree of complementarity.

A genomic library, prepared as described previously, can be screened for the presence of a particular gene of interest by hybridization. The library consisting of bacteriophage or cosmids is grown on plates. A replica copy of each plate is made by transferring the colonies or plaques onto a filter disk, rather like a rubber stamp. The cells/bacteriophage are lysed and their DNA denatured, followed by screening with a probe that has a sequence complementary to the gene of

interest. The probe is labeled with a β-emitting radionuclide (such as phosphorus-32) so that it can be detected easily. The filters are incubated under conditions that favor hybridization of the probe to its complementary sequence (neutral pH, presence of sodium ions to neutralize the negative charge on the DNA, and an elevated temperature). After removing the unhybridized probe, x-ray film is pressed tightly against the filters so that β-particles emitted from the phosphorus-32 expose the film; this is called **autoradiography.** After development, the exposed areas appear as black spots on the film, corresponding to the plaques/colonies that contained the gene of interest.

## Oligonucleotide Probes

If it is possible to obtain a partial or complete amino acid sequence of the protein encoded by the gene under study, the coding sequence derived from these amino acids can be used to synthesize an oligonucleotide, a DNA sequence of a few nucleotides. This can be used as a probe for the gene of interest. A six amino acid sequence can be used to derive a series of 18 nucleotide DNA probes that take into consideration the redundancy of the genetic code. This mixture of oligonucleotides is labeled with a β-emitting radionuclide so that the plaques or lysed bacterial colonies to which it hybridizes in the DNA library can be readily identified by autoradiography.

## Antibody Probes

Antibodies are formed as part of the immune response of animals to the presence of a foreign substance (an antigen).

To make antibodies against a specific protein, the foreign protein is used to immunize a laboratory mouse. B lymphocytes from the animal's spleen are fused with myeloma cells (derived from a mouse bone cancer) to produce hybridomas that are essentially immortal. Individual hybridomas are isolated that produce a monoclonal antibody. This technique is only used to screen a cDNA **expression library.**

# GENE ANALYSES

## Mapping

### Southern Blotting

Southern blotting, named after its discoverer Ed Southern, can be used to study a gene without cloning it. As in library screening, it is based on hybridization. The technique is illustrated in Figure 23-12.

DNA is extracted from a tissue or cell culture of interest, digested with one or more restriction enzymes, and electrophoresed on an agarose gel. The duplex DNA is denatured and transferred to a nitrocellulose filter, a technique called blotting. The filter is then bathed in a solution containing a specific probe labeled with phos-

phorus-32 under hybridization conditions. The radioactive probe hybridizes only to its complementary sequence, and this can be identified by sandwiching the filter against an x-ray film. Exposed regions on the film appearing as dark bands indicate the positions of this sequence on the gel.

Southern blotting is useful for analyzing the sizes of DNA fragments lost in radiation-induced mutations. It is also useful for detecting structural variations in DNA that result in restriction fragments of different lengths, known as restriction fragment length polymorphisms (RFLPs), which can be used as genetic markers to map genes to specific chromosomal locations. The technique of Southern blotting has been exploited by human geneticists to localize and identify a

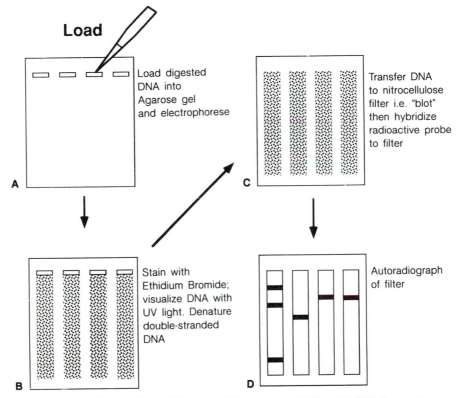

**Figure 23-12.** The technique of Southern blot analysis. (*a*) Digested DNA fragments are loaded into the wells of an agarose gel and subjected to electrophoresis. (*b*) DNA fragments move different distances according to their size and can be visualized under ultraviolet illumination after staining with ethidium bromide. (*c*) The DNA is denatured and then transferred to a nitrocellulose filter by capillary action; that is, a "blot" is made. A probe labeled with a radionuclide is hybridized to the filter. (*d*) An autoradiograph is made of the filter. Bands corresponding to DNA strands to which the probe hybridize are clearly visualized.

number of disease genes and has also been used in "DNA fingerprinting."

### Chromosome Walking

The chromosome walking technique is necessary when a gene of interest has been mapped to a specific arm of a chromosome and it is then desired to isolate the gene. It is *not* needed if the gene of interest is already contained in a discrete DNA fragment obtained from a DNA library. The process is illustrated in Figure 23-13. The starting point is to identify a piece of DNA, a flanking marker, that is close to the gene. This is accomplished by making a genomic library of large DNA fragments (20,000 to 40,000 bp) that includes the gene of interest and identifying flanking markers by mapping or hybridization. Probes are then used to identify an overlapping fragment of DNA from the genomic library that contains the flanking marker (A) and some other identifiable marker (B). The next step is to find a new probe from the genomic library that has marker B at its 5′ end and that includes yet another identifiable marker (C). This process of identifying overlapping probes that span a chromosomal region containing a gene of interest is referred to as *chromosome walking* and is continued until the gene of interest is reached.

### Contiguous Mapping

Mapping refers to the determination of the physical location of a gene or genetic marker on a chromosome. Contiguous mapping refers to the alignment of sequence data from large, adjacent regions of the genome to produce a continuous nucleotide sequence of a region of a chromosome. The basic idea is to orient physical markers, such as RFLPs, on adjacent fragments so that they can be lined up and the nucleotide sequence can be made continuous. If, for example, restriction fragments from a DNA library are sequenced, then relating these sequences to known physical markers would eventually produce the nucleotide sequence of the entire genome. This is the goal of the Human Genome Project, but the task is so massive that it cannot be accomplished without the development of automated sequencing technology and sophisticated computer strategies to store and handle the data.

## DNA Sequence Analyses

### Introns/Exons

It is at once obvious from a comparison of a mature cytoplasmic mRNA transcript with its pa-

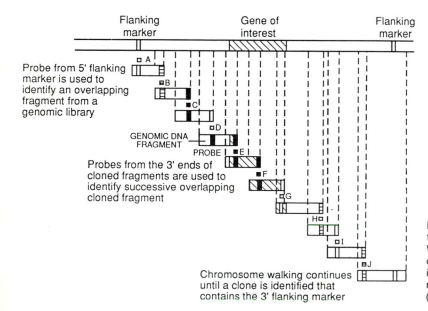

Figure 23-13. Illustration of the technique of chromosome walking. Working from a flanking DNA marker, overlapping clones are successively identified that span a chromosomal region containing a gene of interest. (Courtesy of Dr. Greg Freyer)

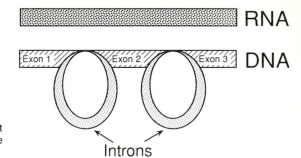

RNA

DNA

Introns

**Figure 23-14.** DNA is made up of nucleotide sequences that are transcribed to mRNA, called exons, and sequences that are excised from pre mRNA during RNA processing, called introns.

rental DNA that the mRNA sequence is not contiguous with the DNA sequence. Some blocks of DNA sequence are represented in the mRNA, while others are not. DNA is transcribed into pre-mRNA. During this process of splicing, large regions called **introns** are removed and the remaining **exons** are joined together. Almost all genes from higher eukaryotes contain introns; genes may have only a few or as many as 100 introns. Typically, introns make up the bulk of the gene. For example, in the gene involved with muscular dystrophy, the mRNA consists of 14,000 bases while the gene spans more than 2 million bp. The way in which exons are transcribed and introns omitted is illustrated in Figure 23-14.

### Sequencing Gel; Chain Termination Method

This technique depends on two characteristics of DNA synthesis:

1. With the availability of the four deoxyribonucleotide triphosphates, dATP, dTTP, dCTP, and dGTP, synthesis of a new strand of DNA will be initiated by DNA polymerase at any point where a short DNA primer hybridizes to a single-stranded DNA template.
2. If the deoxyribonucleotide triphosphates are mixed with *di* deoxyribonucleotide triphosphates, the DNA chain elongation will cease when a *di* deoxyribonucleotide triphosphate is incorporated. The preparation of a sequencing gel is shown in Figure 23-15. Four reaction tubes are set up, each containing in addition to the DNA template to be sequenced, a primer sequence, DNA polymerase, and all four deoxyribonucleotide triphosphates (dATP, dTTP, dCTP, and dGTP), one of which is la-

beled with the radionuclide phosphorus-32. One *di* deoxyribonucleotide triphosphate is added to each of the tubes. The concentration of the *di* deoxyribonucleotide triphosphate is such that it is incorporated in only about 1 in 100 nucleotides, thereby stopping the synthesis of the strand. In the reaction containing *di*dATP, DNA fragments will be made of all lengths terminating in adenine, while in the reaction containing *di*dCTP, all fragment lengths will be made terminating with cytosine.

## DNA + Sequencing Reagents Loaded into Gel

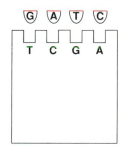

## Autoradiograph of Gel

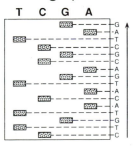

**Figure 23-15.** Illustration of a sequencing gel based on the chain termination method.

After the reactions are completed the newly synthesized DNA fragments are separated on a polyacrylamide gel and an autoradiograph is made from the gel. Since the DNA fragments were of all different lengths, they will have moved different distances under the influence of the electric field. The sequence can then be read, starting at the bottom. An actual gel is shown later to illustrate one of the examples of the use of molecular techniques in radiobiology.

DNA sequencing has been automated as part of the Human Genome Project. With the appropriate equipment, fluorescein-labeled primers are used that can be monitored as they move past a detector at the end of the sequencing gel.

### Deduced Protein Sequences

The "message" in DNA is linear, consisting of combinations of the four bases adenine, thymine, guanine, and cytosine. Proteins have a three-dimensional form. The first step in the production of a protein from the message in the DNA is that the DNA code is **transcribed** in the nucleus into pre-mRNA, which is a complementary version of the DNA code. Next, the pre-mRNA is processed to mRNA by removal of its introns. The mRNA enters the cytoplasm where it associates with a ribosome and the mRNA message is **translated** into "chains" of amino acids. The steps from DNA to protein are illustrated in Figure 23-16. The genetic code is read as triplets. Thus, three nucleotides code for an amino acid. There are 64 possible combinations of the four bases; 61 of these code for the 20 amino acids. Consequently, there is degeneracy, or redundancy, in the code since the same amino acid is coded for by more than one triplet. Nearly all proteins begin with the amino acid methionine, for which the codon is AUG. Consequently, this represents the "start" signal for protein synthesis. The "stop" signal is any one of the three codons for which there is no naturally occurring tRNA, namely UAA, UAG, or UGA. Most proteins contain only one polypeptide chain, characterized by a unique sequence of amino acids. There are, however, other proteins formed through the aggregation of separately synthesized chains that have different sequences.

Since the message in the DNA results in a unique protein, it is clearly possible to go in the reverse direction and deduce the sequence of the gene from the protein(s) expressed by the gene. This is not straightforward since there is redundancy in the code for specifying amino acids from triplet RNA codons. With four bases and triple codons, far more combinations are available than there are amino acids and so in practice the same amino acid corresponds to more than one sequence of bases in the mRNA. There are ways to circumvent this problem, as described earlier in the section on oligonucleotide

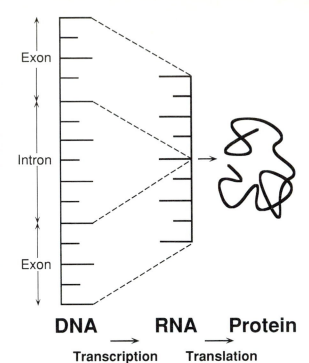

**DNA → RNA → Protein**

**Transcription     Translation**

**Figure 23-16.** Illustration of the process of transcription and translation. The "information" in DNA is linear, consisting of combinations of the four nucleotides adenine, guanine, cytosine, and thymine. The information is transcribed into mRNA (messenger RNA), which in turn is a complementary version of the DNA code. The mRNA message is translated into amino acids. Triplet RNA codons specify each of the 20 amino acids. The sequence of amino acids determines the protein, which ultimately has three-dimensional form.

probes. Once a DNA sequence is obtained, the amino acid sequence of the corresponding protein can be determined.

### Homologies to Known Genes and Proteins

Interpreting a new sequence is no easy matter. An early step is to find an "open reading frame, that is, a sequence that corresponds to a "long" stretch of amino acids and does not contain a stop codon. This is more likely to be part of an active gene since protein coding regions are not interrupted by stop codons.

When a new gene is sequenced the information is entered into various data bases to search for sequence homology with existing genes. These homologies are important in identifying function and the relationship between genes. Typically, when searching a data base, the coding sequences of both the entire gene and also of the cDNA are entered. The cDNA sequence is often more useful because intron sequences diverge rapidly, as do gene flanking sequences, while exon sequences (primarily coding for amino acids) tend to be conserved. It is even more desirable to search for a protein sequence because changes can occur in the DNA sequence that do not lead to changes in the amino acid sequence due to the degeneracy of the genetic code.

## Polymorphisms or Mutations

### Restriction Fragment Length Polymorphisms

Relatively small differences in similar DNA sequences, or polymorphisms as they are called, may result from point mutations, deletions or insertions, or varying numbers of copies of a DNA fragment (so-called tandem repeats). A Southern blot analysis can be used to detect DNA polymorphisms, using a probe that hybridizes to a polymorphic region of the DNA molecule. Other techniques may also be used to detect polymorphisms.

When a particular restriction enzyme is used to cut human DNA, a polymorphic locus will yield restriction fragments of different sizes. These are called restriction fragment length poly-

morphisms (RFLPs). Deletions, insertions, or tandem repeats involving more than about 30 nucleotides can be detected as recognizable shifts in the Southern blot hybridization pattern. Even a point mutation can be detected if the resultant change in sequence removes or adds a new recognition site at which a restriction endonuclease cuts.

### Single-Stranded Conformation Polymorphism

Several methods have been developed to screen for an **unknown** mutation in a gene. Among them, single-stranded conformation polymorphism (SSCP) is particularly useful. A single base-pair difference between two short single-stranded DNA molecules (such as the difference between a wild type gene and one that had suffered a point mutation) results in a difference in conformation between the two strands that, remarkably enough, can be detected by a difference in the molecule's electrophoretic mobilities on a neutral polyacrylamide gel. The same change would go undetected if electrophoresis were carried out under denaturing conditions in which strands separate only according to size, not base composition. This represents a powerful technique to screen for mutations in an oncogene (such as *ras*) or in a tumor suppressor gene (such as p53).

## Expression

### Northern Blotting and Hybridization

In northern blotting, a probe is hybridized to RNA, in contrast to Southern blotting where the probe is hybridized to DNA.

This is the best technique available to monitor mRNA abundance and turnover in cells. The techniques used in northern blotting are essentially similar to those described for Southern blotting except that RNA is used in place of DNA, is all really single stranded, and does not need previous digestion with restriction enzymes. The intensity of the bands on the final autoradiograph reflects the abundance of the "message" and its expression in a particular cell or tissue.

## EXAMPLES OF PROJECTS OF DIRECT OR INDIRECT INTEREST TO RADIOBIOLOGY EMPLOYING MOLECULAR TECHNIQUES

1. *The first repair gene in a mammalian cell identified and cloned by gene transfer* (Rubin et al, 1983; VanDuin et al, 1986)

A mutant line of Chinese hamster ovary (CHO) cells was used that was about 500 times as sensitive to killing by mitomycin C (MMC) as wild type cells (Fig. 23-17). Total genomic DNA from a human cell line (HeLa) was isolated and was transfected by the calcium phosphate precipitation method into the sensitive CHO cells. Cells were grown for several cycles in mitomycin C to select for repair proficient derivatives, and clones were chosen that had a sensitivity to mitomycin C close to the wild type cells (see Fig. 23-17). To demonstrate the successful integration of human DNA, use was made of the fact that the human genome contains a family of highly repetitive *Alu* sequences, which, under stringent hybridization conditions, can be used to establish the presence of human DNA within a CHO background. A Southern blot was used to determine the presence of human sequences. Independently derived transformants contained a common set of human specific DNA restriction fragments, apparently associated with the DNA repair gene. The steps used in these experiments are illustrated in Figure 23-18. The gene was subsequently cloned from resistant derivatives by a different group.

*Techniques:* DNA-mediated gene transfer using the calcium phosphate precipitation technique, restriction fragment length analysis, Southern blotting.

2. *The first ionizing radiation repair gene isolated and sequenced in mammalian cells* (Thompson et al, 1990)

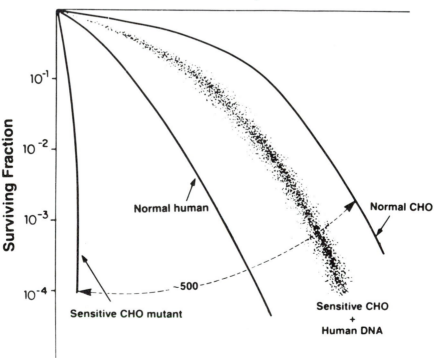

**Dose of Mitomycin-C**

Surviving Fraction

Normal human

Normal CHO

Sensitive CHO mutant

~500~

Sensitive CHO
+
Human DNA

**Figure 23-17.** Dose response curves for mitomycin C (MMC) for wild type Chinese hamster ovary (CHO) cells, for a very sensitive mutant line, for human HeLa cells, and for sensitive CHO cells complemented by DNA fragments from the HeLa cells. (Redrawn and simplified from Rubin JS, Joyner AL, Bernstein A, Whitmore GF: Nature 306:206–208, 1983)

## Identification of Repair Gene for DNA Damage by Mitomycin-C

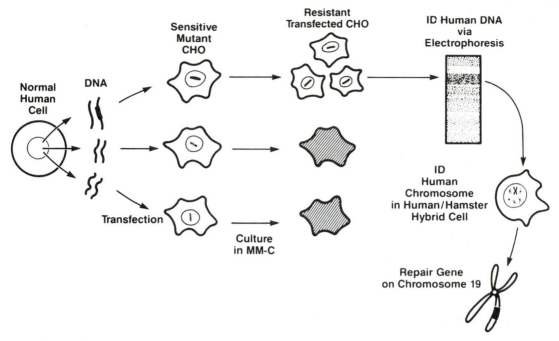

**Figure 23-18.** Illustrating the series of experiments in which DNA-mediated gene transfer was used to complement the repair-deficient CHO cells that were sensitive to mitomycin C. The repair gene from human cells was mapped to human chromosome 19. (From Rubin JS, Joyner AL, Bernstein A, Whitmore GF: Nature 306:206–208, 1983)

This was the first repair gene isolated using ionizing radiation to select for functionally complemented radiosensitive mutant CHO cells. In fact, the radiosensitivity to ionizing radiation of this cell line differs from the wild type by a factor of only 1.8. Much more radiosensitive mutants are known, but, in general, very radiosensitive lines are also defective in double-strand break repair, and it has proven difficult to transfect human DNA stably into these cells, perhaps for this reason.

A human fibroblast cDNA library in a cosmid vector was used to correct the radiation defect. The complementing human gene was cloned from the cosmid library of a transformant. The gene was given the designation XRCCI (x-ray repair cross complementing) and was assigned to the long arm of human chromosome 19.

*Techniques:* cDNA library, gene transfer, sequencing gel, Northern blotting, gene mapping.

**3.** *Molecular checkpoint genes identified and*

*sequenced in yeast* (Murray et al, 1991; Lieberman et al, 1992)

Figure 23-19 shows ionizing radiation survival curves for the wild-type yeast *Schizosaccharomyces pombe* and for cells containing the mutant allele *rad9-192*. The mutant is more sensitive both to ionizing radiation and ultraviolet light by a factor between 10 and 100. The *rad9+* and *rad9-192* genes have been isolated and their DNA sequences determined; there is a single nucleotide base-pair difference: a cytosine-guanine substituting for a thymine-adenine. This would cause the coding for proline in place of leucine in the mutant *rad9*, which probably results in a dramatic change in the three-dimensional structure of the protein. This change has evidently destroyed protein activity and resulted in the dramatic increase in radiosensitivity exhibited by *rad9-192* cells. The alteration of 1 bp in a total of about 1200 bp in the gene leads to this dramatic difference in radiosensitivity. Analysis of PCR-amplified genomic DNA in-

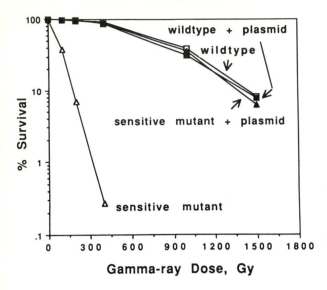

**Figure 23-19.** Gamma ray dose–response curves for the yeast *Schizosaccharomyces pombe*. Data for the wild type are shown as open squares, with those for the radiosensitive mutant shown as open triangles. The closed triangles show data for the radiosensitive strain, into which a plasmid had been transformed containing the *rad9* wild-type gene; wild-type resistance is restored by this means; introducing the cosmid into wild-type cells did not affect radiosensitivity (closed squares). (Redrawn from Lieberman HB, Hopkins KM, Laverty M, Chu HM: Mol Gen Genet 232:367–376, 1992)

cluding the mutated region in *rad9-192* cells, and the corresponding region in wild-type cells, confirms this difference. The sequencing gel is shown in Figure 23-20, and its interpretation is shown in Figure 23-21.

At first it was thought that the *rad9* gene was involved directly in DNA repair, and that the mutant cells were radiosensitive only because they were repair deficient. This is not the case. The *rad9* is a "molecular checkpoint gene."

In the most general terms, the function of checkpoint genes is to ensure the correct order of cell cycle events, that is, to ensure that the initiation of later events is dependent on the completion of earlier events. The particular genes involved in radiation effects halt cells in the $G_2$ phase, so that an inventory of chromosome damage can be taken and repair initiated and completed, before the complex task of mitosis is attempted. Mutant cells that lose this gene function move directly into mitosis with damaged chromosomes and are therefore at a higher risk of dying, hence their greater sensitivity to radiation, or for that matter to many other DNA damaging agents. The first checkpoint control gene of this kind was identified in the yeast *Saccharomyces cerevisiae*, by Weinert and Hartwell (1988), and coincidentally was also named *RAD9*.

*Techniques:* Genomic DNA library, transformation, gene cloning, DNA sequencing, PCR, sequencing gel.

**4.** *p53 as a checkpoint determinant in mammalian cells* (Kuerbitz et al, 1992)

Cell cycle checkpoints appear to be an important factor in determining radiosensitivity, that is, the fraction of cells surviving a given dose of radiation. Although much is known about checkpoint genes in yeast, relatively little is known about similar genes in mammalian cells.

It was found that cells lacking endogenous p53 gene function did not arrest in $G_1$ after irradiation but that transfection of wild type p53 genes restored this property of arresting in $G_1$. It was further hypothesized that the participation of p53 in this pathway suggests a mechanism for the contribution of p53 in tumorigenesis and genetic instability. Additional studies are, however, needed to determine whether p53 participates directly in checkpoint control and also to determine what its precise role might be.

*Techniques:* Transfection of genes, Northern blotting.

**5.** *Altered ras oncogenes in radiation-induced tumors* (Guerrero et al, 1984)

Several studies have attempted to identify activated oncogenes in radiation-transformed cells by various indirect methods. In the first paper from this group on this topic, the authors described the isolation of DNA from γ-radiation–induced thymic lymphoma in mice and were able to show that K-*ras* and N-*ras* were activated in 9 of 24 tumors. Of particular

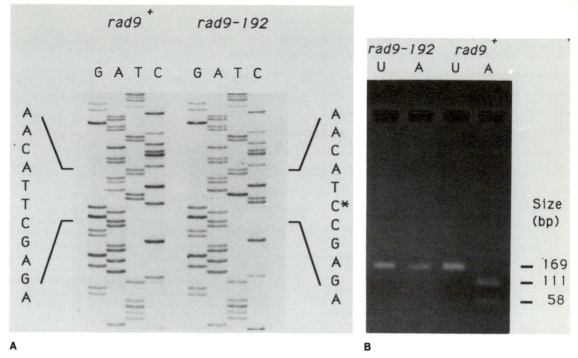

**Figure 23-20.** **(A)** Sequencing gel. Part of a DNA sequencing gel indicating the single base-pair difference between the *S pombe rad9+* and *rad9-192* genes. **(B)** PCR experiment. The single base-pair alteration within *rad9-192* falls within an *Alu*I restriction enzyme cutting site normally found in wild-type genomic DNA. To confirm the sequence, PCR was used to amplify the region directly from wild-type and *rad9-192* mutant cell genomic DNAs. Resulting fragments were treated with *Alu*I (A) or untreated (U) and then run through and visualized in an agarose gel. As can be seen, mutant genomic DNA is missing the *Alu*I site, confirming the existance of the mutation within the *rad9-192*–containing cells. (Courtesy of Dr. H. B. Lieberman and Dr. K.M. Hopkins)

note was that 7 of the tumors involved the **same** mutation. In a later publication, they showed that when neutrons were used, 4 of 25 tumors contained activated *ras*, but all of the mutations were different from one another and from those seen in the γ-ray–induced tumors. Since the activated oncogene could be identified in only a minority of tumors, it was concluded that while this altered gene may be involved in tumor development and progression, it is unlikely to be the sole causative event.

*Techniques:* PCR, Southern blotting.

6. *Characteristic mutations in p53 in lung tumors from uranium miners* (Vahakangas et al, 1992)

The identification of a radiation "signature" has been much discussed. It would clearly be of great importance to be able to say with certainty if a given biological lesion were produced by ionizing radiation as opposed to a chemical, for example, particularly if it was also possible to distinguish between high and low linear energy transfer radiations. "Molecular forensics" may still be a dream, but this paper indicates that it may one day be realized.

The study involved 19 uranium miners who developed lung cancer after prolonged exposure to high levels of radon. Mutations were not found in Ki-*ras*, but nine p53 mutations, including two deletions, were found in 7 miners by direct DNA sequencing after PCR amplification of the tumor DNA. None of the mutations were guanine-cytosine to thymine-adenine transversions in the coding strand of the p53 gene, which is the most frequent base substitution associated with tobacco smoking. The pattern of changes seen in this suppressor gene may reflect the specific products of a high linear energy transfer α-particle and are distinguishable from the other

```
                                                    M   E   F
TCACTGTTTCAAATGTTAATCTTCGGGACCTCGCAAGGATCTTTACAAATCTTTCTAGAATCGATG
  T   V   S   N   V   N   L   R   D   L   A   R   I   F   T   N   L   S   R   I   D   D
ATGCTGTCAACTGGGAAATTAACAAAAATCAGgtgtgttggaactttttcaaaccttactaaaca
  A   V   N   W   E   I   N   K   N   Q
ttgaaactaattggtaaagATAGAGATTACATGTTTAAATTCTTCTAGGTCAGGATTTAGCATGGT
                      I   E   I   T   C   L   N   S   S   R   S   G   F   S   M   V
GACTTTAAAAAAAGGCATTTTTGACAAGTACATTTTTCAGCCGGATTCCGTCCTGTTGACGGGATT
  T   L   K   K   A   F   F   D   K   Y   I   F   Q   P   D   S   V   L   L   T   G   L
GATGACTCCTACAATACGTATTCGTACGCAAGTCAAGCCCATACTATCGTGTTTAGAAACAAAAT
  M   T   P   T   I   R   I   R   T   Q   V   K   P   I   L   S   V   F   R   N   K   I
CTTTGATTTCATCCCGACTGTCGTCACTACCAATAGCAAGAACGGTTATGGCAGTGAATCTGCAAG
  F   D   F   I   P   T   V   V   T   T   N   S   K   N   G   T   G   S   E   S   A   S
CAGAAAAGATGTGATTGTCGAGAATGTTCAAATCTCAATCTCTACTGGTAGCGAGTGTAGGATTAT
  R   K   D   V   I   V   E   N   V   Q   I   S   I   S   T   G   S   E   C   R   I   I
ATTTAAATTCTTATGCAAGCACGgtacgtagtttgtccgtcttattattttatttgctctactaac
  F   K   P   L   C   K   H   G
gtttattcatcaagGAGTGATTAAAAACATATAAAATATCATATGAACAAACCCAAACTTTACACGC
                V   I   K   T   Y   K   I   S   Y   E   Q   T   Q   T   L   H   A
TGTTTTTGATAAATCTCTTAGTCACAATAATTTTCAAATAAACTCAAAAATTCTAAAAGATTTGAC
  V   F   D   K   S   L   N   N   F   Q   I   N   S   K   I   L   K   D   L   T
TGAACATTTTGGTCAGAGAACGGAAGAGC...
  E   H   F   G   Q   R   T   E   E   P   T   I   Q   P   L   Q   E   R   V   L   L   T
AAGTTCACAGAAGAGGTCGTACATAAT...
  S   F   T   E   E   V   V   H   N   Q   P   T   Q   T   T   V   S
CATTGATGGTAAAGAATTTGAACGC...
  I   D   G   K   E   F   E   R   R
TGAATTTCGTGCTGCCGTCATTTT...                                         TGT
  E   F   R   A   A   V   I   L                                       V
CCCAGGAAAACCGATACTTTTAAC...                                         CAT
  P   G   K   P   I   L   L   T                                       I
TCTTGCAACTGTAGTTGGATCAGA...                                         GCA
  L   A   T   V   V   G   S   D                                       H
CAGTTCAACACCAGCTTCTCTGTT...                                         ACA
  S   S   T   P   A   S   L   F   N   S   V   E   R   N   N   S   L   T   A   V   A   H
TAATCCCCTGGATCTATTGGATGGCAAACTGATGTATGTAATTCGGCTTTAGTACTAAGTACAAT
  N   P   P   G   S   I   G   W   Q   T   D   V   C   N   S   A   L   V   L   S   T   I
AATTTATTAACATTAACTTTATAGCAAAGTGACTCATCCAGAATGTTTAATTCTGCGCTTGACCGA
```

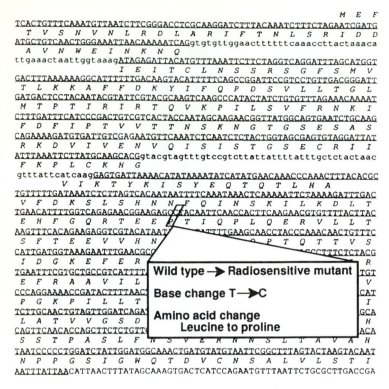

Wild type → Radiosensitive mutant

Base change T → C

Amino acid change
Leucine to proline

Figure 23-21. The radioresistant wild-type *S. pombe* contains the *rad9+* gene. The radiosensitive strain contains the mutant allele *rad 9-192*. Both genes contain a 1092 base-pair open-reading frame. A comparison of the DNA sequence of the two genes reveals a single nucleotide base-pair difference, a cytosine-guanine substituting for a thymine-adenine. This would cause the coding for proline instead of leucine in the mutant gene, promoting a dramatic change in the three-dimensional structure of the protein. Lieberman HB, Hopkins KM, Laverty M, Chu HM: Mol Gen Genet 232:367–376, 1992)

principal cause of lung cancer, namely tobacco smoke.

*Techniques:* PCR, sequencing gel.

**7.** *Parental bias indicating genetic susceptibility to the induction of lung cancer* (You et al, 1992)

The genetic basis of individual susceptibility to induced cancer was dramatically demonstrated in a recent paper involving the induction of cancer in mouse hybrids. A mouse strain with a low lung tumor susceptibility (C3H) was crossed with a strain characterized by a high lung tumor susceptibility. Lung tumors, both spontaneous and chemically induced, were studied in the first-generation hybrids. The appearance of tumors was associated with mutations at codon 12 or codon 61 in the Ki-*ras* oncogene, leading to its activation. In 68 of 70 tumors studied, the mutation occurred in the allele from the susceptible parent. It was possible to identify the parental origin of mutated *ras* because of a characteristic 37-bp deletion in the second intron of the Ki-*ras* allele. This was a fortuitous occurrence that made this study possible.

This study, illustrated in Figure 23-22, dramatically shows that the yield of tumors after a given treatment depends critically on the genetic makeup of the individual exposed.

In the context of radiation protection, the identification of susceptibility genes may allow the classification of both high- and low-risk groups. This may lead to questions of different exposure standards for different persons. At the present time only two special groups are recognized. Exposure of the embryo or fetus is recommended to be controlled more stringently because of the susceptibility to radiation damage, while female astronauts are limited to lower doses than males because of an increased cancer risk associated with a longer life expectancy and radiogenic sites such as the breast. Important and far-reaching ethical considerations would be involved if laboratory tests could be devised to identify susceptible persons, such as ataxia-telangiectasia heterozygotes.

**8.** *Analysis of radiation-induced mutations* (Thacker, 1986; Thacker et al, 1990)

One of the earliest applications of molecular techniques in radiobiology was the use of Southern blotting to analyze mutation spectra in somatic cells cultured in vitro.

The DNA from wild type and mutant cells is digested with several different restriction enzymes and analyzed by the Southern blot technique. Figure 23-23 shows such a blot after cutting DNA with *Bgl*II. There are seven lanes: one for wild-type cells (V79), four for γ-ray–induced mutants (G), one for a spontaneous mutant (S), and a series of markers of known molecular weight (M).

DNA is electrophoresed in a gel, hybridized with the hamster HGPRT gene probe, and then autoradiographed.

In this *Bgl*II digest, DNA from the wild-type cells containing an intact HGPRT gene shows up six bands on the autoradiograph. Mutant G32 shows the same bands; that is it is indistinguishable from the wild-type, indicating that the mutation involves only a small change, possibly a point mutation. Changes of about 30 base-pairs or less are not detectable by this technique. The other γ-ray mutants, G15, G27 and G37, have all lost several bands, indicating the deletion of a significant portion of the gene. The HGPRT gene has been sequenced

and the position at which each restriction enzyme cuts has been mapped. With this information available, it is possible from a Southern blot analysis to show the size and position of partial deletions and rearrangements of the HGPRT gene in a series of mutants produced by γ-rays and α-particles. An example from a 1990 paper by Thacker and his coworkers is shown in Figure 23-24. Some radiation-induced mutations involve a change too small to be detected by Southern blotting, but most involve a sizable deletion of part or all of the gene. Figure 23-24 suggests that the deletions produced by α-particles are larger (on average) than those produced by γ-rays.

*Techniques:* Southern blotting.

**9.** *Oncogenes and radioresistance* (Sklar, 1988; McKenna et al, 1990, 1991)

The first paper to show that transfecting an activating oncogene into cells could result in enhanced radioresistance was published by Sklar in 1988. NIH 3T3 cells were transfected by the calcium phosphate precipitation technique with either genomic DNA containing human c-H-*ras* from bladder cancer or N-*ras* from Hodgkin's disease or HL 60 leukemia or cloned oncogenes including c-H-*ras*, v-H-*ras*,

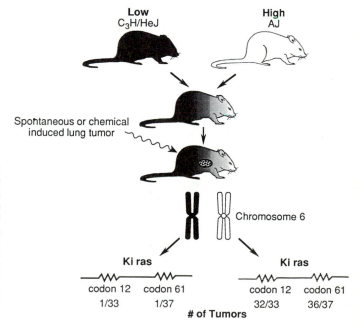

**Figure 23-22.** Illustration of an experiment that demonstrates the genetic basis of susceptibility to cancer. Two strains of mice were mated, one with a high and one with a low susceptibility to lung cancer. The FI hybrids were examined for both spontaneous and chemically induced lung cancers. The tumors were associated with the activation of the Ki-*ras* oncogene, by a mutation in either codon 12 or codon 61. In 68/70 tumors the mutation was in the allele from the susceptible parent. From You M, Wang Y, Stoner G, You L, Maronpot R, Reynolds S, Anderson M: Proc Natl Acad Sci USA 89:5804–5808, 1992)

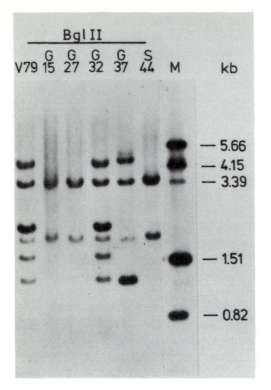

**Figure 23-23.** Hybridization analysis (Southern blot) of genomic DNA from V79 parent cells, four γ-ray–induced mutants, and one spontaneous mutant digested with Bgl II. Pseudogene fragments are at 3.4- and 1.9-kb (Bgl II). M, molecular weight markers. (From Thacker J: Mutat Res 160: 267–275, 1986)

and v-*fms*. With one exception, all *ras* genes were altered by missence mutations at codon 12 or 61; and in all of these cases, the cells showed a large increase in radiation resistance, as illustrated in Figure 23-25. The resistance is expressed as a shallower slope, (ie, a larger $D_0$) as well as a smaller shoulder. There were no significant differences among *ras* genes in their effect on $D_0$ regardless of the type of *ras* gene, the site of the activating mutation, the means of introducing the gene (infection or transfection), the number of copies of the gene, or whether the *ras* gene was introduced as genomic DNA or as a gene cloned in a plasmid.

To check that the increased radiation resistance was not a nonspecific consequence of oncogenic transformation, survival curves were also obtained for cells transformed with an unrelated oncogene v-*fms* and for a cell line transformed with a c-H-*ras* proto-oncogene that had been transformationally activated by linkage with a Moloney retrovirus. Cells transformed by these means showed markedly **less** intrinsic resistance to radiation than cells transformed with the activated *ras* genes.

In a later and more detailed paper, McKenna and his colleagues (1990) investigated the effect of oncogenes on the radiosensitivity of primary rat embryo cells, which have the advantage of being diploid and of being in culture for only a few cell generations. Cell lines were generated from primary rat embryo fibroblasts by DNA-mediated gene transfer of a plasmid bearing the v-*myc* or c-H-*ras* gene, using calcium phosphate precipitation. It was found that the activated H-*ras* oncogene was associated with radiation resistance after transformation but that the effect of the oncogene itself was small and consisted of a change of slope of the radiation survival curve at high doses but little or no change at lower doses in the shoulder region of the curve. By contrast, cells transformed by H-*ras* **plus** v-*myc* were characterized by increased resistance to low doses in the shoulder region of the radiation survival curve as well as a shallower slope at high doses. The v-*myc* oncogene by itself had essentially no effect on radiation survival. This change of inherent radioresistance in the shoulder region is more relevant to the dose range of importance in clinical radiation oncology.

The mechanism for the increased radioresistance conferred by oncogenes is not entirely clear. McKenna and his colleagues have suggested, however, that cells co-transfected with *ras* and *myc* are characterized by a significantly longer $G_2$ phase arrest after irradiation and that this may be the basis of their increased radioresistance.

*Techniques:* DNA mediated gene transfer; genomic library construction; plasmids as vectors.

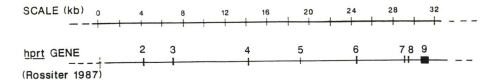

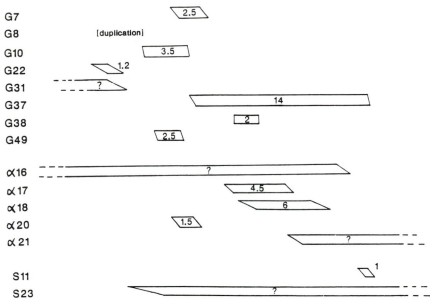

**Figure 23-24.** Size and position of partial deletions/rearrangements of the hamster *hprt* gene in a series of mutants produced by γ-rays (G) or by α-particles (α) or that arose spontaneously (s). A scale with arbitrary positioning is shown at the top, and the next line shows the approximate locations of the known exons of the gene. The mutants analyzed are listed below with the approximate sizes, in kbp, of deletions (*open boxes*) shown where possible; the angles of the vertical lines indicating breakpoints are drawn to include the uncertainties of location. Dashed lines indicate that the deletion extend into flanking DNA. (From Thacker J, Flect EW, Morris T, Rossiter BJF, Morgan TL: Mutat Res 232:163–170, 1990)

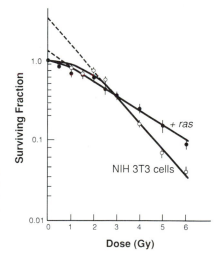

**Figure 23-25.** Radiation survival curves for NIH 3T3 cells (*open symbols*) and similar cells transformed by missence mutation-activated *ras* gene (*closed symbols*). Increase in intrinsic radiation resistance was the same regardless of the source of the *ras* gene, the copy number, or the means of introducing the gene. (Redrawn from Sklar MD: Science 239:645–647, 1988)

# GLOSSARY OF TERMS

**alleles.** Alternate forms of a gene or DNA sequence on the two homologous chromosomes of a pair.

**amino acids.** The 20 basic building blocks of proteins.

**ampicillin.** An antibiotic that prevents bacterial growth.

**amplify.** To increase the number of copies of a DNA sequence by inserting into a cloning vector that replicates within a host cell in vivo or in vitro by the polymerase chain reaction (PCR).

**anneal.** The pairing of complementary DNA or RNA sequences, via hydrogen bonding, to form a double-stranded polynucleotide.

**antibiotic.** Compounds that inhibit the growth of, or kill, microorganisms.

> **antibiotic resistance.** The ability of a microorganism to disable an antibiotic or prevent transport of the antibiotic into the cell.

**antibody.** An immunoglobulin protein produced by B lymphocytes that binds to a specific antigen.

> **monoclonal antibodies.** Immunoglobulin molecules of single-epitope specificity.

> **polyclonal antibodies.** A mixture of immunoglobulin molecules secreted against a specific antigen, each recognizing a different epitope.

**antigen.** Any foreign substance that elicits an immune response by stimulating the production of antibodies.

**bacteriophage.** A virus that infects bacteria. Altered forms are used as vectors for cloning DNA.

**bacterium.** A single-cell prokaryotic organism.

**base pair.** A pair of complementary nitrogenous bases in a DNA molecule: adenine-thymine and guanine-cytosine. It is also a measure of the length of DNA (bp).

**B lymphocyte.** A white blood cell responsible for production of antibodies involved in the humoral immune response.

**cDNA.** *See* DNA.

**cDNA library.** *See* library.

**centromere.** The central portion of the chromosome to which the spindle fibers attach during mitotic and meiotic division.

**codon.** A group of three nucleotides that specifies the addition of one of the 20 amino acids during translation of mRNA into a polypeptide.

> **initiation codon.** The mRNA sequence AUG, which codes for methionine and which initiates translation.

> **termination (stop) codon.** Any of three mRNA sequences (UGA, UAG, UAA) that do not code for an amino acid and thus signal the end of protein synthesis.

**colony.** A group of identical cells derived from a single ancestor cell.

**cosmid.** A plasmid vector containing a COS site that enables it to be packaged into infective bacteriophage particles. It can accommodate DNA sequences of 25,000 to 45,000 bp.

**digest.** To cut DNA molecules with one or more restriction endonucleases.

**DNA (deoxyribonucleic acid).** An organic acid composed of four nitrogenous bases (adenine, thymine, cytosine, and guanine) linked via sugar and phosphate units. DNA is the genetic material of most organisms and usually exists as a double-stranded molecule in which two antiparallel strands are held together by hydrogen bonds between adenine-thymine and cytosine-guanine base pairs.

> **cDNA (copy DNA).** DNA synthesized from an RNA template using reverse transcriptase.

**DNA fingerprint.** A unique pattern of DNA fragments identified by Southern hybridization or by polymerase chain reaction.

**DNA polymorphism.** One or two or more alternate forms of a chromosomal locus that differ in nucleotide sequence or have variable numbers of repeated nucleotide units.

**DNA sequencing.** Procedures for determining the nucleotide sequence of a DNA fragment.

**electrophoresis.** The technique of separating charged molecules in a matrix to which an electrical field is applied.

> **agarose gel electrophoresis.** A matrix composed of purified agar is used to separate larger DNA and RNA molecules ranging from 100 to 20,000 nucleotides.

> **polyacrylamide gel electrophoresis.** Electrophoresis through a matrix composed of a synthetic polymer, used to separate small DNA, or RNA, molecules (up to 1000 nucleotides) or proteins.

> **pulse-field electrophoresis.** The current is alternated between pairs of electrodes set at angles to one another to separate very large DNA molecules of up to 10 million nucleotides.

**electroporation.** High-voltage pulses of electricity are used to open pores in the cell membrane through which foreign DNA can pass.

**Escherichia coli.** A bacterium found in the human

colon that is widely used as a host for molecular cloning experiments.

**ethidium bromide.** A fluorescent dye used to stain DNA and RNA, which intercalates between nucleotides and fluoresces when exposed to ultraviolet light.

**exon.** That portion of a gene expressed in mature mRNA.

**flanking region.** The DNA sequences extending on either side of a specific locus or gene.

**gene.** A locus on a chromosome that encodes a specific protein or several related proteins.

> **dominant gene.** A gene whose phenotype is expressed when it is present in a single copy.
>
> **gene amplification.** The presence of multiple copies of a gene. This is one mechanism by which proto-oncogenes are activated to result in neoplasia.
>
> **gene expression.** The process of producing a protein from its DNA- and mRNA-coding sequences.
>
> **recessive gene.** The phenotype is expressed only when both copies of the gene are mutated or missing.

**genetic code.** The three-letter code that translates a nucleic acid sequence into a protein sequence.

**genome.** The genetic complement contained in the chromosomes of a given organism.

**hybrid.** The offspring of two parents differing in at least one genetic characteristic.

**hybridization.** The hydrogen bonding of complementary DNA and/or RNA sequences to form a duplex molecule.

> **Northern blotting.** A procedure in which RNA fragments are transferred from an agarose gel to a nitrocellulose filter, where the RNA is then hybridized to a radioactive probe.
>
> **Southern blotting.** A procedure in which DNA restriction fragments are transferred from an agarose gel to a nitrocellulose filter, where the denatured DNA is then hybridized to a radioactive probe.

**library.** A collection of cells (usually bacteria or yeast) that have been transformed with recombinant vectors carrying DNA inserts from a single species.

> **cDNA library.** A library composed of complementary copies of cellular mRNAs (ie, the exons without the introns).
>
> **expression library.** A library of cDNAs whose encoded proteins are expressed by specialized vectors.

> **genomic library.** A library composed of fragments of genomic DNA.

**ligase.** An enzyme that catalyzes a reaction that links two DNA molecules by the formation of a phosphodiester bond.

**ligation.** The process of joining two or more DNA fragments.

**microinjection.** Introducing DNA into a cell using a fine microcapillary pipet.

**mitosis.** Replication of a cell to form two identical daughter cells.

**mutation.** An alteration in DNA structure or sequence of a gene.

> **point mutation.** A change in a single base pair in a gene.

**nucleotide.** A building block of DNA and RNA.

> **complementary nucleotides.** Members of the pairs adenine-thymine, adenine-uracil, and guanine-cytosine that have the ability to hydrogen bond to one another.

**oncogene.** A gene that contributes to cancer formation when mutated or inappropriately expressed.

> **cellular oncogene (proto-oncogene).** A normal gene that when mutated or improperly expressed contributes to the development of cancer.
>
> **myc.** A nuclear oncogene involved in immortalizing cells.
>
> **ras.** An oncogene that can induce the malignant phenotype; it converts guanosine triphosphate to guanosine diphosphate, a step in signal transduction.

**plaque.** A clear spot on a lawn of bacteria or cultured cells where cells have been lysed by viral infection and replication.

**plasmid.** A circular DNA molecule, capable of autonomous replication, which may typically carry one or more genes encoding antibiotic resistance.

**polymerase.** An enzyme that catalyzes the addition of multiple subunits to a substrate molecule.

> **DNA polymerase.** Synthesizes a double-stranded DNA molecule using a primer and DNA as a template.
>
> **polymerase chain reaction (PCR).** A procedure that enzymatically amplifies a DNA sequence through repeated replication by DNA polymerase.
>
> **RNA polymerase.** Transcribes RNA from a DNA template.
>
> **Taq polymerase.** A heat-stable DNA polymerase used in PCR.

***primer.*** A short DNA or RNA fragment annealed to single-stranded DNA.

***probe.*** A single-stranded DNA (or RNA) that has been radioactively labeled and is used to identify complementary sequences.

***reading frame.*** A series of triplet condons beginning from a specific nucleotide.

   ***open reading frame.*** A long DNA sequence, uninterrupted by a stop codon, that encodes part or all of a protein.

***recombinant DNA.*** The process of cutting and recombining DNA fragments.

***restriction endonuclease (enzyme).*** A class of endonucleases that cleaves DNA after recognizing a specific sequence.

***restriction fragment length polymorphism (RFLP).*** Differences in nucleotide sequence between alleles that result in restriction fragments of varying lengths.

***retrovirus.*** A class of viruses whose genome consists of RNA and that utilizes the enzyme reverse transcriptase to copy its genome into a DNA intermediate, which integrates into the chromosome of a host cell.

***reverse transcriptase.*** An enzyme that synthesizes a complementary DNA strand from an RNA template.

***RNA (ribonucleic acid).*** An organic acid composed of repeating nucleotide units of adenine, guanine, cytosine, and uracil, whose ribose components are linked by phosphodiester bonds.

   ***messenger RNA (mRNA).*** The class of RNA molecules that copies the genetic information from DNA, in the nucleus, and carries it to ribosomes, in the cytoplasm.

   ***transfer RNA (tRNA).*** Small RNA molecules that transfer amino acids to the ribosome during protein synthesis.

***Saccharomyces cerevisiae.*** Brewer's yeast.

***selectable marker.*** A gene whose expression makes it possible to identify cells that have been trans-formed or transfected with a vector containing the marker gene. It is usually a gene for resistance to an antibiotic.

***somatic cell.*** Any cell other than a germ cell that composes the body of an organism and that possesses a set of multiploid chromosomes.

***stem cell.*** An undifferentiated cell that gives rise to one or more types of specialized cells.

***sticky end.*** A single-stranded nucleotide sequence produced when a restriction endonuclease cleaves off center in its recognition sequence.

***stringency.*** Reaction conditions, such as temperature, salt, and pH, that dictate the annealing of single-stranded DNA/DNA, DNA/RNA, and RNA/RNA hybrids. At high stringency, duplexes form only between strands with perfect one-to-one complementarity: lower stringency allows annealing between strands with less than a perfect match between bases.

***template.*** An RNA or single-stranded DNA molecule upon which a complementary nucleotide strand is synthesized.

***transcription.*** The process of creating a complementary RNA copy of DNA.

***transfection.*** The uptake and expression of foreign DNA by cultured eukaryotic cells.

***transformation.*** In higher eukaryotes, the conversion of cultured cells to a malignant phenotype. In prokaryotes, the natural or induced uptake and expression of a foreign DNA sequence.

***translation.*** The process of converting the genetic information of an mRNA on ribosomes into a polypeptide.

***vector.*** An autonomously replicating DNA molecule into which foreign DNA fragments are inserted and then propagated in a host cell.

***yeast artificial chromosome (YAC).*** A vector used to clone DNA fragments of up to 400.000 bp, which contains the minimum chromosomal sequences needed to replicate in yeast.

► *Summary of Pertinent Conclusions*

---

**Terms and Techniques**

- Restriction endonucleases are enzymes that cleave DNA after recognizing a specific sequence. Those most useful for constructing recombinant molecules leave a "sticky" end, that is, a single-strand overhang of two to four nucleotides that can pair with a complementary strand.

*(continued)*

► *Summary of Pertinent Conclusions* (Continued)

- A **vector** is an autonomously replicating DNA molecule into which foreign DNA fragments are inserted and then propagated in a host cell. Vectors include plasmids, bacteriophage, cosmids, yeast artificial chromosomes, and viruses.

- A **library** is a collection of cells, usually bacteria- or yeast, containing recombinant vectors, carrying DNA inserts from a different species. The inserts may be constructed by using restriction enzyme digested genomic DNA or cDNA.

- A **host** is used to grow (ie, to multiply) or to express a DNA fragment containing a gene of interest.

- In **agarose gel electrophoresis,** DNA or RNA molecules can be separated according to size by causing them to move through a matrix composed of purified agar under the influence of an electric field.

- **Polymerase chain reaction (PCR)** is a procedure that enzymatically amplifies the number of copies of a DNA sequence, up to several thousand base pairs, through repeated replication by DNA polymerase. (A DNA polymerase is an enzyme that catalyzes the addition of nucleotides to a growing DNA molecule.)

- Genes may be cloned by **functional complementation** (ie, putting a functional version of a defective gene into cells to correct the phenotype associated with the defect) by **hybridization** or by making an **antibody probe or oligonucleotide probe.**

- Genes may be "mapped," that is, their position in the genome identified by **in situ hybridization,** by **Southern blotting,** and by **chromosome walking** if a flanking sequence is identified and by **contiguous mapping** if sequence data from large adjacent regions of the genome are aligned.

- Once a gene is isolated, it can be **sequenced** by one of several methods, the most common of which is the **chain termination method**.

- The amino acid sequences within a protein can be determined from the corresponding DNA sequence using the known genetic triplet code.

- A newly acquired sequence can be compared with the international database to seek **homologies** with known genes or proteins.

- Structural variations in DNA caused by point mutations, deletions, or insertions can result in restriction fragments of different lengths, which can often be detected by Southern blotting. These are known as **restriction fragment length polymorphisms (RFLPs),** which can be used as genetic markers to map genes to specific chromosomal locations and identify aberrant genes causing disease.

- A mutation involving only a single base-pair difference between two short single-stranded DNA molecules can be detected by the technique of **single-stranded conformation polymorphism (SSCP).**

*Projects in Radiobiology Employing Molecular Techniques*

- The first **human repair gene** isolated was involved in repairing damage induced by mitomycin C. The techniques of DNA-mediated gene transfer and functional complementation were used; that is, the gene from a human cell (HeLa) was used to correct the repair deficiency in a Chinese hamster cell.

- The **first human ionizing radiation repair gene** was isolated, char-

*(continued)*

► *Summary of Pertinent Conclusions*    (Continued)

acterized, and sequenced by using a human cDNA library in a cosmid vector to correct the radiation repair deficiency in Chinese hamster cells. The gene was assigned to the long arm of human chromosome 19.

- A number of **molecular checkpoint genes** have been identified and sequenced in yeast. These genes function by arresting cells in $G_2$ phase after irradiation to allow repair of damaged DNA before cells enter mitosis; cells in which these genes are not functional exhibit very much more radiosensitivity.

- Human cells that lack endogenous p53 genes did not arrest in $G_1$ phase after irradiation, while transfection of wild-type p53 genes restored this property. It appears that one of the functions of **p53 may be a checkpoint regulator.**

- K-*ras* and N-*ras* were **activated** in 9 of 24 **thymic lymphomas** induced by γ-rays, and 4 of 25 tumors induced by neutrons. Since the activated oncogenes are present in only a minority of tumors, it is likely to be a late step in tumor progression rather than a causative event.

- By direct sequencing of the p53 tumor suppressor gene in lung tumors from Uranium miners, a characteristic spectrum of mutations was observed that was quite different from that produced by tobacco smoke. This may reflect the specific products of high linear energy transfer α-particles, that is, a **radiation "signature."**

- **Genetic susceptibility** to lung cancer, spontaneous or induced, was shown by cross breeding two mouse strains, one with high and one with low susceptibility to lung cancer, and showing that the mutation in the Ki-*ras* oncogene associated with the tumors almost always occurred in the allele from the susceptible parent.

- Southern blot analysis has been used to show that most mutations produced by ionizing radiation (at least in somatic cells cultured in vitro) are large deletions. There is some suggestion that the spectrum of mutations is different for α-particles than for γ-rays, with a preponderance of larger deletions for the densely ionizing radiation.

- By transferring cloned genes and/or genomic DNA from tumor cells, it was shown that **activated oncogenes** could confer **resistance** to cell killing by radiation. The combination of *ras* plus *myc* was more effective than either alone.

# BIBLIOGRAPHY

Guerrero J, Viollasonte A, Corces V, Pellicer A: Activation of a cK-*ras* oncogene by somatic mutation in mouse lymphomas induced by gamma radiation. Science 225:1159–1162, 1984

Kuerbitz SJ, Plunkett BS, Walsh, WV, Kastan MB: Wild-type p53 is a cell cycle checkpoint determinant following irradiation. Proc Natl Acad Sci USA 89:7491–7495, 1992

Lieberman HB, Hopkins KM, Laverty M, Chu HM: Molecular cloning and analysis of *Schizosaccharomyces pombe rad9*, a gene involved in DNA repair and mutagenesis. Mol Gen Genet 232:367–376, 1992

McKenna WG, Weiss MC, Endlich B, Ling CC, Bakanauskas VJ, Kelsten ML, Muschel RJ: Synergistic effect of the v-*myc* oncogene with H-*ras* on radioresistance. Cancer Res 50:97–102, 1990

McKenna WG, Iliakis G, Weiss MC, Bernhard EJ, Muschel RJ: Increased $G_2$ delay in radiation-resistant cells obtained by transformation of primary rat embryo cells with the oncogenes H-*ras* and v-*myc*. Radiat Res 125:283–287, 1991

Micklos DA, Freyer GA: DNA Science: A First Course

in Recombinant DNA Technology. Burlington, NC, Cold Spring Harbor Laboratory Press and Carolina Biological Supply Company, 1990

Murray JM, Carr AM, Lehmoenn AR, Watts Z: Cloning and characterization of the *rad 9* DNA repair gene from *Schizosaccharomyces Pombe*. Nucl Acids Res 19:3525–3531, 1991

Rubin JS, Joyner AL, Bernstein A, Whitmore GF: Molecular identification of a human DNA repair gene following DNA-mediated gene transfer. Nature 306:206–208, 1983

Sklar MD: The *ras* oncogenes increase the intrinsic resistance of NIH 3T3 cells to ionizing radiation. Science 239:645–647, 1988

Sloan S, Newcomb EW, Pellicer A: Ionizing radiation and *ras* oncogene activation. Cancer Res Clin Oncol 116(suppl 808), 1990

Thacker J Fleck, EW, Morris T, Rossites BJF, Morgan TL: Localization of deletion breakpoints in radiation-induced mutants of the hprt gene in hamster cells. Mutation Res 232:163–170, 1990

Thacker J: The nature of mutants induced by ionizing radiation in cultured hamster cells. Mutation Res 160:267–275, 1986

Thompson LH, Brookman KW, Jones NJ, Allen SA, Carrano AV: Molecular cloning of the human XRCC1 gene, which corrects defective DNA strand break repair and sister chromatid exchange. Mol Cell Biol 10:6160–6171, 1990

Vahakangas KH, Samet JM, Metcalf RA, Welsh JA, Bennett WP, Lane DP, Harris CC: Mutations of p53 and *ras* genes in radon-associated lung cancer from uranium miners. Lancet 1(339):576–580, 1992

van Duin M, deWit J, Odijk H, Westerveld A, Yasui A, Koken MHM, Hoeijmakers J, Bootsma D: Molecular cloning and characterization of the human excision repair gene ERCC-1: cDNA cloning and amino acid homology with the yeast DNA repair gene. Radio Cell 44:913–923, 1986

Watson JD, Gilman M, Witkowski J, Zoller M: Recombinant DNA, 2nd ed. New York, Scientific American Books, 1992

Weinert TA, Hartwell LH: The *RAD9* gene controls the cell cycle response to DNA damage in *Saccharomyces cerevisiae*. Science 241:317–322, 1988

You M, Wang Y, Stoner G, You L, Maronpot R, Reynolds SH, Anderson M: Parental bias of Ki-*ras* oncogenes detected in lung tumors from mouse hybrids. Proc Natl Acad Sci USA 89:5804–5808, 1992

*Radiobiology for the Radiologist, Fourth Edition*, by Eric J. Hall
J. B. Lippincott Company, Philadelphia © 1994.

# 24

# *Diagnostic Radiology and Nuclear Medicine: Risk Versus Benefit*

Diagnostic Radiology
Nuclear Medicine

## SOURCES OF RADIATION TO THE HUMAN POPULATION

All humans are exposed inevitably to ionizing radiation. The sources involved are of three general types: unperturbed **natural sources, enhanced natural sources,** where human activity has increased the level of individual exposure, and **man-made sources.**

Natural sources include cosmic radiation from outer space, terrestrial radiation from natural radioactive materials in the ground, and radiation from radionuclides naturally present in the body, inhaled, or ingested.

Enhanced natural sources are sources that are natural in origin but to which exposure is increased as a result of human activity (inadvertent or otherwise). Examples include air travel at high altitude, which increases cosmic-ray levels, and movement of radionuclides on the ground in phosphate mining, which can increase the terrestrial component to persons living in houses built on waste landfills. Radon exposures indoors might be considered in some instances to be an enhanced natural source, inasmuch as it is not natural to live in an insulated house! In a sense, also, all operations of the nuclear fuel cycle, starting with mining, involve natural radionuclides, but these are more generally classified as man-made exposures.

A variety of exposures result from man-made materials and devices. First and foremost are x-rays and radiopharmaceuticals in medicine. Other examples include consumer products containing radioactive materials, such as smoke detectors; atmospheric testing of nuclear weapons; and accidents in nuclear power plants.

## RELATING RADIATION EXPOSURE TO RISK

For the purpose of relating exposure to somatic risk, the most suitable quantity for cancer induction is the **effective dose.**\* This is the weighted sum of the equivalent doses to each of the tissues of the body exposed. This quantity is simple to calculate in the case of a uniform total-body exposure (eg, as from natural background radiation) but more complicated when only certain parts of the body are exposed (as in the case of irradiation of the lung by natural radon-daughter products or most procedures in diagnostic radiology).

For purposes of expressing *genetic* risk, the most suitable quantity is the **genetically significant dose** (GSD). This is the equivalent dose to the gonads weighted for the age and sex distribution in those members of the exposed population expected to have offspring. The GSD is an index of the presumed genetic impact of radiation on the whole population. Only a part of the population, not everyone, receives radiation from a given source, such as medical or dental radiographs, color television, or cosmic rays from flying at high altitudes. The calculation of the GSD attempts to *average* the genetic effects over the whole population. The GSD for the total population is the dose that, if received by every member of the population, might be expected to result in the same total genetic injury to the population as do the actual gonadal doses received by the various persons exposed.

Because the genetic injury is only associated with the offspring of irradiated persons, the gonadal doses received by these persons must be weighted for the probability of their having offspring. Therefore, the measured or calculated gonadal dose for each exposed person is weighted by the expected number of future children for a person of that age and sex. For example, a dose of radiation received by a postmenopausal woman has no impact on the genetic future of

---

\**For the reader unfamiliar with terms such as* effective dose, *it may be necessary to first read the definitions at the end of Chapter 25.*

the human race, and so that weighting factor would be zero. By contrast, healthy teenage patients, with their reproductive life ahead of them, would be weighted to allow for the number of children they would be likely to produce. This is the procedure used in estimating the GSD from medical and dental radiation. For natural background radiation, the GSD is assumed to be the same as the gonadal dose, since exposure is uniformly distributed over all ages. It is somewhat less than the total-body radiation dose because of shielding of the gonads by other body tissues.

It should be emphasized that the GSD is an *index* of genetic impact on an exposed population, but the units are sieverts (Sv) or rems (ie, the units of equivalent dose), so that it is *not* an estimate of the *number* of mutations produced.

## DOSES FROM DIAGNOSTIC RADIOLOGY PROCEDURES

Information concerning the doses of radiation received by the population of the United States from medical radiation is sketchy. Surveys were attempted in 1964, 1970, and 1980, but these are expensive to conduct and of dubious accuracy. Although there are no recent comprehensive national surveys of diagnostic procedures using x-rays or nuclear medicine techniques, there have been a variety of limited surveys for special groups and somewhat larger surveys involving use in hospitals. These were all combined in National Council on Radiation Protection and Measurement (NCRP) report No. 100 published in 1989.

In recent years, too, the Conference of Radiation Control Program Directors, the umbrella organization for state and local radiation control agencies, together with the Food and Drug Administration (FDA), conducts the Nationwide Evaluation of X-ray Trends (NEXT) survey program. Reports have appeared for a few key areas, such as mammography, computed tomography scans of the head, and upper gastrointestinal fluoroscopy.

These various sources are all used in this chapter, but it should be noted that simple look-up tables can lead to dose estimates that

Table 24-1.
**Estimated Total Diagnostic Medical and Dental X-Ray Procedures in the United States**

|  | NUMBER OF EXAMINATIONS (IN MILLIONS) | | |
|  | 1964 | 1970 | 1980 |
|---|---|---|---|
| Medical | 109 | 136 | 180 |
| Dental | 54 | 67 | 101 |
| Total | 163 | 203 | 281 |
| Frequency per 1000 population | 870 | 990 | 1240 |

*(From National Council on Radiation Protection and Measurements: Exposure of the Population in the United States to Ionizing Radiation. Report No. 93. Bethesda, MD, NCRP, 1987)*

may be grossly misleading for the individual patient and are no substitute for dose measurements. Techniques, and the resulting doses, vary enormously between different institutions.

Table 24-1 shows the steady increase in the use of x-rays for diagnostic purposes in the United States during the period when widespread surveys were available. The figures are out-of-date, but it is clear that the number of x-ray procedures is close to the United States population! Table 24-2 shows more recent data on the growth in the use of computed tomography. In addition to the exposure of patients, the Environmental Protection Agency (EPA) estimated that in 1984 about 1.32 million persons in the United States were engaged nominally in radiation work.

Table 24-2.
**Estimated Use of Computed Tomography**

| | NUMBER OF EXAMINATIONS (IN THOUSANDS) | | |
| EXAMINATION | 1981 | 1982 | 1983 |
|---|---|---|---|
| Head | 1755 | 2481 | 2712 |
| Spine | 59 | 141 | 425 |
| Body | 523 | 960 | 1166 |
| Total | 2337 | 3582 | 4303 |

*(Adapted from Evans R, Mettler FA: AJR 144:1077, 1985)*

Table 24-3.
Specific Organ Doses From Diagnostic Radiology*

| EXAMINATION | IMAGES (NUMBER) | ORGAN DOSE (µGy) | | | | | | |
|---|---|---|---|---|---|---|---|---|
| | | Thyroid | Marrow | Lung | Breast | Testes | Ovaries | Embryo |
| Chest | 1.5 | 60 | 40 | 200 | 140 | † | 0.6 | 0.6 |
| Skull | 4.1 | 2200 | 300 | 20 | † | † | † | † |
| Cervical spine | 3.7 | 4000 | 100 | 150 | † | † | † | † |
| Ribs | 3.0 | 1500 | 450 | 3000 | 4100 | † | 4 | 5 |
| Shoulder | 1.8 | 600 | 60 | 350 | 750 | † | † | † |
| Thoracic spine | 2.1 | 800 | 450 | 4000 | 5400 | † | 10 | 1 |
| Cholecystogram | 3.2 | 10 | 650 | 1800 | † | † | 60 | 50 |
| Lumbar spine | 2.9 | 3 | 1200 | 1400 | † | 70 | 4000 | 4100 |
| Upper gastrointestinal tract | 4.3 | 70 | 1200 | 5000 | 550 | 4 | 450 | 500 |
| Kidney-ureter-bladder | 1.7 | 0.1 | 500 | 100 | † | 150 | 2100 | 2600 |
| Barium enema | 4.0 | 2 | 3000 | 500 | † | 600 | 7900 | 8200 |
| Lumbosacral spine | 3.4 | 0.5 | 2200 | 350 | † | 450 | 6400 | 6400 |
| Intravenous pyelography | 5.5 | † | 1200 | 350 | † | 500 | 6400 | 8200 |
| Pelvis | 1.3 | † | 250 | 10 | † | 550 | 1500 | 2000 |
| Hip | 2.0 | † | 150 | † | † | 3700 | 800 | 1300 |
| Mammography | 2.0 | ‡ | ‡ | ‡ | 1000 | ‡ | ‡ | ‡ |
| Urethrocystography | | 50 | 3000 | 200 | 200 | 20000 | 15000 | |
| Hysterosalpingography | | 10 | 1700 | 100 | 50 | | 5900 | |
| Paranasal sinuses | | 7900 | 1200 | 100 | 100 | 10 | 10 | |
| Carotid angiography | | 3000 | 15000 | 100 | 100 | 100 | 100 | |
| Dental | 1.0 | 30 | 10 | 1 | 5 | 0.1 | 0.1 | |
| CT brain | 5.0 | | 1400 | | | 70 | 70 | |
| CT abdomen | 5.0 | | 4900 | | | 400 | 400 | |

*Doses in µGy: divide by 10 for doses in mrad.*
*Data from Laws PW, Rosenstein M: Health Phys 35:629–642, 1978; United Nations Scientific Committee on the Effects of Atomic Radiation: Sources and Effects of Ionizing Radiation. New York, UNSCEAR, 1977; Gregg EC: Radiology 123:447–453, 1977; and Shrivastava PN, Lynn SL, Ting JY: Radiology 125:411–415, 1977)*
*†Less than 0.1 µGy.*
*‡Considered negligible compared with dose to breast.*
*(From Committee on Radiological Units, Standards and Protection: Medical Radiation: A Guide to Good Practice. Chicago, American College of Radiology, 1985)*

This includes the nuclear power industry as well as medical facilities. The average annual equivalent dose was about 1.1 mSv (110 mrems) but only about half received measurable exposures.

The fact that so many persons, representing such a large fraction of the population, receive radiation regularly must be a cause of concern because of the known and much publicized deleterious effects of radiation. It is true that, as the use of radiation has become more and more widespread, the techniques employed and the equipment used have undergone a continuing ev-

olution, so that the dose of radiation required for most procedures has steadily decreased. These improvements in technology balance to some extent the increasing use of radiation in medicine.

There is no direct evidence that small doses of radiation, similar to those used in diagnostic radiology, cause harmful effects in the persons who are exposed. Discussions in this chapter involve *inferences* and *estimates* of the biological effects that *might* occur when a large number of persons are exposed to small doses of radiation, based on extrapolation from the known deleterious effects observed when smaller numbers of persons (or animals) are exposed to much larger doses of radiation. All that can be done for low doses of radiation is to make estimates, based on plausible assumptions, but estimates nevertheless. They are not measurements or observations.

A point frequently made is that many of the new developments in diagnostic imaging involve technologies that do not include ionizing radiations. The principal examples are ultrasound and magnetic resonance imaging (MRI). The proponents of these new imaging devices claim that they are absolutely safe because no x-rays are involved. This, in turn, is an assumption, inasmuch as the possibility that the nonionizing radiations or high magnetic fields involved may cause a biological effect has not been investigated in anything near as much detail as the consequences of x-rays. Only time and much experimentation and observation will tell whether these new technologies are any safer than x-rays.

Table 24-3 lists specific organ doses from representative x-ray examinations. The data do not contain any big surprises. As would be expected,

radiographs of the lumbar spine, pelvis, and hip involve sizable effective total-body doses, because relatively large amounts of radiation are necessary to penetrate these thick regions of the body. The gonadal doses are high, too, because the ovaries or testes are within or close to the field. Large gonadal doses are also inevitable with a barium enema or with an intravenous or retrograde pyelogram. On the other hand, the GSD from dental radiographs is negligible.

The results of the detailed NEXT surveys are of particular interest as they become available, but to date they have been conducted for only a limited number of x-ray procedures. Table 24-4 shows the results of the survey for upper gastrointestinal fluoroscopy examinations, which represents the widest use of fluoroscopy. Table 24-5 shows data from the NEXT survey for CT examinations of the head. Note the wide ranges of doses reported with a given machine.

The evaluation of techniques and practices in mammography is of special interest. The Nationwide Evaluation of X-ray Trends (NEXT) program has shown that mammography underwent the greatest change of any existing radiologic examination during the 1980s. Between 1985 and 1988 image quality improved substantially at the cost of slightly higher glandular doses (1.59 from 0.89 mGy, or 159 from 89 mrems), for screen-film combinations. Techniques in xeromammography

**Table 24-4.**
Nationwide Evaluation of X-ray Trends (NEXT) Survey of Upper Gastrointestinal Fluoroscopy Examinations

**Entrance—Air—Kerma—Rate (mGy*/min)**

|  | WITH PHANTOM | PHANTOM AND SIMULATED BARIUM | UNIT DRIVEN TO MAXIMUM |
|---|---|---|---|
| Average | 38 | 56 | 59 |
| Maximum | 130 | 160 | 160 |
| Minimum | 10 | 10 | 10 |

**Mean Single Spot Film Exposure (mGy)**

| Hospitals | 2.1 | 19 |
|---|---|---|
| Nonhospitals | 4.0 | 22 |

*Doses in mGy can be converted to mrad by multiplying by 100.

**Table 24-5.**
Nationwide Evaluation of X-ray Trends (NEXT) Survey of CT Examinations of the Head: Values for CT Systems With 10 or More Units in 1990

| MANUFACTURER | MODEL | MULTIPLE SCAN AVERAGE DOSE (mGy)* | AVERAGE mAs |
|---|---|---|---|
| GE | 8800 | 42 (17–119) | 586 |
|  | 9800 | 47 (20–140) | 385 |
| Philips | 60 | 35 (23–61) | 348 |
| Picker | 1200 | 49 (23–70) | 333 |
| Siemens | DR | 34 (19–66) | 442 |

*Values in parentheses represent ranges. Doses in mGy can be converted to mrad by multiplying by 100.
(From Conway BJ, McCrohan JL et al: Radiology 184:135–140, 1992)

Table 24-6.
Factors Included in Calculation of Genetically Significant Dose for 1980
by Sex and Examination Type[*]

| SEX | EXAMINATION TYPE | MEAN GONADAL DOSE $\mu Gy$ (mrad) | RELATIVE FREQUENCY ($\times 10^{-3}$) | RELATIVE CHILD EXPECTANCY | GSD FOR EXAMINATION TYPE $\mu Gy$ (mrad) |
|---|---|---|---|---|---|
| Male | Head and neck | — | 40 | 0.57 | — |
| | Chest | 10 (1) | 298 | 0.31 | 0.9 (0.09) |
| | Cervical spine | — | 23 | 0.47 | — |
| | Lumbar spine | 2180 (218) | 59 | 0.15 | 19.3 (1.93) |
| | Hips/pelvis | 6000 (600) | 18 | 0.38 | 41.0 (4.10) |
| | Upper extremities | — | 106 | 0.65 | — |
| | Lower extremities | 150 (15) | 119 | 0.70 | 12.5 (1.25) |
| | Abdomen (kidneys, ureters, bladder) | 970 (97) | 35 | 0.31 | 10.5 (1.05) |
| | Upper gastrointestinal and small bowel | 10 (1) | 28 | 0.22 | 0.1 (0.01) |
| | Barium enema | 1750 (175) | 17 | 0.17 | 5.1 (0.51) |
| | Gallbladder | — | 11 | 0.20 | — |
| | Intravenous pyelogram | 2070 (207) | 18 | 0.24 | 8.9 (0.89) |
| | Head CT | — | 11 | 0.13 | — |
| | Body CT | — | 3 | 0.21 | — |
| | | | | Total | 98 (9.8) |
| Female | Head and neck | — | 32 | 0.41 | — |
| | Chest | 10 (1) | 270 | 0.21 | 0.6 (0.06) |
| | Cervical spine | — | 22 | 0.30 | — |
| | Lumbar spine | 7210 (721) | 56 | 0.21 | 84.8 (8.48) |
| | Hips/pelvis | 2100 (210) | 25 | 0.21 | 11.0 (1.10) |
| | Upper extremities | — | 72 | 0.15 | — |
| | Lower extremities | — | 103 | 0.41 | — |
| | Abdomen (kidneys, ureters, bladder) | 2210 (221) | 35 | 0.38 | 29.4 (2.94) |
| | Upper gastrointestinal and small bowel | 1710 (171) | 39 | 0.26 | 17.3 (1.73) |
| | Barium enema | 9030 (903) | 26 | 0.17 | 39.9 (3.99) |
| | Gallbladder | 780 (78) | 19 | 0.14 | 2.1 (0.21) |
| | Intravenous pyelogram | 5880 (588) | 20 | 0.20 | 23.5 (2.35) |
| | Head CT | — | 13 | 0.33 | — |
| | Body CT | — | 3 | 0.21 | — |
| | | | | Total | 209 (20.9) |

(—) *indicates less than 0.01 $\mu Gy$; GSD, genetically significant dose.*
[*]*There are a number of examination types that are usually included in the category of "others" that have not been included in this table. Inclusion of these types may increase the genetically significant dose by 10% to 20%.*
*(From National Council on Radiation Protection and Measurements: Exposure of the US Population From Diagnostic Medical Radiation. Report No. 100, Bethesda, MD, 1989)*

have changed little over this period of time, although this technique is used much less now. The mean glandular dose for xeromammography was measured to be 4.32 mGy (432 mrems) in 1988, almost three times as large as that for screen-film combinations.

## GONADAL AND GENETICALLY SIGNIFICANT DOSE

For estimates of possible detriment to future generations, two quantities are often reported. These are the gonadal dose and the GSD. The gonadal dose is the calculated dose to the testes or ovaries from a given examination in either an individual patient or a "standard" patient. The GSD is defined as that dose that, if given to every member of the population, would produce the same genetic detriment as the actual doses received by the various persons." The GSD is a weighted dose calculated on the basis of the number of procedures, the gonadal dose, and the age distribution of the population exposed (particularly the number of children expected among that age population). Analysis of the GSD from diagnostic radiological procedures can be used to estimate possible detriment from a specific practice and, to a limited extent, allows diagnostic radiology to be compared with other radiation sources such as nuclear medicine and natural radiation exposure.

Table 24-6 taken from NCRP report No. 100 shows the estimated GSD for various radiologic procedures and the components used in its calculation. The total annual GSD is about 300 mGy (30 mrad), made up of one third from the male and two thirds from the female. The largest contributors to the GSD are examinations of the hips and pelvis of males and examinations of the lumbar spine and barium enemas of females. The GSD contribution from dental x-ray examinations has not been included, because it is so small.

## COLLECTIVE DOSES FROM DIAGNOSTIC RADIOLOGY

Next to be considered is the effect of Diagnostic Radiology on the population as a whole, rather than on one person. The relevant quantity here is the **collective effective dose,** that is, the sum of the product of the effective dose and the number of persons exposed.

Several attempts have been made to estimate the collective effective dose for diagnostic radiology; such estimates are fraught with difficulties and can only result in ball-park figures. Table 24-7 shows the collective effective dose from all diagnostic procedures performed in hospitals and doctors' offices in the United States in 1980. The total amounts to 92,000 person Sv (9.2 million man-rems). This results in a per caput effective dose of 0.4 mSv (40 mrems). This estimate is probably low for the 1990s because of the greatly increased use of CT scans. The results of a worldwide survey of collective dose and per caput doses (ie, average individual doses) are shown in Tables 24-8 and 24-9. This survey indicates that the per caput dose for the United States is now as high as 1.3 mSv (130 mrems), which is intermediate among the developed industrialized countries (see Table 24-8). This survey also shows that the collective dose is high in countries with plenty of doctors and low in countries where physicians are few—a not surprising result (see Table 24-9).

The values of the collective effective dose in Table 24-7 should be reduced because the population receiving diagnostic x-rays is substantially skewed with regard to age distribution compared with the general population. Over half are older than 45 years of age, and a fourth are older than 64. This has an impact on the possible detriment as defined by the International Commission on Radiological Protection, as discussed in Chapter 25. Detriment includes contributions of years of life lost, as well as compromised quality of life, as a consequence of exposure to radiation, and these factors will be different in an older population.

Table 24-10, taken from NCRP report No. 100, compares the total collective effective dose with a weighted value, allowing for the fact that patients receiving medical radiation tend to be older than the general population; this reduces the collective effective dose from 73,000 to 46,000 person-Sv, or by about 37%. These data relate to diagnostic radiology in US **hospitals;** comparable figures are not available for procedures performed in physicians' offices. If we make the assumption that the same age distribu-

Table 24-7.
Collective Effective Dose From Diagnostic Medical X-rays: United States 1980

| EXAMINATION TYPE | EFFECTIVE DOSE (mSv)* | EXAMINATIONS (IN THOUSANDS) | COLLECTIVE EFFECTIVE DOSE (PERSON-Sv)† |
|---|---|---|---|
| CT (head and body) | 1.11 | 3,300 | 3,660 |
| Chest | 0.08 | 64,000 | 5,120 |
| Skull | 0.22 | 8,200 | 1,800 |
| Cervical spine | 0.20 | 5,100 | 1,020 |
| Biliary | 1.89 | 3,400 | 6,430 |
| Lumbar spine | 1.27 | 12,900 | 16,400 |
| Upper gastrointestinal | 2.44 | 7,600 | 18,500 |
| Abdomen (kidneys, ureters, bladder) | 0.56 | 7,900 | 4,420 |
| Barium enema | 4.06 | 4,900 | 19,900 |
| Intravenous pyelogram | 1.58 | 4,200 | 6,640 |
| Pelvis | 0.44 ⎫ 0.64 | | |
| Hip | 0.83 ⎭ | 4,700 | 3,010 |
| Extremities | 0.01 | 45,000 | 450 |
| Other | 0.50 | (8,400) | 4,200 |
| Rounded total | | | 92,000 |

*1 mSv = 100 mrem.
†1 person-Sv = 100 man-rem.
(Adapted from National Council on Radiation Protection and Measurements: Exposure of the US Population From Diagnostic Medical Radiation. Report No. 100. Bethesda, MD, NCRP, 1989)

Table 24-8.
Annual per Caput Doses From Diagnostic Radiology*

| COUNTRY | PER CAPUT DOSE (mSv) |
|---|---|
| Poland | 1.7 |
| France | 1.6 |
| USSR | 1.4 |
| Japan | 1.3 |
| United States | 1.3 |
| Italy | 0.8 |
| Spain | 0.8 |
| Finland | 0.7 |
| Sweden | 0.6 |
| United Kingdom | 0.2 |

*Doses in mSv can be converted to mrem by multiplying by 100.
(From Bennett BG: Exposures from medical radiation worldwide. Radiat Protect Dosimetry 36:237–242, 1991)

Table 24-9.
Diagnostic Radiology Exposures Worldwide*

| REGION | NUMBER OF PATIENTS PER PHYSICIAN | PER CAPUT DOSE (mSv) | COLLECTIVE DOSE ($10^3$ PERSON Sv) |
|---|---|---|---|
| I | 1000 | 1.0 | 1300 |
| II | 1000–3000 | 0.2 | 350 |
| III | 3000–10,000 | 0.06 | 80 |
| IV | >10,000 | 0.03 | 20 |

*mSv can be converted to mrem, or person-Sv to man-rem, by multiplying by 100.
(Adapted from Bennett BG: Radiat Protect Dosimetry 36:237–242, 1991)

Table 24-10.
## Collective Effective Dose and Collective Weighted Dose From Diagnostic Radiology During 1980 in United States Hospitals

| EXAMINATION TYPE | COLLECTIVE EFFECTIVE DOSE (PERSON-Sv)*† | COLLECTIVE WEIGHTED DOSE (PERSON-Sv)*† |
|---|---|---|
| Chest | 4,339  (5.9) | 2,650  (5.7) |
| Skull and face | 1,560  (2.1) | 1,280  (2.8) |
| Cervical spine | 630  (0.8) | 430  (0.9) |
| Biliary‡ | 6,660  (9.1) | 3,820  (8.3) |
| Lumbar spine | 5,340  (7.3) | 3,580  (7.8) |
| Upper gastrointestinal‡ | 15,770 (21.5) | 9,030 (19.6) |
| Abdomen (kidneys, ureters, bladder) | 3,730  (5.1) | 3,470  (7.5) |
| Barium enema‡ | 15,400 (21.0) | 7,470 (16.3) |
| Intravenous pyelogram | 7,910 (10.8) | 6,630 (14.5) |
| Pelvis | 5,460  (7.4) | 4,280  (9.3) |
| Hip | 2,730  (3.7) | 1,560  (3.4) |
| Extremities | 200  (0.3) | 110  (0.2) |
| Computed tomography | 3,660  (5.0) | 1,700  (3.7) |
| Rounded total | 73,000 (100) | 46,000 (100) |

*1 person-Sv = 100 person-rem.
†Numbers in parentheses are the percent of total.
‡Includes fluoroscopic component as well as radiographic.
(Adapted from National Council on Radiation Protection and Measurements: Exposure of the US Population from Diagnostic Medical Radiation. Report No. 100. Bethesda, MD, NCRP, 1984)

tion applies to all patients receiving diagnostic x-rays, then the total collective effective dose in Table 24-6 should be reduced by 37% too, from 92,000 person-Sv to about 58,000 person-Sv (5.8 million man-rems). This is the figure used later in the chapter to assess the **risk** of diagnostic radiology to be weighed against its undoubted benefits.

## DOSES FROM NUCLEAR MEDICINE

The first person to suggest using radioactive isotopes to label compounds in biology and medicine was the Hungarian chemist Hevesy, whose work, beginning before World War I, earned him a Nobel Prize in 1943 (Fig. 24-1). The concept of using radioactive tracers in medicine could not be exploited until the means to produce artificial isotopes were readily available. The cyclotron was invented by Ernest Lawrence in the 1930s and has been used to produce short-lived isotopes and positron emitters (Fig. 24-2). Nuclear reactors were developed during World War II and are used to produce most medically used radioactive isotopes that have an excess of neutrons and that consequently are electron and γ-ray emitters.

For these reasons nuclear medicine was a late starter compared with radiation therapy and x-ray diagnosis. Radiopharmaceuticals of adequate quality and consistency were not available until 1946, but since then nuclear medicine has grown into a specialty in its own right and was one of the most rapidly growing areas of medicine until slowed by the advent of computed tomography and magnetic resonance imaging. A broad array of pharmaceuticals, coupled with the development of sophisticated hardware, has made possible a widening diversity of applications. Table 24-11 shows the growth and distribu-

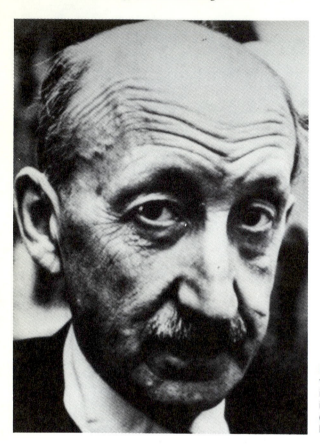

**Figure 24-1.** The great Hungarian chemist Hevesy, whose work beginning before World War I earned him a Nobel prize in 1943. He was the first to conceive of using radioactive isotopes to label compounds for biology and medicine. (Courtesy of the University of California Lawrence Berkeley Laboratory)

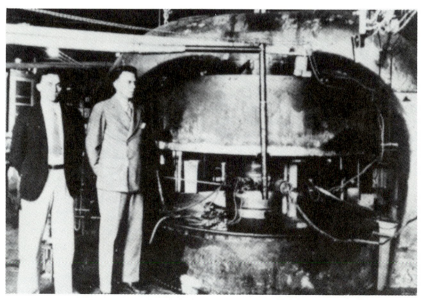

**Figure 24-2.** The concept of using radioactive isotopes as tracers in medicine was not fully explored until the invention of the cyclotron in 1931. Its inventor, Ernest O. Lawrence, is seen here (*right*) with his second cyclotron in 1934. Many short-lived isotopes are made with a device of this sort. (Courtesy of the University of California Lawrence Berkeley Laboratory)

Table 24-11.
**Estimated Number of Diagnostic Radionuclide in Vivo Examinations in the United States (in thousands)**

| EXAMINATION | YEAR | | | | | | | |
|---|---|---|---|---|---|---|---|---|
| | 1972 | 1973 | 1975 | 1978 | 1980 | 1980 | 1981 | 1982 |
| Brain | 1250 | 1510 | 2120 | 1546 | 870 | 1176 | 1038 | 812 |
| Hepatobiliary | 26 | — | — | — | — | — | 109 | 179 |
| Liver | 455 | 535 | 676 | 1302 | 1180 | 1399 | 1445 | 1424 |
| Bone | 81 | 125 | 220 | 1160 | 1270 | 1307 | 1613 | 1811 |
| Respiratory | 332 | 417 | 597 | 1053 | 830 | 898 | 1095 | 1191 |
| Thyroid* | 356 | 460 | 627 | 699 | 650 | 506 | 664 | 677 |
| Urinary | 108 | 122 | 154 | 205 | 200 | 164 | 402 | 236 |
| Tumor | 10 | 14 | 22 | 166 | 130 | — | 125 | 121 |
| Cardiovascular | 25 | 33 | 49 | 160 | 580 | 558 | 708 | 950 |
| Other | 405 | 294 | 338 | 115 | 110 | 368 | — | — |
| Rounded total | 3300 | 3500 | 4800 | 6400 | 5800 | 6400 | 7000 | 7400 |

*Scans and uptakes.
(Adapted from Mettler FA, Moseley RD: Medical Effects of Ionizing Radiation. Orlando, FL, Grune & Stratton, 1985)

tion of procedures in nuclear medicine from 1972 to 1982. In the 1990s, it is estimated that there are more than 10,000 physicians in the United States licensed to administer radiopharmaceuticals to patients for diagnostic and therapeutic purposes, and it is estimated that 10 to 12 million doses are administered each year.

Nuclear medicine would have grown even faster if it were not for the reservations felt by many physicians about administering radioactive materials to humans, especially to young persons with their reproductive life ahead of them. The fears may not be especially rational, but they are nonetheless real. Even when a nuclear medicine procedure results in a radiation dose that is actually *lower* than that involved in an alternative x-ray examination, the latter may be recommended or preferred by many physicians because of their reluctance to administer a radioactive material to humans.

The use of radiopharmaceuticals for diagnosis or therapy is based on the accumulation or concentration of the isotope in the organ of interest, which is referred to as the *target organ*. A radiopharmaceutical may have an affinity for a certain organ that is not necessarily the organ of interest, in which case it is termed the *critical organ*. Often the dose to a critical organ will limit the amount of radioisotope that may be administered. The risk to which the patient is subjected is clearly a function of the dose received and must be balanced against the expected advantages and benefits that the procedure confers. The calculation of the dose absorbed from a radiopharmaceutical can represent a tricky problem, since it may vary with a number of factors. These factors include the following:

1. The distribution of the radionuclide within the body and its uptake in certain critical organs
2. *Inhomogeneous* distribution of the nuclide even within the critical organ
3. The biological half-life of the nuclide, which may vary with the patient's age and may be modified by disease or pathologic conditions

The use of radionuclides in medicine is rather sharply divided into diagnostic and therapeutic procedures. There may be a thousandfold difference in the amounts of radioactive material used and therefore in the doses absorbed, depending on whether a given isotope is used to aid diag-

(text continues on page 433)

Table 24-12.
Radiation Doses for Selected Nuclear Medicine Procedures

| RADIO-PHARMACEUTICALS | STUDY | AGE (YEARS) | MEAN DOSE (rad/mCi ADMINISTERED) | | | | | | | | | | |
|---|---|---|---|---|---|---|---|---|---|---|---|---|---|
| | | | Gastrointestinal | Gonads | | Kidneys | Liver | Lungs | Marrow (Red) | Spleen | Thyroid | Total Body | Other |
| | | | | Testes | Ovaries | | | | | | | | |
| $^{51}$Cr chromate red blood cells | Red blood cell survival time or volume | A | — | 0.23 | 0.29 | — | — | — | 0.31 | 14 | — | 0.28 | 0.3—blood |
| $^{57}$Co vitamin B$_{12}$ | Vitamin B$_{12}$ absorption | A | 0.13 (SI) 0.25 (ULI) 0.6 (LI) | 1.1 | 1.6 | — | 110 | — | 2 | — | — | 10 | — |
| $^{67}$Ga citrate | Tumor and abscess imaging | A 10 1 N | 0.22 (ST) 0.56 (ULI) | 0.26 0.44 0.93 2.6 | | 0.41 | 0.45 | — | 0.58 | 0.6 1 2.6 8 | — | 0.16 0.28 0.57 1.4 | 0.44—bone |
| $^{81m}$Kr | Lung ventilation | A | — | 0.002 $\frac{mrad}{mCi\ min}$ | 0.002 $\frac{mrad}{mCi\ min}$ | — | — | 2.5 $\frac{mrad}{mCi\ min}$ | — | — | — | 0.05 $\frac{mrad}{mCi\ min}$ | — |
| $^{99m}$Tc DTPA | Renal imaging (dynamic) | A 10 1 N | — | 0.020 0.110 0.132 0.170 | 0.027 0.049 0.110 0.330 | 0.085 0.144 0.318 0.828 | — | — | 0.010 | — | — | 0.016 0.029 0.062 0.170 | 0.45—bladder wall |
| $^{99m}$Tc MAG3, mertiatide | Renal imaging function | A | 0.016 (SI) 0.019 (ULI) 0.033 (LLI) | 0.016 | 0.026 | 0.014 | 0.004 | — | 0.005 | — | — | 0.007 | 0.48—urinary bladder wall |
| $^{99m}$Tc disofenin, mebrofenin | Hepatobiliary | A | 0.22 (SI) 0.30 (LIW) | — | — | — | 0.05 | — | 0.03 | — | — | 0.020 | 0.50—gallbladder wall (jaundice) 0.09—gallbladder wall (normal) |
| $^{99m}$Tc glucoheptonate | Renal imaging | A | — | 0.0038 | 0.0069 | 0.3 | — | — | 0.012 | — | — | 0.01 | — |
| $^{99m}$Tc macroaggregates | Perfusion study | A 10 1 N | — | 0.007 0.038 0.046 0.06 | 0.009 0.016 0.038 0.11 | 0.16 | 0.017 | 0.2 0.35 1.0 3.1 | 0.015 | 0.017 | 0.008 | 0.015 0.028 0.064 0.18 | 0.29—bladder wall |

(continued)

| Radiopharmaceutical | Application | | | | | | | | | | | | Critical organ (mGy/MBq) |
|---|---|---|---|---|---|---|---|---|---|---|---|---|---|
| $^{99m}$Tc pertechnetate | Thyroid imaging | A | 0.25 (ST); 0.012 (ULI); 0.20 (LLI) | 0.012 | 0.017 | — | 0.015 | — | 0.022 | — | 0.20 | 0.013 | 0.053—bladder (resting); 0.085—bladder (active); 0.013—brain |
| | Thyroid imaging or ectopic gastric mucosa imaging | 10; 1; N | 0.33; 0.67; 1.9 | 0.066; 0.079; 0.1 | 0.032; 0.076; 0.22 | — | — | — | — | — | 0.48; 1.3; 3.4 | 0.024; 0.055; 0.15 | — |
| $^{99m}$Tc pyrophosphate, methylene diphosphate | Bone imaging | A; 10; 1; N | — | 0.015 | 0.015 | 0.03 | 0.01 | — | 0.035 | — | — | 0.013; 0.025; 0.057; 0.15 | 0.05—bone; 0.089—bone; 0.2—bone; 0.64—bone; 0.13—bladder (2-h void) |
| $^{99m}$Tc exametazime | Brain imaging | A | 0.04 (SIW); 0.08 (ULIW); 0.05 (LLIW) | 0.007 | 0.023 | 0.13 | 0.054 | — | 0.013 | — | 0.10 | 0.013 | 0.19—gallbladder wall; 0.26—lachrymal glands |
| $^{99m}$Tc cardiolite | Myocardial imaging | A | 0.10 (SI); 0.18 (ULI); 0.13 (LLI) | 0.010 | 0.050 | 0.066 | 0.020 | 0.010 | 0.017 | — | 0.023 | 0.017 | 0.07—gallbladder wall; 0.07—urinary bladder wall; 0.02—heart wall |
| $^{99m}$Tc cardiotec | Myocardial imaging | A | 0.07 (SI); 0.12 (ULI); 0.09 (LLI) | 0.010 | 0.036 | 0.020 | 0.062 | 0.028 | 0.017 | 0.015 | 0.011 | 0.017 | 0.10—gallbladder wall; 0.03—urinary bladder wall; 0.02—heart wall |
| $^{99m}$Tc MUGA | Myocardial imaging | A | 0.03 (SI); 0.03 (ULI); 0.03 (LLI) | 0.012 | 0.022 | — | 0.020 | — | 0.022 | 0.018 | 0.040 | 0.016 | 0.07—bladder wall; 0.02—heart wall |
| $^{99m}$Tc red blood cells | Blood pool imaging | A | 0.027 (SW); 0.032 (ULIW); 0.029 (LLIW) | 0.012 | 0.021 | — | 0.019 | — | 0.023 | 0.018 | 0.041 | 0.017 | 0.34—bladder wall (8-h void); 0.028—bladder wall; 0.053—blood |
| $^{99m}$Tc $Sb_2$ $Sb_3$ colloid | Lymphoscintigraphy | A | — | 0.052 | — | 0.016 | 0.016 | — | — | 0.027 | — | — | 0.052—bladder wall |

## 24-12. Radiation Doses for Selected Nuclear Medicine Procedures *(Continued)*

| RADIO-PHARMA-CEUTICALS | STUDY | AGE (YEARS) | Gastroin-testinal | Gonads — Testes | Gonads — Ovaries | Kidneys | Liver | Lungs | Marrow (Red) | Spleen | Thyroid | Total Body | Other |
|---|---|---|---|---|---|---|---|---|---|---|---|---|---|
| $^{99m}$Tc sulfur colloid | Liver, spleen, bone marrow imaging | A | — | 0.019 | 0.023 | — | 0.34—nl<br>0.21—ei<br>0.16—id | — | 0.027—nl<br>0.045—ei<br>0.079—id | 0.21—nl<br>0.28—ei<br>0.42—id | — | 0.019<br>0.018<br>0.016 | — |
| | | 10 | | 0.1 | 0.014 | | 0.56 | | | 0.6 | | 0.027 | |
| | | 1 | | 0.13 | 0.097 | | 1.3 | | | 1.2 | | 0.056 | |
| | | N | | 0.16 | 0.28 | | 2.9 | | | 2.7 | | 0.14 | |
| $^{111}$In platelets | Clot scanning | A | — | 0.2 | 0.4 | 1.4 | 2 | — | 1 | 33.5 | — | 0.6 | |
| $^{113m}$In DTPA | Brain imaging (static and dynamic) | A | — | 0.005 | 0.009 | 1.9 | — | — | 0.011 | — | — | 0.01 | 0.4—bladder |
| | | 10 | | | | | | | | | | 0.015 | 0.82—bladder |
| | | 1 | | | | | | | | | | 0.04 | 2.2—bladder |
| | | N | | | | | | | | | | 0.13 | 7.1—bladder |
| | Renal imaging (dynamic) | A | — | | 0.027 | | 0.5 | — | — | — | — | 0.01 | 0.4—bladder |
| $^{123}$I iodide | Thyroid imaging | A | 0.23 (ST) | 0.025<br>0.021<br>0.017 | 0.034 (5% uptake)<br>0.029 (15% uptake)<br>0.024 (25% uptake) | | 0.03 | | 0.044<br>0.04<br>0.035 | | 2.4 (5% uptake)<br>7.5 (15% uptake)<br>13 (25% uptake) | 0.03 | |
| | | 10 | | | 0.051 | | | | | | 30 | 0.051 | |
| | | 1 | | | 0.12 | | | | | | 110 | 0.13 | |
| | | N | | | 0.35 | | | | | | 160 | 0.35 | |
| | | A | | | 0.025 | | | | | | 55 (administered 24 hours after production) | | 3—bladder |
| $^{133}$Xe gas | Ventilation | A | | | 0.0012 | | | 0.011 | 0.0015 | | | 0.0014 | |
| $^{133}$Xe gas | Perfusion-ventilation or perfusion only | | | | 0.0018 | | | 0.016 | 0.0022 | | | 0.0021 | |
| $^{201}$Tl chloride | Myocardial imaging | A | 0.4 (STW)<br>0.38 (SI)<br>0.25 (ULI) | 0.52 | 0.47 | 1.2 | 0.57 | | | | 0.14 | 0.21 | 0.5—heart wall |

MEAN DOSE (rad/mCi ADMINISTERED)

*A, adult; N, newborn; nl, normal liver; ei, early to intermediate diffuse parenchymal disease; id, intermediate to advanced diffuse parenchymal disease. (Courtesy of Dr. J. Kereiakes, unpublished data, 1993)*

nosis or for therapy. Consequently, therapeutic uses are discussed later under a separate heading.

In general, there are three doses that are of interest after the administration of a given amount of a radiopharmaceutical:

1. The total-body dose, since this will largely determine the risk of leukemia
2. The dose to the critical organ, since this may be many times larger than the total-body dose and it is known that certain tissues are particularly susceptible to radiation-induced cancer
3. The gonadal dose, since this is a measure of the genetic hazard

When the radiation doses that are delivered from nuclear medicine procedures are compared with those from diagnostic x-rays, it must be remembered that the *dose rates* are usually much lower with radionuclides, since the dose is accumulated slowly and continuously over a period of time. In general, biological effects are dependent on the dose rate, at least for sparsely ionizing radiations, such as x- or γ-rays. The consequences of a given dose are *reduced* if the radiation is spread out over a period of time in comparison with a single acute exposure, because of the potential for repair. This is certainly true of genetic effects, for which, at least in mice, there is a significant dose-rate effect. The situation is not as clear for carcinogenesis, and there are conflicting data, but in general, for a given absorbed dose, lower dose rates result in less damage.

Organ doses from a few selected radiopharmaceuticals are listed in Table 24-12, while gonad doses characteristic of selected procedures are listed in Table 24-13.

Of more general interest and concern are the GSD and the collective effective dose to the US population shown in Tables 24-14 and 24-15, respectively. The age-weighted collective effective dose for nuclear medicine is reduced by an even larger factor than for diagnostic x-rays to account for the fact that the patient population is skewed toward older ages. The biggest contributors to the collective effective dose are brain, bone, thyroid, and cardiovascular procedures. These figures are used later in the chapter to assess the risks of nuclear medicine to be offset against the benefits.

# DOSES FROM NATURAL BACKGROUND RADIATION

Natural background radiation comes from three sources: cosmic radiations that reach the earth from space, radioactivity in the earth's crust and in the building materials from which houses are made, and internal deposits of radionuclides in the body that have been inhaled or ingested. This is illustrated in Figure 24-3.

## Cosmic Radiation

Cosmic rays are made up of radiations from outside the galaxy and charged particles emanating from the surface of the sun. The intensity of cosmic rays arriving at the earth's surface varies with both latitude and altitude above sea level. The variation with latitude is a consequence of the magnetic properties of the earth: cosmic rays are charged particles that are deflected away from the equator and funneled into the poles. This is illustrated in Figure 24-4. The *aurora borealis*, or northern lights, result from charged particles spiraling down the lines of magnetic field into the polar regions. Consequently, cosmic-ray intensity is least in equatorial regions and rises toward the poles. There is an even larger variation in cosmic-ray intensity with altitude, since at high elevations above sea level there is less atmosphere to absorb the cosmic rays, and so their intensity is greater. For example, the average cosmic-ray annual dose equivalent in the United States is about 0.26 mSv (26 mrems) at sea level. This essentially doubles for each 2000-meter increase in altitude in the lower atmosphere. Latitude, solar cycle variations, and other factors can only modify exposures by about 10%.

## Natural Radioactivity in the Earth's Crust

Naturally occurring radioactive materials are widely distributed throughout the earth's crust, and as a consequence, humans are exposed to the γ-rays from them. There is a big variation between areas such as Colorado where the rocks and soil contain radioactive thorium and uranium

Table 24-13.
Administered Activity and Gonadal Doses

| EXAMINATION TYPE | ESTIMATED ADMINISTERED ACTIVITY PER EXAMINATION* | GONADAL DOSE FOR EACH RADIOPHARMACEUTICAL (mGy)† | | GONADAL DOSE WEIGHTED AVERAGE (mGy)† | |
|---|---|---|---|---|---|
| | | Male | Female | Male | Female |
| Brain | 740 MBq$^{99m}$Tc DTPA (50) | 2.2 | 4.4 | 1.9 | 4.4 |
| | 740 MBq$^{99m}$Tc O$_4$ (50) | 1.5 | 4.4 | | |
| Hepatobiliary | 185 MBq$^{99m}$Tc iminodiacetic acid (IDA)(10) | 0.2 | 1.7 | 0.2 | 0.5 |
| | 185 MBq$^{99m}$Tc sulfur colloid (90) | 0.2 | 0.4 | | |
| Bone | 740 MBq$^{99m}$Tc phosphate | 3.7 | 4.4 | 3.7 | 4.4 |
| Respiratory | | | | 0.3 | 0.3 |
| Perfusion | 185 MBq$^{99m}$Tc macroaggregated albumin (MAA) (66) | 0.4 | 0.4 | | |
| Ventilation | 370 MBq$^{133}$Xe gas (34) | 0.1 | 0.1 | | |
| Thyroid | 185 MBq$^{99m}$Tc O$_4$ (80) | 0.4 | 1.1 | | |
| | 3.7 MBq$^{131}$I (10) | < 0.1 | 0.1 | 0.3 | 0.9 |
| | 11.1 MBq$^{123}$I (10) | < 0.1 | 0.1 | | |
| Renal | 740 MBq$^{99m}$Tc DTPA (60) | 2.2 | 4.4 | 1.3 | 2.7 |
| | 9.25 MBq$^{131}$I hippuran (40) | < 0.1 | < 0.1 | | |
| Abscess/tumor | 111 MBq$^{67}$Ga citrate | 7.2 | 8.4 | 7.2 | 8.4 |
| Cardiovascular | 740 MBq$^{99m}$Tc labeled red blood cells (40) | 0.2 | 0.8 | | |
| | 111 MBq$^{201}$T1 chloride (40) | 45.5 | 11.1 | 18.9 | 5.7 |
| | 740 MBq$^{99m}$Tc phosphate (20) | 3.2 | 4.4 | | |

*Number in parentheses is the estimated percent of examination type with a particular radiopharmaceutical.
†1 mGy = 100 mrad.
(Adapted from National Council on Radiation Protection and Measurements: Exposure of the US Population From Diagnostic Medical Radiation. Report No. 100. Bethesda, MD, NCRP, 1984)

and areas such as the Atlantic seaboard where radioactivity is low. This is shown in Figure 24-5.

### Internal Exposure

Small traces of radioactive materials are normally present in the human body, ingested from the tiny quantities present in food supplies or inhaled as airborne particles. Radioactive thorium, radium, and lead can be detected in most persons, but the amounts are small and variable and the figure usually quoted for the dose rate resulting from these deposits is less than 10 mSv/y (1 mrem/y). Only radioactive potassium-40 makes an appreciable contribution to human exposure from ingestion. The dose rate is about 0.2 mSv/y (20 mrems/y), which cannot be ignored as a source of mutations in humans.

It is instructive to compare the external natural background radiation between Denver, Colorado, and New York City. The dose rate from radioactivity in food is much the same across the United States at 0.2 mSv/y (20 mrems/y). Since Denver is at an elevation of 1 mile above sea level the dose from cosmic rays amounts to about 0.5 mSv/y (50 mrems/y) and at the same time the component from the earth's crust amounts to about 0.9 mSv/y (90 mrems/y) as a consequence of the thorium and uranium content of the rocks in the area. By contrast, New York City is at sea level so that the cosmic-ray

Table 24-14.
Genetically Significant Dose (GSD) to the US Population in 1980
From Diagnostic Nuclear Medicine Procedures

| SEX | TYPE OF EXAMINATION | GONADAL DOSE (mGy)* | RELATIVE FREQUENCY OF EXAMINATION ($\times 10^{-3}$) | RELATIVE CHILD EXPECTANCY† | GSD FOR EXAMINATION TYPE (µGy)‡ |
|------|--------------------|---------------------|--------------------|--------------------|--------------------|
| Male | Brain | 1.85 | 4.63 | 0.165 | 1.41 |
| | Hepatobiliary | 0.19 | 5.68 | 0.124 | 0.13 |
| | Bone | 3.70 | 4.74 | 0.123 | 2.16 |
| | Lung | 0.28 | 3.50 | 0.116 | 0.11 |
| | Thyroid | 0.31 | 0.77 | 0.259 | 0.06 |
| | Renal | 1.34 | 0.70 | 0.197 | 0.19 |
| | Cardiovascular | 18.92 | 2.86 | 0.084 | 4.55 |
| | Abscess/tumor | 7.22 | 1.33 | 0.235 | 2.26 |
| | | | | Subtotal | 10.87 |
| Female | Brain | 4.44 | 5.32 | 0.136 | 3.21 |
| | Hepatobiliary | 0.50 | 5.94 | 0.077 | 0.23 |
| | Bone | 4.44 | 5.92 | 0.071 | 1.87 |
| | Lung | 0.30 | 4.11 | 0.111 | 0.14 |
| | Thyroid | 0.91 | 3.26 | 0.207 | 0.62 |
| | Renal | 2.68 | 0.54 | 0.192 | 0.28 |
| | Cardiovascular | 5.65 | 1.87 | 0.042 | 0.44 |
| | Abscess/tumor | 8.44 | 1.21 | 0.158 | 1.61 |
| | | | | Subtotal | 8.40 |
| | | | | Total | 19.27 µGy |

*1 mGy = 100 mrad.
†Relative child expectancy refers to the number of children expected for the average person undergoing this examination.
‡1 µGy = 100 µrad.
(Adapted from National Council on Radiation Protection and Measurements: Exposure of the US Population From Diagnostic Medical Radiation. Report No. 100. Bethesda, MD, NCRP, 1984)

component is only 0.25 mSv/y (25 mrems/y) and the component from the earth's crust is low, too, at 0.20 mSv/y (20 mrems/y) because the rock formations are old on the Atlantic and Gulf coastal plain. As a consequence, the background radiation level in New York City (0.68 mSv/y or 68 mrems/y) is less than half the comparable figure in Denver (1.6 mSv/y or 160 mrems/y).

The annual average natural background level is usually quoted to be about 1 mSv (100 mrems); the third report of the Committee on the Biological Effects of Ionizing Radiation (BEIR III) suggests about 0.78 mSV (78 mrems). This is a consequence of the fact that most big cities housing the majority of the population are close

to sea level and about halfway between the equator and the poles. These include London, New York, and Tokyo. There are no major cities at very high altitudes or close to the poles, where background levels would be high.

A source of natural radiation ignored until recently is radon gas, which leads to irradiation of the surface of the lungs when the gas and its daughter products are inhaled. Radon levels in houses vary enormously, but the average concentration in the United States appears to be about 37 mBq/L (1 pCi/L) in the living area and much much more in the basement. The average annual dose to the bronchial epithelium from α-particles emitted by radon and its daughter

Table 24-15.
Comparison of Collective Effective Dose vs. Age-Weighted Collective Dose
for US Nuclear Medicine Procedures in 1982

| EXAMINATION | EFFECTIVE DOSE (mSv) | EXAMS (× 10³) | COLLECTIVE EFFECTIVE DOSE (PERSON-Sv)* | AGE-WEIGHTED COLLECTIVE DOSE (PERSON-Sv)* |
|---|---|---|---|---|
| Brain | 6.5 | 813 | 5,300 | 2,200 |
| Hepatobiliary | 3.7 | 180 | 700 | 300 |
| Liver | 2.4 | 1,424 | 3,400 | 1,300 |
| Bone | 4.4 | 1,811 | 8,000 | 2,900 |
| Pulmonary | 1.5 | 1,203 | 1,800 | 800 |
| Thyroid | 7.5 | 530 | 4,000 | 2,400 |
| Renal | 3.1 | 236 | 700 | 400 |
| Tumor | 12.2 | 121 | 1,500 | 600 |
| Cardiovascular | 7.1 | 961 | 6,800 | 2,600 |
| Total | | | 32,100 | 13,500 |
| Per caput | | | 140 µSv (14 mrem) | 59 µSv (5.9 mrem) |

*1 Sv = 100 rem.
*(Adapted from National Council on Radiation Protection and Measurements: Exposure of the US Population From Diagnostic Radiation. Report No. 100. Bethesda, MD, NCRP, 1989)*

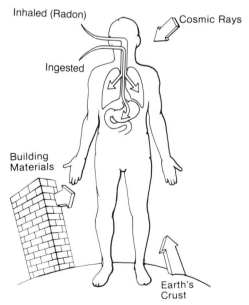

**Figure 24-3.** Three principal components of natural background radiation: (1) cosmic rays from solar flares in the sun or from outer space; (2) ingested radioactivity, principally potassium-40 in food and inhaled radioactivity, principally radon, and (3) radiation from the earth's crust, which in practice means from building materials, since most persons spend much of their lives indoors.

products is of the order of 5 mSv (500 mrems). This translates into an annual effective dose equivalent (Table 24-16) of about 2 mSv (200 mrems) because, of course, only the lungs are irradiated by this source, and an appropriate weighting factor is involved. Nevertheless, radon is by far the largest component of natural background radiation.

**Areas of High Natural Background**

There are several inhabited areas of the world where background radiation is considerably elevated because of radioactivity in rocks or soil or in building materials from which houses are made. These areas are in Brazil, France, India, Niue Island in the Pacific, and Egypt.

In Brazil, some 30,000 persons who live in coastal areas are exposed to dose rates of 5 mSv/y (500 mrems/y). About one sixth of the population of France, largely in the Burgundy wine-growing district, live in areas where the rocks are principally granite and receive 1.8 to 3.5 mSv/y (180 to 350 mrems/y) from background radiation. Undoubtedly, the highest back-

Figure 24-4. **(A)** The earth behaves like a giant magnet. Showers of charged particles from solar events on the surface of the sun are deflected away from the equator by the magnetic field of the earth; most miss the earth altogether, while others are funneled into the polar regions. This explains why cosmic-ray dose is low near the equator and high in the polar regions. It is also the basis of the *aurora borealis*, or northern lights; intense showers of cosmic-ray particles spiral down the lines of magnetic field into the poles. **(B)** Viewed from above the poles, the earth is ringed with lines of magnetic force. Because of the spin of the earth, charged particles are trapped by the lines of magnetic field and form regions of high radiation dose known as the van Allen belts. Man could not live for long in the dose rates characteristic of these belts. To leave earth, spaceships passed quickly through the van Allen belts; the space shuttle orbits well below them.

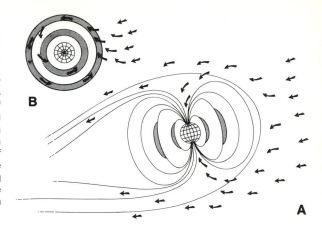

ground is in Kerala, India, where more than 100,000 persons receive an annual dose of about 13 mSv (1300 mrems). On Niue Island in the Pacific a combination of volcanic soil and an unusually high radioactive content of plants results in a few thousand persons being exposed to an external dose rate of 10 mSv/y (1000 mrems/y), in addition to their ingesting significant amounts of radioactivity from plant material. In the northern Nile delta, a densely populated area of Egypt, dose rates of 3 to 4 mSv/y (300 to 400 mrems) have been noted in several villages.

Many studies have been made of these human populations, who have lived for many generations in areas of high natural background radiation. So far, no excess incidence of cancer or genetic anomalies has been observed that can reasonably be attributed to the radiation. Such studies are, of course, beset with difficulties. To begin with, the number of persons who live in these areas of high natural radiation is relatively small and they tend to live in closed communities, so that the level of congenital anomalies is unusually high anyway from consanguinity. In addition, their life-style is very different.

Nevertheless, in spite of the obvious difficul-

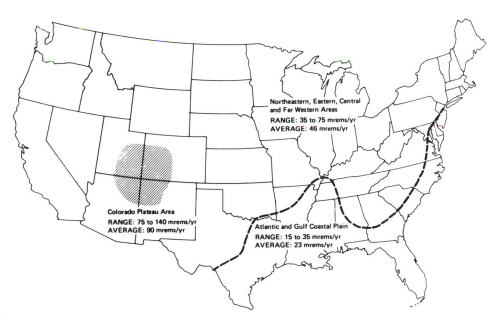

Figure 24-5. The variation of the component of natural background radiation originating from the earth's crust. (From the BEIR III Report, National Academy of Sciences, 1980)

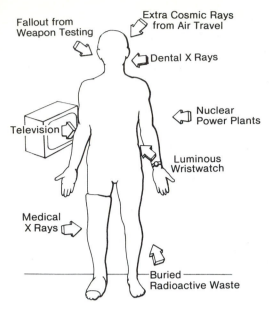

**Figure 24-6.** The various sources of man-made radiation to which the human population is exposed. In developed countries the effective dose is dominated by medical radiation.

ties involved in making comparisons, it is an important and significant fact that human populations who have lived for generations at levels of background radiation that differ by an order of magnitude do not show noticeable differences in the incidence of cancer or genetic disorders. This is the basis for believing that as long as man-made radiation does not exceed the average background value, it is unlikely to produce any detectable deleterious effects on the world's population. This is an important point and is referred to again later in this chapter when risk versus benefit is discussed.

## COMPARISON OF RADIATION DOSES TO THE HUMAN POPULATION FROM NATURAL AND MAN-MADE SOURCES

In addition to natural background radiation, the human population is exposed to a variety of

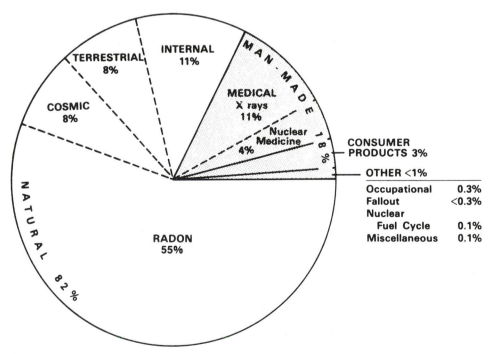

**Figure 24-7.** This pie diagram, which appeared in 1987 (NCRP report # 93) showed for the first time that the *average effective dose* to the population of the United States is dominated by indoor radon daughter products. The effective dose, of course, is the dose in gray (or rads) multiplied by the radiation weighting factor ($W_R$), which is 20 for the α-particles emitted by radon daughter products, and multiplied by the tissue weighting factor ($W_T$), which is about 0.12 for the lungs. The annual effective dose to the US population is about 6.46 mSv (646 millirems). More than half of this is due to radon, and altogether 82% comes from natural sources. Medical x-rays contribute only 11% and nuclear medicine 4%.

man-made or enhanced natural sources, as illustrated in Figure 24-6.

Radiation doses to the US population from natural and man-made sources are summarized in Figure 24-7 and in somewhat more detail in Table 24-16. The average annual effective dose from all sources amounts to 3.6 mSv (360 mrems). There is a large extra dose to the bronchial epithelium in smokers from naturally occurring radionuclides in tobacco products, but it is difficult to estimate with any precision.

## The Most Significant Exposures

The data in Figure 24-7 and Table 24-16 indicate that the greatest contribution to the effective dose for nonsmokers in the US population comes from natural sources. Inhaled radon-daughter products make the largest contribution to the effective dose but make little or no contribution to the GSD. In the past, exposures from "natural" sources have been regarded as inevitable, but it is now appreciated that indoor radon results in significant doses and may conceivably be responsible for a substantial number of lung cancer deaths. It is also clear that the target organ for radiation exposure of the public, nonsmokers as well as smokers, is the lungs.

Among man-made or man-enhanced sources of radiation, medical exposures represent the largest contribution, an annual average effective dose of 0.39 mSv (39 mrems) for diagnostic radiology and 0.14 mSv (14 mrems) for nuclear medicine. These are different in character from

Table 24-16.
## Annual Effective Dose in the US Population Circa 1980–1982

| SOURCE | NUMBER OF PERSONS EXPOSED (THOUSANDS) | AVERAGE ANNUAL EFFECTIVE DOSE IN THE EXPOSED POPULATION (mSv)* | ANNUAL COLLECTIVE EFFECTIVE DOSE (PERSON-Sv)† | AVERAGE ANNUAL EFFECTIVE DOSE IN THE US POPULATION (mSv)* |
|---|---|---|---|---|
| Natural sources | | | | |
|   Radon | 230,000 | 2.0 | 460,000 | 2.0 |
|   Other | 230,000 | 1.0 | 230,000 | 1.0 |
| Occupational | 930‡ | 2.3 | 2,000 | 0.009 |
| Nuclear fuel cycle | —‖ | — | 136 | 0.0005 |
| Consumer products | | | | |
|   Tobacco§ | 50,000 | — | — | — |
|   Other | 120,000 | 0.05–0.3 | 12,000–29,000 | 0.05–0.13 |
| Miscellaneous environmental sources | ~25,000 | 0.006 | 160 | 0.0006 |
| Medical | | | | |
|   Diagnostic x-rays | —¶ | — | 91,000 | 0.39 |
|   Nuclear medicine | —‖ | — | 32,000 | 0.14 |
| Rounded total | 230,000 | — | 835,000 | 3.6 |

*1 mSv = 100 mrem.
†1 person-Sv = 100 person-rem.
‡Those nominally exposed total 1.68 × 10⁶.
§Effective dose equivalent difficult to determine; dose to a segment of bronchial epithelium estimated to be 0.16 Sv/y (16 rem/y).
‖Number of persons exposed is not known. Number of examinations was 7.4 million and effective dose per examination 4,300 µSv.
¶Number of persons exposed is not known. Number of examinations was 180 million and effective dose per examination 500 µSv.
(Data from National Council on Radiation Protection and Measurements: Exposure of the Population in the United States to Ionizing Radiation. Report No. 93. Bethesda, MD, NCRP, 1987)

inadvertent exposures, since they contribute directly to the benefit of the persons receiving them.

It is of interest to view the doses from other man-made sources in the context of medical exposures. The doses for fallout from 1959 to 1962, when above-ground testing of nuclear weapons was at its peak, never reached more than a small fraction of those from medical diagnosis. The radiation dose to the general population from nuclear power stations is also very small. A significantly larger contribution, especially to those of younger age groups who travel a good deal, comes from flying in commercial jetliners. A transatlantic flight from the United States to Europe, for example, involves a dose of about 50 μSv (5 mrems) from cosmic radiation. The pilot and crew of a jetliner, making regular transatlantic or transcontinental flights on northern routes, can easily accumulate more than 5 mSv/y (500 mrems/y), which makes them, technically, radiation workers.

There are several obvious conclusions to be drawn from this summary of doses from various sources. First, medical diagnostic x-rays represent by far the largest source of man-made radiation. Second, the overall effective dose from medical radiation is less than half that from natural background, excluding radon, and only one sixth of background if radon is included. Third, the GSD from diagnostic x-rays and nuclear medicine combined is about 0.33 mSv,[†] that is, about one third of that due to background radiation (1 mSv).

There are three potential hazards that can result from medical radiation: (1) heritable effects may be increased in future generations because half of the population receive x-rays annually; (2) the risk of cancer or leukemia may be increased in the patients themselves who receive multiple x-rays; and (3) anomalies and/or malignancies may be produced in children irradiated in utero. These three biological effects of radiation have been described in detail in previous chapters but are now to be discussed briefly in the context of the doses associated with medical radiation.

---

[†]*300 μGy for diagnostic x-rays from Table 24-6 plus 30 μGy for nuclear medicine from Table 24-14.*

# DIAGNOSTIC RADIOLOGY: RISK VERSUS BENEFIT

## The Risk of Radiation-Induced Cancer and Heritable Effects

The medical use of radiation involves the offsetting of a risk against a benefit. The risk–benefit equation is particularly hard to balance in the case of heritable effects, because those who receive the benefits and those who run the risks are not the same persons. The x-ray examination confers an immediate benefit (it is hoped) on the patient, while the risk of deleterious effects falls on future unborn generations. Consequently, it is incumbent on radiologists to minimize the number of x-ray examinations that are performed and to reduce the dose per film to the absolute minimum consistent with adequate diagnostic film quality. In the future, as in the past, the GSD from medical diagnostic procedures will dwarf all other sources of man-made radiation, including nuclear power. (To preclude the immediate reaction that this radiation is necessary and beneficial, it should be added that several independent estimates have indicated that about one third of all radiographs are not based on medical requirements but relate either to the generation of income or to *defensive* practices based on medicolegal requirements!)

There are three ways to look at these data. The first is to compare the GSD for radiology with the estimated doubling dose for mutations in humans. The GSD is about 0.3 mSv, while the estimated doubling dose is 1 Sv. So long as the GSD is 3000 times smaller than the doubling dose, the genetic effects of medical radiation are unlikely to pose a worrisome problem.

Second, it is the opinion of many experts in this field that there is no immediate cause for alarm as long as the GSD to the population from all man-made sources combined is not allowed to exceed the average background level. This is certainly the case at the present time. So long as this is true, then it is certain that the additional genetic burden will be less in quantity and no different in kind from what has been experienced throughout human history. For this reason, committees that suggest guidelines for public exposure are not alarmed at the present levels of man-made radiation as far as genetic consequences are concerned. To some extent, this view is based on the study of persons who live in areas of high natural background radiation, referred to earlier in this chapter. These sizable populations of humans have lived for generations at a background level that is three to ten times higher than the average for the United States, with no obvious ill effects in terms of an elevated incidence of congenital anomalies. From this it is argued that as long as the doses from man-made radiation do not exceed natural background levels, then they are unlikely to produce any detectable genetic changes in the human population.

To illustrate the point in a more parochial fashion, it is possible to live in Washington, DC, or New York City and have several x-ray procedures each year, while still accumulating less of a radiation dose than that received naturally by everyone who lives in Denver. Since the persons in Denver do not appear to suffer any ill effects from this background radiation, there is some justification for assuming that a few medical radiographs on the east coast will not be too harmful.

The risk–benefit equation is different in the case of cancer induction since the person who receives the benefit is also the person at risk. The risk is also more substantial than is the case for heritable effects.

It is possible to make a quantitative estimate of the consequences of exposure to diagnostic radiology in terms of cancers and heritable effects. Two pieces of data are required:

1. The annual collective effective dose due to diagnostic radiology in the United States, which was estimated earlier in this chapter to be 58,000 person-Sv (5.8 million man-rems)
2. The risk of deleterious effects, or the "detriment" from radiation. This is discussed in detail in Chapters 19 and 20 and summarized again in Chapter 25. For the general population exposed to low doses or low dose-rate, the detriment is estimated to be
   Fatal cancer 4%/Sv
   Nonfatal cancer 0.8%/Sv
   Heritable effects (mutations) 0.8%/Sv

The "detriment" includes an allowance for loss of quality of life as well as for death. It is calculated by multiplying the risk by the collective effective dose.

Based on these figures, the practice of diagnostic radiology in the United States for 1 year may result in

2320 fatal cancers (4% of 58,000)
464 nonfatal cancers (0.8% of 58,000)
464 serious heritable defects (0.8% of 58,000)

This possible risk of a few thousand cases of cancer and a few hundred cases of heritable defects must be weighed against the benefit that millions of persons in the United States received from improved diagnosis. No amount of radiation, however small, is justified unless a benefit is conferred; but it is not difficult to draw the conclusion that—for a patient who is sick and in need of medical care—the tiny risk of cancer 10 to 30 years in the future is a small price to pay for an accurate and speedy diagnosis. In other words, so long as there is a real and tangible immediate benefit to the person or society, the small risk is acceptable. This is almost always the case when the request for a radiologic procedure is part of the diagnosis of an unidentified ailment, ignoring for the moment the statistic quoted already that one third of all diagnostic procedures are not based on medical need but on generation of income or as part of the practice of defensive medicine.

A different argument applies, however, to x-rays that are used for screening purposes, when a large number of perfectly healthy persons will of necessity be irradiated needlessly to pick up the occasional case of ill health. The most striking example is mammography. The breast is one of the body tissues known to be particularly susceptible to radiation-induced cancer. There is no question that mammography is an effective method of screening and that some breast tumors may be detected by this means at an earlier stage than they would be otherwise. An appreciable dose of radiation is, however, involved in mammography. When the technique is used for screening millions of women, a small proportion of those examined receive a benefit in the form of an early diagnosis of a malignant disease, but the majority are perfectly healthy young women unnecessarily exposed to x-rays. Inevitably, the screening procedure involves a risk of *producing* cancer, as well as *detecting* it. Indeed, it has been estimated that if mammography is used indiscriminately to screen young women, when the natural incidence of breast cancer is low and the sensitivity to radiation-induced breast cancer is high, then the radiation used for the examination may *induce* more tumors than the procedure *detects*! For this reason mammography is recommended only in older women or special high-risk groups in whom the natural incidence of the disease is higher. In this case, a larger potential benefit can be offset against the undoubted risk.

Other screening procedures, such as routine chest films, may be questioned on the same premises. Another case in point is the widespread use of routine dental films. Many dentists regularly take a full set of x-ray films at each 6-month checkup. This may involve up to 12 exposures, each of which involves an entrance dose of about 10 mGy (1 rad). In a typical patient, adding up all of these exposures means that the entire oral cavity may receive a dose of 50 mGy (5 rads) per examination. The major hazard may be the small scattered dose to the thyroid, which is probably the tissue most sensitive to the induction of a malignancy by radiation, especially in children. About half the population of the United States receives a dental x-ray examination each year. There is little doubt that some number of a malignancies are induced as a result, and this is a compelling argument against the indiscriminate taking of dental radiographs, especially in children. The hazard of heritable effects from dental radiographs is negligibly small, but it is by no means certain that the risk of carcinogenesis is also negligible, involving as it does a tissue as sensitive as the thyroid.

## The Risk to the Developing Embryo and Fetus

Numerous studies with rats and mice have shown that x-rays, in sufficient doses, can lead to a variety of adverse effects, depending on the stage of gestation at which the radiation is delivered. Data in the human come from more than a thousand children exposed in utero at Hiroshima and Nagasaki, and to a lesser extent from a small number of children exposed in utero to therapeutic doses of radiation. The only reported effect for exposure during preimplantation (0 to 10 days after conception) is early prenatal death,

which in humans constitutes early unrecognizable abortion. Anomalies and growth retardation are not seen. Thus, if there is an effect during this early stage of pregnancy, the patient is unlikely to be aware that she had been pregnant.

In animals, gross structural anomalies, neonatal death, or growth retardation are observed after exposure during organogenesis. Growth retardation is the principal effect seen in animals irradiated in the fetal period. These end points appear to be deterministic effects; some authors suggest a threshold of about 0.1 Sv (10 rems), although changes in the embryo and fetus can be detected at doses below this.

In humans, the principal effects of radiation to the developing embryo and fetus appear to be reduced head diameter and mental retardation. Severe mental retardation was not observed after exposure before 8 weeks of gestation and reached a maximum between 8 and 15 weeks with a risk coefficient of 40% per Gy (40% per 100 rads). The risk was about four times lower at 16 to 25 weeks. In addition, IQ tests suggested the loss of about 30 points per 1 Gy (100 rads). As discussed in detail in Chapter 21, the incidence of severe mental retardation appears to increase linearly with dose; if there is a threshold, it is not larger than 0.2 Gy (20 rads). Since the cause of the mental retardation is thought to be due to radiation effects on cell migration within the brain during critical periods of development, a small threshold would not be unexpected, that is, this is a **deterministic** rather than a **stochastic** effect.

There is also the possible association between diagnostic x-rays in utero and the subsequent development of leukemia or other childhood malignancies. As discussed in an earlier chapter, the unborn child appears to be very sensitive to radiation carcinogenesis since a few diagnostic x-ray exposures increases the natural risk of leukemia and other childhood malignancies by a factor of 1.5 to 2.0.

To summarize the animal and human data, malformations including mental retardation have been observed during organogenesis (ie, from the 10th day after conception) through to the 25th week. An increased susceptibility to carcinogenesis may be an additional risk.

The problem faced in the clinical practice of radiology is that it is never possible to prove an association between an individual anomaly and a radiation exposure. About 5% of all children born have a defect of some sort, and the anomalies produced by radiation are no different from those that occur spontaneously. Consequently, every effort should be made to avoid the inadvertent exposure of a developing embryo or fetus.

Despite the most careful precautions, instances occasionally occur when a woman discovers that she is pregnant after receiving a whole series of x-rays to the pelvis. To make matters worse, as likely as not, the dose was delivered during the most sensitive period. The first step is to enlist the help of a radiologic physicist to make as accurate an estimate as possible of the dose involved—including measurements if necessary. In most instances the dose to the embryo or fetus will be less than 10 to 20 mGy (1 to 2 rads), which involves a risk that is small compared with all of the other risks of childbearing. It has been suggested that a therapeutic abortion might be considered if the unborn child received a dose in excess of 100 mGy (10 rads) during a sensitive period. This dose level is debatable, and the recommendation to abort must depend on many factors of each individual case; the dose level does, however, serve as a guideline.

## Conclusion

No one knows for certain whether there is a significant risk, either to the population or to the person, associated with the use of radiation for diagnostic purposes in medical practice. Effects cannot be observed directly. The estimates of heritable effects (mutations) and carcinogenesis in this chapter are extrapolations from the unequivocal observed effects at high doses. These estimates use the best available data and are based on plausible assumptions, but they are *estimates* nevertheless and must be viewed as such. They are *not* measurements or observations and should be afforded limited credibility. If there is a risk to patients from medical radiation, it is numerically very small. Even so, prudence dictates that the *potential* for adverse effects of radiation, even from small doses, should be recognized. It is the responsibility of the practicing radiologist to conduct each examination such

that radiation risk is minimized and in the spirit of "no risk, no benefit!"

The bottom-line risk versus benefit equation for diagnostic radiology in the United States may be written as follows: About half the population receives medical x-rays each year and stands to benefit by an improved diagnosis. The balancing risk is that a few thousand cases of cancer and a few hundred heritable effects (mutations) may be induced.

It is never possible, either, in an individual case, to associate the birth of an anomalous child with the irradiation of the mother with diagnostic x-rays during pregnancy. All that can be said is that radiation increases the risk. Every effort should be made to avoid the inadvertent exposure of the unborn child, but on the rare occasions when it occurs a therapeutic abortion may be considered if the dose exceeds 0.1 Gy (10 rads) during a sensitive period of gestation. This dose must be flexible and the difficult decision influenced by many social factors.

## NUCLEAR MEDICINE: RISK VERSUS BENEFIT

The potential risks and biological consequences of nuclear medicine procedures are basically the same as for any other use of radiation, namely, *carcinogenesis, heritable effects (mutations)* and *effects on the developing embryo and fetus*. These possible hazards can only be presumed, since there are no good data linking radiation doses from diagnostic procedures in nuclear medicine with deleterious effects. An absence of proof does not mean that a correlation does not exist; when many millions of persons are irradiated annually, there must be a price tag.

### Dose Reduction

The trend in radiopharmaceutical development is to use radionuclides that emit γ-rays and few, if any, β-particles. In this way the amount of information that is of diagnostic value is maximized, while the useless tissue dose is minimized. The best example of such a radionuclide is technetium-99m. Another way to reduce the dose is to use radionuclides with a shorter half-life. An example is iodine-123, which has largely replaced the longer-lived iodine-131.

In parallel with the development of better radiopharmaceuticals, methods of imaging are continually being improved. More sensitive detectors, better data storage and retrieval, and the use of computers for image subtraction techniques all aim to provide more diagnostic information from a smaller quantity of administered radioactivity.

## The Risk of Heritable Effects and Cancer

The risk of heritable effects is not to the exposed person but to future unborn generations. The annual GSD for nuclear medicine is about 0.03 mSv (the sum of 10.87 mGy to the male and 19.27 mGy to the female, from Table 24-14). This is about one tenth of the GSD for diagnostic x-rays and one thirtieth of the GSD for natural background radiation. The contribution of nuclear medicine to the genetic load, therefore, is very small indeed. This is due to two factors. First, only a relatively small proportion of the total population is exposed to nuclear medicine procedures. Second, young persons of childbearing age—the genetically significant population—are often not exposed to radiation from radionuclides because of the frequently repeated warning that radiopharmaceuticals are contraindicated in young persons with their reproductive life ahead of them.

It is possible to make an estimate of the "detriment" from nuclear medicine in the same way as for diagnostic x-rays. Two pieces of data are required:

1. The annual collective effective dose from nuclear medicine in the United States. This is listed as 13,500 person-Sv in Table 24-15. Note that the age-weighted collective dose is reduced much more in the case of nuclear medicine (13,500 from 32,100 person-Sv) than in the case of diagnostic x-rays, reflecting the older age distribution of patients receiving radionuclides.
2. The risk of deleterious effects, that is, the "detriment" from radiation. This was discussed

in detail in Chapters 19 and 20 and summarized again in Chapter 25. For the general population exposed to low doses or low dose rate, the detriment is estimated to be

Fatal cancer 4%/Sv
Nonfatal cancer 0.8%/Sv
Heritable effects (mutations) 0.8%/Sv

Based on these figures, the practice of nuclear medicine in the United States for 1 year may result in

540 fatal cancers (4% of 13,500)
108 nonfatal cancers (0.8% of 13,500)
108 serious heritable effects (0.8% of 13,500)

This possible risk of a few hundred fatal cancers, and about 100 nonfatal cancers and heritable defects, must be weighed against the benefit that about 10 million patients receive in terms of diagnosis.

## Pediatric Nuclear Medicine

Of prime consideration in pediatric nuclear medicine is the possibility of late effects from low dose levels, even when delivered at low dose rate. The hazards associated with using radiopharmaceuticals in children are basically the same as in adults—namely, cancer and heritable effects (mutations)—except for the possibility that the risks associated with a given absorbed dose of radiation are higher because of an increased sensitivity in younger persons. There is some evidence for this. The most widely studied neoplasm has been leukemia, and for the Japanese children who were exposed to the A-bomb the risks of developing this malignancy may be increased as compared with adults. The same appears to be true of thyroid cancer, for which the incidence per unit dose is probably higher in childhood. The most reliable estimates for thyroid cancer come from children irradiated externally with x-rays for a supposedly enlarged thymus and from children irradiated in the course of treatment of tinea capitis. In both cases the thyroid received a dose of radiation (as little as 60 mGy [6 rads], in the children with tinea capitis), and within 20 years an elevated incidence of thyroid cancer was evident. The risk estimate is perhaps three times higher for children irradiated when younger than 10 years of age.

The effect of prenatal irradiation on the induction of leukemia and cancer is less clear. In a much discussed series of papers, Stewart and her associates reported an increase in the frequency of pelvimetric or other obstetric irradiation in the mothers of children who later developed leukemia compared with the frequency of maternal irradiation in mothers of matched controls. These and other similar retrospective studies indicated that the relative cancer risk was increased by a factor of 1.5 to 2 as a consequence of x-rays in utero, which amounted to a dose of 5 to 20 mGy (0.5 to 2 rads).

In pediatric nuclear medicine the general principle is that radiation exposures should be kept to the lowest practical level. In each case the expected benefit must clearly be shown to exceed the risk. More importantly, nuclear medicine procedures should not be used for screening purposes in children—the indications for each test should be clearly stated before the procedure is begun. The implication of the review of biological effects on humans is that any amount of radiation, no matter how small, has a deleterious effect. Because the effect cannot be detected in a finite number of patients does not mean that it does not exist. The conclusion is based on the assumption of a linear, nonthreshold, dose-effect model that has been adopted by most standard-setting bodies as the most conservative basis for risk estimates. This philosophy requires that the physician have some reasonable indications that the potential gain for the patient from the use of a procedure in nuclear medicine will exceed the potential risks. The demand for nonessential repetitive examinations and the use of children in poorly planned "research" studies or poorly conceived survey tests are examples of nonproductive uses of radiation.

## Nuclear Medicine and the Pregnant Woman

The effect of radionuclides on the developing embryo or fetus has not been studied as extensively as the consequences of externally administered x-rays. This is unfortunate, since the situation is much more complex in the case of administered radionuclides. The biological effects may depend on many factors, including the chemical form of the isotope, the type and energy of the radiation emitted, whether the compounds containing the radioactivity cross the placenta, and whether they tend to be concentrated in specific target organs.

In the early years of nuclear medicine, radioactive isotopes of iodine were commonly used. There is justification for carefully avoiding their use if a pregnancy is suspected, since the fetal thyroid takes up iodine from the 10th week onward and does so more avidly than the maternal gland. Organic iodine crosses the placenta readily, and while iodine attached to proteins or hormones is less likely to do so, there is probably no radioactive iodine compound that does not release some iodine into the circulation, and this can end up in the fetal thyroid. Since there is the possibility of inducing thyroid cancer by prenatal exposure to even small amounts of radioactive iodine, it is prudent to avoid its use during pregnancy, except in extreme cases when there is no alternative. Technetium-99m is much less hazardous in this connection and is now the most important radionuclide for diagnostic imaging. Its usefulness depends on its optimal $\gamma$-ray energy (140 keV), while its short half-life (6 hours) and the fact that it does not emit $\beta$-rays account for the much lower dose of radiation delivered to the patient when this radionuclide is used as compared with the same procedures carried out with radioactive iodine. Technetium-99m-pertechnetate is trapped to some extent by the thyroid gland, but it is not incorporated into thyroid hormones.

Although pregnant women receive diagnostic x-rays occasionally, it is rare for them to be given radioactive isotopes. In general, physicians and patients alike are much more wary and cautious about nuclear medicine procedures than about diagnostic x-rays, even when dose levels may be similar. Never is this more true than in the case of pregnant or potentially pregnant women.

Table 24-17 includes estimates of the dose to the embryo for selected radiopharmaceuticals, and Table 24-18 shows calculated doses to the fetal thyroid as a function of fetal age from intakes by the mother of radionuclides of interest.

Table 24-17.
Dose Estimated to Embryo
From Radiopharmaceuticals

| RADIOPHARMACEUTICAL | EMBRYO DOSE (RAD/mCi ADMINISTERED) |
|---|---|
| $^{67}$Ga-citrate | 0.25 |
| $^{75}$Se-methionine | 3.8 |
| $^{99m}$Tc-DTPA | 0.035 |
| $^{99m}$Tc-human serum albumin | 0.018 |
| $^{99m}$Tc-lungaggregate | 0.035 |
| $^{99m}$Tc-polyphosphate | 0.036 |
| $^{99m}$Tc-sodium pertechnetate | 0.037 |
| $^{99m}$Tc-stannous glucoheptonate | 0.04 |
| $^{99m}$Tc-sulfur colloid | 0.032 |
| $^{123}$I-sodium iodide (15% uptake) | 0.032 |
| $^{131}$I-sodium iodide (15% uptake) | 0.1 |
| $^{123}$I-rose bengal | 0.13 |
| $^{131}$I-rose bengal | 0.68 |

*(Courtesy of Dr. J. Kereikes, unpublished data, 1984)*

Table 24-18.
Thyroidal Radioiodine Dose of the Fetus

| GESTATION PERIOD | FETAL/ MATERNAL RATIO (THYROID GLAND) | DOSE TO FETAL THYROID (rad/μCi)* |
|---|---|---|
| 10–12 weeks | — | 0.001 (precursors) |
| 12–13 weeks | 1.2 | 0.7 |
| Second trimester | 1.8 | 6 |
| Third trimester | 7.5 | — |
| Birth imminent | — | 8 |

*Rad/μCi of $^{131}$I ingested by mother.*
*(Courtesy of Dr. J. Keriakes, unpublished data, 1984)*

# THE THERAPEUTIC USE OF RADIONUCLIDES

Radioactive iodine-131 is widely used for the treatment of hyperthyroidism. Since this radionuclide first became generally available in 1946, there has been a gradual shift in the selection of definitive therapy for hyperthyroidism. In the late 1940s and early 1950s iodine-131 was reserved for patients deemed to be poor surgical risks. By the 1960s the situation had been completely reversed. Radioactive iodine had become the preferred modality, with thyroidectomy being reserved for the young and for those patients whose clinical evaluation suggested the desirability of surgery to allow an examination of the gland. As a rough estimate, 250,000 patients have now received at least one therapeutic dose of radioactive iodine. Hyperthyroidism is probably the major benign disease for which radiation is the treatment of choice.

A therapeutic treatment with iodine-131 involves an absorbed dose to the thyroid gland that varies with the person and is very nonuniform within the tissue itself but is on the order of many tens of gray (thousands of rads). In addition, there is a total-body dose of typically 50 to 150 mGy (5 to 15 rads), which is due to the isotope circulating in the blood. Because radiation is known to be a potent carcinogen, the possibility of the production of leukemia after iodine-131 therapy has been appreciated from the outset and has been carefully looked for. There is also the risk of thyroid cancer, since the isotope is concentrated in the thyroid, and a large dose is delivered there. These are discussed in turn.

There is no question that thyroid cancer can be induced by external x-irradiation. In the case of children treated for a supposedly enlarged thymus, a few gray (a few hundred rads) of x-rays resulted in a clearly elevated incidence of thyroid cancer. In children epilated with x-rays for the treatment of tinea capitis, cases of thyroid cancer have been reported, although the dose to the gland was alleged to be only 60 mGy (6 rads). Also, in the Japanese who were younger than 20 years of age when exposed to the A-bomb explosion, cancer is a legacy of the radiation received. By contrast, no excess of thyroid cancer has been observed in adults after the iodine-131 treatment of hyperthyroidism. The failure of radiation to induce thyroid cancer in this instance is probably due to the high doses involved, which are far above the optimal level for cellular transformation. The presumed explanation for a decrease in oncogenicity of radiation at high levels, which has been observed in many experimental animal systems as well as in humans, is that the radiation injury is so severe as to kill the cells or render them incapable of sustained proliferation. The fact that hypothyroidism often follows 5 to 10 years after treatment of hyperthyroidism with iodine-131 suggests that the doses of radiation involved are sufficient to cause extensive death of thyroid cells. In rats, the carcinogenic effectiveness of iodine-131 per rad of absorbed dose is about one tenth that of x-rays. Of course the radiation from iodine-131 and x-rays differs in dose rate, quality, and (probably most important) distribution within the gland.

Because of isolated reports of patients who developed leukemia after treatment with iodine-131 for hyperthyroidism, the Cooperative Thyrotoxicosis Therapy Follow-up Study was initiated in 1961 under the sponsorship of the US Bureau of Radiological Health. The study included 36,000 patients in 26 medical centers in the United States who were treated for hyperthyroidism either by radioiodine or surgery. The mean bone marrow doses from the iodine-131 treatments were in the range of 70 to 150 mGy (7 to 15 rads). The incidence of leukemia was in fact slightly *higher* in the group treated by thyroidectomy than in the group receiving iodine-131, although the difference was not statistically significant. In other words, the data failed to reveal an excess of leukemia from the radioiodine treatment per se. It is of interest to note that the age-adjusted death rate from leukemia in *both* treatment groups was one and a half times higher than expected on the basis of figures for the general population, from which it was concluded that patients with hyperthyroidism have an enhanced risk of leukemia, regardless of the way in which they are treated.

Although the results of this study do not demonstrate leukemogenesis from treatment with iodine-131, it is still not possible to say that such treatments do not induce leukemia, since the sample size is too small to detect the excess incidence from a total-body dose of 0.1 Gy (10 rads) even if it were there.

In the practice of nuclear medicine therefore it must be assumed that a small risk of leukemia will accompany the therapeutic use of iodine-131 for hyperthyroidism. It is, however, a risk that is more than counterbalanced by the benefit. The clinician, when selecting treatment for a hyperthyroid patient, must balance the known hazards of surgery, treatment with antithyroid drugs, or uncontrolled hyperthyroidism against a possible risk of leukemia from iodine-131, which may amount to about 5 cases per 10,000 patients treated. It is no wonder that the radionuclide is the treatment of choice in an ever-increasing number of cases. The administration of a general anesthetic alone involves a risk of death several times higher.

Pregnancy is, of course, an absolute contraindication to treatment of hyperthyroidism with iodine-131. Even the relatively small doses delivered to the developing embryo or fetus by iodine-131 in the circulating blood is undesirable because of the extreme sensitivity of the embryo for the production of malformations. Also, radioiodine passes the placental barrier, so that its hazard is increased, because after the first trimester the sensitive fetal thyroid concentrates iodine. Treatment of fertile women should be preceded by the taking of a careful history and should be delayed if necessary to eliminate the possibility of treatment during pregnancy.

In the treatment of thyroid cancer many hundreds of millicuries of iodine-131 may be given, which results in a total-body dose sufficient to cause severe depression of the bone marrow. For example, $3.7 \times 10^3$ MBq (100 mCi) of iodine-131 will deliver 0.5 to 1 Gy (50 to 100 rads) to the hematopoietic tissue. The effect of such doses on the circulating blood elements is similar to the effect of total-body exposure to external radiation. Ultimately, bone marrow depression may limit the treatment. Since the treatment of thyroid cancer involves the use of such large and repeated quantities of iodine-131, with the attendant total-body doses, it is not surprising that a few cases of myeloid leukemia have been reported in patients who have received this form of therapy. This is the risk entailed whenever therapeutic doses of radiation are involved; it is usually acceptable because of the serious and malignant character of the disease under treatment.

## COMPARING THE RISKS

Life in an industrialized society involves a multitude of risks. Some are obvious and dramatic, like the risk of an automobile accident or an airplane crash. Others are more subtle and insidious, such as the high cancer rates in certain industrialized areas. Most persons judge the speed, comfort, and convenience of air travel to be worth the risk of death that amounts to about 1 in 1 million per flight. The convenience of driving an automobile is considered to be worth much higher levels of risk. Sometimes judgments are not especially rational: millions of Americans continue to smoke cigarettes despite the warning of risk to their health that is printed on each pack. In general, the hazards in an industrialized society are all associated directly or indirectly with an improved standard of living. Driving automobiles, flying in airplanes, living in heated houses, and enjoying the mass-produced consumer products of factories all represent a step forward from primitive life in a bygone age. But each advantage carries with it the small, but finite, risk of death as a result of human error, mechanical malfunction, or environmental pollution. The use of ionizing radiations in medicine is no exception. X-rays have the potential for great good; they can also be the cause of distress and suffering if used excessively.

So far in this chapter a serious attempt has been made to introduce the concept of a risk balanced against a benefit. The man in the street is not used to thinking in these terms and instead classifies activities as either "safe" or "unsafe." In a modern industrialized society few things are as simple or clear cut as this, and the hazards associated with the use of radiation are no exception.

In an attempt to put into perspective the risk of leukemia and cancer associated with the use of radiation in medicine, it is instructive to make a comparison with the other risks to which persons are subjected in our society, for instance, smoking cigarettes or driving an automobile. About 50,000 persons a year die of lung cancer in the United States, almost all of whom are smokers. Fifty million Americans smoke an average of 20 cigarettes per day, and if it is assumed that there is a linear relationship between the risk of cancer and the number of cigarettes smoked, then it may be calculated that one person dies of lung cancer for every 7.3 million cigarettes smoked. This is a gross oversimplification, but it is no more a distortion of the truth than is applying a linear extrapolation to the cancer data from the Japanese survivors who received an average of 0.6 Gy (60 rads) to deduce risk estimates for patients who receive a dose of a few milligray (a few hundred mrem).

Statistics indicate that about 56,000 persons a year are killed in vehicular accidents on US highways. About half of the population (100 million) drive automobiles, and the average driver covers 10,000 miles per year. From these figures it can be calculated that there is one fatality on the road for every 18 million miles driven. These risk estimates are summarized in Table 24-19 together with the risk of radiation-induced fatal cancer, taken to be 4% per sievert for low doses or low dose rate. On the basis of the risk estimates given in Table 24-19, which are admittedly very crude, it is possible to compare the risk of death from radiation-induced cancer with other risks faced in society.

To illustrate the risk involved in diagnostic radiology, a barium enema, a chest radiograph, and a skull examination will be considered as representative of high, low, and intermediate dose procedures. The effective dose for each procedure is shown in Table 24-20, calculated from the appropriate organ doses listed in Table 24-3 and using the tissue weighting factors ($W_T$) recommended by ICRP and listed in Table 25-2. For example, a skull series of 4 images involves

Table 24-19.
**Comparing the Risks: Radiation, Driving, and Smoking**

**Cigarette Smoking**

50,000 lung cancer deaths each year per 50 million smokers consuming 20 cigarettes a day, or one death per 7.3 million cigarettes smoked, or $1.37 \times 10^{-7}$ deaths per cigarette

**Highway Driving**

56,000 deaths each year per 100 million drivers, each covering 10,000 miles, or one death per 18 million miles driven, or $5.6 \times 10^{-8}$ deaths per mile driven

**Radiation-Induced Fatal Cancer**

4% per Sv for exposure to low doses or low dose rate

Table 24-20.
Comparing the Risks: Radiation, Driving, and Smoking

| PROCEDURE | EFFECTIVE DOSE (Sv) | RISK OF FATAL CANCER | EQUIVALENT TO NO. OF CIGARETTES SMOKED | EQUIVALENT TO NO. OF HIGHWAY MILES DRIVEN |
|---|---|---|---|---|
| Chest radiograph (1.5 images) | $3.2 \times 10^{-5}$ | $1.3 \times 10^{-6}$ | 9 | 23 |
| Skull examination (4.1 images) | $15 \times 10^{-5}$ | $6 \times 10^{-6}$ | 44 | 104 |
| Barium enema (male) (4 images) | $5.4 \times 10^{-4}$ | $2 \times 10^{-5}$ | 148 | 357 |
| Bone scan | $4.4 \times 10^{-3}$ | $1.8 \times 10^{-4}$ | 1300 | 3200 |

a dose of 2.2 mGy to the thyroid with a weighting factor of 0.05, 0.3 mGy to the bone marrow, which has a weighting factor of 0.12, and 0.02 mGy to the lung, with a weighting factor of 0.12; this amounts to a total effective dose of about $15 \times 10^{-5}$ Sv. The representative procedure for nuclear medicine is a bone scan, which according to Table 24-15 is the most common procedure performed in the United States and involves one of the largest effective doses at 4.4 mSv.

The next step is to use the effective dose to estimate the risk of inducing a fatal cancer, based on the figure of 4% per sievert quoted earlier; the risk varies from a little over 1 in 1 million for a chest radiograph, to 2 in 100,000 for a barium enema, to about 2 in 10,000 for a bone scan.

In Table 24-20 these risks from radiation are compared with the comparable risks from smoking or driving a car. For example, a chest radiograph involves the same risk of a fatality as smoking 9 cigarettes or driving 23 miles on the highway; that is, the risk of having the radiograph is about the same as the risk of driving to the hospital! On the other hand, a barium enema, which involves the largest effective dose of any radiologic procedure, involves a risk of death from cancer about equivalent to the hazards of 1 week of average highway driving (357 miles) or 1 week of average cigarette smoking (148 cigarettes). The effective dose is largest for a bone scan, since a larger proportion of the body is exposed; this translates into a risk of fatality comparable to smoking 1300 cigarettes or driving 3200 miles on the highway.

► *Summary of Pertinent Conclusions*

- Everyone is exposed to radiation from

  1. Unperturbed natural sources
  2. Enhanced natural sources
  3. Man-made sources including medical sources

*(continued)*

► *Summary of Pertinent Conclusions* (Continued)

- Heritable risks are expressed in terms of the genetically significant dose (GSD)—the gonad dose weighted for the age and sex of the exposed population.
- The cancer risk is expressed in terms of the effective dose, the equivalent dose to the various organs and tissues exposed, multiplied by the appropriate tissue weighting factors $(W_T)$.
- About 180 million medical and about 101 million dental x-ray examinations are performed each year in the United States.
- About 10 million doses of radiopharmaceuticals are administered each year in the United States.
- Natural background radiation comes from cosmic rays, terrestrial radiation from the earth's crust, and inhaled or ingested radioactivity.
- Cosmic-ray levels vary with altitude and latitude.
- Terrestrial radiation levels vary widely with locality.
- Radon and its daughter products result in irradiation of lung tissue with $\alpha$-particles; this is the largest source of natural radiation.
- Diagnostic radiology is the largest man-made source of radiation contributing to the GSD.
- The genetically significant dose (GSD) for diagnostic radiology is about 0.3 mSv (30 mrems). This is about 3000 times smaller than the estimated doubling dose for mutations in the human (1 Sv or 100 rems).
- The biggest contributors to the GSD in diagnostic radiology are radiographs of the hip and pelvis in men and of the lumbar spine and lower gastrointestinal tract in women. These examinations account for 50% of the GSD.
- The contribution of dental radiographs to the GSD is negligible.
- The contribution of radiotherapy to the GSD is likewise very small.
- The GSD for nuclear medicine is 0.03 Sv, that is, ten times smaller than for diagnostic radiology.
- Annual average *total* effective doses, to the US population are

| | | | |
|---|---|---|---|
| Natural background, radon | 2 | mSv | 200 mrems |
| Natural background, other | 1 | mSv | 100 mrems |
| Medical diagnostic x-rays | 0.39 | mSv | 39 mrems |
| Nuclear medicine | 0.14 | mSv | 14 mrems |
| Consumer products | 0.12 | mSv | 12 mrems |
| Rounded total | 3.6 | mSv | 360 mrems |

- The annual collective effective dose to the US population from diagnostic x-rays is 58,000 person Sv (5.8 million man-rems). This is the weighted value, allowing for the fact that the patient population is skewed with regard to age compared with the general population.
- The weighted annual collective effective dose for nuclear medicine is 13,500 person Sv (1.35 million man-rems). An even bigger allowance is necessary to correct for the older age distribution for nuclear medicine patients than for patients receiving diagnostic radiology.
- The "detriment" from diagnostic radiology and nuclear medicine may be calculated from the collective effective dose and the risk estimate of 4%

*(continued)*

► **Summary of Pertinent Conclusions**   *(Continued)*

per sievert for fatal cancer, 0.8% per sievert for nonfatal cancer and 0.8% per sievert for serious heritable effects.

- Detriment includes an allowance for loss of quality of life as well as death.
- The practice of diagnostic radiology for 1 year in the United States may benefit about half of the population but may result in several thousand fatal cancers, several hundred nonfatal cancers, and several hundred heritable effects (mutations).
- The practice of nuclear medicine for 1 year in the United States may benefit 10 million patients but may result in several hundred fatal cancers, about 100 nonfatal cancers, and about 100 serious heritable effects.
- For irradiation of the human in utero, the risk of severe mental retardation as a function of dose is apparently linear, with a risk coefficient as high as 40% per Sv (40% per 100 rems) at 8 to 15 weeks after conception and about four times lower at 16 to 25 weeks. If there is a threshold, it is not larger than 0.2 Sv (20 rems).
- Loss of IQ is estimated to be about 30 points per sievert (30 points per 100 rems).
- Every precaution should be taken to avoid exposure of a conceptus.
- Many x-ray exposures involve doses too small to pose a significant risk to the embryo or fetus.
- In the event of an accidental exposure of an unsuspected conceptus, the dose should be estimated carefully. Some believe that a dose exceeding 0.1 Sv (10 rems) during a sensitive period of gestation may be grounds for a therapeutic abortion. This dose is flexible and depends on many social factors.
- The effects of radionuclides on the developing embryo and fetus have been studied less than the effects of x-rays and are likely to be much more complex. Special care should be taken to avoid this problem.
- In the treatment of hyperthyroidism with iodine-131, the risk of death from radiation-induced leukemia or cancer is less than the risk of death from a general anesthetic if surgery is used.
- The risks posed by diagnostic x-rays and nuclear medicine procedures are small compared with other hazards in an industrialized society, such as smoking cigarettes or driving an automobile.

# BIBLIOGRAPHY

Brent RL, Gorson RO: Radiation exposure in pregnancy. Curr Probl Radiol 2:1–48, 1972

Bureau of Radiological Health: Gonad Doses and Genetically Significant Doses From Diagnostic Radiology, US, 1964 and 1970. Publication No. (FDA) 76-8034. Washington, DC, Department of Health, Education and Welfare, 1976

Comar CL: An individual looks at the implications of the BEIR report. Pract Radiol 1:40–44, 1973

Committee on Biological Effects of Ionizing Radiations: The Effects on Populations of Exposure to Low Levels of Ionizing Radiation (BEIR I). Washington, DC, National Academy of Sciences, 1971

Committee on Biological Effects of Ionizing Radiations: The Effects on Populations of Exposure to Low Levels of Ionizing Radiation (BEIR II). Washington, DC, National Academy of Sciences/National Research Council, 1972

Committee on the Biological Effects of Ionizing Radiations: Health Effects of Exposure to Low Levels of

Ionizing Radiation. Washington, DC, National Academy of Sciences/National Research Council, 1990

Committee on Radiological Units, Standards and Protection: Medical Radiation: A Guide to Good Practice. Chicago, American College of Radiology, 1985

Department of Health, Education and Welfare: Organ Doses in Diagnostic Radiology. Publication No. (FDA) 76-8030. Washington, DC, US Government Printing Office, 1976

Fabrikant JI: The BEIR III controversy. Radiat Res 84:351–368, 1980

Friedman LM, Johnson PM: Clinical Scintillation Imaging. New York, Grune & Stratton, 1975

Fullerton GD, Kopp DT, Waggener RG, Webster EW (eds): Biological Risks of Medical Irradiations. Med Phys Monogr No. 5. New York, American Institute of Physics, 1980

Gibbs SJ: Biological effects of radiation from dental radiography. J Am Dent Assoc 105:275–281, 1982

Gregg EC: Radiation risks with diagnostic x-rays. Radiology 123:447–453, 1977

International Commission on Radiological Protection: Recommendations. ICRP publication No. 9. New York, Pergamon Press, 1965

International Commission on Radiological Protection: Re-examination of dose limits. Lancet 2:1158, 1972

International Commission on Radiological Protection: Recommendations. ICRP publication No. 26. Ann ICRP 1:1–53, 1977

International Commission or Radiological Protection: Recommendations. ICRP publication No. 60. New York, Pergamon Press, 1991

Jablon S, Kato H: Childhood cancer in relation to prenatal exposure to atomic-bomb radiation. Lancet 2:1000–1003, 1970

Langham WH (ed): Radiobiological Factors in Manned Space Flight. Washington, DC, National Academy of Sciences, 1967

Laws PW, Rosenstein M: A somatic dose index for diagnostic radiology. Health Phys 35:629–642, 1978

Modan B, Mart H, Baidatz D, Steinitz R, Levin SG: Radiation-induced head and neck tumors. Lancet 1:277–279, 1974

National Council on Radiation Protection and Measurements: Exposure of the US Population From Diagnostic Medical Radiation. Report No. 100. Bethesda, MD, NCRP, 1989

Radford EP: Human health effects of low doses of ionizing radiation: The BEIR II controversy. Radiat Res 84:369–394, 1980

Refetoff S, Harrison J, Karanfilski BI, Kaplan E, DeGroot LJ, Bekerman C: Continuing occurrence of thyroid carcinoma after irradiation to the neck in infancy and childhood. N Engl J Med 292:171–175, 1975

Rossi HH: Comments on the somatic effects section of the BEIR III report. Radiat Res 84:395–406, 1980

Rossi HH, Kellerer AM: Radiation carcinogenesis at low doses. Science 175:200–202, 1972

Shrivastava PN, Lynn SL, Ting JY: Exposures to patient and personnel in computed axial tomography. Radiology 125:411–415, 1977

Smith PG, Doll R: Mortality from cancer and all causes among British radiologists. Br J Radiol 54:187–194, 1981

Stewart A, Webb J, Giles D, Hewitt D: Malignant disease in childhood and diagnostic irradiation in utero. Lancet 2:447, 1956

Stewart A, Webb J, Hewitt D: A survey of childhood malignancies. Br Med J 1:1495–1508, 1958

Sufa AM, Schumacher OP, Rodriquez-Antunez A: Long-term follow-up results in children and adolescents treated with radioactive iodine ($^{131}$I) for hypertension. N Engl J Med 292:167–170, 1975

Ulrich H: Incidence of leukemia in radiologists. N Engl J Med 234:45–46, 1946

United Nations Scientific Committee on the Effects of Atomic Radiation: Sources and Effects of Ionizing Radiation. New York, UNSCEAR, 1977

United Nations Scientific Committee on the Effects of Atomic Radiation: Sources and Effects of Ionizing Radiation. New York, UNSCEAR, 1982

United Nations Scientific Committee on the Effects of Atomic Radiation: Sources and Effects of Ionizing Radiation. New York, UNSCEAR, 1986

Wyckoff HO: The international system of units. Radiology 128:833–835, 1978

*Radiobiology for the Radiologist, Fourth Edition*, by Eric J. Hall
J. B. Lippincott Company, Philadelphia © 1994.

# 25

# *Radiation Protection*

Diagnostic Radiology
Nuclear Medicine
Radiation Therapy

This chapter was written in 1992 in the light of the 1990 recommendations for quantities and definitions of the International Commission of Radiological Protection (ICRP) contained in ICRP publication 60 and on report No. 116 of the National Council of Radiological Protection and Measurements (NCRP). The chapter is written for students coming to the subject de novo, and consequently no historical preamble or description of the development of the quantities is given at the outset. At the end of the chapter, a glossary is provided devoted to a comparison of old and new terminology. The changes are confusing, and some think capricious, since those who are not new to radiation protection must struggle with yet another set of new definitions before the ink was properly dry on the last.

## ORGANIZATIONS

The organization of radiation protection, and the interrelation of the various committees whose reports will be quoted, deserves a brief explanation.

First, there are the committees that summarize and analyze data and suggest risk estimates for radiation-induced cancer and genetic effects. At the international level there is the United Nations Scientific Committee on the Effects of Atomic Radiation, usually known as UNSCEAR. This committee has wide international representation. Reports appeared in 1958, 1966, 1972, 1977, 1982, with the latest report in 1988. The United States committee is appointed by the National Academy of Sciences (NAS) and is known as the BEIR committee, an acronym which stands for the Biological Effects of Ionizing Radiations. The first report appeared in 1956 when it was known as the BEAR committee (Biological Effects of Atomic Radiation). Subsequent reports appeared in 1972 (BEIR II), 1980 (BEIR III), and 1990 (BEIR V).

These committees are "scholarly" committees in the sense that when information is not available on a particular topic they do not feel compelled to make a recommendation. Since they do not serve an immediate pragmatic aim, they are not obliged to make a best "guess estimate" when data are uncertain. For example, both committees declined to choose a value for the dose-rate effectiveness factor for carcinogenesis in the human (for which there are not data) and simply quoted a range of 2 to 10 based on animal studies.

Second, there are the committees that formulate the concepts for use in radiation protection and recommend maximum permissible levels. These committees serve more pragmatic aims and must therefore make best estimates even when good data are unavailable. At the international level there is the International Commission of Radiological Protection (ICRP), which (together with the International Commission on Radiological Units and Measurements [IRCU]) was established in 1928 after a decision by the Second International Congress of Radiology. In 1950, this commission was restructured and given its present name. The ICRP often takes the lead in formulating concepts in radiation protection and in recommending dose limits. As an international body it has no jurisdiction over anyone and can do no more than recommend; it has established considerable credibility, however, and its views carry great weight. Its most recent report is ICRP publication 90, published in 1991.

In the United States there is the National Council on Radiological Protection and Measurement (NCRP), chartered by Congress to be an "impartial" watchdog and consisting of 70 experts from the radiation sciences who are, therefore, not impartial at all! The NCRP often, but not always, follows the lead of ICRP. Their most recent report on dose limits (NCRP report No. 116 published in 1992) differs from ICRP in several important respects. The ICRP and NCRP suggest dose limits and safe practices, but in fact neither body has any jurisdiction to enforce their recommendations.

In the United States, the Environmental Protection Agency (EPA) has responsibility for providing guidance to federal agencies, and it is the

EPA for example that sets the action level for radon. Each state can formulate its own regulations for x-rays and radiations from other than reactor-produced sources. In agreement states, the Nuclear Regulatory Commission (NRC) formulates rules for by-product materials from reactors; in other states this responsibility falls on the US Occupational Safety and Health Administration (OSHA). The Department of Energy (DOE) is responsible for radiation safety regulations at all of its facilities operated by contractors. Up to the present time, the various regulating bodies in the United States have accepted, endorsed, and used the reports issued by the NCRP, but they are not obligated to do so.

## QUANTITIES AND UNITS

The quantity used to measure the "amount" of ionizing radiation is the *absorbed dose*. This is defined to be the energy absorbed per unit mass, and its unit is the joule per kilogram, which is given a special name, gray (Gy). The unit used in the past was the rad, defined to be an energy absorption of 100 ergs per gram. Consequently, one Gy = 100 rads.

## RADIATION WEIGHTING FACTORS

The probability of a stochastic effect, such as the induction of cancer or of heritable events, depends, not only on the dose but also on the type and energy of the radiation; that is, some radiations are biologically more effective, for a given dose, than others. This is taken into account by weighting the absorbed dose by a factor related to the quality of the radiation. The weighting factors recommended by the ICRP for different types of radiations, such as protons, neutrons, and α-particles, are listed in Table 25-1. A radiation weighting factor ($W_R$) is a dimensionless multiplier used to place biological effects (risks) from exposure to different types of radiation on a common scale. Radiation weighting factors are chosen by commissions such as the ICRP as representative of relative biological effectiveness, applicable to low doses and low dose rates, and for biological endpoints relevant to stochastic late

**Table 25-1.**
**Radiation Weighting Factors**

| TYPE AND ENERGY RANGE | RADIATION WEIGHTING FACTOR ($W_R$) |
|---|---|
| Photons, all energies | 1 |
| Electrons and muons, all energies | 1 |
| Neutrons, energy <10 keV | 5 |
| 10 keV to 100 keV | 10 |
| >100 keV to 2 MeV | 20 |
| >2 MeV to 20 MeV | 10 |
| >20 MeV | 5 |
| Protons, other than recoil protons, energy >2 MeV | 5 |
| α-Particles, fission fragments, heavy nuclei | 20 |

*(Data from International Commission on Radiological Protection: Recommendations. ICRP publication No. 60. New York, Pergamon Press, 1991)*

effects. They can be traced ultimately to experimentally determined RBE values, but a large judgmental factor is involved in their choice.

## EQUIVALENT DOSE

In radiologic protection, the equivalent dose is the product of the absorbed dose averaged over the tissue or organ and the radiation weighting factor ($W_R$) selected for the type and energy of radiation involved. Thus,

$$\text{Equivalent dose} = \text{absorbed dose} \times \text{radiation weighting factor}$$

When absorbed dose is measured in gray (Gy), the equivalent dose is in sieverts (Sv). When the absorbed dose is in rads, the equivalent dose is in rems. While 1 Gy of neutrons does not produce the same biological effect as 1 Gy of x-rays, 1 Sv of either neutrons or x-rays does result in equal biological effects.

When a radiation field is made up of a mixture of radiations, the equivalent dose is the sum of the individual doses of the various types of radiations, each multiplied by the appropriate radiation weighting factor. Thus, if a tissue or organ were exposed to 0.15 Gy of cobalt-60 γ-rays, plus 0.02 of 1-MeV neutrons, the equivalent dose would be

$$0.15 \times 1 + 0.02 \times 20 = 0.55 \text{ Sv}$$

## EFFECTIVE DOSE

When the body is uniformly irradiated, the probability of the occurrence of stochastic effects (cancer and heritable mutations) is assumed to be proportional to the equivalent dose, and the risk can be represented by a single value. In fact, truly uniform total-body exposures are rare, particularly when irradiation is from radionuclides deposited in tissues and organs. Sometimes, equivalent doses to various tissues differ substantially, and it is well established that different tissues vary in their sensitivity to radiation-induced stochastic effects. For example, it is difficult to produce heritable effects by irradiation of the head or hands! On the other hand, the thyroid and breast appear to be particularly susceptible to radiation-induced cancer. To deal with this situation, the ICRP introduced the concept of the tissue weighting factor ($W_T$), which represents the relative contribution of each tissue or organ to the total detriment resulting from uniform irradiation of the whole body. Table 25-2 lists the tissue weighting factors recommended by the ICRP.

The sum of all of the weighted equivalent doses in all the tissues or organs irradiated is called the *effective dose*.

The effective dose is

$$\Sigma \text{ absorbed dose} \times W_R \times W_T$$

for all tissues or organs exposed.

## COMMITTED EQUIVALENT DOSE

In the case of external irradiation the absorbed dose is delivered at the time of exposure; but for irradiation from internally deposited radionuclides, the total absorbed dose will be distributed in time, as well as in different tissues in the body. The dose rate will fall off, depending on the physical and biological half-lives of the radionuclide.

To take into account the varying time distributions of dose delivery, the ICRP defined the **committed equivalent dose** as the integral over 50

**Table 25-2.**
**Tissue Weighting Factors**

| TISSUE OR ORGAN | TISSUE WEIGHTING FACTOR ($W_T$) |
|---|---|
| Gonads | 0.20 |
| Bone marrow (red) | 0.12 |
| Colon | 0.12 |
| Lung | 0.12 |
| Stomach | 0.12 |
| Bladder | 0.05 |
| Breast | 0.05 |
| Liver | 0.05 |
| Esophagus | 0.05 |
| Thyroid | 0.05 |
| Skin | 0.01 |
| Bone surface | 0.01 |
| Remainder | 0.05 |

*(Data from International Commission on Radiological Protection: Recommendations. ICRP publication No. 60. New York, Pergamon Press, 1991)*

years of the dose equivalent in a given tissue after intake of a radionuclide. This time is chosen to correspond to the working life of a person. For radionuclides with effective half-lives up to about 3 months, the committed equivalent dose is essentially equal to the annual equivalent dose in the year of intake, but for radionuclides with longer effective half-lives it will be greater, because it reflects the dose that will accrue over future years.

## COMMITTED EFFECTIVE DOSE

If the committed equivalent doses to individual organs or tissues resulting from the intake of a radionuclide are multiplied by the appropriate tissue weighting factors and then summed, the result will be the **committed effective dose.**

## COLLECTIVE EQUIVALENT DOSE

The quantities referred to earlier all relate to the exposure of a person. They become appropriate for application to the exposure of a group or population by the addition of the term **collec-**

tive. Thus the **collective equivalent dose** is the product of the average equivalent dose to a population and the number of persons exposed. There appears to be some confusion about the accepted name of the unit for collective dose equivalent in the new SI system of units. Some use *man-sievert*, presumably agreeing with the judgment of Sir Winston Churchill that "man embraces woman." The more liberated prefer the term *person-sievert*, which will be used here. (The old unit was the man-rem.)

## COLLECTIVE EFFECTIVE DOSE

The **collective effective dose** is likewise the product of the average effective dose to a population and the number of persons exposed. The unit is again the person-sievert (man-rem). An example is in order here. If 100 persons receive an average effective dose of 0.3 sievert (30 rems), the collective effective dose is 30 person-sieverts (3000 man-rems).

These collective quantities can be thought of as representing the total consequences of exposure of a population or group. For example, the annual collective effective dose to the US population from diagnostic radiology is about 100,000 person-sieverts (10 million man-rems). Such collective quantities are much beloved by the bureaucrats because they make it possible to compare different activities or accidents inasmuch each can be described by a single number. The danger is that the next step is to convert the collective dose into the number of cancers or heritable effects produced, which, of course, assumes proportionality between dose and biological effect, which is seldom true. The quantities certainly are widely used to give a rough guide to the probability of cancer and hereditary effects in a population exposed to radiation and, in particular, can be used to compare approximately the impact of different types of radiation accidents in terms of the number of health effects that might arise in that population.

## COLLECTIVE EFFECTIVE DOSE COMMITMENT

In the case of a population ingesting radionuclides that deposit their dose over a prolonged period of time, the integral of the effective dose over the entire population out to a period of 50 years is called the **collective effective dose commitment.**

## SUMMARY OF QUANTITIES AND UNITS

Table 25-3 is a summary of quantities and units described earlier, showing how they build logically one on another. If on reading this section the reader gains the impression that the bureaucrats have taken over, it is because they have!—at least in the field of radiation protection. An elaborate set of definitions has been produced based on the assumption of linearity between risk and dose. The whole business needs to be taken with a generous pinch of salt, since it is like a house of cards built as an inverted pyramid, based on somewhat shaky and flimsy premises that cannot be tested.

The concept of collective effective dose does allow a rough and quick estimate to be made of the potential health hazards to a population from, for example, an accidental release of radioactivity from a nuclear reactor. It must be emphasized again that these concepts can only be used under conditions in which it is *reasonable to assume linearity between risk and dose;* that is, that risks are directly proportional to the summation of doses from different sources. Exposures that are within the administratively allowed dose limits may cause an increased incidence of stochastic effects, such as cancer and genetic mutations, but are much below the thresholds for early deterministic effects. In the case of larger accidental releases, in which doses to some persons might be high enough to exceed these thresholds to the point of causing early death, collective effective dose is an inappropriate quantity.

## OBJECTIVES OF RADIATION PROTECTION

As stated by the NCRP the objectives of radiation protection are (1) to prevent clinically significant radiation-induced **deterministic** effects by adhering to dose limits that are below the apparent or practical threshold and (2) to limit the risk of

Table 25-3.
Quantities and Units Used in Radiation Protection

| QUANTITY | DEFINITION | UNIT New | UNIT Old |
|---|---|---|---|
| Absorbed dose | Energy per unit mass | gray | rad |
| **For Individuals** | | | |
| Equivalent dose | Average dose × radiation weighting factor | sievert | rem |
| Effective dose | Sum of equivalent doses to organs and tissues exposed, each multiplied by the appropriate tissue weighting factor | sievert | rem |
| Committed equivalent dose | Equivalent dose integrated over 50 years (relevant to incorporated radionuclides) | sievert | rem |
| Committed effective dose | Effective dose integrated over 50 years (relevant to incorporated radionuclides) | sievert | rem |
| **For Populations** | | | |
| Collective effective dose | Product of the average effective dose and the number of individuals exposed | person-sievert | man-rem |
| Collective effective dose committed | Integration of the collective dose over 50 years (relevant to incorporated radionuclides) | person-sievert | man-rem |

**stochastic** effects, (cancer and heritable effects) to a reasonable level in relation to societal needs, values, and benefits gained. These objectives can be achieved by reducing all exposure to as low as reasonably achievable (ALARA) and by applying dose limits for controlling occupational and general public exposures. For radiation protection purposes, it is assumed that the *risk of stochastic effects are strictly proportional to dose without threshold, throughout the range of dose and dose rates of importance in radiation protection.* Furthermore, the probability of response (risk) is assumed to accumulate linearly with dose. This will not be true at higher doses characteristic of accidents where more complex (nonlinear) dose–risk relationships may apply.

Given the above assumptions, any selected dose limit will have an associated levels of risk. Consequently, it is necessary to justify any use of radiation in terms of a benefit to a person or to society.

## BASIS FOR EXPOSURE LIMITS

Exposure limits have changed over the years in step with evolving information about the biological effects of radiation and with changes in the social philosophy within which recommended exposure limits are developed.

In the 1930s, the concept of a **tolerance dose** was used, a dose to which workers could be exposed continuously without any evident deleterious acute effects such as erythema of the skin.

By the early 1950s, the emphasis had shifted to late effects. The maximum permissible dose was designed to ensure that the probability of the occurrence of injuries was so low that the risk would be readily acceptable to the average person. At about that time, based on the results of genetic studies in *Drosophila* and mice, the occupational limit was substantially reduced and a limit for exposure of the public introduced. Subsequently, the genetic risks were found to be smaller and cancer risks larger than were thought at the time.

By the 1980s, the NCRP was comparing the probability of radiation-induced cancer mortality in radiation workers with annual accidental mortality in "safe" industries. Exposure standards therefore are necessarily based on a mixture of observed effects and judgments.

## LIMITS FOR OCCUPATIONAL EXPOSURE

The NCRP recommends the following:

### Stochastic Effects
1. The individual worker's lifetime effective dose should not exceed age in years × 10 mSv (age in years × 1 rad), and no occupational exposure should be permitted until age 18 years.
2. The effective dose in any one year should not exceed 50 mSv (5 rems).

These limits apply to the sum of the effective dose from external radiation and the committed effective dose from internal exposures and are summarized in Table 25-4.

### Deterministic Effects
1. 150 mSv (15 rems) for the lens of the eye
2. 500 mSv (50 rems) for localized areas of the skin and the hands and feet

These additional limits are required since the weighting factors for, for example, the hands and the feet are so small that huge doses could be given before cancer induction became a problem. Other deterministic effects are limiting at lower doses.

Table 25-4.
Summary of Recommended Dose Limits

| | NCRP | ICRP where different |
|---|---|---|
| **Stochastic effects** | | |
| Effective dose limits (cumulative) | 10 mSv × age | 20 mSv y$^{-1}$ averaged over 5 years |
| Effective dose limited (annual) | 50 mSv y$^{-1}$ | |
| **Deterministic effects** | | |
| Dose equivalent limits for tissues and organs (annual) | | |
| Lens of eye | 150 mSv y$^{-1}$ | |
| Skin, hands, and feet | 500 mSv y$^{-1}$ | |
| **Embryo or fetus exposure** | | |
| Effective dose limit | 0.5 mSv month$^{-1}$ | Total of 2 mSv to abdomen surface |
| **Public exposures (annual)** | | |
| Effective dose limit, continuous or frequent exposure | 1 mSv y$^{-1}$ | |
| Effective dose limit, infrequent exposure | 5 mSv y$^{-1}$ | Averaged over 5 years Must be 1 mSv y$^{-1}$ |
| Dose equivalent limits for lens of eye, skin, and extremities | 50 mSv y$^{-1}$ | |
| **Education and training exposures (annual)** | | |
| Effective dose limit | 1 mSv y$^{-1}$ | No statement |
| Dose equivalent limit for lens of eye, skin, and extremities | 50 mSv y$^{-1}$ | No statement |
| Negligible individual dose (annual) | 0.01 mSv y$^{-1}$ | No statement |

*(Based on National Council on Radiation Protection and Measurement: Recommendations on Limits for Exposure to Ionizing Radiation. Bethesda, MD, NCRP Report No. 116, 1993, and International Commission on Radiation Units and Measurements. ICRP publication No. 60. New York, Pergamon Press, 1991)*

## AS LOW AS REASONABLY ACHIEVABLE (ALARA)

The dose limits referred to earlier are all *upper* limits and subject to the concept of **ALARA,** *as low as reasonably achievable.* The recommendation that standard-setting committees would like to make for personnel protection is zero exposure. This is not feasible, however, if society is to realize the enormous benefits derived from the uses of radiations and radioactive materials.

Radiation is potentially harmful, and exposure to it should be continually monitored and controlled. No unnecessary exposure should be allowed. Equipment and facilities should be designed so that exposure of personnel and the public is kept to a minimum and not up to a standard. No exposure at all should be permitted without considering the benefits that may be derived from that exposure and the relative risks of alternative approaches.

Of course the ultimate problem is what is "reasonable." How much expense is justified to reduce the exposure of personnel by a given amount? As a rule-of-thumb in the nuclear power industry in the United States, ALARA has a cash value of about $1000 per 10 mSv (1 rem). If the exposure of one person to 10 mSv (1 rem) can be avoided by the expenditure of this amount of money, it is considered to be reasonable. If the cost is more, it is considered to be unreasonable, and the exposure is allowed. The figure of $1000 per 10 mSv (1 rem) applies to low doses, when the risk involves an objective health detriment. At higher dose levels, when the accumulation of an additional exposure may threaten a worker's job if the life-time dose limit is approached, the cash value of saving 10 mSv (1 rem) may be closer to $10,000. This sort of choice seldom has to be made in a hospital setting, except in the purchase of remote afterloading equipment for brachytherapy.

## PROTECTION OF THE EMBRYO/FETUS

The NCRP recommends a monthly limit of 0.5 mSv (0.05 rem) to the embryo or fetus once the pregnancy is declared. Once pregnancy has been declared, the ICRP recommends a limit of 2 mSv to the surface of the woman's abdomen (lower trunk) for the remainder of the pregnancy. These recommendations are essentially similar and are designed to limit the risk of mental retardation, other congenital malformations, or carcinogenesis. The NCRP and ICRP no longer recommend specific controls for occupationally exposed women *until* a pregnancy is declared.

Internally deposited radionuclides pose special problems for protection of the embryo or fetus. Some remain in the body for long periods of time, and the doses delivered to fetal organs are not well known for all radionuclides. Consequently, particular care should be taken to limit the intakes of radionuclides by pregnant women so that the equivalent dose to the embryo or fetus would not exceed the recommended limit.

## EMERGENCY OCCUPATIONAL EXPOSURE

Under normal conditions, only actions involving life saving justify acute exposures in excess of the annual effective dose limit. The use of volunteers for exposures during emergency actions is desirable. When possible, older workers with low lifetime accumulated effective doses should be chosen from among the volunteers. Exposure during emergency actions that do not involve life saving should, to the extent possible, be controlled to the occupational exposure limits. When this cannot be accomplished the NCRP and ICRP recommendation of 0.5 Sv (50 rems) should be applied.

When, for life saving or equivalent purposes, the exposure may approach or exceed 0.5 Sv (50 rems) to a large portion of the body, the worker needs to understand not only the potential for acute effects but should also have an appreciation of the substantial increase in his or her lifetime risk of cancer. If the possibility of internal exposures also exists, these should be taken into account.

## EXPOSURE OF PERSONS YOUNGER THAN 18 YEARS OF AGE

For educational and training purposes it may be necessary and desirable to accept occasional exposure of persons younger than the age of 18 years, in which case an annual effective dose limit of 1 mSv (0.1 rem) should be maintained.

## EXPOSURE OF MEMBERS OF THE PUBLIC (NONOCCUPATIONAL LIMITS)

The limitation of radiation exposure of members of the public from man-made sources is inevitably arbitrary, because it cannot be based on direct experience. The variety of risks faced by members of the public every day vary greatly; the number ranges from $10^{-4}$ to $10^{-6}$ per year. Depending on their nature, these risks seem to be accepted without much thought. At the same time, everyone is exposed to natural background radiation of about 1 mSv (100 mrems) annually, excluding radon, which may result in a mortality risk of $10^{-4}$ to $10^{-5}$ annually.

Based on these considerations, the recommended levels for man-made sources other than medical are as follows: for continuous (or repeated) exposure the annual effective dose equivalent should not exceed 1 mSv (0.1 rem). It is clear, however, that larger exposures to more limited groups of persons are not especially hazardous, provided they do not occur often to the same groups. Consequently, a maximum permissible annual effective dose equivalent of 5 mSv (0.5 rem) is recommended as a limit for infrequent exposure. Medical exposures are excluded from these limitations because it is assumed that they confer personal benefit to the exposed person and are extremely variable from one person to another.

Because some organs and tissues are not necessarily protected against deterministic effects in the calculation of effective dose, the hands and feet, localized areas of the skin, and the lens of the eye are also subject to an annual dose limit of 50 mSv (5 rem).

## EXPOSURE TO INDOOR RADON

Many homes in the United States and Europe contain an appreciable quantity of radon gas, which originates from the earth and enters the house through the basement. Insulating and sealing houses as a result of the escalating cost of heating oil in the 1970s exacerbated the radon problem, since a well-sealed house allows fewer exchanges of air with the outside and consequently results in a greater concentration of radon. Radon is a noble gas and is itself relatively nonhazardous since, if breathed in, it is breathed out again without being absorbed. In a confined space such as a basement, however, the decay of radon leads to the accumulation of daughter products that are solids, which stick to particles of dust or moisture, and tend to be deposited on the bronchial epithelium. These daughter products emit α-particles and cause intense local irradiation.

Radon levels vary enormously with different localities, depending on the composition of the soil and the presence of cracks, or fissures, in the ground, which allows radon to escape to the surface. There is the famous example of the man who wanted to work in a nuclear power station but was turned away because the radiation monitors were set off as he entered the plant by the accumulation of radon daughter products deposited in his body and on his clothes that came from his home!

Indoor radon is currently perceived to be the most important problem involving radiation exposure of the public. In the United States and most European countries the mean radon concentration in homes is in the range 20 to 60 Bq/m³ (0.5 to 1.6 pCi/L) with higher mean values of about 100 Bq/m³ (2.7 pCi/L) in Finland, Norway, and Sweden. Converting radon concentrations into dose to the bronchial epithelium involves many uncertainties because it depends on the model used and the assumptions made. One widely used conversion factor equates an air concentration of 20 Bq/m³ with an effective dose to the bronchial epithelium of 1 mSv/y (0.5 pCi/L corresponding to 100 mrems/y).

The EPA has set the "action level" at about 160 Bq/m³ (4 pCi/L), suggesting that remedial action should be taken to reduce radon levels if they are higher than this. The action level is about four times the average radon concentrations in homes. About 1 in 12 homes in the United States—about 6 million in all—have radon concentrations above this action level. This is the most stringent action level in the world. In Germany and Great Britain the action level is more than double this figure, while in Finland, Sweden, and Canada it is five times higher. This action level translates into an effective dose to the bronchial epithelium of about 8 mSv/y (800 mrems/y) and a cancer risk of $4 \times 10^{-4}$/y. This is almost **ten** times higher than the cancer risk associated with the dose limits recommended for the public from man-made radiation. There are two reasons for this ambivalent attitude. First, the lung cancer risk estimates for radon are based on extrapolation from uranium miners, for whom there were other contributing factors, such as dust and heavy smoking. If these risk estimates were applied to naturally occurring radon in homes, it would appear that this is the cause of a large proportion of all human lung cancer. The question is, do these risk estimates apply? Second, if the radiation safety levels applicable to external radiation were applied to radon, millions of homes in the United States and Europe would be declared unsafe. This is a problem that no one knows how to handle, and the above recommendations are liable to revision.

## DE MINIMUS DOSE AND NEGLIGIBLE INDIVIDUAL DOSE

Collective dose to a population has little meaning without the concept of *de minimus dose*. The idea is to define some very low threshold below which it would make no sense to make any additional effort to reduce exposure levels further. For example, suppose there is a release of radioactivity from a reactor that dissipates into the atmosphere, blows around the world, and eventually exposes many hundreds of millions of persons to very low doses. The doses may be so low that the biological effects are negligible, but because the number of persons involved is so large, the product of dose times number of persons would dominate the collective dose. The term *de minimus* comes from the legal saying *De minimus non curat lex*, which roughly translates to "The law does not concern itself with trifles."

Dr. Merril Eisenbud in an NCRP publication quotes this poem of dubious origin:

> There was a young lawyer named Rex
> Who was very deficient in sex
> When charged with exposure
> He said with composure
> *De minimus non curat lex.*

The concept of *de minimus* dose has been espoused by the NCRP in the form of *negligible individual dose*, defined here to be the dose below which further efforts to reduce radiation exposure to the person is unwarranted.

The NCRP considers an annual effective dose of 0.01 mSv (1 mrem) to be a negligible individual dose (NID). This dose is associated with a risk of mortality between $10^{-6}$ and $10^{-7}$, which is considered to be *trivial* compared with the risk of fatality associated with ordinary and normal societal activities and can therefore be dismissed from consideration of additional radioprotective measures.

## RISKS ASSOCIATED WITH CURRENT RECOMMENDED LIMITS

Risk estimates for radiation-induced cancer and hereditary effects were discussed in Chapters 19 and 20. They are summarized in Table 25-5. The possible deleterious effects of long-term occupational exposure to radiation include the reduction of life expectancy (a combination of the probability of developing a fatal cancer and the number of years lost if it occurs) as well as the morbidity, that is, decreased quality of life, associated with nonfatal cancers and hereditary effects. The ICRP has coined the term *detriment* to cover all of these effects. The best estimate for the risk of fatal cancer in a working population exposed to a uniform total-body equivalent dose of 1 Sv at low dose rate is $4 \times 10^{-2}$. The contributions from nonfatal cancers and hereditary effects are more difficult to assess; the ICRP suggests 20% of the detriment from fatal cancers for each, that is, $0.8 \times 10^{-2}$/Sv.

The total detriment (life lost and quality of life impaired) amounts to about $5.6 \times 10^{-2}$/Sv. Recent surveys indicate that the average annual equivalent dose to monitored radiation workers with measurable exposures is about 2 mSv, which results in a total detriment per year of less than $2 \times 10^{-4}$. This is comparable to the average death rate from fatal accidents in what are considered to be "safe" industries, such as trade and government service (Table 25-6). For those few persons who might receive doses close to the limit over an entire working life, the total detriment reaches 3.6% and is comparable to less safe industries such as construction or working in mines or quarries.

Table 25-5.
Risk Estimates for Cancer and Hereditary Effects

| EXPOSED POPULATION | DETRIMENT ($10^{-2}$ Sv$^{-1}$) | | | |
| --- | --- | --- | --- | --- |
| | Fatal Cancer | Nonfatal Cancer | Severe Hereditary Effects | Total |
| Adult workers | 4.0 | 0.8 | 0.8 | 5.6 |
| Whole population | 5.0 | 1.0 | 1.3 | 7.3 |

*(Data from International Commission on Radiation Units and Measurements. ICRP publication No. 60. New York, Pergamon Press, 1991)*

## NCRP AND ICRP COMPARED

At the present time, there is a difference in the recommendations of the national and international bodies regarding the maximum permissible effective dose for occupational exposure (stochastic effects). The differences are highlighted in Table 25-4.

Both bodies recommend a maximum of 50 mSv (5 rems) in any one year, but the NCRP adds a lifetime cumulative limit of age × 10 mSv (age × 1 rem) while the ICRP adds a limit of 20 mSv (2 rems) per year averaged over defined periods of 5 years.

Table 25-6.
Trends in Fatal Accident Rates (1976–1989) for Workers in the United States

| | MEAN RATE 1976 ($10^{-6}$ y$^{-1}$) | MEAN RATE 1989 ($10^{-6}$ y$^{-1}$) |
| --- | --- | --- |
| All groups | 142 | 90 |
| Trade | 64 | 40 |
| Manufacture | 89 | 60 |
| Service | 86 | 40 |
| Government | 111 | 90 |
| Transport and public utilites | 313 | 240 |
| Construction | 568 | 320 |
| Mines and quarries | 625 | 430 |
| Agriculture (1973–1980) | 541 | 400 |

*(Based on National Safety Council: Accident Facts 1976 Chicago, National Safety Council, 1977, and National Safety Council: Accident Facts 1989 Chicago, National Safety Council, 1990)*

The practical consequence of this difference is that a radiation worker starting at, for example, age 18 can accumulate more dose under the NCRP recommendations in the early years up to 32 years of age but later in life could accumulate more dose under the ICRP recommendations. Under NCRP recommendations, a new radiation worker could receive 50 mSv (5 rems) in each of several consecutive years until the age × 10 mSv (age × 1 rem) limit kicks in. Under ICRP rules, the average cannot exceed 20 mSv (2 rems) per year over a 5-year period, so one or two 50 mSv (5 rems) years would have to be followed by several years at very low exposure levels. If persons were exposed throughout their working lives to the maximum permissible dose, the excess risk of stochastic effects (cancer and hereditary effects) would be about the same under NCRP or ICRP recommendations. Under NCRP, a person occupationally exposed from 18 to 65 years of age could receive a total dose of 650 mSv (65 rems). Under the ICRP the same person could receive 940 mSv (94 rems), but less would be received between 18 and 32 years of age and more at later ages.

The NCRP scheme is less restrictive for a few workers in the nuclear power industry who tend to receive large effective doses in their early years while working on nuclear reactors. Later in life, these persons tend to occupy supervisory or administrative positions and receive little if any dose. To cope with those who do not, NCRP has added the extra recommendation that this limit, age × 10 mSv (age × 1 rem) can be relaxed *in individual cases after counseling*, if implementation of the recommendation would mean loss of a job!

It should be emphasized that few persons exposed occupationally in a medical setting receive doses anywhere near the limits recommended. Some interventional radiologists may well receive more than 50 mGy (5 rad) per year to a monitor worn outside the lead rubber apron or to a monitor worn at neck level or on the forearm. But the recommended maximum permissible levels refer to **effective dose,** which take into account the parts of the body exposed.

## GLOSSARY OF TERMS

**absorbed dose.** The energy imparted to matter by ionizing radiation per unit mass of irradiated material at the place of interest. The unit is the gray (Gy), defined to be an energy absorption of 1 joule/kg. The old unit was the rad, defined to be an energy absorption of 100 ergs/g.

**ALARA.** As low as reasonably achievable, economic and social factors being taken into account. This is identical to the principle of optimization of protection used by the ICRP.

**annual limit on intake (ALI).** The activity of a radionuclide taken into the body during a year that would provide a committed equivalent dose to a person, represented by *reference man*, equal to the occupational dose limit set by recommending and regulating bodies. The ALI is normally expressed in becquerel (Bq).

**becquerel (Bq).** The special name for the unit of activity. 1 Bq = $3.7 \times 10^{10}$ Bq = 1 Curie.

**collective effective dose.** Applies to a group of persons and is the sum of the products of the effective dose and the number of persons receiving that effective dose.

**collective equivalent dose.** Applies to a group of persons and is the sum of the products of the equivalent dose and the number of persons receiving that equivalent dose.

**committed effective dose.** The sum of the committed organ or tissue equivalent doses resulting from an intake multiplied by the appropriate tissue weighting factors.

**committed equivalent dose.** The equivalent dose averaged throughout a specified tissue in the 50 years after intake of a radionuclide into the body.

**deterministic effects.** Effects for which the severity of the effect in affected persons varies with the dose and for which a threshold usually exists. These were formerly known as nonstochastic effects. An example is a cataract.

**effective dose.** The sum over specified tissues of the products of the equivalent dose in a tissue and the appropriate tissue weighting factor for that tissue ($W_T$)

**equivalent dose.** A quantity used for radiation-protection purposes that takes into account the different probability of effects that occur with the same absorbed dose delivered by radiations of different quality. It is defined as the product of the averaged absorbed dose in a specified organ or tissue and the radiation weighting factor ($W_R$). The unit of equivalent dose is the sievert (Sv).

**genetically significant dose (GSD).** The dose to the gonads weighted for the age and sex distribution in those members of the population expected to have offspring. The GSD is measured in sieverts (rems).

**gray (Gy).** The special name for the SI unit of absorbed dose, kerma, and specific energy imparted. 1 Gy = 1 J kg$^{-1}$. 1 Gy also equals 100 rads.

**negligible individual dose (NID).** A level of effective dose that can be dismissed as insignificant and below which further efforts to improve radiation protection are not justified. The recommended NID is 0.01 mSv/y$^{-1}$

**nonstochastic effects.** Previous term for deterministic effects.

**nuclide.** A species of atom having a specified number of neutrons and protons in its nucleus.

**optimization.** This has the same meaning as ALARA.

**organ or tissue weighting factor ($W_T$).** A factor that indicates the ratio of the risk of stochastic effects attributable to irradiation of a given organ or tissue to the total risk when the whole body is uniformly irradiated. Organs that have a large $W_T$ are those that are susceptible to radiation-induced carcinogenesis (such as the breast or thyroid) or to heritable effects (the gonads).

**rad.** The old unit for absorbed dose, kerma, and specific energy imparted. One rad is 0.01 joule absorbed per kilogram of any material (also defined as 100 ergs/g). The term is being replaced by *gray:* 1 rad = 0.01 Gy.

**radiation weighting factor ($W_R$).** A factor used for radiation-protection purposes that accounts for differences in biological effectiveness between different radiations. The radiation weighting factor, $W_R$, is independent of the tissue weighting factor, $W_T$.

**relative biological effectiveness (RBE).** A ratio of the absorbed dose of a reference radiation to the absorbed dose of a test radiation to produce the same level of biological effect, other conditions being equal. It is the quantity that is measured experimentally.

**rem.** The old unit of dose equivalent. It is the product of the absorbed dose in rads and modifying factors and is being replaced by the sievert.

**sievert (Sv).** The unit of dose equivalent in the SI system. It is the product of absorbed dose in gray and quality factor; 1 Sv = 100 rem.

**stochastic effects.** Effects for which the probability of their occurring, rather than their severity, is a function of radiation dose without threshold. More generally, stochastic means random in nature.

**working level (WL).** The amount of potential α energy in a cubic meter of air that will result in the emission of $2.08 \times 10^{-5}$ joules of energy.

**working level month (WLM).** A cumulative exposure, equivalent to exposure to one working level for a working month (170 hours), that is, $2 \times 10^{-5}$ $Jm^{-3} \times 170$ h = $3.5 \times 10^{-3}$ $Jhm^{-3}$.

► *Summary of Pertinent Conclusions*

- Radiation weighting factors ($W_R$) are approximate values of the relative biological effectiveness (RBE), applicable to low doses and relevant to carcinogenesis and hereditary effects. Radiation weighting factors are chosen by the ICRP based on experimental RBE values with a large judgmental factor.

- Equivalent dose is the product of absorbed dose and radiation weighting factor. The units are sieverts or rems for an absorbed dose in gray or rads.

- Tissue weighting factors ($W_T$) reflect the susceptibility of different organs or tissues to carcinogenesis or hereditary effects.

- Effective dose is the sum of the weighted equivalent doses for all irradiated tissues and organs; the weighting factors represent the different risks of each tissue or organ for cancer or hereditary effects.

- Committed equivalent dose is the integral over 50 years of the equivalent dose after the intake of a radionuclide.

- Collective effective dose is a quantity for a population and is the sum of effective doses to all members of that population. The unit is person-sievert (man-rem).

- The objectives of radiation protection are to prevent clinically significant *deterministic* effects by keeping doses below the practical threshold and to limit the risk of *stochastic* effects (cancer and heritable effects) to a reasonable level in relation to societal needs, values, and benefits gained.

- All radiation exposures are governed by the ALARA principle (as low as reasonably achievable).

- The individual worker's lifetime effective dose should not exceed

  Age in years × 10 mSv (age in years × 1 rad)

- No occupational exposure should be permitted before 18 years of age.

- The effective dose in any one year should not exceed 50 mSv (5 rems).

- To limit deterministic effects, the dose limit to the lens of the eye is 150 mSv (15 rems) and the dose limit to localized areas of the skin, hands, and feet is 500 mSv (50 rems).

- Once a pregnancy is declared, the NCRP recommends a monthly limit of 0.5 mSv (0.05 rem) to the embryo or fetus.

- Specific controls for occupationally exposed women are no longer recommended until a pregnancy is declared.

*(continued)*

► *Summary of Pertinent Conclusions* (Continued)

- Internally deposited radionuclides pose a special problem for protection of the embryo or fetus; particular care should be taken to limit intake.

- Emergency occupational exposures normally justify doses in excess of the recommended limits only if life-saving actions are involved. Volunteers from among older workers with low life-time accumulated effective doses should be chosen in emergencies where the exposure may be up to 0.5 Sv (50 rems). When the exposure may exceed 0.5 Sv (50 rems) the worker should be counseled about the short-term and long-term possible consequences.

- For educational or training purposes it may sometimes be desirable to accept radiation exposures of persons younger than 18 years of age, in which case the annual effective dose limit of 1 mSv (0.1 rem) should be maintained.

- The annual effective dose limit for *members of the public* is 1 mSv (0.1 rem) except infrequent exposures when the limit may be 5 mSv (0.5 rem). Medical x-rays are excluded from these limitations because they are assumed to confer personal benefit.

- For deterministic effects, the dose limits for members of the general public are 50 mSv (5 rems) to the hands and feet, to localized areas of the skin, or to the lens of the eye.

- Indoor radon is perceived to be the most important problem involving radiation exposure of the general public. Remedial action in homes is recommended by the EPA if the radon concentration exceeds 160 Bq/m$^3$ (4 pCi/L). This represents a much higher cancer risk than the general public is allowed from other radiation sources and illustrates the equivocal views on radon.

- Negligible individual dose (NID) is the dose below which further expenditure to improve radiation protection is unwarranted. The NID is an annual effective dose of 0.01 mSv (1 mrem), which carries a risk of between $10^{-6}$ and $10^{-7}$ of carcinogenesis or heritable effects.

- A uniform whole body equivalent dose of 1 Sv to a working population is assumed to result in a total *detriment* of about $5.6 \times 10^{-2}$/Sv. This is made up of a risk of fatal cancer of $4 \times 10^{-2}$, a risk of severe hereditary effects of $0.8 \times 10^{-2}$/Sv and a risk of nonfatal cancer of $0.8 \times 10^{-2}$/Sv.

- The average annual equivalent dose to monitored radiation workers is about 2 mSv. This involves a total detriment of about $2 \times 10^{-4}$, which is comparable to the annual risk of a fatal accident in a "safe" industry, such as trade or government service.

- The NCRP and ICRP differ in two important recommendations:

  1. *The effective dose limit for occupational exposure (stochastic effects).* The NCRP recommends a lifetime cumulative limit of age × 10 mSv (age × 1 rem) with a limit in any year of 50 mSv (5 rems), while the ICRP recommends a limit of 20 mSv (2 rems) per year averaged over defined periods of 5 years, with a limit in any year of 50 mSv (5 rems).
  2. *The dose limit to the developing embryo or fetus once a pregnancy is declared.* The NCRP recommends a monthly limit of 0.5 mSv (0.05 rem) to the embryo or fetus. The ICRP recommends a limit of 2 mSv (0.2 rem) to the surface of the woman's abdomen for the remainder of pregnancy.

# BIBLIOGRAPHY

Burkhart RL, Gross RE, Jans RG, McCrohen JL Jr, Rosenstein M, Reuter FA (eds): Recommendations for Evaluation of Radiation Exposure From Diagnostic Radiology Examinations. Springfield, VA, Food and Drug Administration, Health and Human Services publication No. 85-8247. National Technical Information Service, 1985

Committee on the Biological Effects of Ionizing Radiations: The Effects on Populations of Exposure to Low Levels of Ionizing Radiation. Washington DC, National Academy Press, 1980

Committee on the Biological Effects of Ionizing Radiations: Health Effects of Exposure to Low Levels of Ionizing Radiation. Washington, DC, National Academy Press, 1990

International Commission on Radiological Protection: Recommendations. ICRP Report No. 26. New York, Pergamon Press, 1977

International Commission on Radiological Protection: Quantitative Bases for Developing a Unified Index of Harm. Report No. 45. New York, Pergamon Press, 1985

International Commission on Radiological Protection: Recommendations. Report No. 60. New York, Pergamon Press, 1991

International Commission on Radiation Units and Measurements: Determination of Dose Equivalent Resulting From External Radiation Sources. Report No. 39. Bethesda, MD, ICRU, 1985

International Commission on Radiation Units and Measurements: The Quality Factor of Radiation Protection: Report of a Joint Task Group of the ICRP and ICRU to the ICRP and ICRU. Report No. 40. Bethesda, MD, ICRU, 1986

Kato H, Schull WJ: Studies of the mortality of A-bomb survivors: 7. Mortality, 1950–1978: I. Cancer mortality. Radiat Res 90:395, 1982

National Council on Radiation Protection and Measurements: Radiation Protection in Educational Institutions. Report No. 32. Bethesda, MD, NCRP, 1966

National Council on Radiation Protection and Measurements: Basic Radiation Protection Criteria. Report No. 39, Bethesda, MD, NCRP, 1971

National Council on Radiation Protection and Measurements: Review of NCRP Radiation Dose Limit for Embryo and Fetus in Occupationally-Exposed Women. Report No. 53, Bethesda, MD, NCRP, 1977

National Council on Radiation Protection and Measurements: Evaluation of Occupational and Environmental Exposure to Radon and Radon Daughters in the United States. Report No. 78. Bethesda, MD, NCRP, 1984

National Council on Radiation Protection and Measurements: Comparative Carcinogenicity of Ionizing Radiation and Chemicals. Report No. 96. Bethesda, MD, NCRP, 1989

National Council on Radiation Protection and Measurements: Recommendations on Limits for Exposure to Ionizing Radiation. Report No. 91, Bethesda, MD, NCRP, 1987

National Council on Radiation Protection and Measurements: Implementation of the Principle of As Low As Reasonably Achievable (ALARA) for Medical and Dental Personnel. Report No. 107. Bethesda, MD, NCRP, 1990

United Nations Scientific Committee on the Effects of Atomic Radiation: Sources and Effects of Ionizing Radiation. Report to the General Assembly, with Annexes, publication No. E.77.IXI. New York, UNSCEAR, 1977

United Nations Scientific Committee on the Effects of Atomic Radiation: Ionizing Radiation: Sources and Biological Effects. Report to the General Assembly, with Annexes, publication No. E.82.IX8. New York, UNSCEAR, 1982

United Nations Scientific Committee on the Effects of Atomic Radiation: Biological Effects of Pre-Natal Irradiation. Presented before the 35th Session of UNSCEAR. New York, UNSCEAR, 1986

# *Index*

Numbers followed by an *f* indicate a figure; *t* following a page number indicates tabular material; *n* indicates information in a footnote.

## A

Aberrations
  chromatid, 19
  chromosome, 19, 355-356
    exchange-type, and cell lethality, 40*f*
    in human lymphocyctes, 25-26, 25*f*
    by premature condensation and fluorescent in situ hybridization, 249-250
    radiation-induced, 18-19
Absolute risk model, in assessing carcinogenesis, 328
Absorbed dose, 455, 464
Accelerated repopulation, 219, 220*f*, 221
Accelerated treatment, 221-222
  choice between hyperfractionation and, 222
  design of, 252-253
  and $T_{pot}$, 222-223*f*
Acentric fragment, 19
Acute hypoxia, 139-140, 142*f*
Adenine, 352
Agarose gel electrophoresis, 396, 413
Age-response function, 111
  implications of, in radiotherapy, 103
  mechanisms for, 103
  for tissue in vivo, 101-102*f*
Alkylating agents, 291-293
Alleles, 412
α/β, values of, for early- and late-responding tissues, 217, 218*t*
α/β ratio
  in calculating effective doses, 224
  definition of, 215
  inferring, from multifraction experiments in nonclonogenic systems, 64-65*f*
α-particles, 6*f*, 10, 11
  charge-to-mass ratio for, 154

American Society of Therapeutic Radiology and Oncology, 223
Americium-241, in brachytherapy, 125
Amifostine
  clinical use of, 189
  as radioprotector, 186, 187-189, 188*f*,*t*
Amino acids, 412
Ampicillin, 412
Amplify, 412
Anaphase, 18
Anaphase bridge, 22, 23*f*
Angstrom, 4*n*
Animals
  carcinogenesis in laboratory, 327-328, 327*f*
  determinations of cell loss in, 202-203, 202*t*
  growth fraction of, 201*t*, 205
  proportion of hyponic cells in, 142-145, 144*f*
  spontaneous tumors in domestic, 277
  transplantable solid tumor systems in experimental, 76
Anneal, 412
Annual limit on intake (ALI), 464
Antibiotic resistance, 412
Antibiotics, 293, 412
Antibody, 412
Antibody probes, 398
Antigen, 412
Antimetabolites, 293-294
Apoptosis, 46, 68, 87-88, 202
Arrhenius plot, 261*f*, 270
As low as reasonably achievable (ALARA), 458, 460, 464
Ataxia-telangiectasia (AT), 236, 343-345, 344*t*
Atomic number, 7*n*
Autoradiography, 92, 93*f*, 94*f*, 398
5-Azacytidine, 294

## B

Bacteriophage, 412
  as vectors, 388
Bacterium, 412
Barium enema, risks from radiation in, 449
Base pair, 412
Becquerel (Bq), 464
Becqueri, Antoine Henri, 2
Berkeley, Lawrence, Laboratory, 6-8*f*
β-particles, 92-93
Biological effect, correlation of temperature and, 271
Biologically effective dose, 224
Bioreductive drugs, 175
  dual-function nitroheterocyclic compounds, 176-177, 176*f*
  Mitomycin C, 175
  organic nitroxides, 175-176
Bleomycin, 148, 174
  and oxygen effect, 297
Bleomycin sulfate (Blenoxane), 293
Blobs, 17
Bone cancer, and radiation carcinogenesis, 331, 332*f*
Bone marrow assay, death, 46-47, 312
Bone marrow stem cells, dose-response relationship in, 56*f*, 57*f*, 58
Bone marrow transplantation
  and near lethal dose ($LD_{50}$), 316-317*f*,*t*
  in treating radiation accident victims, 318, 319*f*, 320*f*
Bone scan, risks from radiation in, 449
Boron neutron capture therapy, 237
  clinical trials in, 238
  compounds in, 237-238
  sources in, 238
Brachytherapy
  interstitial, 122-123*f*, 122*f*, 124*f*

Brachytherapy
  interstitial, (*continued*)
    permanent implants, 124-125*t*
  intracavitary radiotherapy, 121-122
Bragg peak, 238-240
Brazil, radiation exposure in, 436-437
Breast cancer, and radiation
    carcinogenesis, 330, 331*f*
Breathing frequency, assay of, 62, 64*f*
Broad-beam radiotherapy, 240
Bromodeoxyuridine
  in assessment of cell cycle, 193
  in cell labeling, 93-94*f*
  side effects of, 167
5-bromodeoxyuridine, 166
Burkitt's lymphoma, 24
Busch, W., 258
Buthionine sulfoximine, 300

**C**

Calcium phosphate precipitation,
    394-395*f*
Cancer. *See also* Radiation
    carcinogenesis
  bone, 331, 332*f*
  breast, 330, 331*f*
  childhood, after irradiation in utero,
    337, 373-374, 373*t*
  lung, 330-331, 341
  radiolabeled immunoglobulin
    therapy for, 125-126
    clinical results, 126-127
    dosimetry, 127
    radionuclides, 126
    targeting, 126
    tumor target visualization, 126
  risks of nuclear medicine, 444
  skin, 332
  thyroid, 329, 446-447
Carbon monoxide, as radioprotectors,
    184
Carcinogenesis
  and heat, 276-277
  radiation. *See also* Radiation
    carcinogenesis
Casaret's classification, of tissue
    radiosensitivity, 68-70, 69*t*
Cataracts, 380. *See also* Radiation
    cataractogenesis
cDNA, 412
cDNA library, 391, 405, 413
Cell adhesive matrix assay, 248-249,
    250*f*
Cell age, sensitivity to heat as func-
    tion of, in mitotic cycle, 262
Cell cultures
  in generating survival curve, 31, 32*f*
  synchronously dividing, 95-97
    effect of x-rays on, 97*f*, 98*f*,
      99-100, 99*f*
Cell cycle, 92-95, 92*f*, 93*f*, 94*f*, 192*f*
  and cell loss, 201-202
  effect of oxygen at various phases
    of, 101
  and growth fraction, 201*t*
  measurement of potential tumor
    doubling time, 199-201, 200*f*

progression of, molecular check-
    point genes in controlling,
    100-101
  and pulsed photo cytometry,
    198-199*f*
  quantitative assessment of con-
    stituent parts of, 192-193*f*
Cell-cycle nonspecific, 291
Cell-cycle specific, 291
Cell cycle times, 92
  comparison of cells of solid
    tumors and their normal
    counterparts, 206-207
  experiment measurements of, in
    vivo and in vitro, 196-198*f,t,*
    197*f*
Cell death, 30
  programmed, 46, 202
Cell division, and chromosomes, 17-18*f*
Cell killing, mechanism of, 39-40, 39*f*
Cell labeling techniques, 93*f*
Cell lethality, and exchange-type
    chromosal aberrations, 40*f*
Cell lines, radiosensitivity of, 246-247
Cell loss, 201-202
  determination of, in experimental
    tumors, 202-203, 202*t*
Cell loss factor, 201-202
  for human tumors, 205
Cell survival curve, 30
  calculations of tumor cell kill, 37-38
  and concentration of oxygen,
    137-138*f*
  dilution assay technique for
    obtaining, 79-81*f*, 80*f*
  effective, for multifraction regimen,
    37, 38*f*
  and exchange-type chromasomal
    aberrations and cell lethality,
    40*f*
  and intrinsic radiosensitivity and
    predictive assays, 36
  mechanism of cell killing in, 39-40,
    39*f*
  and oncogenes and radioresistance,
    38-39
  shape of, 32-34, 33*f*
  for various mammalian cells in
    culture, 35-36, 35*f*, 37*f*
  in vitro, 30-31*f*, 32*f*
Cellular oncogene (proto-oncogene),
    413
Cellular response to heat, 260-262,
    260*f*, 261*f*
Centromere, 18, 412
Cerebrovascular syndrome, 312,
    313-314
Cesium-137, in intracavitary
    radiotherapy, 121-122
Chain termination method, 401-402
Charge-to-mass ratio, for α-particles,
    154
Chemopotentiation, 174-175
Chemotherapeutic agents
  adjunct use of, with radiation,
    303-304, 303*f*
  comparison of, 300, 302-303, 302*f*
  and heat, 274-276, 274*t*, 275*f*

Chemotherapy, 290-291
  adjunct use of chemotherapeutic
    agents with radiation,
    303-304, 303*f*
    with hyperthermia, 304
  assays for sensitivity of individual
    tumors, 304
  biological basis of, 291
  classes of agents and mode of
    action, 291, 292*t*
    alkylating agents, 291-293
    antibiotics, 293
    cisplatin, 294-295
    5-fluorouracil, 294
    hydroxyurea, 294
    nucleoside analogues, 294
    procarbazine, 294
  coining of term, 290
  combination, 290
  comparison of chemotherapeutic
    agents with radiation,
    300-302, 302*f*
  dose-response relationships,
    295-296, 295*f*
  drug resistance, 298
  oxygen effect and chemothera-
    peutuc agents, 297*f*
  proliferating and nonproliferating
    cells, 297-298, 299*f*
  and radioprotectors, 189
  and second malignancies, 304-305*t*
  sublethal and potentially lethal
    damage repair, 296-297, 296*f*
Chernobyl accident victims, treatment
    of, 316, 319
Childhood cancer, after irradiation in
    utero, 337, 373-374, 373*t*
Chlorambucil (Leukeran), 292
Chromatid aberrations, 19
Chromosomal rearrangement or
    translocation, 338
Chromosome aberrations, 19, 355-356
  exchange-type, and cell lethality, 40*f*
  in human lymphocytes, 25-26, 25*f*
  by premature condensation and
    fluorescent in situ
    hybridization, 249-250
  radiation-induced, 18-19
Chromosome breakage, 355
Chromosome imbalance, 355
Chromosome painting, 24, 26
Chromosomes
  and cell division, 17-18*f*
  definition of, 352
Chromosome walking, 400
Chronic hypoxia, 139, 140*f*, 141*f*
Cisplatin, 174, 294
Clonogenic, 30
Clonogenic assays
  dose-response curves for, 59, 60*f*
  for dose-response relationships, 46
Clonogenic endpoints, clones
    regrowing in situ
    crypt cell of the mouse jejunum,
      49*f*, 50*f*, 51, 52*f*
    kidney tubules, 51, 54*f*, 55*f*, 56
    skin colonies, 47-49, 47*f*
    testes stem cells, 51, 53*f*, 54*f*

ISBN 0-397-51248-1

90000
9 780397 512485